Piezo-

elastium
mechanism.

Cochlear Mechanisms

Structure, Function, and Models

NATO ASI Series

Advanced Science Institutes Series

A series presenting the results of activities sponsored by the NATO Science Committee, which aims at the dissemination of advanced scientific and technological knowledge, with a view to strengthening links between scientific communities.

The series is published by an international board of publishers in conjunction with the NATO Scientific Affairs Division

A	**Life Sciences**	Plenum Publishing Corporation
B	**Physics**	New York and London
C	**Mathematical and Physical Sciences**	Kluwer Academic Publishers
D	**Behavioral and Social Sciences**	Dordrecht, Boston, and London
E	**Applied Sciences**	
F	**Computer and Systems Sciences**	Springer-Verlag
G	**Ecological Sciences**	Berlin, Heidelberg, New York, London,
H	**Cell Biology**	Paris, and Tokyo

Recent Volumes in this Series

Volume 158—Biocompatibility of Co-Cr-Ni Alloys
edited by Hartmut F. Hildebrand and Maxime Champy

Volume 159—Biologically Based Methods for Cancer Risk Assessment
edited by Curtis C. Travis

Volume 160—Early Influences Shaping the Individual
edited by Spyros Doxiadis

Volume 161—Research in Congenital Hypothyroidism
edited by F. Delange, D. A. Fisher, and D. Glinoer

Volume 162—Nematode Identification and Expert System Technology
edited by Renaud Fortuner

Volume 163—Leishmaniasis: The Current Status and New Strategies for Control
edited by D. T. Hart

Volume 164—Cochlear Mechanisms: Structure, Function, and Models
edited by J. P. Wilson and D. T. Kemp

Series A: Life Sciences

PREFACE

Great advances have been made in understanding hearing in recent years. In particular, the mechanical function of the cochlea has become the focus of intense interest. This started in one direction, with the discovery of otoacoustic emissions in 1978, which required active mechanical amplification processes, as first postulated by Gold in 1948. Direct evidence for the role of this mechanism in sharpening-up the otherwise poor, basilar membrane tuning properties, was provided in 1982; and in 1983, motility was shown in outer hair cells. In parallel, an immense amount of work has been done on the electrophysiology of hair cells, following the first intracellular recordings in 1977.

Over a longer time scale, models of basilar membrane motion have been developed and refined, and recently much effort has been put into incorporating active mechanisms and non-linear processes. It seemed an opportune time to bring together the leading workers in these various areas, to take stock of the whole field and to stimulate further progress.

This book represents the proceedings of a NATO ARW on the Mechanics of Hearing held at the University of Keele, 3-8 July, 1988. The conception of the meeting owes much to earlier meetings held in Boston in 1985 (*Peripheral Auditory Mechanisms*, Eds. J.B. Allen, J.L. Hall, A. Hubbard, S.T. Neely and A. Tubis, Springer-Verlag, Berlin, 1986) and Delft in 1983 (*Mechanics of Hearing*, Eds. E. de Boer and M.A. Viergever, Delft University Press, 1983) and also London in 1980 (*Nonlinear and Active Mechanical Processes in the Cochlea*, Eds. D.T. Kemp and S.D. Anderson, Hearing Research, 2 (3/4)). In this meeting, however, we have departed from previous practice by omitting middle ear measurements. This was necessitated by the very rapid and exciting growth in the field of micromechanics and hair cell motility. Furthermore, to broaden the understanding of this field, it appeared advantageous to introduce some of the recent ultrastructural findings. The editors received much encouraging feedback during the meeting, both from modellers and morphologists, that this had been a popular and fruitful decision.

In addition to the main papers we have included extra material as "comments", either sent in beforehand, presented as posters, or written up during the meeting. The edited discussions are also included, and, in a much less heavily edited form, the two main discussion sessions, which by default, have not necessarily been approved by the authors concerned.

We were fortunate in having so many of the pioneer workers in this field, present at the workshop, and in addition, two eminent scientists from other fields, who had interesting contributions to make. Professor Thomas Gold, FRS, the cosmologist and astronomer, had made predictions about active feedback mechanisms within the cochlea, forty years ago, and it was intriguing to hear about auditory research of that era, and to wonder how different the development of hearing might have been if his attempts at that time, to measure spontaneous otoacoustic emissions, had been successful; and Sir James Lighthill, FRS, who was able to relate, as guest of honour at the dinner, some of the background to the earlier meetings, particularly that at Delft for which he was on the organising committee. As chairman of the modelling discussion session, he showed how his expertise in fluid dynamics can be applied to energy flow problems within the cochlea.

The editors would like to thank the members of the International Organising Committee for many useful suggestions which have helped shape the meeting, the Chairmen of Sessions, and the members of the Local Organising Committee who contributed so much to the smooth running of the meeting. These are all named following the list of participants. We would also like to thank NATO for so generously supporting the workshop in administrative costs, and in providing accommodation and travel support for participants who needed it.

Plans were made at the end, to hold another workshop in 1990, probably in the US Mid West.

J.P. Wilson and D.T. Kemp October, 1988

CONTENTS

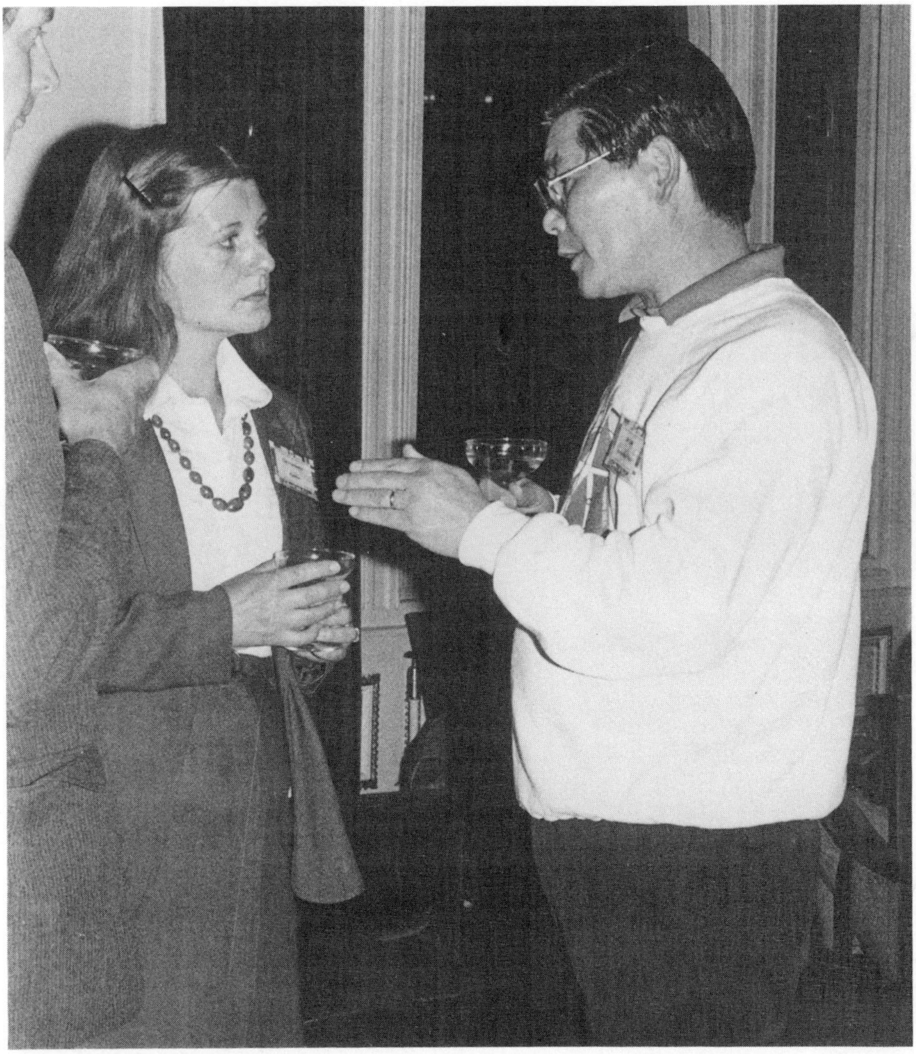

C.M. Hackney and D.J. Lim

1. HAIR CELL ULTRASTRUCTURE

STRUCTURAL ORGANIZATION OF THE MAMMALIAN AUDITORY HAIR CELLS IN RELATION TO MICROMECHANICS

D.J. Lim, Y. Hanamure, and Y. Ohashi

Otological Research Laboratories
The Ohio State University
456 West 10th Avenue
Columbus, Ohio 43210, U.S.A.

Introduction

The mammalian auditory sensory cells are mechano-receptors characterized by sensory stereocilia, the cuticular plate, and the polarized cell body, innervated by the afferent and efferent nerve endings. The auditory sensory cells in mammals are further specialized into two functional groups (inner hair cells vs. outer hair cells) that are morphologically distinct from each other with differing innervation patterns. There is good evidence to suggest that the inner hair cells are largely responsible for auditory sensitivity and the outer hair cells are responsible for auditory tuning (Liberman & Kiang, 1984). The role of the outer hair cell in frequency selectivity is thought to be the result of its interaction with the inner hair cell. Recent evidence suggests that the outer hair cell of the cochlea is motile. It has been suggested that this outer hair cell motility is responsible for generating the otoacoustic emission and tuning of the auditory sensory response by exerting influence on the micromechanical environment of the inner hair cell stereociliary bundles. Thus, motile activity of the outer hair cell may have a direct bearing on the micromechanics of the cochlea. This paper is an attempt to review the current data of the sub-structural organization of the mammalian auditory hair cell that are relevant to the sensory transduction process and cell motility.

Hair Cell Ultrastructures

1. STEREOCILIARY ORGANIZATION IN INNER AND OUTER HAIR CELLS

An important observation made in recent years is the existence of the gradation of the stereocilary stiffness along the cochlear length (Strelioff & Flock, 1984). The stereocilia is made up of polymerized F actin cables bundled by linking protein fimbrin, and such molecular organization provides the stereociliary stiffness. The stereociliary stiffness may be dictated by the gradation of the ciliary length, the thickness of the stereocilia, the geometric arrangement of the stereociliary bundle, the difference in height of the first and second row, as well as the degree of the lateral connecting linkage system.

A unique feature of the auditory sensory stereociliary bundles in many species is the presence of *tip links* (Pickles et al., 1984). The tip links are observed in both inner and outer hair cell stereocilia. According to the concept of Hudspeth (1982), the bending of the stereociliary bundle to the excitatory direction would open the transduction channel allowing the K^+ ion to pass through, while the bending of the hair bundles toward an inhibitory direction would close the ion channels. It has been suggested that the tip links may be related to these transduction channels. However, the nature of this tip link is not yet established.

2. MOLECULAR ORGANIZATION OF THE CUTICULAR PLATE AND MICROMECHANICS

Stereocilia are stiff rods that pivot at their bases when deflected. The rootlet of the stereocilia is held by lock-wheel-like filaments that are attached to the crisscrossing actin filaments and arranged in opposing directions in the cuticular plates (Hirokawa & Tilney, 1982). Such an arrangement may be designed to regulate the stereociliary stiffness by adjusting the rootlet-anchoring tension. The stiffness of the stereociliary tension can be modulated by the increase of intracellular calcium and ATP (Orman & Flock, 1983). The exact mechanism for this stereociliary stiffness modulation is not fully understood, although Nielsen and Slepecky (1986) suggested that the cytoskeletal and contractile proteins present in the cuticular plates directly affect the stereocilia stiffness in both inner and outer hair cells. It is conceivable that the stereociliary stiffness may modulate the micromechanics of the transduction system.

3. ORGANIZATION OF THE OUTER HAIR CELL

As mentioned, there are several lines of evidence to indicate that the outer hair cell is motile. There are two types of motile activities reported: slow contraction (e.g. induced by high K+ concentration in the medium or by acetylcholine) (Brownell, 1983; Flock et al., 1986; Zenner, 1988) and fast contraction/relaxation induced by alternating hyper- or hypopolarizing currents (Ashmore, 1987; Zenner et al., 1987; Kachar et al., 1986; Evans & Warner, 1987). Contrary to this, the inner hair cell does not show any evidence of motility. Thus, in order to shed light on the cellular and molecular basis for motile activity of the outer hair cell, a critical examination and comparison of the fine morphology of the outer hair cell and that of the inner hair cell is needed.

One of the remarkable features of the outer hair cell is the presence of well organized cisternae which are considered to be specialized endoplasmic reticulum. These are *subsurface cisternae*, encircling the entire inner circumference of the body of the hair cell; *sub-synaptic cisternae* that are apposing to the efferent nerve endings as a collapsed double layer; and *apical cisternae*, which appear dome-shaped, encircling the basal body in the cuticle-free area of the hair cell (Lim, 1986) (Fig. 1). Outer hair cell subsurface cistern, by virtue of their intimate association with mitochondria, suggest that its function requires a high level of energy consumption.

The subsurface cisternae are firmly attached (or anchored) to the inner leaflet of the plasma membrane by means of an amorphous "*subplasma lamina*" resembling the basal lamina of the epithelial cells (Lim, 1986), and

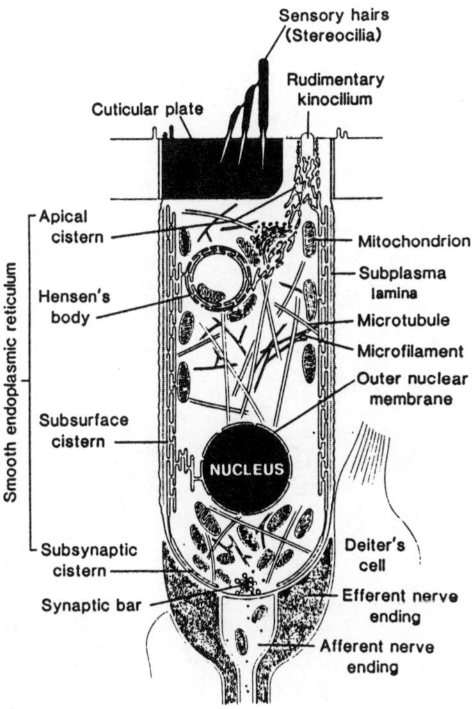

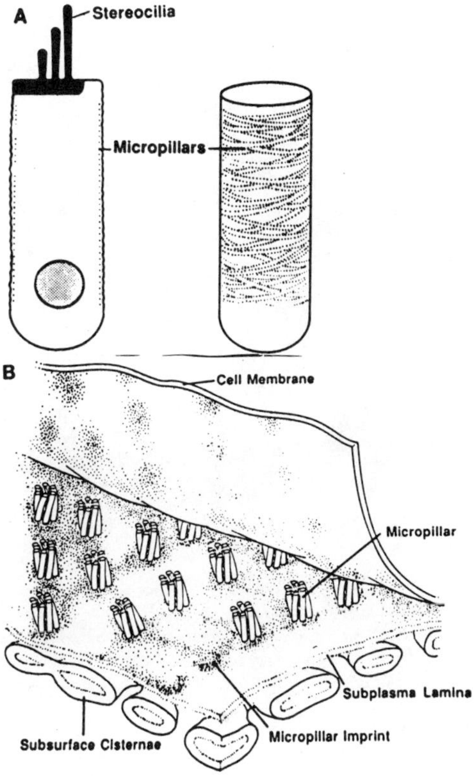

FIGURE 1. (Left) A schematic representation of the substructures of the outer hair cell.

FIGURE 2A. (Right) An artistic conception of the subsurface cisternal associated "micropillars" which are arranged in parallel arrays in a criss-cross fashion.

FIGURE 2B. An artistic conception of the subplasma lamina associated with micropillars which bridge between the hair cell plasmalemma and the subsurface cisternae.

the subplasma lamina associated "*micropillars*" which anchor the outermost layer of the subsurface cisternae to the inner leaflet of the cell wall (Figs. 2, 3, 4). The micropillars have been described as "short pillars" (Flock et al., 1986) and "circumferential filaments" (Holley and Ashmore, 1988b).

In our concept, the micropillars are arranged in parallel arrays embedded in the subplasma lamina in a criss-cross fashion encircling the entire inner surface of the outer hair cell (Fig. 3A). In a high magnification view, the single micropillar appears to be formed of multiple units (6-8) of slightly helical filaments forming a tubular opening in the center (Fig. 3B) (Flock - personal communication). Sections of Triton-extracted outer hair cells prepared for transmission electron microscopy revealed a circumferential lattice composed of filaments 5-8nm thick and 40-50nm apart (Holley & Ashmore, 1988b).

The subplasma lamina appears as a sheet and is closely associated with the outer leaflet of the subsurface cisternae. This amorphous lamina, with a parallel array of indented marks that approximate the circumferential parallel array of micropillars, is well-preserved in freeze-fractured and osmium digested specimens (Fig. 3A & B). This can be interpreted to suggest that the micropillars were partly embedded in the subplasma

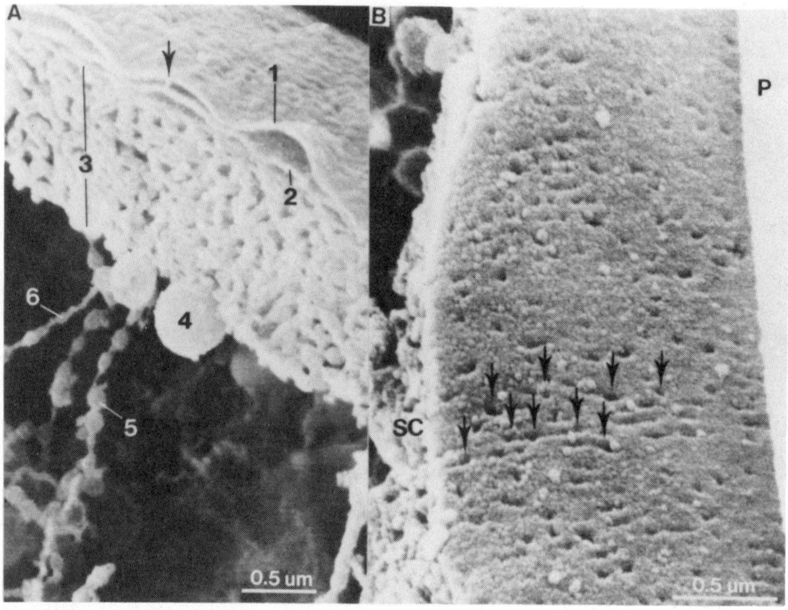

FIGURE 3A. A high resolution SEM photograph of chinchilla outer hair cell showing plasmalemma (1), subplasma lamina (2), subsurface cisternae (3), mitochondria (4), and tubulovesicles (5) attached to the microtubules (6). A micropillar-like structure ? (arrow) is seen.

FIGURE 3B. A close-up view of the subplasma lamina covering the subsurface cisternae (SC) showing parallel arrays of indentations (arrows).

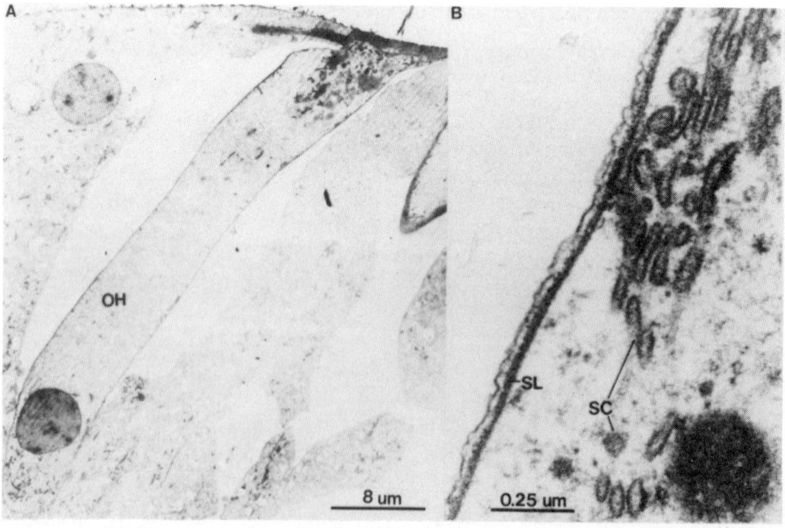

FIGURE 4A. A TEM micrograph of guinea pig outer hair (OH) maintaining its cell shape even when the subsurface cisternae are lost by kanamycin ototoxicity.

FIGURE 4B. A portion of the lateral wall of the guinea pig outer hair cell, which also maintains its cell shape following acoustic trauma, showing well preserved and thickened subplasma lamina (SL) with a few detached subsurface cisternae (SC).

lamina, but dissolved away by the osmium digestion procedure. Holley and Ashore (1988b) also described connecting fibrils between micropillars, which may also exist to provide additional circumferential strength of the cell wall.

The subplasma lamina often remained intact (or even became thicker) following severe disruption or disappearance of most of the subsurface cisternae due to acoustic trauma or aminoglycoside ototoxicity (Fig. 4A & B). Such cells, although they look empty, are remarkably able to maintain their cell shape, suggesting that this amorphous lamina may be a critical backbone for maintaining the cell shape.

Although the functions of the micropillars are not yet known, Flock et al. (1986) suggested they are similar to T-tubules of the sarcoplasmic reticulum of the skeletal muscle fibers. They also observed using the immuno-gold technique the localization of actin (in the general vicinity of the micropillars) and suggested that these structures may be involved in the contraction and elongation of the outer hair cells.

Holley and Ashore (1988a) also postulated that the "circumferential filaments" (micropillars) of the outer hair cell is related to the force generation of the outer hair cells. The helical pattern of cross-linked circumferential filaments (or micropillars) is suggested to be best suited for maintaining the cylindrical shape of the outer hair cell, while allowing limited change in cell length and diameter. In their recent study, Holley and Ashmore (1988b) demonstrated that the dissociated outer hair cell shape was retained following extraction with Triton X-100 in a buffer designed to stabilize the cytoskeleton. When a dissociated outer hair cell was placed in the hyperosmotic extraction buffer without Triton, the cell collapsed but recovered its original cell shape within seconds when Triton was added. Assuming that their "circumferential filaments" are integral parts of the subplasma lamina, their finding is in line with our observation that the outer hair cell maintains its shape when the subplasma lamina complex is preserved, although the subsurface cistern is lost following cell injuries.

4. ORGANIZATION OF THE INNER HAIR CELL

In contrast to the well-organized and specialized cisternal system in the outer hair cell, the inner hair cell has a well developed tubulo-vesicular cytoplasmic membrane system which fills the entire body of the hair cell. Mitochondria are scattered more or less evenly in the hair cell body. As the tubulovesicular system may be related to the neuro-transmitter vesicles and membrane turnover, this finding may suggest that the inner hair cell is better equipped with the neurotransmitter vesicle production.

Flock et al. (1986) examined the subsurface cisternae of the inner hair cell and found no micropillars. However, recently Forge (1988) in this meeting described the presence of "circumferential trabeculae" in the inner hair cell. This structure in the inner hair cells is also associated with a poorly developed single lamina of the subsurface cistern. It appears that the subsurface cistern is not found consistently, and even when found, they do not cover the entire length of the inner hair cell body, leaving a large portion of the lower part devoid of such structure. Because systematic studies on the subsurface cisternal system of the inner hair cells have not yet been done, it is difficult to conclude with any certainty the role this system plays in cell shape maintenance and/or sensory transduction in the inner hair cell. However, the fact that large number of mitochondria are intimately attached to the surface of the subsurface cisternae of the outer hair cell but not the inner hair cell subsurface cistern (when present) suggests that they may have different energy requirements and different specialized functions.

It is interesting to note that, in the inner hair cell, most of the efferent nerve endings of the medial system do not directly synapse with the sensory cell body, but rather establish synapses with afferent fibers. This finding would imply that, unlike the outer hair cell body, which is directly influenced by the lateral efferent nerve (mediated through the subsurface cisternae), the inner hair cell body is largely not under direct efferent neural influence. Although some efferent nerve endings may make direct contact with the inner hair cell, they are only a few.

5. CYTOSKELETAL ORGANIZATION OF THE HAIR CELLS

Many cytoskeletal and contractile proteins are found in the sensory cells (Drenckhahn et al., 1985; Zenner, 1986; Nielsen & Slepecky, 1986). They may play an important role for modulating stereociliary stiffness, length of the outer hair cells, and motile activity of the outer hair cells, thus contributing to the tuning of the auditory organ. For a hair cell to rapidly change its cell shape, it must have a cellular mechanism to support the motile activity. While the information is far from clear as to the molecular organization of the lateral cell wall as well as the complex cytosole of the hair cells, many investigators have attempted to characterize and localize the cytoskeletal/contractile proteins in the hair cells in order to better understand the cellular micromechanics of the auditory hair cells. (Flock et al., 1982, 1986; Drenckhahn et al., 1985; Zenner, 1988; Slepecky & Chamberlain, 1985; Slepecky et al., 1988.)

Microtubules are important cytoskeletal proteins that often determine the polarized cell shape (particularly during development) and determine the distribution of actin filaments and intermediate filaments. Antibodies to *tubulin* labeled a network of microtubules in the outer hair cell in the supranuclear (Slepecky et al., 1988a), infranuclear, and cuticular plate associated regions (Hackney & Furness, 1988). Under a high resolution SEM, the freeze-fractured, osmium-digested outer hair cell shows supranuclear and infranuclear groups. The supranuclear group consists largely of bundles of microtubules and microfilaments that run centrally and longitudinally, and attach to the nuclear envelope, and run radially, linking the subsurface cisternae. In the basal group, orientation of microtubules is irregular: some running oblique to the cell surface and some run in a right angle to it. It appears that microtubular systems are better developed in the outer hair cell, and the number of microtubules present varies considerably among specimens. When the dissociated guinea pig outer hair cell was incubated in the medium containing microtubule de-polymerizing agent colchicine, it had no effect on the cell shape (Zenner et al., 1985). Thus, these microtubular systems do not appear to provide the structural framework of the mature outer hair cell. In high resolution SEM small vesicles are often found attached to the microtubule (Lim et al., unpublished data), suggesting that the microtubules may serve as a guide for transporting microvesicles as in other cells (Kachar et al., 1987).

Actins are also major cytoskeletal proteins and are involved in cell shape maintenance or change by assembling the actin from the labile pool or disassembling them when not needed. Antibody to *smooth-muscle actin* diffusely stained the outer hair cell body and the stereocilia and cuticular plate, but the inner hair cell body was not stained (Slepecky et al., 1988). Antibodies to *non-muscle actin* labeled the lateral wall of the outer hair cell as well as the stereocilia, cuticular plate, and central core (Slepecky et al., 1988). Immune electron microscopy showed discrete localization of actin along the circumferential spotty protruded areas of the inner side of the outer hair cell plasmalemma (Flock et al., 1986). These actins may provide a structural framework of the outer hair cell and may play a role in the active process of the outer hair cells.

Myosins are contraction-producing proteins and actin-activated ATPase. Although antibodies to *smooth-muscle myosin* failed to stain the organ of Corti, antibodies to *non-muscle myosin* positively labeled cuticular plates of both the inner and outer hair cells (Drenckhahn et al., 1985), and possibly the lateral side of the outer hair cell (their Figure 14). The non-muscle myosin can mediate contraction of cells by interacting with actin filaments in a Ca^{2+}-dependent manner. The presence of myosin together with actin in the lateral surface of the outer hair cell raises the possibility that actin-myosin interaction is involved in certain types (slow) of outer hair cell motility.

Discussion

Molecular organization of the various cell components of the auditory hair cells may have direct bearings on the micromechanics of the auditory sensory system. These include the stereociliary stiffness, cuticular plate rigidity, and motile activity of the hair cell body. The stereociliary stiffness can be affected by the stereociliary length, size, and thickness, molecular organization of hair cell bundles, and interciliary linkages, and the tension (or rigidity) of the cuticular plate into which the rootlet is inserted. The tensile strength of the tectorial membrane may also play a role in the micromechanics of the sensory transduction. The modulation of stiffness of the stereociliary bundles and/or tectorial membrane and the outer hair cell length all will directly and indirectly influence the micromechanics of the auditory sensory transduction process.

While many of cytoskeletal/contractile proteins and specialized membrane structures described in the outer hair cell may be related to both the fast and slow motility of the outer hair cells, it is difficult to explain the fast motility that is not dependent on Ca^{2+} or ATP with the commonly known cellular mechanisms. Recently Kachar et al. (1986) proposed electro-osmosis as a possible mechanism for fast motility of the hair cell. Obviously future studies concerning the clarification of the molecular organization of the sensory cells are crucial in better elucidating the active micromechanical regulatory process in auditory sensory cells.

Acknowledgements

Supported, in part, by the Distinguished Scholar Award of the Ohio State University.

References

Ashmore, J.F. (1987) A fast motile response in guinea-pig outer hair cells: The cellular basis of the cochlear amplifier. J. Physiol. 388, 323-347.

Brownell, W.E. (1983) Observations on a motile response in isolated hair cells. In: Mechanisms of Hearing (Eds. Webster, W.R. and Aitken, L.M.), Monash University Press, Clayton, Australia, pp. 5-10.

Drenckahn, D., Schafer, T., and Prinz, M. (1985) Actin, myosin, and associated proteins in the vertebrate auditory and vestibular organs: Immunocytochemical and biochemical studies. In: Auditory Biochemistry (Ed. Drescher, D.G.), Charles C. Thomas, Springfield, IL, pp. 317-335.

Evans, B.N. and Warner, R.L. (1987) Frequency response analysis of isolated outer hair cells to sinusoidal and step function stimuli. In: Abstracts of the Tenth Midwinter Research Meeting, Association for Research in Otolaryngology, Feb. 1-5, Clearwater Beach, Florida, p. 25.

Flock, Å., Bretscher, A. and Weber, K. (1982) Immunohistochemical localization of several cytoskeletal proteins in inner ear sensory and supporting cells. Hear. Res. 6, 75-89.

Flock, Å., Flock, B. and Ulfendahl, M. (1986) Mechanisms of movement in outer hair cells and a possible structural basis. Arch. Otorhinolaryngol. 243, 83-90.

Forge, A. (1988) The lateral walls of inner and outer hair cells. In: Cochlear Mechanisms: Structure, Function and Models, eds. J.P. Wilson and D.T. Kemp, Plenum, NY.

Hackney, C.M. and Furness, D.N. (1988) Observations on the Cytoskeleton and Related Structures of Mammalian Cochlear Hair Cells. Abstracts of the Mechanics of Hearing 1988 Advanced Research Workshop, July 4-8, University of Keele, England.

Hirokawa, N. and Tilney, L. (1982) Interactions between actin filaments and between actin filaments and membranes in quick-frozen and deeply etched hair cells of the chick ear. J. Cell Biol. 95, 249-261.

Holley, M.C. and Ashmore, J.F. (1988a) On the mechanism of a high-frequency force generator in outer hair cells isolated from the guinea pig cochlea. Proc. R. Soc. London B232, 413-429.

Holley, M.C. and Ashmore, J.F. (1988b) A cytoskeletal spring for the control of cell shape in outer hair cells isolated from the guinea pig cochlea. In: Abstracts of the Inner Ear Biology Workshop, Sept. 4-7, University College, London.

Hudspeth, A.J. (1982) Extracellular current flow and the site of transduction by vertebrate hair cells. J. Neurosci. 2, 1-10.

Kachar, B., Albanesi, J.P., Fujisaki, H. and Korn, E.D. (1987) Extensive purification from Acanthamoeba castellanii of a microtubule - dependent translocator with microtubule - activated Mg^{2+} - ATPase activity. J. Biol. Chem. 33, 16180-16185.

Kachar, B., Brownell, W.E., Altschuler, R. and Fex, J. (1986) Electrokinetic shape changes of cochlear outer hair cells. Nature 322(6077), 365-367.

Liberman, M.C. and Kiang, N.Y.S. (1984) Single-neuron labeling and chronic cochlear pathology. IV. Stereocilia damage and alterations in rate- and phase-level functions. Hear. Res. 16, 75-90.

Lim, D.J. (1986) Functional structure of the organ of Corti: A review. Hear. Res. 22, 117-146.

Nielsen, D.W. and Slepecky, N. (1986) Stereocilia. In: Neurobiology of Hearing: The Cochlea (Eds. Altschuler, R.A., Bobbin, R.P. and Hoffman, D.W.), Raven Press, New York, 23-46.

Pickles, J.O., Comis, S.D. and Osborne, M.P. (1984) Cross-links between stereocilia in the guinea pig organ of Corti, and their possible relation to sensory transduction. Hear. Res. 15, 103-112.

Orman, S. and Flock, Å. (1983) Active control of sensory hair mechanics implied by susceptibility to media that induce contraction in muscle. Hear. Res. 11, 261-266.

Slepecky, N., Ulfendahl, M. and Flock, Å. (1988) Effects of caffeine and tetracaine on outer hair cell shortening suggest intracellular calcium involvement. Hear. Res. 32, 11-22.

Strelioff, D. and Flock, Å. (1984) Stiffness of sensory-cell hair bundles in the isolated guinea pig cochlea. Hear. Res. 15, 19-28.

Zenner, H.P. (1986) Molecular structure of hair cells. In: Neurobiology of Hearing: The Cochlea (Eds. Altschuler, R.A., Bobbin, R.P. and Hoffman, D.W.), Raven Press, New York, 1-21.

Zenner, H.P. (1988) Motility of outer hair cells as an active, actin-mediated process. Acta Otolaryngol. (Stockh) 105, 39-44.

Zenner, H.P., Zimmerman, U. and Gitter, A.H. (1987) Fast motility of isolated mammalian auditory sensory cells. Biochem. and Biophys. Res. Com. 149(1), 304-308.

Zenner, H.P., Zimmerman, U. and Schmitt, U. (1985) Reversible contraction of isolated mammalian cochlear hair cells. Hear. Res. 18, 127-133.

OBSERVATIONS ON THE CYTOSKELETON AND RELATED STRUCTURES OF MAMMALIAN COCHLEAR HAIR CELLS

C.M. Hackney and D.N. Furness

Department of Communication and Neuroscience
University of Keele Staffs ST5 5BG, UK

Introduction

The cytoskeleton of sensory hair cells is of particular interest since it is likely to affect the characteristics of mechano-electrical transduction in the cochlea, either indirectly, by maintaining the cellular morphology which results in precise tensions or stiffnesses, or directly, by modifying these features. At least one class of hair cell, the outer hair cell, can undergo both slow and rapid length changes (Brownell, 1985; Ashmore, 1987; Zenner et al., 1987), and the rootlets of stereocilia have been suggested to change in length after noise exposure (Liberman and Dodds 1987). Which cytoskeletal components are involved in these structural changes is not yet known. Ultrastructural differences between outer hair cells (OHCs) and inner hair cells (IHCs) have been proposed to result in differences in function - certain structures have been suggested to occur exclusively in one or other of the two cell types and related to motility as a consequence, e.g., the pillars which link the subsurface cistern to the plasmalemma (Flock et al., 1986). Other structures which occur in both OHCs and IHCs have been suggested to underly the process of transduction itself, e.g. the tip links on stereocilia (Pickles et al., 1984). It is therefore of interest to continue to make ultrastructural observations on the morphology of the hair cells which may be relevant to the mechanics of the cochlea.

Methods

For transmission electron microscopy (TEM), cochleae from pigmented guinea pigs were fixed with 2.5% glutaraldehyde in 0.1M sodium cacodylate and 2mM calcium chloride buffer for 2h, and postfixed in 1% osmium tetroxide (in the same buffer) for 1h, then dehydrated and embedded in Spurr resin as described previously (Furness and Hackney, 1985). For scanning electron microscopy (SEM), cochlear segments were prepared using the osmium thiocarbohydrazide (OTOTO) technique (which makes gold coating unnecessary), then dehydrated and critical point dried (see Furness and Hackney, 1986a, for details). All specimens were examined in a JEOL 100CX electron microscope with an ASID.4D scanning attachment.

Results and Discussion

STEREOCILIA - FILAMENTS AND LINKAGES

It is well known that stereocilia contain parallel arrays of longitudinally orientated actin microfilaments (Flock and Cheung, 1977; and Figs. 1a, b). There is also a ring of intermediate filaments around the central actin bundle towards the base of the stereocilium (Furness and Hackney, 1988). In transverse sections of the ankle region, the actin filament bundle is enclosed by a peripheral dense zone (Fig. 1c). As the stereocilium broadens out, individual profiles of 10-12 nm diameter filaments can be seen (Fig. 1d). Similar structures appear to be present in both IHC and OHC stereocilia. The composition of these filaments is unknown, but they could represent actin filaments in association with tropomyosin, which has already been reported to occur in the rootlet region (Flock, 1985; Slepecky and Chamberlain, 1985). An alternative possibility for the composition of these filaments is myosin, which has been demonstrated immunocytochemically in stereocilia (Macartney et al., 1980) although there has been a suggestion that the staining was non-specific (Drenkhahn et al., 1982). Whatever the explanation, the presence of these thicker filaments in association with rootlet region is intriguing as they may be involved in stiffness or even length changes of the stereocilium.

In addition to observations on intracellular filaments we have also accumulated many observations on extracellular linkages between stereocilia. Considerable attention has been focussed on these since Pickles et al. (1984) suggested that one category of link running from the tip of each short stereocilium to the side of the taller stereocilium behind was in an appropriate position to be involved in the transduction process by mechanically affecting the ion channels. We noticed that not only is there dense material under the membrane at the apex of each stereocilium (Engstrom and Engstrom, 1978), and thus at one end of the tip link, but also a submembraneous density associated with the other end of the link (Figs. 1a, b), on the side of the tall stereocilium (Furness and Hackney, 1985). This would seem to support the suggestion that these linkages have a specific function. However, our observations on the linkage systems differ in several important respects from those of Pickles' group.

Firstly, we see linkages in well-osmicated material, both in TEM and in SEM (Fig. 2; Furness and Hackney, 1986a). This differs from the results obtained by Osborne et al. (1984) which suggest that the links are osmium sensitive and from which it has been implied that they may be composed of actin (Pickles et al., 1988). (In our TEM material the tip-to-side links are finer (2-3nm) in diameter than the intrastereociliary actin filaments - Fig. 1a, b). The extent and appearance of the side-to-side linkages can be modified by the presence or absence of calcium ions (Hackney and Furness, 1985), so perhaps the routine addition of 2mM $CaCl_2$ to our fixation media improves the preservation of these structures in our hands. Secondly, we have observed tip-to-side links in animals treated chronically with high levels of kanamycin (Fig. 2b), even on hair cell bundles with fused stereocilia (Furness and Hackney, 1986b), a result which suggests that they are resistant to this particular ototoxic agent. This also differs from the findings of Pickles et

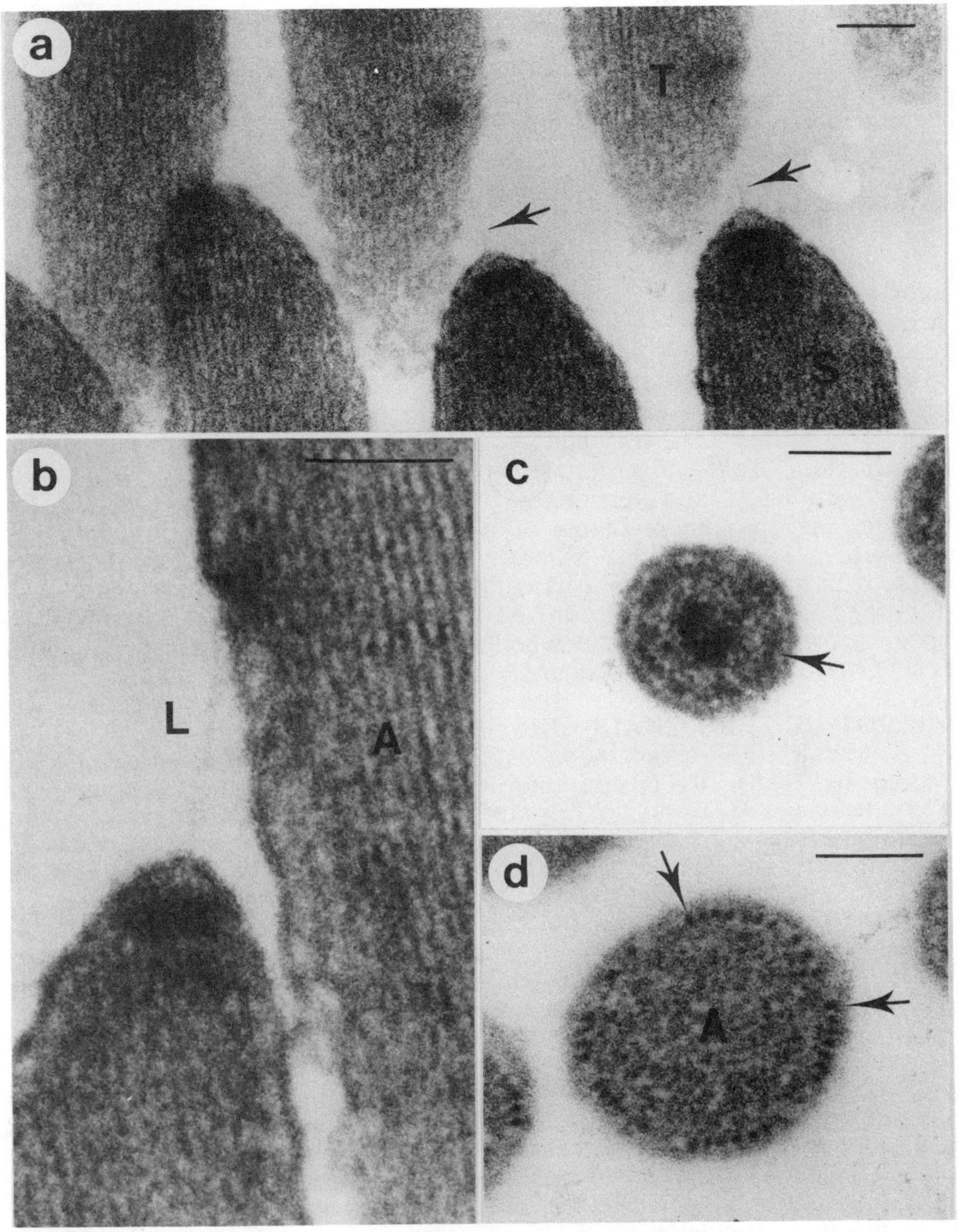

FIGURE 1 (a) Tangential section of OHC stereocilia showing the tip-to-side links in face view (arrows) between tall stereocilia (T) and shorter stereocilia (S) of adjacent rows. Note the dense patches at either end of the links. (b) Longitudinal section of OHC stereocilia showing a tip-to-side link (L). Electron dense material underlies the membrane at either end of the link. The appearance and dimensions of the linkage filament differ from that of intracellular actin filaments (A) within the stereocilia. (c) Cross-section of the ankle region of a stereocilium. A peripheral densely-staining zone (arrow) encloses the actin filament bundle and the central rootlet. (d) Cross-section of the shaft region of a stereocilium. An incomplete peripheral ring of densely-staining thick (ca. 10 nm diameter) filaments (arrows) surrounds the bundle of thinner (4-7 nm diameter), more lightly-stained actin filaments (A). Bars = 100 nm.

al., (1987), who suggest that the links are sensitive to kanamycin. Thirdly, we have seen side-to-side links running intercellularly, between adjacent IHCs (Fig. 2c), and between adjacent OHCs. Side-to-side linkages have been suggested to hold the stereocilia in appropriate positions for transduction during displacement. If this is so, the intercellular linkages, which may occur between 70% of IHCs (Hackney and Furness, 1986), might be expected to result in movements of adjacent IHC bundles. Since no-one has so far reported observing this during experimental manipulations, the proposed function seems unlikely. In addition to intercellular side-to-side linkages, we have seen tip-to-side links in unexpected positions, e.g., running between closely opposed IHCs (Fig. 2d). They also occur on hair cells which have their bundles rotated from their normal position and on the strial-facing side of bundles which have short stereocilia in the appropriate position (Hackney et al., 1988, in press). Thus, they seem to be found where the appropriate stereociliary geometry arises rather than necessarily in appropriate sites for transduction. Taken together with recent work on the glycocalyx by Lim (1986) and Santi and Andersen (1987), these results suggest that the linkages may be the remnants of a more extensive glycocalyx which is best-preserved in regions where the stereocilia are closely opposed, perhaps in association with particular ion channels. In the absence of any published physiological data on the function of the linkage systems, it is now important to investigate whether their presence is indeed necessary for normal transduction to occur.

MICROTUBULES IN HAIR CELLS

Although the organization of the microtubule systems of the supporting cells has been studied in detail (e.g., Slepecky and Chamberlain, 1983), only a few authors discuss the microtubule systems of hair cells (e.g., Ekstrom von Lubitz, 1982 ; Morup Jorgensen, 1982; Lim, 1986). The function of the microtubule systems in hair cells is unknown - they may represent mechanical strengthening, be used to transport neurotransmitter vesicles or represent a substrate for movement or tension changes. We are reconstructing serial sections in TEM to determine microtubular organisation in relation to other cytoskeletal structures, e.g., the cuticular plate.

In IHCs the upper surface of the cuticular plate is frequently grooved, and lies adjacent to the apical plasma membrane except for a belt of cytoplasm around the periphery of the apex. This belt is widest on the side of the cells facing the strial wall of the *scala media*, and is continuous with the channel between the upper and lower surfaces of the plate (Fig. 3a). The lower surface of the cuticular plate follows the contours of the upper surface centrally and at the edge is extended downwards, particularly on the strial side. There are many microtubules in the cytoplasm surrounding the cuticular plate, following its contours. Three main groups can be identified on the basis of position and orientation (Fig. 3a). These are: (1) as a ring just on the edge of the cuticular plate, and lining the channel through it (in which the basal body is often found); (2) as a meshwork below the central lower surface of the cuticular plate; (3) in a ring just inside the lateral lower extensions of the plate. Microtubules are also found running in an apex to base direction

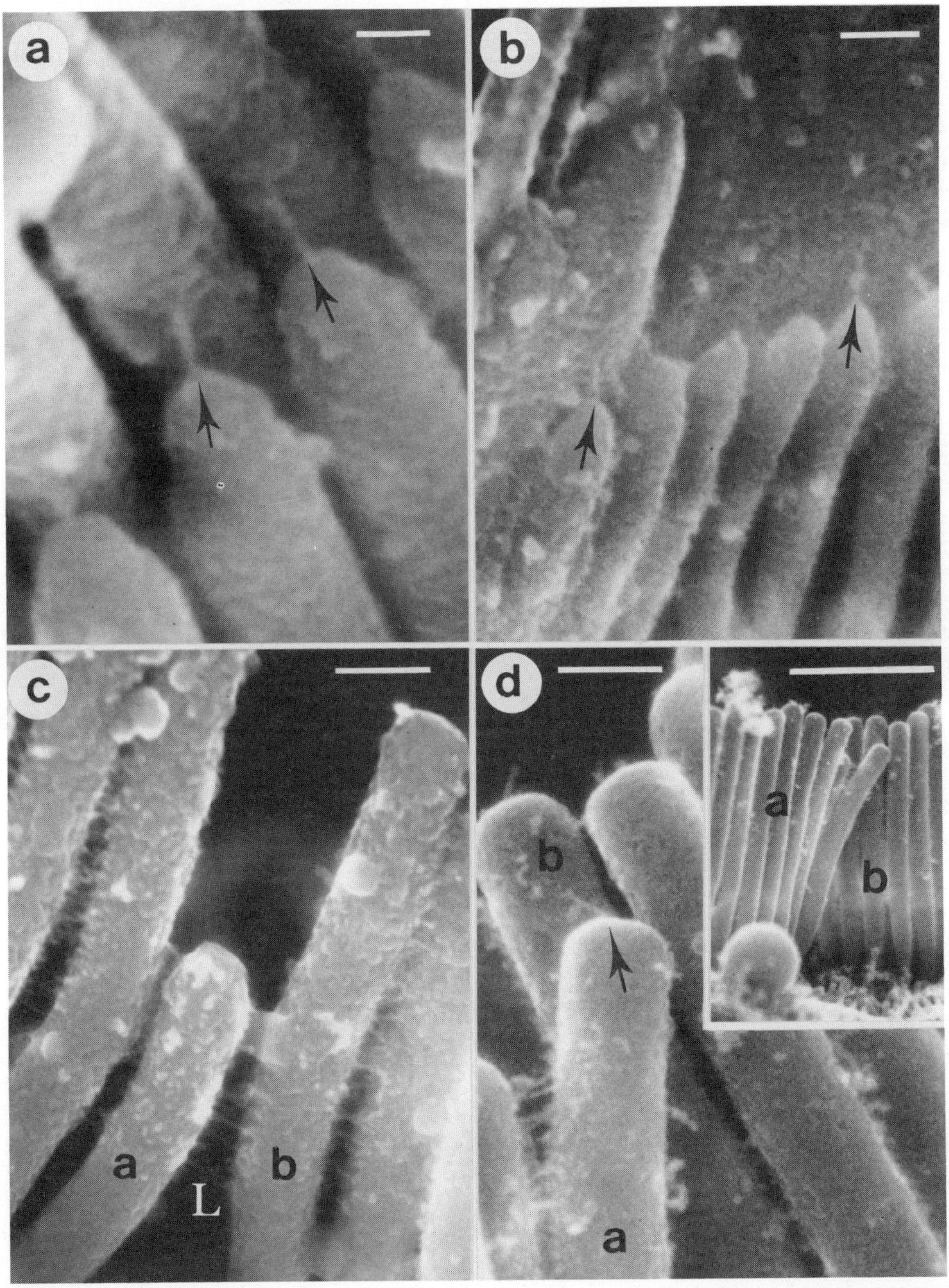

FIGURE 2 (a) OHC stereocilia in a specimen treated with high levels of osmium during the OTOTO preparation procedure, showing tip-to-side links (arrows). Bar = 0.1 μm. (b) OHC stereocilia in a specimen from a kanamycin-treated guinea pig. Tip links are still present despite considerable fusion of several stereocilia (arrows). OTOTO preparation, bar = 0.2 μm. (c) IHC stereocilia from two adjacent bundles (a, b) showing intercellular lateral links (L). OTOTO preparation, bar = 0.5 μm. (d) IHC stereocilia from two adjacent bundles (a, b) showing an intercellular tip-to-side link (arrow). Bar = 0.5 μm. Inset: Low magnification view of the two bundles (a, b) between which the link runs. OTOTO preparation, bar = 2 μm.

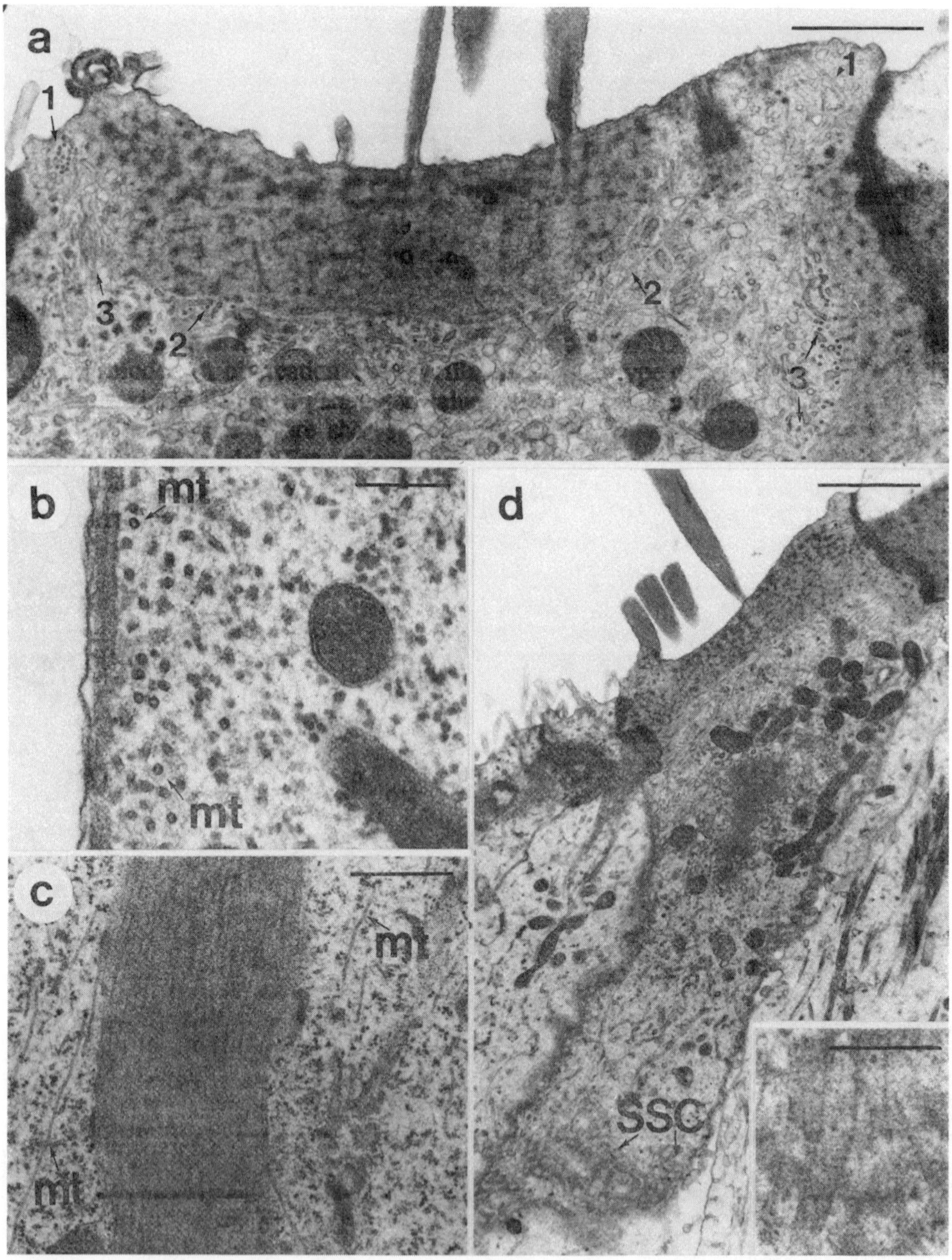

FIGURE 3 (a) Radial section of the apex of an IHC showing three main groups of microtubules (numbered as in the text) around the cuticular plate. Bar = 1 µm. (b) Section through the basal region of an OHC showing microtubules (mt) running just below the subsurface cisternae. Bar = 0.25 µm. (c) Detail of the downward extension of the cuticular plate in an OHC from the cochlear apex, showing the filamentous structure surrounded by microtubules (mt). Bar = 1 µm. (d) Glancing section of IHC showing the subsurface cistern (SSC). Bar = 2 µm. Inset: Detail of the IHC cistern showing structures resembling the pillars seen in OHCs. Bar = 0.5 µm.

in the cell body in bundles or groups, and are present in the synaptic region of the cell. The OHCs show a similar pattern of microtubular distribution but at the apex the microtubules tend to be fewer in number. Many microtubules are found towards the base of the OHCs, running around the hair cell body just below the subsurface cisternae (Fig. 3b), with others forming a cytoplasmic network below the nucleus. They are also found around a downward extension of the cuticular plate which has been reported previously in cells from the apex of the cochlea (Thorne et al, 1988), which can be seen to contain microfilaments and dense strands (Fig. 3c). Immunofluorescent studies at the light microscope level using an anti-tubulin antibody agree well with these electron microscopic observations (Furness et al., 1988).

CISTERNAL SYSTEMS

The structure of the subsurface cistern in OHCs has been well-described by previous authors (see Lim, 1986, for a review). This system has recently been suggested to play a role in both the slow contractions performed by these cells (Flock et al., 1986) and the faster ones (Brownell, 1986) which appear unaffected by blockers of acto-myosin interactions (Holley and Ashmore, 1988). Flock et al. (1986) suggested that the 'pillars' which occur in rows between the outermost membrane of the subsurface cistern and the plasmalemma, resemble structures associated with the T-tubules of muscle and that the mechanism underlying OHC motility was similar to that found in muscle. It is therefore relevant to point out that not only do IHCs have a subsurface cistern (Kimura, 1975), although it is generally less-developed than that of the OHCs, but that this is also connected to the plasmalemma by structures resembling the OHC pillars in position, dimensions and track-like pattern (Fig. 3d). It has been noted by Smith (1978) that the numbers of stacked cisternae in the OHCs varies from species to species. It would be of interest to know whether OHCs from cats or primates where there are fewer cisternae exhibit motility, or whether this is independent of the numbers of cisternae, as is perhaps indicated by the presence of the subsurface cistern with its associated pillars in the apparently non-motile IHCs. (Supported by the Wellcome Trust and MRC.)

References

Ashmore, J.F. (1987) A fast motile response in the guinea pig outer hair cells: the cellular basis of the cochlear amplifier. J. Physiol. 388, 323-347.

Brownell, W.E. (1985) Evoked mechanical responses of isolated cochlear outer hair cells. Science 227, 194-196.

Brownell, W.E. (1986) Outer hair cell motility and cochlear frequency selectivity. In: Auditory Frequency Selectivity (Eds: Moore, B.J.C. and Patterson, R.D.) Plenum Press, New York and London, pp. 109-116.

Drenkhahn, D., Kellner, J., Mannherz, H.G., Groschel-Steward, U., Kendrick-Jones, J. and Scholey, J. (1982) Absence of myosin-like immunoreactivity in stereocilia of cochlear hair cells. Nature 300, 531-532.

Ekstrom von Lubitz, D.K.J. (1981) Sub-surface tubular system in the outer sensory cells of the rat cochlea. Cell. Tiss. Res. 220, 787-795.

Engstrom, H. and Engstrom, B. (1978) Structure of the hairs on cochlear sensory cells. Hearing Res. 1, 49-66.

Flock, A. (1985) Contractile and structural proteins in the auditory organ. In: Auditory Biochemistry (Eds: Drescher, D. and Thomas, C.C.) Springfield, Illinois, pp. 310-316.

Flock, A. and Cheung, H.C. (1977) Actin filaments in sensory hairs of inner ear receptor cells. J. Cell. Biol. 75, 339-343.
Flock, A., Flock, B. and Ulfendahl, M. (1986) Mechanisms of movement in outer hair cells and a possible structural basis. Arch. Oto.-Rhino.-Laryngol. 243, 83-90.
Furness, D.N. and Hackney, C.M. (1985) Cross-links between stereocilia in the guinea pig cochlea. Hearing Res. 18, 177-188.
Furness, D.N. and Hackney, C.M. (1986a) High-resolution scanning electron microscopy of stereocilia using the osmium thiocarbohydrazide coating technique. Hearing Res. 21, 243-249.
Furness, D.N. and Hackney, C.M. (1986b) Morphological changes to the stereociliary bundles in the guinea pig cochlea after kanamycin treatment. Brit. J. Audiol. 20, 253-259.
Furness, D.N. and Hackney, C.M. (1988) Cytoskeletal organisation in the apex of cochlear hair cells. Symposium on Auditory Pathway - Structure and Function (In press).
Furness, D.N., Steyger, P.S. and Hackney, C.M. (1988) The organization of microtubules in cochlear hair cells. Abstr. of the Eleventh Midwinter Research Meeting, Ass. for Res. in Otolaryngol. p. 141.
Hackney, C.M. and Furness, D.N. (1985) The ultrastructural effects of altering calcium levels during preparation of mammalian hair cells for electron microscopy. Abstracts of the XXII Workshop on Inner Ear Biology, p. 16.
Hackney, C.M. and Furness, D.N. (1986) Intercellular cross-linkages between the stereociliary bundles of adjacent hair cells in the guinea pig cochlea. Cell Tiss. Res. 245, 685-688.
Hackney, C.M., Furness, D.N. and Sayers, D.L. (1988) Stereociliary cross-links between adjacent inner hair cells. Hearing Res. (In press).
Holley, M.C. and Ashmore, J.F. (1988) On the mechanism of a high frequency force generator in outer hair cells isolated from the guinea pig cochlea. Proc. Roy. Soc. London. B. 78.
Kimura, R.S. (1975) The ultrastructure of the organ of Corti. Int. Rev. Cytol. 42, 173-222.
Liberman, M.C. and Dodds, L.W. (1987) Acute ultrastructural changes in acoustic trauma, serial section reconstruction of stereocilia and cuticular plates. Hearing Res. 26, 45-64.
Lim, D.J. (1986) Functional structure of the organ of Corti: a review. Hearing Res. 22, 117-146.
Macartney, J.C., Comis, S.D. and Pickles, J.O. (1980) Is myosin in the cochlea a basis for active motility? Nature 288, 491-492.
Morup Jorgensen, J. (1982) Microtubules and laminated structures in inner ear hair cells. Acta Oto.-Laryngol. 94, 241-248.
Osborne, M.P., Comis, S.D. and Pickles, J.O. (1984) Morphology and cross-linkage of stereocilia in the guinea pig labyrinth examined without the use of osmium as a fixative. Cell Tissue Res. 237, 43-48.
Pickles, J.O., Comis, S.D. and Osborne, M.P. (1984) Cross-linkages between stereocilia in the guinea pig organ of Corti, and their possible relation to sensory transduction. Hearing Res. 15, 103-112.
Pickles, J.O., Comis, S.D. and Osborne, M.P. (1987) The effect of chronic application of kanamycin on stereocilia and their tip links in hair cells of the guinea pig cochlea. Hearing Res. 29, 237-244.
Pickles, J.O., Brix, J. Gleich, O., Manley, G.A., Osborne, M.P. and Comis S.D. (1988) The fine structure and organization of tip links on hair cell stereocilia. Basic Issues in Hearing - 8th International Symposium. (In Press).
Santi, P.A. and Anderson, C.B. (1987) A newly identified surface coat on cochlear hair cells. Hearing Res., 27, 47-66.
Slepecky, N. and Chamberlain, S.C. (1983) Distribution and polarity of actin in inner ear supporting cells. Hearing Res. 10, 359-370.
Slepecky, N. and Chamberlain, S.C. (1985) Immuno-electron-microscopic and immunofluorescent localization of cytoskeletal and muscle-like contractile proteins in inner ear sensory hair cells. Hearing Res. 20, 245-260.
Smith, C.A. (1975) The inner ear: its embryological development and microstructure. In: The Nervous System. Vol. 3: Human Communication and Its Disorders. (ed. Turner, D.B.,) Raven Press, New York, pp. 1-18.
Zenner, H.P., Zimmerman, U. and Gitter, A.H. (1987) Fast motility of isolated mammalian auditory sensory cells. Biochem. Biophys. Res. Comm. 149, 304-308.

Comments and Discussion

HOLLEY

You state that fast outer hair cell length changes were not affected by blockers of acto-myosin interactions (Holley and Ashmore, 1988). In that paper we did not apply such blockers. Our arguments against an acto-myosin mechanism were based on experiments suggesting that fast length changes are independent of calcium and ATP, and that they are too fast to involve the biochemical steps required for muscle contraction.

HACKNEY

Thank you for your comment clarifying the conclusions of your paper. Our intention here was merely to indicate that it has been suggested that the fast motility is independent of acto-myosin mechanisms. With regard to your specific point perhaps a more appropriate reference here would be Zenner et al. (1987, Biochemical and Biophysical Research Communications, vol. 149, pp. 304-308) in which he states, with regard to outer hair cell responses which follow the stimulus up to at least 1 kHz: "Control experiments in the presence of cytochalasin B, phalloidin and dinitrophenol excluded actomyosin as a molecular basis of the high frequency motility".

PICKLES

Your paper raises a number of points in relation to our own work.

1. Although the central filament of the tip link has an appearance rather similar to that of an actin filament, we are careful to state that we have no detailed knowledge of its composition (see also our contribution, this volume).

2. The point of the OTOTO method is that it reduces the amount of osmium tetroxide that reacts directly with the tissue. It is therefore commonly used to preserve osmium-sensitive material. However, following further discussions, it does appear that there may well be genuine differences between the results of our different groups in the osmium-sensitivity and kanamycin-sensitivity of tip links prepared by our different methods, and this deserves further investigation.

3. We disagree strongly with the suggestion that the links we observe are simply the remains of a collapsed glycocalyx. There are four main lines of evidence supporting our view:

(i) There is a very great regularity in the organization of the tip links, with the great majority of the tip links (over 99% in the hair cells that we have examined) running parallel to the axis of bilateral symmetry. Our paper in the present volume shows further examples from the starling. If the links are merely condensation products, then the regular organization of this 99% of links is difficult to explain.

(ii) The submembrane specialisations associated with the links are difficult to account for on the basis of a condensation of extracellular material (as also suggested here by Hackney and Furness).

(iii) The links (both side-to-side and tip links) survive digestion by chondroitinase, hyaluronidase, keratonase and amylase, all of which would be expected to digest components of the glycocalyx. However, the links are readily digested by crude protease or by trypsin, wich suggests that there is an essential protein component (Osborne et al., in preparation). Interestingly, tip links survive digestion in collagenase, in the concentrations and for the periods used to extract functionally-viable hair cells for electrophysiological investigations (Brix and Pickles, to appear at Inner Ear Biology Meeting, September, 1988). This is consistent with the hypothesis that the tip links are indeed involved in transduction.

(iv) The explanation of tip links as condensation products does not account for the fine structure of the links, with a fine central filament and a surrounding variable coat, which we see consistently (Pickles et al., this volume).

A COMPARATIVE STUDY OF ACTIN FILAMENTS IN COCHLEAR HAIR CELLS: OUTER HAIR CELLS IN THE APEX OF THE GUINEA PIG COCHLEA CONTAIN A UNIQUE ULTRASTRUCTURAL FEATURE

L. Carlisle*, P.R. Thorne, G. Zajic***, R.A. Altschuler***, J. Schacht***.**

**Dept. of Audiology, Institute of Laryngology & Otology, London*
***Dept. of Pathology, Univ. of Auckland Medical School, New Zealand*
****Kresge Hearing Research Institute, Univ. of Michigan, USA*

Rhodamine-labelled phalloidin, a specific marker for filamentous actin, was used to describe the distribution of F-actin in the hair cells of the organs of Corti of guinea pigs, hooded rats, chinchillas and squirrel monkeys using surface preparations, cryosections, and isolated outer hair cells. The stereocilia and cuticular plates of all inner and outer hair cells were labelled, as were the lateral margins of outer hair cells of all species. In the outer hair cells of the apical turns of the guinea pig organ of Corti, an additional labelled structure was present in the apical cytoplasm of the cell. This infracuticular network of F-actin was never observed in outer hair cells of the basal turn of the guinea pig, nor in outer hair cells at any location in the organs of Corti of the other species examined.

Introduction

The function of the outer hair cells of the organ of Corti has been a subject of interest since Spoendlin (1969) described the paucity of afferent innervation to these cells. Subsequent physiological experimentation has attributed two functional properties to the outer hair cells (OHC); firstly, the ability to 'fine tune' information processing in the organ of Corti (LePage and Johnstone, 1980; Davis, 1983; Neely and Kim, 1986), and secondly, the ability to generate various types of cochlear emissions (Kemp, 1978; Zurek, 1981). The identification of contractile proteins in OHC, (Flock and Cheung, 1977; Tilney et al, 1980; Zenner, 1980; Slepecky and Chamberlain, 1985; Flock et al, 1986; Zenner et al, 1985; Zenner, 1986; Zenner and Drenkhahn, 1986) coupled with the demonstration that isolated OHC *in vitro* will contract either in response to electrical stimulation (Brownell et al, 1985; Kachar et al, 1986; Ashmore 1986) or in the presence of depolarizing concentrations of potassium or calcium and ATP (Flock, 1986; Zenner, 1986), suggests that OHC motility may be responsible for the active processes and tuning mechanisms described *in vivo*.

Physiological and structural differences exist in OHC at different locations along the organ of Corti. Base to apex gradients in cell length (Smith, 1968, Bohne and Carr, 1985) the number and length (Wright, 1984) and stiffness of stereocilia (Strelioff and Flock, 1984) as well as in the efferent innervation (Spoendlin, 1969) and the afferent innervation (Pujol, 1987) have been described. The observation that OHC in the base of the cochlea do not produce DC receptor potentials to high frequency stimulation except at very high sound levels suggests that basal OHC are not depolarized by sound stimulation at threshold (Russell and Cody, 1985; Dallos, 1985a). One interpretation of these functional and structural differences is that apical OHC act more as sensory receptor cells but basal OHC act predominately as effector cells (Dallos, 1985b).

Because contractile proteins may be the structural components involved in certain functions attributed to the OHC, and because differences exist in the response properties of OHC of both apical and basal regions of the organ of Corti, it would be interesting to know if a base to apex gradient existed for the presence and distribution of contractile proteins in the organ of Corti, particularly in the OHC. Actin, a major contractile protein, has been identified in the stereocilia, cuticular plates and synaptic regions of OHC (Flock and Cheung, 1977; Tilney et al, 1980; Slepecky and Chamberlain, 1985; Flock et al, 1986), and actin filaments have been observed extending from beneath the cuticular plate to the perinuclear region (Zenner, 1980; Flock et al, 1982; Drenkhahn and Zenner, 1986; Thorne et al, 1988; Carlisle et al, 1988) and along the lateral margins of OHC (Flock et al, 1986). The purpose of this study was to describe the distribution of the filamentous form of actin in the organ of Corti of several mammalian species.

Materials and Methods

Guinea pigs, chinchillas, hooded rats and squirrel monkeys were included in the study. Rhodamine-labelled phalloidin (Molecular Probes, Inc, USA), a specific marker for filamentous (F)-actin, was used to identify actin in surface preparations, cryosections, and isolated hair cells which were studied by light microscopy (Leitz Orthomat) using bright field and epifluorescence optics (460-470 nm excitation filter and 510-550 nm objective filter) and 25 - 100x oil immersion objectives. Rhodamine-labelled alpha-bungarotoxin (Molecular Probes, Inc.) was used as a control for non-specific rhodamine staining.

Surface preparations

Animals were anaesthetised (sodium pentobarbitone, 50 mg/kg), decapitated and the auditory bullae were rapidly removed and opened. Fixative (4% paraformaldehyde and 0.1% glutaraldehyde in 0.1M phosphate buffer at pH 7.4) was perfused through the round and oval windows of the cochleae. Cochleae were immersed in fixative for 1 hour, washed in phosphate buffer and then partially dissected in phosphate buffered saline (PBS). The otic capsule, spiral ligament and tectorial membrane were removed. The organ of Corti, still attached to the modiolus, was immersed in 330 nM phalloidin in PBS and incubated for 24 hours in the dark at room temperature with gentle rotation. In some cases the incubation time was increased to 48 - 72 hours or 0.1% Triton X-100 was added to the phalloidin. After washing in PBS the organ of Corti was dissected from the modiolus, mounted as a surface preparation on glass slides in 1:3 PBS/glycerol and covered with cover slips.

Cryosections

The fixation of cochleae for cryosectioning proceeded as described for surface preparations. Following removal of the otic capsule the cochleae were decalcified for 16 - 48 hours in 2% ethylene diamine tetracetic acid (EDTA) in PBS with 6% sucrose as a cryoprotectant. Ten micron mid-modiolar sections of frozen cochleae were mounted on glass slides and incubated with 330 nM phalloidin for 24 hours in the dark then washed in PBS and mounted in PBS/glycerol under cover slips.

Isolated hair cells

For isolating outer hair cells the technique described by Zenner et al (1985) and Zajic and Schacht (1987) was used. Anaesthetised animals were decapitated and the auditory bullae were removed. Selected turns of the organ of Corti were quickly dissected and placed in tissue culture medium (Hanks' balanced salt solution (HBSS); osmolarity adjusted to 300 mOsm) with 1 mg collagenase/ml at room temperature. After 10 minutes of incubation in this medium the organ of Corti was transferred into fresh HBSS and the OHC were teased away from the basilar membrane using fine tungsten probes. The isolated hair cells were transferred via a syringe to a glass well-slide and incubated in 33 nM phalloidin in HBSS for 20 minutes in the dark at room temperature, then washed in HBSS and covered with a cover slip. Some cells were pre-treated with saponin (12 ug/ml HBSS) or Triton X-100 in calcium-free media.

Results

Surface preparations of the entire length of the organ of Corti were examined. The stereocilia and cuticular plates of both inner and outer hair cells were labelled (Figure 1). Two different patterns of phalloidin labelling were seen in the cuticular plates of OHCs. In most cases the entire apical surface of the OHC was labelled, with the exception of an area at the lateral margin of the cell. In some guinea pig and squirrel monkey OHC phalloidin labelling only extended to the margin of the cell at discrete points resulting in a scalloped appearance (Figure 2). Phalloidin was present around the circumference (Figure 3) and at the base of OHCs. Inner and outer pillar cells were labelled as were all of the junctional complexes in the reticular lamina. In the Deiters cells beyond the third row OHC radiating filaments were labelled (Figure 1). Organs of Corti incubated with phalloidin-labelled a-bungarotoxin showed no fluorescence indicating the absence of non-specific reactions with phalloidin.

Some of the OHC in the guinea pig organ of Corti contained an additional labelled structure. When viewed in surface preparations, these OHC contained a cluster of phalloidin labelled 'dots' (Figure 3) which were first visible below the cuticular plate near the lateral margin of the cell and projected towards the nucleus. In cryosections (Figure 4) and

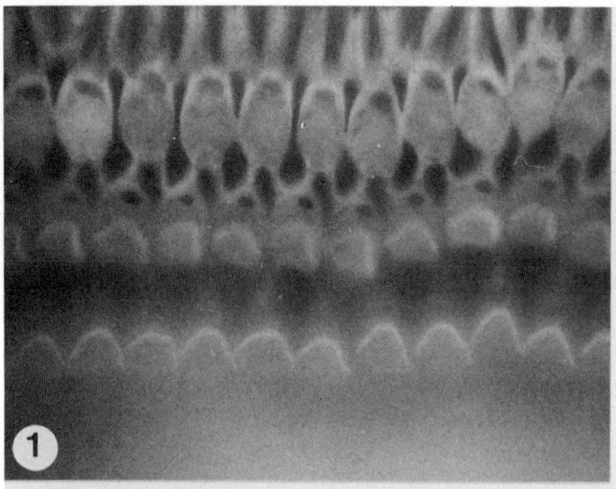

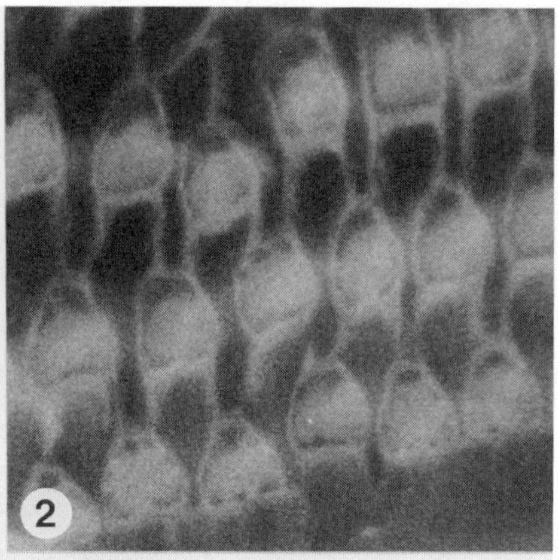

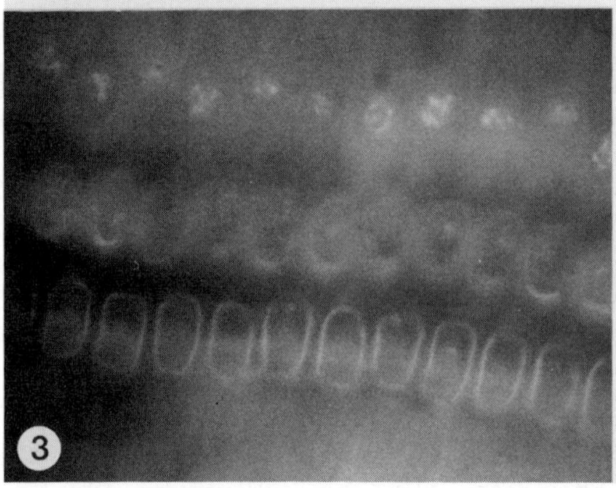

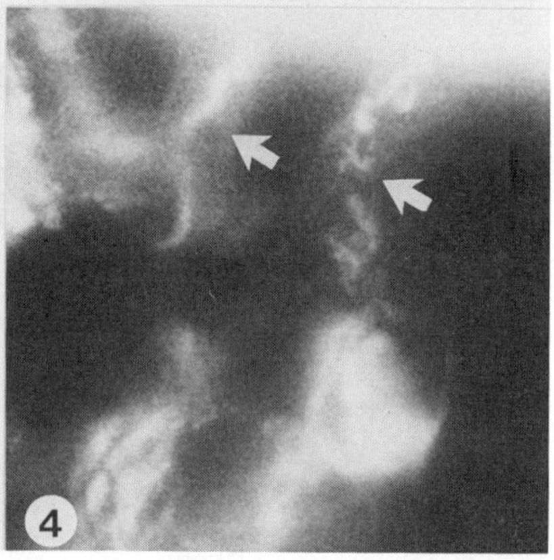

Figure 1. Surface preparation, apical guinea pig organ of Corti, showing phalloidin labelling of stereocilia and cuticular plates of OHC. Also labelled are the junctional complexes between sensory and supporting cells in the reticular lamina, as well as filaments in the Deiters cells beyond the third row OHC.

Figure 2. Surface preparation, squirrel monkey organ of Corti. The pattern of phalloidin staining in the cuticular plate results in a scalloped appearance, particularly in the first row OHC.

Figure 3. Apical guinea pig organ of Corti, same location as in Figure 1 at a deeper level of focus. Highly fluorescent 'dots' of phalloidin are visible, particularly in third row OHC. Phalloidin labelling of the circumference of first and second row OHC is also observed.

Figure 4. Cryosection of apical guinea pig organ of Corti, showing phalloidin labelling of the infracuticular network (arrows) in a second and third row OHC.

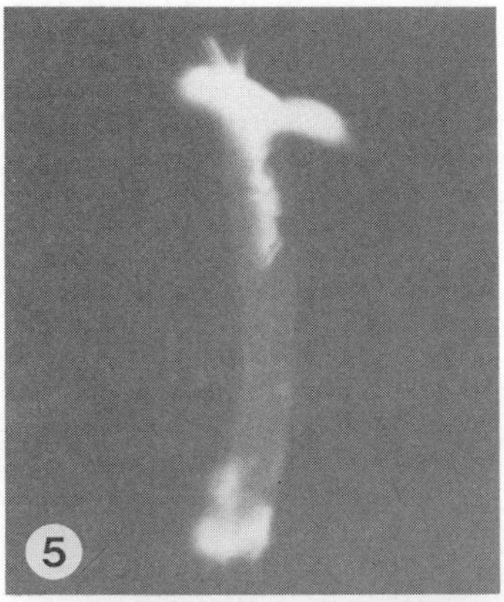

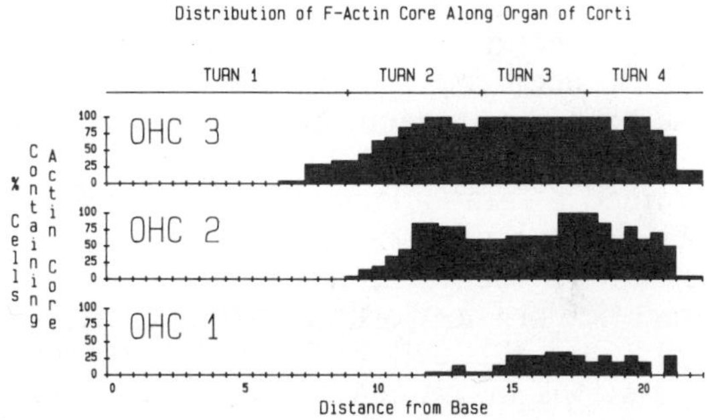

6

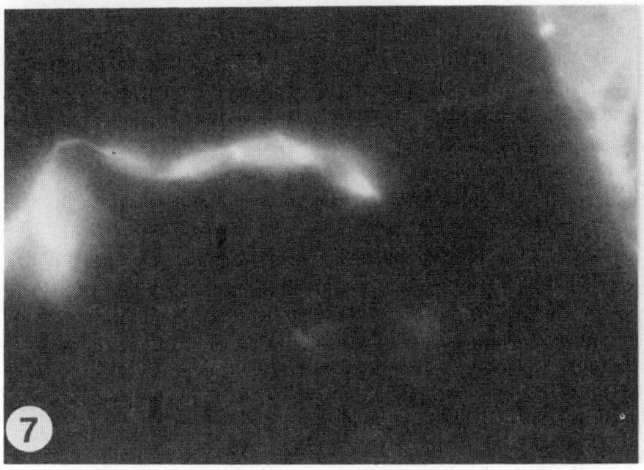

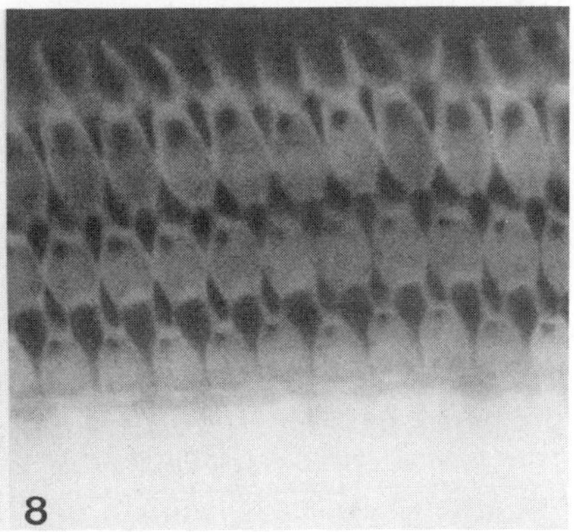

Figure 5. Isolated OHC, permeabilized with Triton X-100, with phalloidin labelling in the cuticular plate, stereocilia, infracuticular network and at the base of the cell. The lateral membrane of the OHC is also faintly labelled.

Figure 6. Quantitative analysis of the distribution of OHC containing the infracuticular network (see text for details).

Figure 7. Cryosection of apical rat organ of Corti. The reticular lamina and the bases of the OHC are labelled with phalloidin, but no evidence of an infracuticular network is present.

Figure 8. Surface preparation of apical chinchilla organ of Corti. Although the cuticular plates and junctional complexes are labelled with phalloidin, no evidence of an infracuticular network is observed.

isolated hair cell preparations (Figure 5) this structure was identified as the infracuticular network of F-actin previously described (Zenner, 1980; Flock et al, 1982). The distribution of this infracuticular network was quantified by recording its presence in OHCs and plotting the results as a function of distance along the organ of Corti, as shown in Figure 6. The infracuticular network first appeared 8mm from the basal end of the organ of Corti in the third row OHC, increased in frequency so that by 12mm from the basal end it was visible in virtually every third row OHC. In the second row OHCs the first appearance of the infracuticular network occurred 10mm from the basal end, the percentage of cells containing the infracuticular network was lower and the labelling was less intense than in third row OHCs. First row OHCs only occasionally contained a faintly labelled infracuticular network. The same pattern was observed in cryosections of guinea pig cochlea; the infracuticular network was not present in basal turn OHC and in the apical turns the infracuticular network was most intensely labelled and extended most deeply into the cell body in the third row OHC. In isolated hair cell preparations of guinea pig cochlea, the infracuticular network was never observed in any OHC isolated from the basal coil but it was present in some OHCs isolated from the apical turns.

In careful examination of the entire lengths of the organs of Corti from chinchillas, hooded rats and squirrel monkeys no structure analogous to the infracuticular network could be observed in OHC of any row or turn, either in cryosections (Figure 7) or surface preparations (Figure 2, Figure 8), even when phalloidin incubation time was increased to 72 hours and 0.1% Triton X-100 was used to permeabilize the cell membranes. Isolated OHC from chinchilla and rat were devoid of an infracuticular network even when saponin was used as a permeabilizing agent.

Discussion

Outer hair cell motility has been attributed to two ultrastructural features which are known to contain actin (Flock et al, 1986; Zenner, 1986). A submembranous contractile apparatus or cortex system, based on the lateral sub-surface cisternae and structures which extend from the cisternae to the plasma membrane, has been likened to the contractile mechanism in skeletal muscle fibers (Flock et al, 1986). Actin and calmodulin, a calcium binding protein involved in smooth muscle contractility and non-muscle cell motility, have been identified in a central core or infracuticular network (Zenner, 1986; Flock et al, 1986). Possibly, receptor current initiates a sequence of events across the cell membrane which leads to the release of calcium ions. This calcium release triggers a contractile response in the cortex system, and the diffusion of calcium through the cytoplasm stimulates the polymerization of the central core of actin. Support for this hypothesis comes from biochemical manipulations of permeabilized isolated OHCs (Zenner, 1986). Reversible contractions were elicited by ATP and calcium and inhibited by bisphosphate, an ATP competitor, and by cytochalasin, which prevents the polymerization of actin filaments.

We can confirm the presence of F-actin in the cortex system in OHC since the circumference of OHCs of all species were labelled by phalloidin. However, this study has demonstrated that the F-actin core or infracuticular network appears to be unique to OHC in the apical turns of the guinea pig cochlea. It is not present in basal guinea pig OHC or in OHC of chinchillas, hooded rats or squirrel monkeys. The base to apex distribution of the infracuticular network in the guinea pig has been confirmed in other laboratories (Flock, pers. comm.) and the absence of an infracuticular network has been noted by other investigators in the rabbit (Flock, pers. comm.) and in the mouse (Richardson, pers. comm.). The absence of the infracuticular network in OHC of most species argues against the involvement of this structure in OHC contractility.

The reason for the differences in actin in the cytoplasm of these various OHC populations is speculative. In non-muscle cells, the balance between unpolymerized and polymerized actin is controlled by regulatory proteins (Alberts et al, 1983). External signals can lead to a weakening of the bonds between actin molecules and regulatory proteins and stimulate a rapid polymerization of actin. When actin filaments so formed are no longer needed they depolymerize. Phalloidin binds to actin filaments and inhibits their depolymerization (Alberts et al, 1983). It is possible that apical OHC of the guinea pig contain a large amount of depolymerized actin not present in other species which responds to an external trigger resulting in the formation of actin filaments in the cytoplasm. Zenner and Drenkhahn (1986) observed that phalloidin fluorescence was enhanced following potassium-induced OHC contraction, which supports this interpretation, but this observation was not confirmed in other studies (Ulfendahl and Slepecky, 1988). It is also possible that the infracuticular network of actin filaments is a permanent part of the cytoskeleton of apical guinea pig OHC.

Most studies of the contractile properties of OHC have used cells from the apical turns of the guinea pig organ of Corti. This study has shown that those OHC contain a structure which was not found in OHCs from the basal turn of the guinea pig or in OHCs of other species. The functional significance of the infracuticular network of F-actin remains to be established; however, the results of the present study emphasize the need for comparative studies of isolated OHCs.

References

Alberts, B., Bray, D., Lewis, J., Raff, M., Roberts, K. and Watson, J.D. (1983): Molecular Biology of the Cell, Garland Publishing, Inc. New York, 571-572.

Ashmore, J.F. (1986): The cellular physiology of isolated outer hair cells: implications for cochlear frequency selectivity. In: Auditory Frequency Selectivity. B.C.J. Moore and R.J. Patterson, ed. New York, Plenum Press, pp. 103-108.

Bohne, B.A. and Carr, C.D. (1985): Morphometric analysis of hair cells in the chinchilla cochlea. J. Acoust. Soc. Am. 77, 153-158.

Brownell, W.E., Bader, C.R., Bertrand, D. and de Ribaupierre, Y. (1985): Evoked mechanical responses of isolated cochlear outer hair cells. Science 227, 194-196.

Dallos, P. (1985a): Response characteristics of mammalian cochlear hair cells. J. Neurosci. 5, 1591-1608.

Dallos, P. (1985b): The role of outer hair cells in cochlear function. In: Contemporary Sensory Neurobiology, M.J. Correia and A.A. Perachio, eds. Alan Liss, New York, pp. 207-230.

Davis, H. (1983): An active process in cochlear mechanics. Hearing Res. 9, 79-90.
Drenkhahn, D., Schafer, T. and Prinz, M. (1985): Actin, myosin and associated proteins in the vertebrate auditory and vestibular organs: Immunocytochemical and biochemical studies. In: Auditory Biochemistry, D. G. Drescher, ed. Thomas, Springfield, Il. pp. 310-316.
Flock, A. and Cheung, H.C. (1977): Actin filaments in sensory hairs of inner ear receptor cells. J. Cell. Biol. 75, 339-343.
Flock, A., Bretscher, A. and Weber, K. (1982): Immunohistochemical localization of several cytoskeletal proteins in inner ear sensory and supporting cells. Hear. Res. 6, 75-89.
Flock, A., Flock, B. and Ulfendahl, M. (1986): Mechanisms of movement in outer hair cells and a possible structural basis. Archiv. Otorhinolargyngol. 243, 83-90.
Kachar, B., Brownell, W.E., Altschuler, R.A. and Fex, J. (1986): Electrokinetic shape changes of cochlear outer hair cells. Nature 322, 365-367.
Kemp, D.T. (1978): Stimulated acoustic emission from within the human auditory system. J. Acoust. Soc. Am. 64, 1386-1391.
LePage, E.W. and Johnstone, B.M. (1980): Non-linear mechanical behavior of the basilar membrane in the basal turn of the guinea pig cochlea. Hearing Res. 2, 183-189.
Neely, S.T. and Kim, D.O. (1986): A model for active elements in cochlear biomechanics. J. Acoust. Soc. Am. 79, 1472-1480.
Pujol, R. and Gil-Loyzaga, P. (1987): Distribution of the two types of afferent dendrite in the developing cochlea: a kainic acid study. Abstr. Assoc. Res. Otolaryngol. 10, p. 122.
Russell, I.J. and Cody, A.R. (1985): Transduction in cochlear hair cells. In: Peripheral Auditory Mechanisms: J.B. Allen, J.L. Hall, A. Hubbard, S.T. Neely and A. Tubis, eds. Springer-Verlag, New York, pp. 349-360.
Slepecky, N. and Chamberlain, S.C. (1985): Immunoelectron microscopic and immunofluorescent localization of cytoskeletal and muscle-like contractile proteins in inner ear sensory hair cells. Hearing Res. 20, 256-260.
Smith, C.A. (1968): Ultrastructure of the organ of Corti. Adv. Sci. 24, 419-433.
Spoendlin, H. (1969): Innervation patterns on the organ of Corti of the cat. Acta Otolaryngol. (Stockh.) 67, 239-254.
Strelioff, D. and Flock, A. (1984): Stiffness of sensory-cell hair bundles in the isolated guinea pig cochlea. Hear. Res. 15, 19-28.
Tilney, L.G., DeRosier, D.J. and Mulroy, M.J. (1980): The organization of actin filaments in the stereocilia of cochlear hair cells. J. Cell Biol. 86, 244-259.
Ulfendahl, M. and Slepecky, N. (1988): Ultrastructural correlates of inner ear sensory cell shortening. J. Submicrosc. Cytol. Pathol. 20 (1), 47-51.
Wright, A. (1984): Dimensions of the cochlear stereocilia in man and the guinea pig. Hear. Res. 13, 89-98.
Zajic, G. and Schacht, J. (1987): Comparison of isolated outer hair cells from five mammalian species. Hearing Res. 26, 249-256.
Zenner, H.P. (1980): Cytoskeletal and muscle like elements in cochlear hair cells. Arch. Otorhinolaryngol. 230, 82-92.
Zenner, H.P., Zimmerman, U. and Schmitt, U. (1985): Reversible contraction of isolated mammalian cochlear hair cells. Hearing Res. 18, 127-133.
Zenner, H.P. (1986): Motile responses in outer hair cells. Hear. Res. 22, 83-90.
Zenner, H.P. and Drenkhahn, D. (1986): Active motile events in guinea pig outer hair cells. Abstr. Assoc. Res. Otolarygol. 9, 1.
Zurek, P.M. (1981): Spontaneous narrowband acoustic signals emitted by human ears. J. Acoust. Soc. Am. 69, 514-523.

THE LATERAL WALLS OF INNER AND OUTER HAIR CELLS

Andrew Forge

Dept of Audiology and EM Unit, Institute of Laryngology and Otology 330-332, Gray's Inn Road, London WC1X 8EE

Outer hair cells (OHCs) are thought to play a role in influencing cochlear micromechanics and have been shown to be actively motile; inner hair cells (IHCs) are presumed to be mechanically passive receptor cells and there is no evidence that they are able to contract. A detailed examination of the structural differences and similarities between IHCs and OHCs may provide clues as to particular specialisations of OHCs which are relevant to cochlear micromechanics. Some evidence has suggested that such specialisation is associated with the lateral wall of the OHC (i.e. the lateral plasma membrane and underlying lateral cisternae) (Flock et al., 1986; Holley and Ashmore, 1988). In the work to be presented here, thin sections, freeze-fracture and freeze-etching have been used to to examine the lateral walls of IHCs and OHCs in the intact organ of Corti of the guinea pig, the the gerbil and the mouse. Some preliminary data on freeze-fractured isolated OHCs of the guinea pig is also presented.

Methods

For examination of the intact organ of Corti, the tissue was first fixed in 2.5% glutaraldehyde in 0.1M cacodylate buffer by direct perfusion of the cochlea with fixative. Pieces of the organ of Corti were dissected out under 0.1M buffer. Samples for freeze-fracture were impregnated with 25% (v/v) glycerol and frozen in freon 22 cooled by liquid nitrogen. Those to be etched were briefly washed in 15% aqueous methanol, and rapidly frozen by plunging into a stirred mixture of propane:isopentane (3:1) cooled in liquid nitrogen; subsequently, fractured surfaces were etched for between 1 and 3 minutes. For thin sections, tissue was post-fixed in 1% OsO_4 with 1mg ml^{-1} $K_3Fe(CN)_6$ before dehydration and embedding. Isolated hair cells were prepared from the apical turn of the guinea pig cochlea using methods described by Zajic and Schacht (1987). They were frozen directly without any pretreatment, neither fixative nor cryoprotectives. Small (1µl) droplets of hair cells in Hanks' Balanced Salt Solution were sandwiched between two thin copper support plates and rapidly plunge frozen in propane:isopentane as above.

Results

IHCs. In the lateral wall of the IHC, freeze-fracture predominantly exposed the lateral plasma membrane (Fig. 1a). Only small areas of the underlying lateral cisternae were revealed. Where the cisternae could be seen in face view (Fig. 1b) they appeared as a network of tubules or as a fenestrated sheet. The cisternal system was only one layer deep as was also seen in thin sections. The fracture faces of the lateral plasma membrane (Fig. 1a) were characterised by the presence a) of large particles in square array ('plaques') and b) of particles organised in rows. The plaque regions appeared to occupy a greater area of the lateral membrane in the IHCs of gerbils than in those of the guinea pig. As discussed previously (Forge, 1987), the plaque regions show morphological features reminiscent of the sites of transmembrane channels.

The particle rows also showed a degree of order (Figs. 1a & c). Within a single row particles were quite regularly spaced about 30-40nm apart and often rows were parallel to each other separated by ca. 50 nm. As shown previously (Forge, 1987) the plaque regions on the IHC membrane are present on areas of membrane beneath which lateral cisternae are absent; the particles rows correspond to areas overlying the cisternae. In thin sections, where the section grazed the membrane (i.e. ran almost parallel to the plane of the membrane providing a face view of the membrane) parallel rows of electron dense points were seen to be in register with the tubules forming the cisternal system (Fig. 1d). The spacing of points was ca. 30-35nm. This grazing section view is similar to that seen in OHCs cut in the same way (Flock et al., 1986) and suggests the possibility of linking strands between the cisternae and the plasma membrane in IHCs. In freeze-etched samples, strands crossing the gap between the cisterna and the plasma membrane could indeed be identified (Fig. 1e). However, they were not regularly arranged and so far it has not been possible to demonstrate any direct connection of these strands with any particular feature on the lateral membrane of the cell.

OHCs. Thin sections of the OHCs showed the characteristic lateral cisternae on the lateral wall of the cell (Fig. 2a). In guinea pigs, and gerbils the cisternae formed several concentric layers (2-6 in guinea pigs, up to 6 in gerbils). In the mice, however, there was only one layer. OHC of the gerbil also often showed a peculiarity where the cisternae were locally involuted and separated from the lateral membrane, but where this occurred the outermost cisternal layer (i.e. that closest to the lateral membrane) did not deform and a single layer of the cisternal system was closely associated with the plasma membrane (Fig. 2b). Strands or 'pillars' (Flock et al., 1986) interconnecting the outermost lateral cistern and the plasma membrane were readily recognisable in the guinea pig (Fig. 2a), though less so in the gerbil (Fig. 2b), but grazing sections of OHCs of both species showed the regularly arranged (ca. 30nm spacing) electron dense spots interpreted as representing the 'end-on' view of the pillars (Fig. 2c).

Following freeze-fracture, the pattern of fracture in OHCs was different from that of the IHCs. Predominantly, fracture occurred in the membranes of the cisternae revealing large face views of these membranes whereas the plasma membrane was usually cross-fractured and only rarely

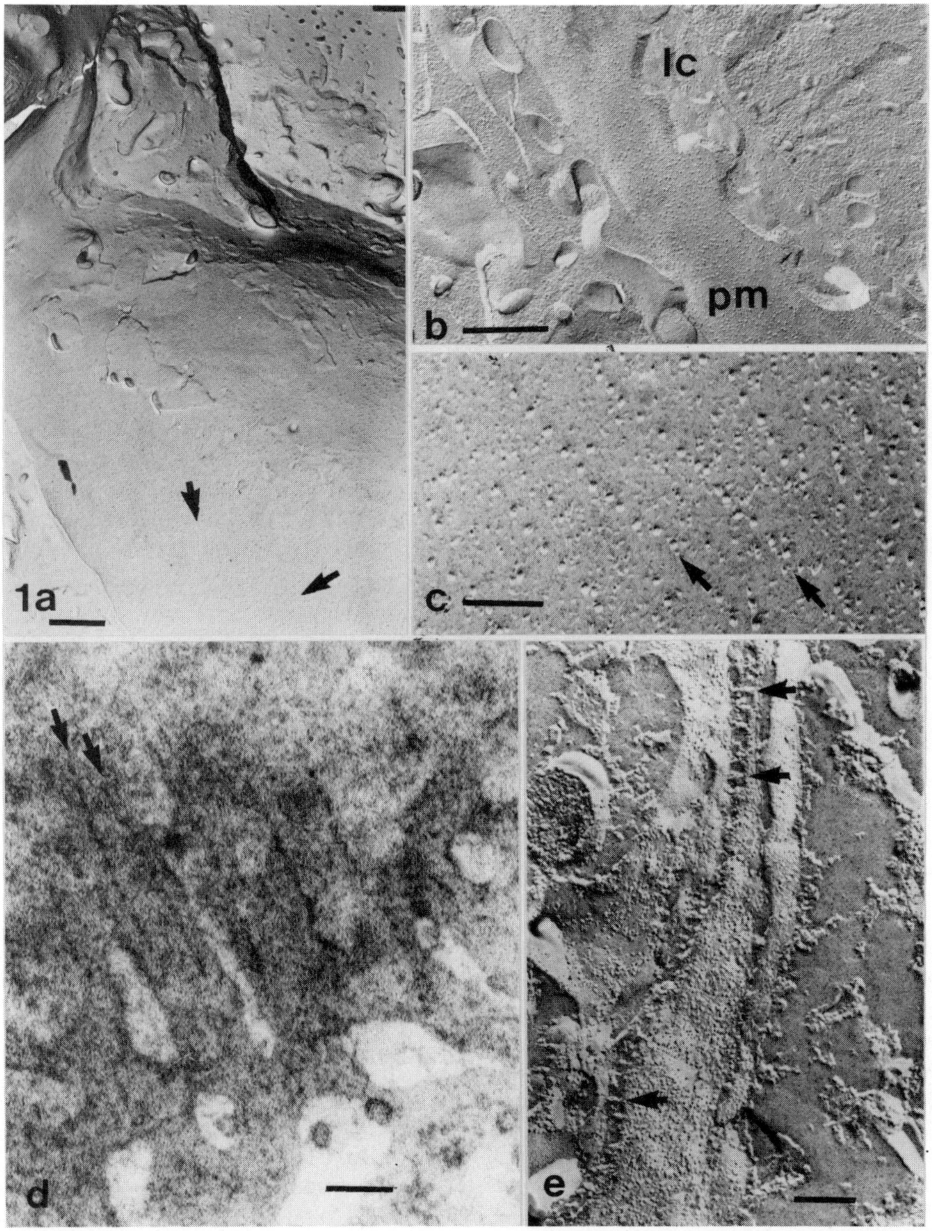

FIGURE 1. Inner hair cells. a). Freeze-fracture showing extensive fracture within the lateral plasma membrane in gerbil. The cell apex is at top left. Arrows indicate particle rows. Large plaque region of particles in square array can also be seen. b). Fracture revealing lateral cisterna (lc) as fenestrated sheet; pm = plasma membrane. c). Lateral plasma membrane at high power. d). Grazing section of IHC lateral wall. Arrows indicate parallel rows of points overlying cisternal tubules. e). Freeze-etch replica showing elements (arrowed) linking the plasma membrane and the lateral cisterna. Scale bars: a&b, 0.5µm; c&d, 0.1µm; e, 0.2µm.

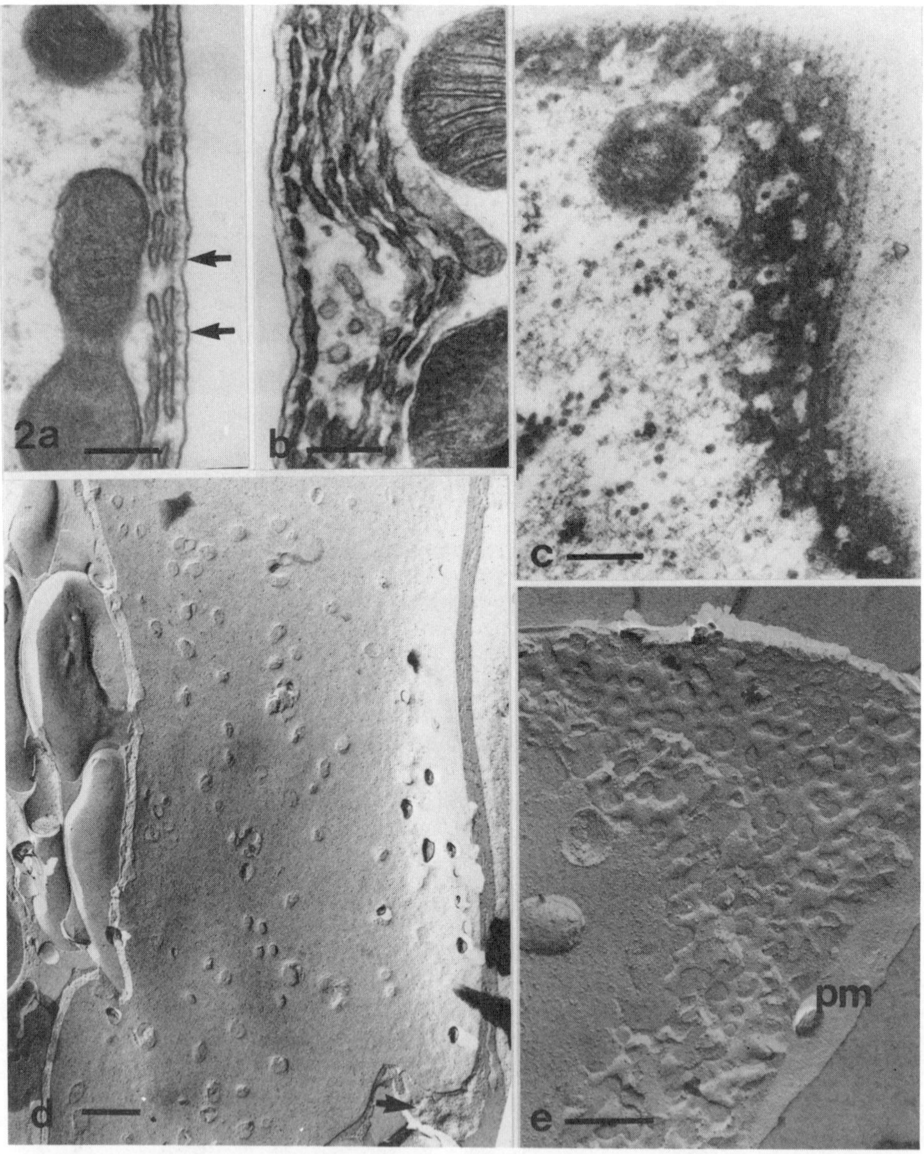

FIGURE 2. Outer hair cell. a). Thin section of guinea pig showing cisternal layers and (arrowed) "pillars" in sub-plasmallemal space. b). Gerbil OHC showing localised involution of cisternae with a single cisternal layer maintained close to the plasma membrane. c). Grazing section showing arrays of points overlying tubules of lateral cisternae. d). Freeze-fracture. Fracture has occurred within the lateral cisternae which in this elongated cell appear as fenestrated sheets. Only a small area of the plasma membrane has been exposed in face view (arrow). e). Freeze-fracture exposing cisternae as tubules. pm = e-face of the plasma membrane. Scale bars: a-c, 0.2μm; d&e, 0.5μm.

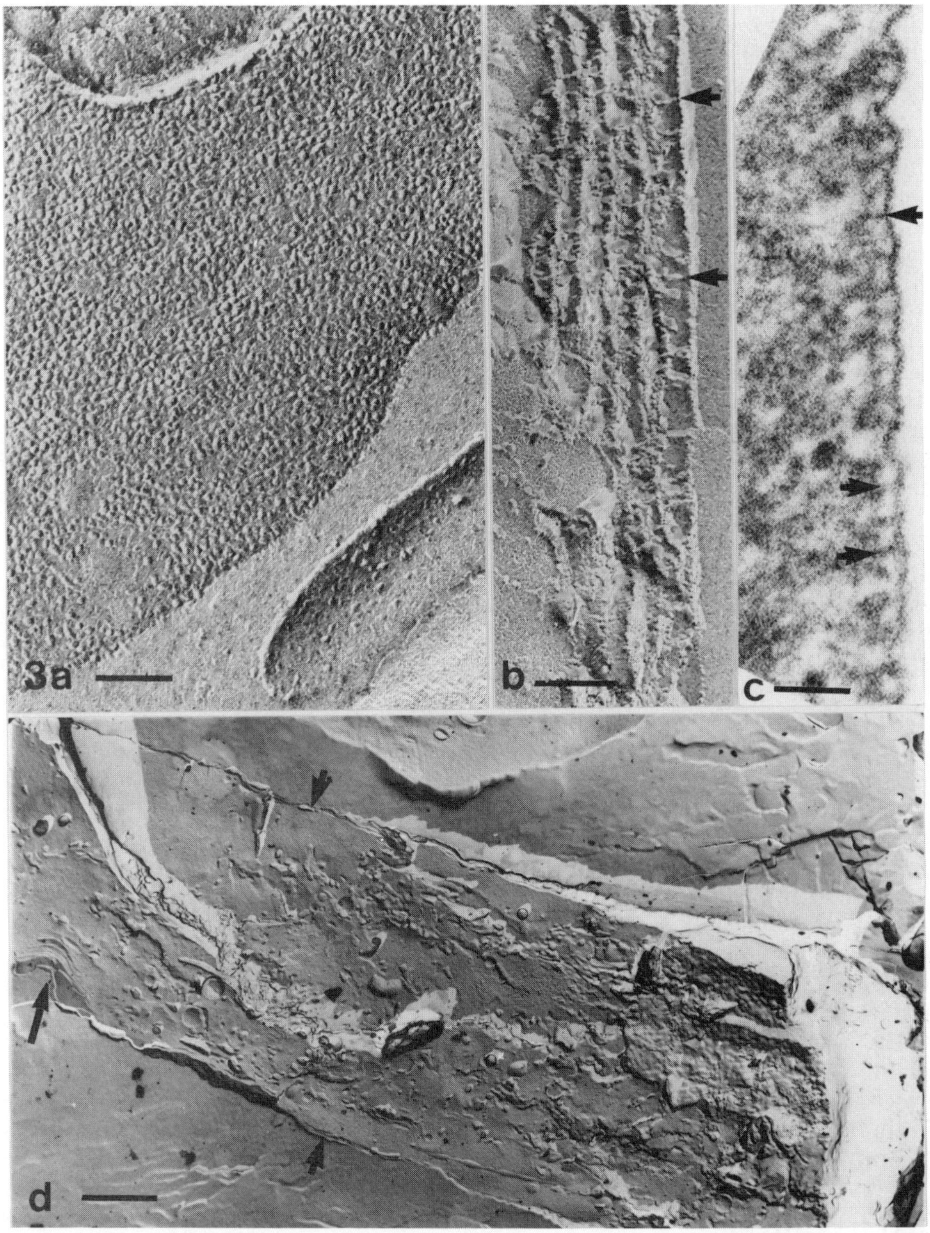

FIGURE 3. a). Lateral plasma membrane of the OHC in a gerbil. The fracture face is covered with closely packed large particles; no obvious ordered arrangements are apparent. b). Freeze-etch replica showing pillar-like structures (arrowed) crossing the gap between the plasma membrane and the cisternae. c). Thin section of lateral wall of OHC following lipid extraction. A plasma membrane-like image is retained but the cisternae have been destroyed. Pillar-like structures (arrowed) also appear to have been retained. d). Freeze-fractured, rapidly fresh-frozen isolated outer hair cell. The elongated cell form has been maintained but lateral cisternae appear to have been disorganised; there are neither sheet-like forms nor tubular cisternae. However, the large arrow indicates a localised stack of cisterna-like membranes and at the small arrows a single layer of cisterns close to and parallel with the plasma membrane is apparent. Scale bars: a, 0.1μm; b, 0.2μm; c, 0.05μm; d, 2.5μm.

was the lateral plasma membrane exposed *en face* (Figs. 2d & e). The cisternae of the guinea pig appeared as either fenestrated sheets (Fig. 2d) or a network of tubules (Fig. 2e). The sheet-like form was most prevalent in the outermost cisternal layer and occurred more frequently in longer cells. In both the gerbil and the mouse the cisternae always appeared as a network of interconnecting tubules; sheet-like forms were not seen. In preparations of the organ of Corti treated with filipin, a probe to localise membrane cholesterol, the membranes of the lateral cisternae showed scattered clumps of filipin-induced lesions in a pattern reminiscent of that associated with the sarcoplasmic reticulum of skeletal muscle cells (Sommer et al., 1980).

The p-fracture face of the lateral membrane of the OHC was characterised by the presence of large numbers of densely packed large particles (Fig. 3a). Neither plaque-like regions nor ordered rows of particles like those found on IHC membranes could be discerned. Similarly, e-fracture faces of the OHC lateral membrane showed no recognisable ordered features. So far, on the fracture faces of OHC lateral membranes, no feature which might represent an associaton of the sub-plasmallemal pillars with the plasma membrane has been recognised. However, freeze-etched preparations of OHCs revealed the presence of pillar-like structures in the gap between the membrane and the outermost cisternal layer (Fig. 3b). These appeared very similar to the pillars seen in thin sections but it has not yet been possible to determine their relationship, if any, with the features on the membrane fracture faces.

The inability of the lateral membrane to carry the fracture plane and the presence of large numbers of particles on the fracture face both suggest that the OHC lateral membrane has a high protein content. This was further suggested by examination of thin sections of tissue from which lipids had been extracted with chloroform-methanol following fixation. In these preparations, the lateral plasma membrane retained a membrane-like image but the lateral cisternae were almost entirely destroyed. Interestingly, sub-plasmallemal pillar-like structures were still present and grazing sections again showed regularly organised, electron dense points (Fig. 3c).

Isolated OHCs. In fresh-frozen, isolated OHCs of the guinea pig (Fig. 3d), lateral cisternae were disorganised. Neither sheet-like forms nor an interconnecting tubule network were recognised. At some localised points around the cell stacks of cisternae were present and the fracture faces of these showed regularly organised particles. In other areas of the cell a single tubule of cisterna running parallel to the lateral membrane was present.

Discussion

The most obvious difference between IHCs and OHCs at the level of the lateral wall is in the structure of the plasma membrane. The OHC membrane appears to be very rich in protein. This may provide some degree of rigidity to the cell. It is of note that isolated cells which have been ruptured and washed free of cell contents retain their original elongated shape (Holley and Ashmore, 1988) and that in the organ of Corti of gentamicin damaged cochleae, OHC remnants are present which consist of no more than the lateral membrane and a single layer of the cisternal system, yet retain an elongated cell form (Forge, unpublished). These observations attest to the rigidity of the lateral wall of the OHC.

It is also apparent that organisation of elements on the lateral walls of OHC and of IHCs may not be very different. Although in some animals there may be multiple concentric cisternae in the OHC, other animals show only one. Where cisternae become distorted (as in the gerbil) or disorganised (as seems to occur in isolated guinea pig OHCs) a single cisternal layer is maintained close to the membrane. This might indicate that only one cisternal layer is of primary significance in the OHC and that this is closely associated with the lateral membrane. This is the situation in the IHC. Furthermore, there appears to be in the IHC some kind of linking element between the cisterna and the lateral membrane which superficially appears similar to that in the OHC. It is of interest that the IHC membrane bears features which could be the points of insertion of this linking element into the lateral whereas a similar feature is not readily recognisable in the OHC lateral membrane. There may be several explanations for this, but clearly further work is necessary.

The differences in the organisation of the cisternal system in the different species studied is also of some interest. The formation of cisternae into extended, fenestrated sheet-like forms appears to be a peculiarity of the more apical cells in the guinea pig. Such cells are those most commonly used in studies of isolated OHCs. Although it is probable that this structural form represents an extreme in the variation in the organisation of the the cisternae, as suggested elsewhere (Carlisle, et al., this meeting), OHCs from the apex of the guinea pig cochlea may not be typical of OHCs generally. Also, it would appear that procedures used in isolating such cells may cause disorganisation of the cisternal system. However, whether this is likely to have a significant effect on the cells' function is not clear; even in the isolated cells a single cisternal layer is apparently maintained close to the lateral membrane.

Acknowledgements

Thanks are due to Stephen Davies for excellent technical assistance, to Gary Zajic for isolation of hair cells and to Dr Karen Steel for the provision of cochleae from mice. Apologies too, to David Kemp and Pat Wilson. The work was supported in part by the Medical Research Council and the Wellcome Trust and by equipment grants from the Hearing and Speech Trust (HAST) and the SmithKline Foundation.

References

Flock,A., Flock,B. and Ulfendahl,M. (1986) Mechanisms of movement in outer hair cells and a possible structural basis. Arch. Otorhinolaryngol. 243, 83-90.

Forge,A. (1987) Specialisations of the lateral membrane of inner hair cells. Hearing Res. 31, 99-110.

Holley,M.C. and Ashmore,J.F. (1988) On the mechanism of a high frequency force generator in outer hair cells isolated from the guinea pig cochlea. Proc. R. Soc. Lond. B 232, 413-429.

Sommer,J.R., Dolber,P.C. and Taylor,I. (1980) Filipin-cholesterol complexes in the sarcoplasmic reticulum of frog skeletal muscle. J. Ultrastruct. Res. 72, 272-285.

Zajic,G. and Schacht,J. (1987) Comparison of isolated outer hair cells from five mammalian species. Hearing Res. 26, 249-256.

TIP-LINK ORGANIZATION IN RELATION TO THE STRUCTURE AND ORIENTATION OF STEREOVILLAR BUNDLES

J.O. Pickles, M.P. Osborne, S.D. Comis, C. Köppl*, O. Gleich*, J. Brix*, G.A. Manley*

Department of Physiology
University of Birmingham, Birmingham B15 2TJ, UK
**Institut für Zoologie, Technische Universität München*
D-8046 München, FDR

Introduction

The linkages between stereovilli (stereocilia) of hair cells have been implicated both in the mechanical properties of the bundles and in the transmission of stimulus-induced movements to the individual mechanotransducer channels (e.g. Flock and Strelioff, 1984; Pickles et al., 1984; Hudspeth, 1985). Here, we describe new observations on the fine structure of the tip links between stereovilli. We also show that the spatial organization of the tip links in bundles of different conformations in a variety of species is appropriate for a role in transduction.

Methods

For transmission electron microscopy, temporal bones were extracted from anaesthetized guinea pigs. The bones were perfused with fixative as described previously (Pickles et al., 1987). Specimens were fixed for 0.5 h at 4° C in 2.5% glutaraldehyde containing 2% tannic acid and buffered with 0.05 M BES (NN-bis[2-Hydroxyethyl]-2-aminoethane sulfonic acid), adjusted to pH 7.4 with NaOH. After fixation tissues were postfixed in 1% OsO_4 in the same buffer for 5 min, followed by soaking in 2% tannic acid in distilled H_2O, with the pH adjusted to 7.0 with NaOH. Dehydration was accomplished with ethanol and the material stained *en bloc* with uranyl acetate and phosphotungstic acid before embedding in an Epon Araldite resin mixture (Mollenhauer, 1964). Sections were stained in methanolic uranyl acetate and lead citrate before examination in a JEOL 120 CXII transmission microscope operated at 80 kV.

For scanning electron microscopy in guinea pigs, the temporal bones were extracted as described above and fixed with 2.5% glutaraldehyde in 0.05 M BES buffer. For scanning electron microscopy in European lizards (*Podarcis muralis* and *P. sicula*), chicks (*Gallus gallus*), pigeons (*Columba livia*) and starling (*Sturnus vulgaris*), the animals were anaesthetized and perfused either transcardially or directly through the oval or round windows with fixative (pigeon: 2.5% glutaraldehyde in 0.1 M phosphate buffer; chick, starling and lizard 1% or 2.5% glutaraldehyde and 15% saturated picric acid in 0.1 M phosphate buffer). Specimens were stored in 2% glutaraldehyde in 0.05 or 0.1 M phosphate buffer until further treatment. They were then dehydrated in acetone, dried by the critical-point technique with liquid CO_2, and sputter-coated with platinum to a nominal depth of 25 nm. Specimens were examined in a JEOL 120 CXII microscope with a scanning attachment at 40 kV, and images were observed by a secondary-electron detector.

Results

THE FINE STRUCTURE OF TIP-LINKS IN GUINEA PIG HAIR CELLS

A fine, straight filament was visible in the centre of each tip link (Fig. 1). In many cases the fine central filament was surrounded by amorphous material, which had a variable conformation (Fig. 2). Similar material was also visible on the surface membranes of the stereovilli (Fig. 2). The fine central filament often appeared more lightly-staining than the surrounding material. Its mean diameter measured in sections taken at a range of original magnifications of 29,000 to 100,000 had a value of 5.5 nm (n=16), the same as the diameter of the actin filaments in the central core of the stereovilli measured in the same sections.

In sections cut perpendicular to the cuticular plate and perpendicular to the rows of stereovilli on an outer hair cell, the bundles had a triangular shape in lateral view, the stereovilli being closely apposed at the tips. The central filaments of the tip links running between the stereovilli of the three rows were nearly coaxial with each other, and also nearly coaxial with the shortest of the three stereovilli in the cross section (Fig. 3). In such sections, therefore, the two tip links and the shortest stereovillus lay along a nearly straight line. Moreover, in those sections where the rootlets were visible, each rootlet continued along the axis of the stereovillus (Fig. 4).

In addition to tip links, a broad band of links was visible running laterally between the rows of stereovilli, particularly visible between the tallest and second-tallest stereovilli in the bundle (arrowheads, Figs 3 and 4).

At its point of attachment on the taller of two stereovilli, the central filament of the tip link ran to the centre of an electron-dense area, which formed a bridge between the external plasma membrane and the central actin filaments of the stereovillus (arrowheads, Figs 1 and 2). At its lower end, the central filament met the plasma membrane at the tip of the shorter stereovillus, which was often pulled out into a point. This point overlay a clear area, with a denser cap over the ends of the actin filaments immediately underneath, visible in sections cut in a suitable plane. In some sections, fine filaments could be seen connecting the plasma membrane to the underlying density. The dense cap was only visible at the ends of the actin filaments immediately underlying the tip link: the other filaments ended without any obvious association with an electron-dense area. This was particularly apparent in the tips of stereovilli of the second tallest row on inner hair cells, which ended with a wider tip.

TIP-LINK ORGANIZATION IN RELATION TO THE HAIR-CELL AXIS

We have previously suggested that tip links on guinea pig inner and outer hair cells are organized such that the horizontal component in their orientation runs parallel to the hair cell axis of bilateral symmetry (Pickles et al., 1984; Comis et al., 1985). This axis defines the axis for excitatory and inhibitory deflections of the stereovilli (Flock, 1965). We have further investigated the point in bird and lizard basilar papillae, where the hair bundles show a quite different conformation and, sometimes, a systematically-varying orientation with respect to the papillar edge (Miller, 1980; Gleich and Manley, 1988).

In micrographs of bundles viewed perpendicular to the cuticular plate, the stereovilli were hexagonally packed (Fig. 5). The tip links were oriented along a 1,0 axis of the hexagon, parallel to the axis of bilateral symmetry, and at right angles to the long axis of the bundle as a whole (arrows: Fig. 5). The stereovilli were therefore organized into columns, running parallel to the hair-cell axis of bilateral symmetry. These observations were made consistently in bundles from lizards and all birds.

In micrographs of bundles viewed at an acute angle to the cuticular plate, the organization of stereovilli into columns, connected by tip links, was also obvious (Fig. 6). In some bundles, within the general gradation in height of the stereovilli from shortest on one side of the bundle to tallest on the opposite side, all the stereovilli in one column were a little taller, or a little shorter, than the corresponding stereovilli in adjacent columns (e.g. arrows, Fig. 6). Examples of this behaviour were found in all ears examined and in all regions of the papillae.

Where bundles had separated, perhaps due to mechanical trauma during preparation of the specimen, the stereovilli separated most commonly into columns running parallel to the axis of bilateral symmetry of the hair cell (Fig. 7). These are the columns defined in the previous paragraphs on the basis of the tip-link connections. When this occurred, there was no obvious debris on the upper ends of the separated, lateral, surfaces of the stereovilli in the gap (Fig. 7).

Discussion

The present observations on the fine structure of tip links suggests that the links have a fine central filamentous core, surrounded by an amorphous coat. We do not have information on the nature of the central filament, although it may well be protein. Like actin, the central filament reacts poorly with positive stains. Moreover, its diameter is similar to that of a single actin filament. On the other hand, the amorphous surrounding coat may well be an extension of the coat on the surface of the individual stereovilli, and may therefore consist of glycocongugates (Santi and Anderson, 1987).

One or both ends of the tip links are possible sites for the transducer channels, on the hypothesis that stretch of the tip links opens the transducer channels (Pickles et al., 1984). The densities associated with the ends of the filament probably represent anchorage points at which the forces are coupled to the internal cytoskeleton. At its lower end, the tip link joins to a conical extension of the membrane at the tip of the shorter

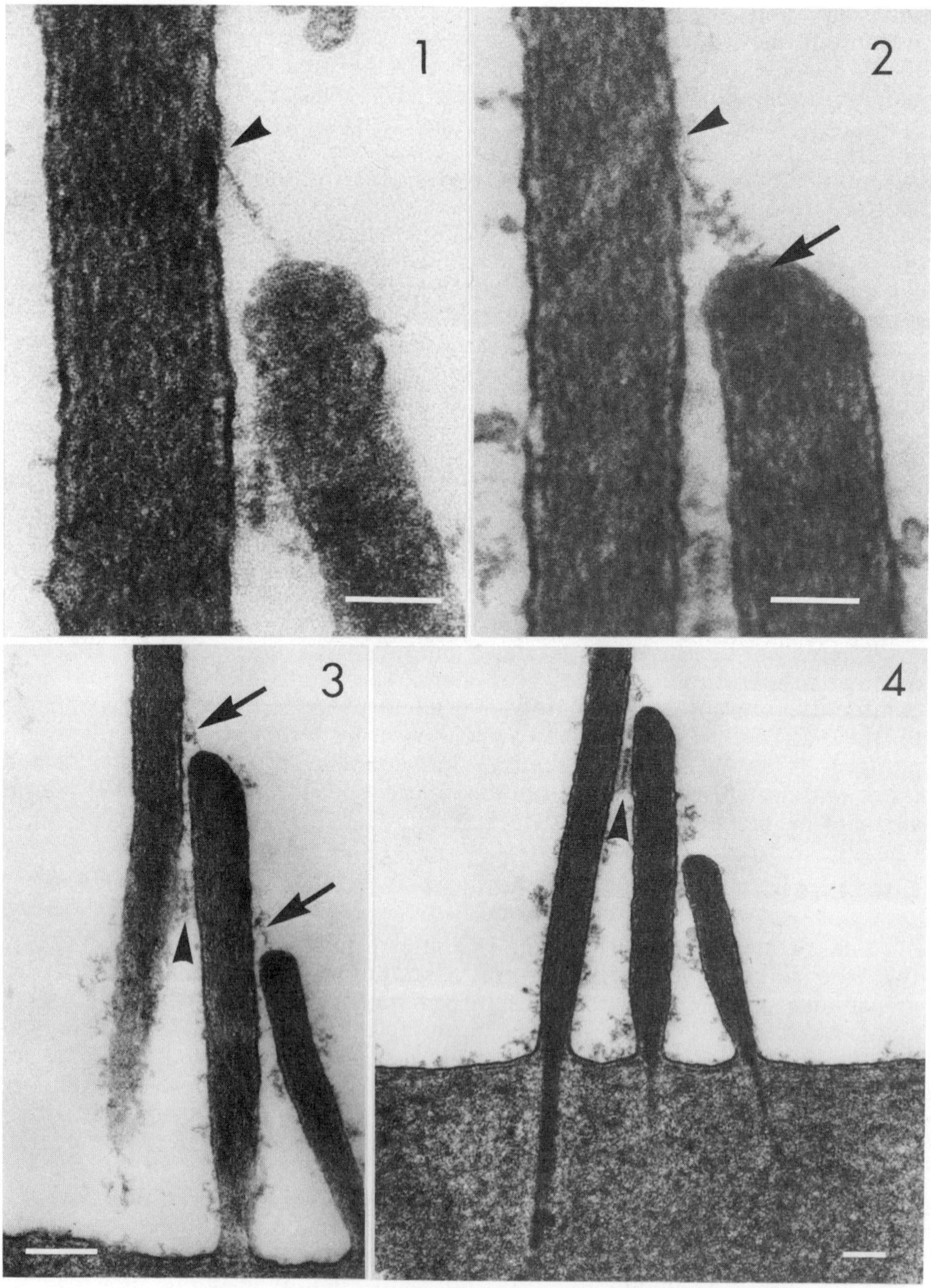
1
2
3
4

Fig. 1. Tip link on guinea pig outer hair cell, showing central filament. Arrowhead: upper dense point of attachment. Scale bar: 100 nm.

Fig. 2. Tip link on guinea pig outer hair cell, showing variable thickness of amorphous material attached to central filament of tip link. Arrowhead: upper dense point of attachment. Arrow: site of lower density under the surface membrane of the stereovillus. Scale bar: 100 nm.

Fig. 3. Tip links on guinea pig outer hair cell, showing that the tip links between the different rows are nearly coaxial, and coaxial with the shortest stereovillus on the bundle. Arrows: tip links. Arrowhead: lateral (inter-row) links. Scale bar: 200 nm.

Fig. 4. Guinea pig outer hair cell, showing that the rootlets are coaxial with the individual stereovilli, and that the stereovilli slope towards each other at their tips. Arrowhead: sideways (inter-row) links. Scale bar: 200 nm.

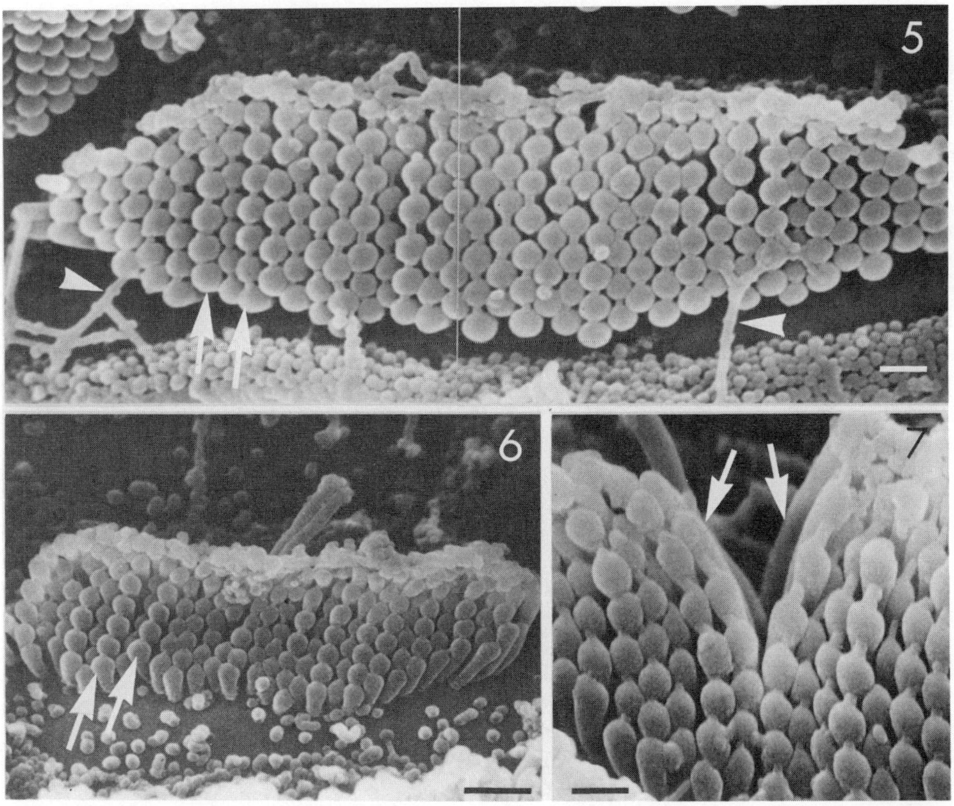

Fig. 5. Hair cell from neural edge of starling basilar papilla, viewed nearly perpendicular to the cuticular plate. Arrows indicate the axes of columns formed by the tip links. The tallest stereovilli in the bundle are at the top of the bundle. Arrowheads: extraneous material, perhaps from tectorial membrane, lying over stereovilli. Scale bar: 500 nm.

Fig. 6. Hair cell of starling basilar papilla. Arrows indicate two columns of stereovilli, joined by tip links. the stereovilli in these columns are a little taller than those in the adjacent columns. Neural edge of papilla. Scale bar: 1 μm.

Fig. 7. Hair cell of starling basilar papilla, showing separation of bundle along the columns defined by the tip links. No debris is visible on the lateral, separated, walls of the stereovilli (arrows). Scale bar: 500 nm.

stereovillus. Fine strands connect the membrane to the underlying dense cap over the ends of the actin filaments. The conical extension of the membrane is one possible site for the transducer channel(s). It is interesting that the conical extension of the membrane at the tips of shorter stereovilli, with the underlying density, was first noted by Flock (1965). The association of densities with attachment sites at both ends of the tip links was first noted by ourselves (Pickles, Osborne and Comis, Society for Experimental Biology, 5 January, 1984).

The geometrical arrangement shown in Figs 1 and 2 would be expected to produce a stretch of the tip links, in response to an angular deflection of the stereovilli. Indeed, the arrangement shown would tend to couple the deflections into the tip links with minimal stretch or compression of the other links, for instance of the lateral links which in guinea pigs join the stereovilli of the different rows just below their tips. This arrangement would therefore be efficient at coupling stimulus energy to the tip links, as opposed to other structures of the hair bundle.

The fine filament within each tip link is ideal for transmitting the stimulus-induced forces to a minute area of membrane. This would be mandatory if energy is to be coupled efficiently to the small number of transducer channels, perhaps between one and four, thought to exist on each stereovillus (Russell, 1983; Holton and Hudspeth, 1986). Calculations from the effective collecting area of the ear (Rosowski et al., 1986), the number of hair cells per mm of cochlear duct (Ulehlova et al., 1987), our own counts of the number of tip links on human inner and outer hair cells, and the critical bandwidth expressed as a length of cochlear duct (Greenwood, 1961), lead us to conclude that the forces collected from the acoustic wavefront would be concentrated onto the central filaments of tip links which have a total cross-sectional area which is smaller by a factor of 10^8 times.

The orientation of the tip links parallel to the axis of bilateral symmetry of the hair cell, and so parallel to the excitatory-inhibitory axis (Flock, 1965), is particularly obvious in the compact, hexagonally-packed bundles of birds and lizards. In addition, the observation of strict orientation of the tip links along the axis of bilateral symmetry of the individual bundle, irrespective of the bundle's orientation within the epithelium, is consistent with the hypothesis that the tip links are associated with the transduction process. This association of the direction of the tip links with the axis of bilateral symmetry of the hair cell was found even though in birds all orientations of hair cell axis could be seen, ranging from 0° to 90° with respect to the neural edge, depending upon position in the papilla.

The fact that stereovilli tend to separate into columns connected by tip links suggests that any sideways connections between different columns are weaker than the connections running within each column. Moreover, when the stereovilli had separated into columns, no debris was visible on the lateral surfaces of stereovilli near their upper ends. This suggests that there are no, or only sparse, lateral links connecting the stereovilli of the different columns in this region. It is likely therefore that the upper end of the bundle is relatively weakly braced against deflections which are oblique to the axis of bilateral symmetry. Again, this would be appropriate if the main mechanical input was parallel to the axis of bilateral symmetry, i.e. parallel to the excitatory-inhibitory axis. At the moment, we do not know if the apparently stronger intra-column connections result only from the tip links, or whether there is a contribution from lateral links running below the tips of the stereovilli. On the other hand, where it was possible to look deep into the gaps where stereovilli had separated, it was possible to see remains of lateral links at the lower ends of the stereovilli, consistent with the rich lateral network of links in this region, as previously reported by Csukas et al. (1987) for the lizard.

Sometimes the stereovilli within one column were, within the general gradation in height of the stereovilli, all a little taller, or a little shorter, than the stereovilli in adjacent columns. This suggests that a factor which governs the heights of the stereovilli during development has a component which is expressed along each column, the column being as defined above on the basis of the tip links connections. It appears therefore that the heights of the stereovilli and tip link orientation are closely related by common factors in development.

Acknowledgements

The skilled technical assistance of T.L. Hayward and L.M. Tomkins is gratefully acknowledged. This research was supported by the Medical Research Council of the UK, and the Deutsche Forschungsgemeinschaft within the programme of the SFB 204 "Gehör".

References

Comis, S.D., Pickles, J.O. and Osborne, M.P. (1985) Osmium tetroxide postfixation in relation to the cross linkage and spatial organization of stereocilia in the guinea-pig cochlea. J. Neurocytol. 14, 113-130.

Csukas, S.R., Rosenquiest, T.H. and Mulroy, M.J. (1987) Connections between stereocilia in auditory hair cells of the alligator lizard. Hearing Res. 30, 147-156.

Flock, A. (1965) Electron microscopic and electrophysiological studies on the lateral line canal organ. Acta Otolaryngol. Suppl. 199 1-90.

Flock, A. and Strelioff, D. (1984) Studies on hair cells in isolated coils from the guinea pig cochlea. Hearing Res. 15, 11-18.

Gleich, O. and Manley, G.A. (1988) Quantitative morphological analysis of the sensory epithelium of the starling and pigeon basilar papilla. Hearing Res., in press.

Greenwood, D.D. (1961) Critical bandwidth and the frequency coordinates of the basilar membrane. J. Acoust. Soc. Am. 33, 1344-1356.

Holton, T. and Hudspeth, A.J. (1986) The transduction channel of hair cells from the bull-frog characterized by noise analysis. J. Physiol. 375, 195-227.

Hudspeth, A.J. (1985) The cellular basis of hearing: the biophysics of hair cells. Science 230, 745-752.

Miller, M.R. (1980) The reptilian cochlear duct. In: Comparative Studies of Hearing in Vertebrates (Eds: Popper, A. N. and Fay, R. R.) Springer-Verlag, New York, Heidelberg, Berlin, pp. 169-204.

Mollenhauer, H.H. (1964) Plastic embedding mixtures for use in electron microscopy. Stain Tech. 39, 111-114.

Pickles, J.O., Comis, S.D. and Osborne, M.P. (1984) Cross-links between stereocilia in the guinea pig organ of Corti, and their possible relation to sensory transduction. Hearing Res. 15, 103-112.

Pickles, J.O., Comis, S.D. and Osborne, M.P. (1987) The effect of chronic application of kanamycin on stereocilia and their tip links in hair cells of the guinea pig cochlea. Hearing Research 29, 237-244.

Rosowski, J.J., Carney, L.H., Lynch, T.J. and Peake, W.T. (1986) The effectiveness of external and middle ears in coupling acoustic power into the cochlea. In: Peripheral Auditory Mechanisms (Eds: Allen, J.B. Hall, J.L., Hubbard, A., Neely S.T., and Tubis, A.) Springer, Berlin, pp. 3-12.

Russell, I.J. (1983) Origin of the receptor potential in inner hair cells of the mammalian cochlea - evidence for Davis' theory. Nature 301, 334-336.

Santi, P.A. and Anderson, C.B. (1987) A newly identified surface coat on cochlear hair cells. Hearing Res. 27, 47-65.

Ulehlova, L., Voldrich, L. and Janisch, R. (1987) Correlative study of sensory cell density and cochlear length in humans. Hearing Res. 28, 149-151.

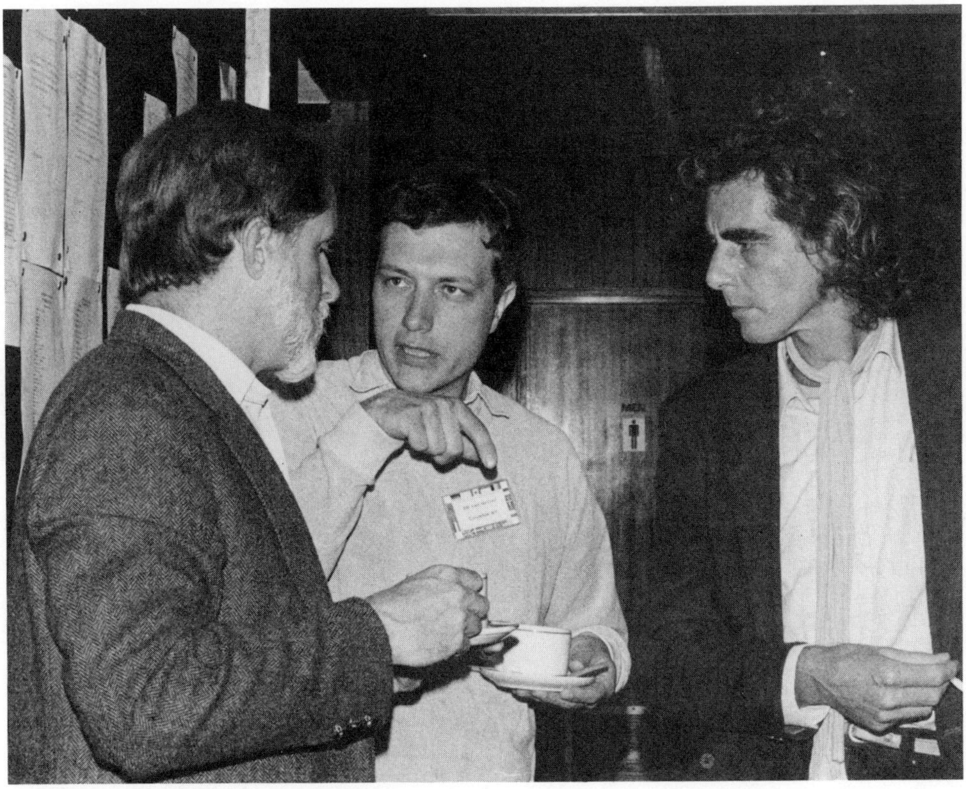

A.J. Hudspeth, S.M. van Netten and A.B.A. Kroese

2. MICROMECHANICAL MEASUREMENTS AND MODELS

HAIR CELL MECHANICS CONTROLS THE DYNAMIC BEHAVIOUR OF THE LATERAL LINE CUPULA

Sietse M. van Netten[1,3] and Alfons B.A. Kroese[2,3]

[1]*Department of Otolaryngology, College of Physicians and Surgeons, Columbia University New York, 630 West 168th street, New York, N.Y. 10032, USA*
[2]*Department of Medical Physics, University of Amsterdam, Academic Medical Center Meibergdreef 15, 1105 AZ Amsterdam, The Netherlands*
[3]*Department of Biophysics, Laboratory for General Physics University of Groningen, Westersingel 34, 9718 CM Groningen, The Netherlands*

Introduction

The direct stimulus for vertebrate sensory hair cells is, in general, provided by fluid surrounded macrostructures that are coupled mechanically to the hair bundles. The dynamic behaviour of these accessory structures is determined by their hydrodynamic and mechanical characteristics. A considerable part of the mechanical suspension of these structures is probably provided by the hair bundles. The micromechanical properties of the hair cells are therefore thought to contribute significantly to the mechanical characteristics of these accessory structures and to influence their motion (Khanna and Leonard, 1982; Flock and Strelioff, 1984; Strelioff et al., 1984). In the mammalian cochlea, for instance, hair cell properties are assumed to be responsible for the sharp tuning of the basilar membrane (Khanna and Leonard, 1986).

In a previous study on the fish lateral line organ *in vivo*, measurements of the motion of the accessory structure, the cupula, have shown that in response to mechanical stimulation of the organ the cupula slides over the sensory epithelium without bending. The results of this study also indicated that the stiffness resisting the sliding motion of the cupula results directly from the stiffness of the pivoting ciliar bundles of the sensory hair cells (van Netten and Kroese, 1987, 1988; van Netten, 1987). In order to obtain further evidence for a contribution of hair bundle micromechanics to the motion of the cupula, we have now studied the effects of an aminoglycoside antibiotic on the mechanical frequency response of the cupula in the fish lateral line. There is strong indirect (Kroese and van den Bercken 1980, 1982) and direct (Howard and Hudspeth, 1988; Richardson et al. 1988) evidence that the aminoglycosides affect the micromechanical properties of sensory hair bundles.

The main finding of this study is that the frequency response of the cupula changes considerably as a result of the effects of the aminoglycoside on the hair cells. Further, the action of the drug on hair bundle micromechanics is studied by the use of a hydrodynamic model of cupular motion.

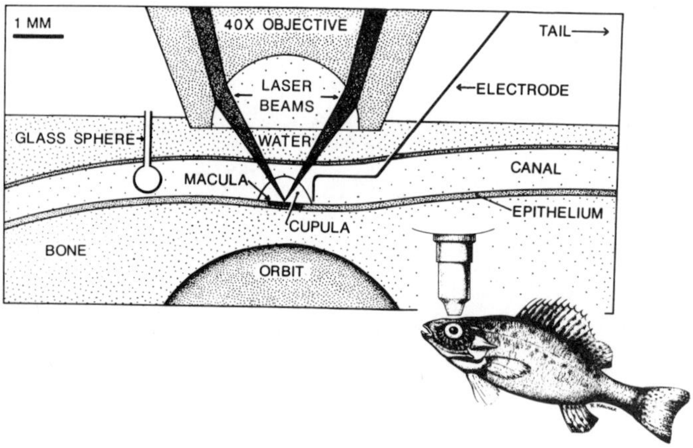

Fig.1. Schematic drawing of the lateral line preparation. Bottom right: the fish is placed below the waterimmersion objective of the microscope. Enlarged area: underneath the waterimmersion objective and just below the skin of the head runs the lateral line canal. The bony bottom of the canal is covered by a thin layer of epithelium. The canal organ consists of a sensory epithelium, or macula, covered by the cupula, in which the hair bundles of the sensory hair cells are embedded. The glass sphere for mechanical stimulation, the laser beams of the interferometer used to measure cupular displacements and the electrode for recording of extracellular receptor potentials are indicated.

Methods

Experiments were performed on neuromasts in the lateral line canal on top of the head of the ruff (*Acerina cernua* L.). Fish were anaesthetized with an intraperitoneal injection (24 mg/kg) of Saffan (Glaxovet), respired artificially by a flow of tapwater (0.4 l/min; 15.5 $\pm$0.5 °C) through the mouth and held rigidly in place by head and body clamps. Canal organs were revealed by removing carefully the overlying skin and bony bridge. Incident light polarization microscopy (ILPM) was used to visualize the sensory hair cells and hair bundles, as described earlier (Kroese and van Netten, 1987) and depicted in Fig.1. Sinusoidal canal fluid displacements in the direction of the longitudinal axis were produced under near field conditions by a piezoelectrically driven glass sphere (ϕ = 0.8 mm) in the canal. More details on the preparation can be found elsewhere (van Netten and Kroese, 1987).

Submicroscopic displacements of the transparent cupula were measured with a heterodyne laser interferometer (van Netten, 1988a) which was coupled to the microscope (Fig.1). A small light scattering polystyrene bead (ϕ = 1.15 µm) was placed under visual control in the cupula near the tips of the sensory hair bundles. Backscattered phase modulated laser light of the bead containing the information about the motion of the cupula was directed to a photodetector and demodulated. Amplitude and phase of the signal were measured with a pair of lock-in amplifiers. The accuracy of the amplitude measurements is within 1 dB, and the phase measurements have an accuracy within 10°.

Extracellular receptor potentials, representing the summed response of all hair cells in the macula, were recorded with a silver wire electrode (ϕ = 100 µm), insulated except at the tip, which was placed near the base of the cupula (see Fig.1). Amplitude and phase of the signal were measured with a pair of lock-in amplifiers. The results of the present experiments were obtained during cupular displacements of less than 60 nm. In this range the extracellular receptor potentials are linearly related to cupular motion (van Netten, 1987; Kroese and van Netten, 1988). Because the cupular displacement is also linearly related to the stimulus amplitude over a range of at least 60 dB (van Netten and Kroese, 1987) the system under study can be considered as linear. Since individual lateral line hair cells in this organ have identical transfer properties (Kroese and van Netten, 1988), after analysis the extracellular receptor potentials depict single hair cell properties.

DHSM (dihydrostreptomycin sulphate; Sigma) was freshly dissolved in tapwater in the desired concentration (12.5 µg/ml; approx. 21 µM) and applied to the fish tank by switching the perfusion flow from standard tapwater to that containing DHSM. The conditions of water supply and drain of the fish tank were such that the concentration of DHSM in the tank increased slowly after switching and reached 99% of the final concentration (12.5 µg/ml) after about 10 min.

In each experiment, measurements of cupular motion in response to 1 min of mechanical stimulation with a single frequency were made with intervals of about 3 min. Five different stimulus frequencies were used, selected to cover adequately the frequency response of the neuromast under study. In addition, extracellular receptor potentials evoked by a 1 min stimulation at 80 Hz were measured regularly (see Fig. 2). The effects of 12.5 µg/ml DHSM were completely reversible (see Fig. 2). The values of the frequency responses of cupular motion depicted in Fig. 3 were obtained in the period immediately before application of DHSM (control), in the presence of DHSM after the effects had reached a stable level (see Fig. 2a) and in the period when, after switching back to tapwater, the responses had become stable again (control).

Results

EFFECTS OF DHSM ON CUPULAR MOTION

The effect of 12.5 µg/ml DHSM on the cupular motion evoked by stimulation with 80 Hz is shown in Fig.2a. DHSM caused a decrease in the amplitude of cupular motion, which after about 30 to 40 min reached a level that remained constant for as long as the drug was present. The phase of cupular displacement with respect to sphere displacement in the presence of DHSM showed a phase lag in comparison with the control situation. Perfusion with fresh tapwater caused the amplitude and phase of the response to return to their original level. Similar effects of DHSM were found in 5 other experiments. By means of visual control over the neuromast, provided by ILPM, it was determined that application of DHSM did not cause any shrinkage or change in the shape of the cupula. These results demonstrate unequivocally that DHSM influences the motion of the cupula.

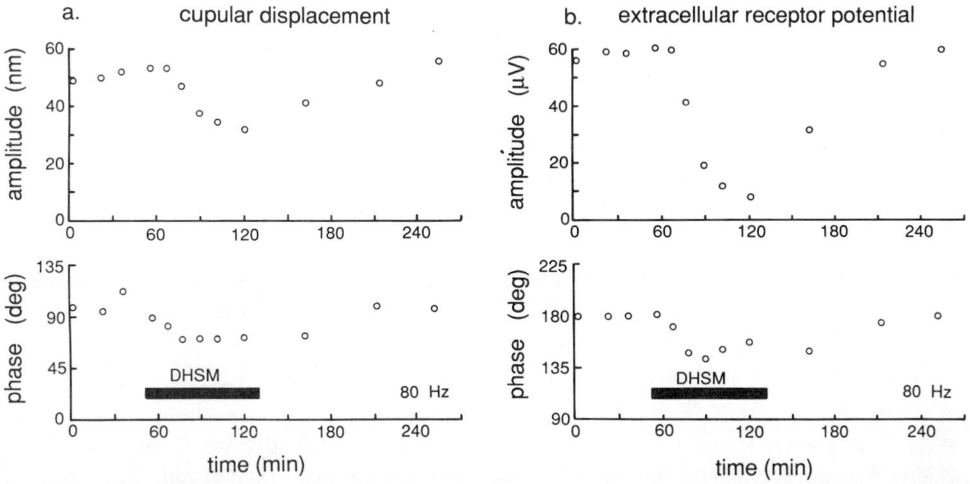

Fig.2 Effects of DHSM on amplitude (above) and phase (below) of cupular displacement (a) and extracellular receptor potentials (b) of a neuromast in the supraorbital canal lateral line of the ruff, evoked by 80 Hz stimulation. The phase of the responses is given with respect to sphere displacement. DHSM (12.5 µg/ml) was applied to the tapwater in the fish tank during the 78 min period indicated by the horizontal bar.

EFFECTS OF DHSM ON EXTRACELLULAR RECEPTOR POTENTIALS

Application of DHSM in a concentration of 12.5 μg/ml markedly affected the extracellularly recorded hair cell receptor potentials evoked by 80 Hz stimulation. DHSM caused a depression of the amplitude and a phase lag in the receptor potentials. As for cupular motion, these effects reached a constant value within about 30 to 40 min after application and were completely reversible. A representative example of this action, obtained in the same experiment as from which results are depicted in Fig. 2a, is shown in Fig. 2b.

Application of DHSM in a higher concentration (25 μg/ml) caused similar but larger effects on cupular motion and receptor potentials than those reported here. The effects of the higher concentration were found to be only partly reversible.

Comparison of the magnitude of the effects of DHSM on cupular motion and on receptor potentials reveals that the reduction in receptor potential amplitude can be only explained partly by the reduction in cupular motion. Thus, these results are in accordance with the finding in earlier studies that aminoglycosides affect the functioning of the sensory hair cells (see e.g. Wersäll and Flock, 1964; Kroese and van den Bercken, 1982; Hudspeth and Kroese, 1983; Ohmori, 1985; Kroese et al., 1988).

FREQUENCY DEPENDENCE OF EFFECTS OF DHSM

The frequency responses of cupular motion as measured in 6 experiments under control conditions were all very well comparable to those reported in an earlier study on this preparation (van Netten and Kroese, 1987, 1988). The effects of DHSM on cupular motion were found to depend on the stimulus frequency, as can be seen in Fig.3. Application of DHSM reduced the amplitude of cupular motion at stimulus frequencies in the range where the cupular motion under control conditions shows a maximum in amplitude (Fig.2a), while at low stimulus frequencies the amplitude of cupular motion increased. The cupular motion in response to high stimulus frequencies was not affected by DHSM. The changes induced by DHSM in the amplitude of cupular displacement were at all stimulus frequencies accompanied by a phase lag. A similar frequency dependence of the effects of DHSM and other aminoglycosides on extracellular receptor potentials and on afferent response properties of the superficial lateral line organ of *Xenopus* has been reported previously (Kroese and van den Bercken, 1980; 1982).

MODEL

The experimental data were compared with the results of a hydrodynamic model of cupular motion. This model (van Netten, 1988b), which incorporates a frequency dependent boundary layer driving the cupula, describes the frequency response of the cupula under physiological (control) conditions (van Netten and Kroese, 1987) in terms of a sliding stiffness of the cupula, the density and viscosity of the canal fluid, and the cupular diameter. The sliding stiffness of the cupula results directly from the stiffness of the pivoting hair bundles coupled to the cupular base (van Netten and Kroese, 1987; van Netten, 1988b). The results of a fit to the present control measurements were very close to the average values of the parameters found previously (e.g. van Netten and Kroese, 1987).

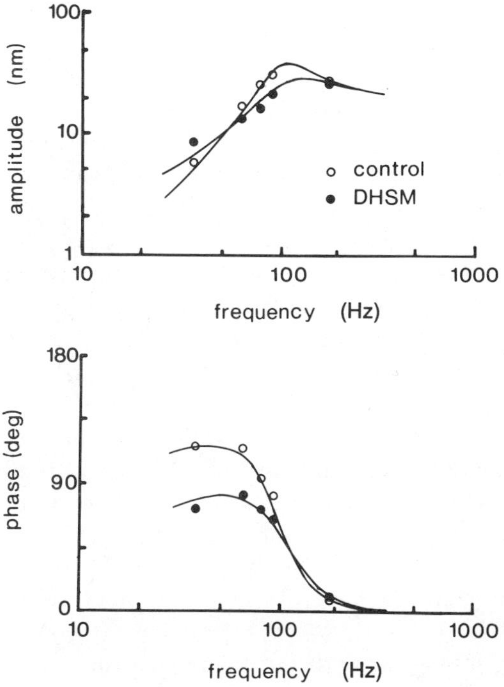

Fig.3 Frequency response of the cupula measured during control conditions (o), and during application of DHSM (•). The solid lines give the results of a hydrodynamic model of cupular motion for two different values of the resistant component R assumed to be present in the hair bundle micromechanics (See Fig.4). The values used for R in the hydrodynamic model (associated with the total of hair cell contributions) are: 1.9 $mN{\cdot}s{\cdot}m^{-1}$ for the control situation and 0.42 $mN{\cdot}s{\cdot}m^{-1}$ for the DHSM exposed situation. The other (summed) parameters used for both the control and DHSM exposed situations are: S1 = 9 $mN{\cdot}m^{-1}$, S2 = 108 $mN{\cdot}m^{-1}$, cupular radius = 0.3 mm, and canal fluid viscosity = $4.8 \cdot 10^{-3}$ $kg{\cdot}m^{-1}{\cdot}s^{-1}$.

The response of the hydrodynamic model, however, could not be fitted properly to the frequency response of the cupula measured during exposure of the organ to DHSM. The finding that variation of the cupular diameter and of the fluid viscosity failed to provide a fit to the data is not surprising since the cupular diameter did not change during exposure to DHSM, and the concentration of the drug applied is too low to cause a significant change in viscosity.

The most obvious changes in the frequency response due to exposure to DHSM are the phase lag at the lowest frequencies and the disappearance of the maximum in the amplitude (Fig.3). These changes, together with the fact that the model could not be fitted by variation of the sliding stiffness, suggest that an extra resistive element, not apparent under the control conditions, is present in the hair bundle micromechanics.

A mechanical model of the hair bundle that meets these requirements consists of a resistance (R) in series with a stiffness (S2) placed in parallel to a stiffness (S1) already assumed to be present in the hair bundle micromechanics (Fig.4). This mechanical

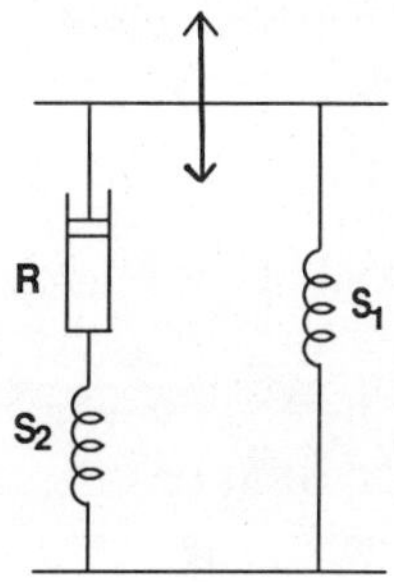

Fig.4 Micromechanical model of the hair bundle; a resistive element R in series with a compliance S2 in parallel to a compliance S1. The arrows indicate the motion of the stereocilium. A decrease of the resistive component R accounts for the changes observed in cupular dynamic behaviour during application of DHSM.

model has also been proposed to account for the mechanical adaptation observed in hair cells of the sacculus of the frog (Howard & Hudspeth, 1987).

The expression of the hair bundle impedance of Fig.4 was incorporated in the closed form solution of the hydrodynamic model. To fit the model response to both the DHSM and control situation, S1, S2, R and the fluid viscosity were varied, while the cupular radius was kept constant. The best fits for both situations were found when S2 was chosen much larger than S1 (S1 =9 $mN \cdot m^{-1}$, S2 =108 $mN \cdot m^{-1}$) and when the viscosity of the fluid was set to about the same value as before ($4.8 \cdot 10^{-3}$ $kg \cdot m^{-1} \cdot s^{-1}$, see van Netten and Kroese, 1987). The difference between the control and DHSM exposed situation is the value of parameter R, which was found to be 1.9 $mN \cdot s \cdot m^{-1}$ under control conditions and 0.42 $mN \cdot s \cdot m^{-1}$ under DHSM exposed conditions. The results of the model with these parameters are added to Fig.3 and describe the measured data satisfactorily.

The values found for S1, S2 and R apply to the summed contribution of all hair cells underlying the cupula and should therefore be corrected for the number of haircells (about 1000) to be compared with those of a single hair cell. Also, due to the contribution to cupular motion of two oppositely oriented hair cell populations in a lateral line neuromast, these values may represent an average of possible directional mechanical asymmetries such as reported in other hair cells (Flock and Strelioff, 1984; Howard and Ashmore, 1986).

We conclude that the measured change in cupular dynamic behaviour induced by DHSM can be accounted for by a change in the resistive component of the hair bundle impedance.

Discussion

The experimental results show unequivocally that the dynamic behaviour of the cupula in the lateral line is affected reversibly by the application of DHSM. Since no mechanical parameters of the organ other than those relating to the micromechanics of the hair bundle can be changed by DHSM, these *in vivo* measurements demonstrate directly that sensory hair cell micromechanics is reflected in the dynamic response of the accessory macrostructure that drives the sensory hair cells.

Before reaching this conclusion, however, we must exclude explanations for the changes in cupular dynamic behaviour that are unrelated to hair bundle micromechanics. There is evidence that aminoglycosides affect hair cell transduction by a selective blockage of the transduction channels (Hudspeth and Kroese, 1983; Ohmori, 1985; Kroese et al., 1988) and by changing the mechanical properties of the hair bundles (Kroese and van den Bercken, 1980; 1982; Howard and Hudspeth, 1988). In the present study we did not find any evidence for a direct effect of DHSM on the cupula. Further, the mechanical coupling between the hair bundles and the cupula is very tight (e.g. Flock, 1971; van Netten and Kroese, 1988) and any damage to that coupling by DHSM would not be easily reversible. Therefore, it is concluded that the action of DHSM on cupular motion results from a direct effect on the hair cells. Since in the experiments the fish were anaesthetized with Saffan and a very low concentration of DHSM was used, the possibility that the hair bundle mechanics was affected indirectly, by changes in efferent activity as a result of a central nervous system action of DHSM, seems higly unlikely.

The micromechanical model of the hair bundle shown in Fig.4 is a simple configuration that explains the measured data in terms of reactive and resistive components. The action of DHSM on the hair cells in this model is a decrease of the coupling (R) of stereociliar motion to spring S2, thereby causing an increase in the energy dissipation in R. This change in hair bundle mechanics results in a broader resonance peak of the frequency response of the cupula and a decrease of the phase lead at low frequencies. From a calculation of the ratio of the reactance and the resistance using the parameters found, it can be seen that during the control situation the hair bundle impedance is dominated by the reactive (stiffness) component. This is consistent with the assumption of a pure stiffness contribution of the hair cells to cupular mechanics under physiological conditions in the frequency range used (van Netten and Kroese, 1987; van Netten, 1988b). During exposure of the organ to DHSM, however, the resistive component of the hair bundle impedance cannot be neglected anymore.

It is interesting that the micromechanical model used also accounts for mechanical adaptation of hair cells and relates the ratio of R to S2 to the adaptation time constant (Howard and Hudspeth, 1987). For the present results R/S2 yields about 20 ms for the control situation and about 4 ms for the DHSM exposed hair cells. A time constant of 20 ms is consistent with the highpass filter characteristics found in the electrical responses of lateral line hair cells under control conditions (van Netten, 1987; Kroese and van Netten, 1988) and with that found by Howard and Hudspeth in hair cells in the sacculus of the frog (Howard and Hudspeth, 1987). These authors associate the spring S2 with elements that gate the transduction channels (Howard and Hudspeth, 1988) which are possibly located near the tip links (Pickles et al., 1984) between the stereocilia. The present results indicate that the mechanical coupling (R) of stereociliar motion to the transduction gating spring S2 is loosened by aminoglycosides. It has indeed been shown that chronic application of aminoglycosides to the cochlea of the guinea pig causes the loss of tip links between the stereocilia of outer hair cells (Pickles et al., 1987). The changes of cupular response caused by DHSM may therefore reflect an early, reversible stage of damage to the mechanical elements that gate the opening and closing of the transduction channels in sensory hair cells.

The results of this study provide strong support for the concept that hair cell micromechanics contributes significantly to the mechanical behaviour of accessory structures in more complex systems such as the mammalian cochlea (Flock and Strelioff, 1984; Strelioff et al., 1984; Khanna and Leonard, 1986).

Acknowledgements

We are grateful to Mr. Rob C.B. Kreuger for skillfully producing Fig.1. The use of facilities at the Dept. of Biophysics in Groningen is gratefully acknowledged. This work was supported by the Netherlands Organization for the advancement of Pure Research (Z.W.O.), and by a Z.W.O. -NATO Science Fellowship (SvN).

References

Flock, Å. (1971) Sensory transduction in hair cells. In: Handbook of sensory physiology Vol.I (Ed: Loewenstein, W.R.) Springer Verlag, Berlin, pp. 396-441.

Flock, Å and Strelioff, D. (1984) Graded and nonlinear mechanical properties of sensory hairs in the mammalian hearing organ. Nature 310, 597-599.

Howard, J and Ashmore, J.H. (1986) Stiffness of sensory hair bundles in the sacculus of the frog. Hearing Res. 23, 93-104.

Howard, J. and Hudspeth, A.J. (1987) Mechanical relaxation of the hair bundles mediates adaptation in mechanoelectrical transduction by the bullfrog's saccular hair cell. Proc. Natl. Acad. Sci. USA 84, 3064-3068.

Howard, J. and Hudspeth, A.J. (1988) Compliance of the hair bundle associated with gating of mechanoelectrical transduction channels in the bullfrog's saccular hair cell. Neuron. 1, 189-199.

Hudspeth, A.J. and Kroese, A.B.A. (1983) Voltage-dependent interaction of dihydrostreptomycin with the transduction channels in bullfrog sensory hair cells. J.Physiol. 345, 66P.

Khanna, S.M. and Leonard, D.G.B. (1982) Basilar membrane tuning in the cat cochlea. Science 215, 305-306.

Khanna, S.M. and Leonard, D.G.B. (1986) Relationship between basilar membrane tuning and hair cell condition. Hearing Res. 23, 55-70.

Kroese, A.B.A. and Bercken, J. van den (1980) Dual action of ototoxic antibiotics on sensory hair cells. Nature 283, 395-397.

Kroese, A.B.A. and Bercken, J. van den (1982) Effects of ototoxic antibiotics on sensory hair cell functioning. Hearing Res. 6, 183-197.

Kroese, A.B.A. and Netten, S.M. van (1987) The application of incident light polarization microscopy for the visualization of sensory hair cells *in vivo*. J. Microsc. 145, 309-317.

Kroese, A.B.A. and Netten, S.M. van (1988) Sensory transduction in lateral line sensory hair cells. In: Neurobiology and evolution of the lateral line. (Eds: Coombs, S., Görner, P. and Münz, H.) Springer Verlag, New York. In press.

Kroese, A.B.A. Das, A. and Hudspeth, A.J. (1988) Blockage of the transduction channels of hair cells in the bullfrog's sacculus by aminoglycoside antibiotics. Submitted for publication.

Netten, S.M. van (1987) Laser interferometric study of the mechanosensitivity of the fish lateral line. Thesis, University of Groningen, Groningen.

Netten, S.M. van (1988a) Laser interferometer microscope for the measurement of nanometer vibrational displacements of a light-scattering microscopic object. J. Acoust. Soc. Am. 83, 1667-1674.

Netten, S.M. van (1988b) Hydrodynamics of the excitation of the cupula in the fish canal lateral line. Submitted for publication.

Netten, S.M. van and Kroese, A.B.A. (1987) Laser interferometric measurements on the dynamic behaviour of the cupula in the fish lateral line. Hearing Res. 29, 55-61.

Netten, S.M. van and Kroese, A.B.A.(1988) Dynamic behaviour and micromechanical properties of the cupula. In: Neurobiology and evolution of the lateral line. (Eds: Coombs, S., Görner, P. and Münz, H.) Springer Verlag, New York. In press.

Ohmori, H. (1985) Mechano-electrical transduction currents in isolated vestibular hair cells of chick. J.Physiol. 359, 189-217.

Pickles, J.O. Comis, S.D. and Osborne, M.P. (1984) Cross-links between stereocilia in the guinea pig organ of Corti, and their possible relation to sensory transduction. Hearing Res. 15, 103-112.

Pickles, J.O. Comis, S.D. and Osborne, M.P. (1987) The effect of chronic application of kanamycin on stereocilia and their tip links in hair cells of the guinea pig cochlea. Hearing Res. 29, 237-244.

Richardson, G.P., Russell, I.J., Wasserkort, R. and Hans, M. (1988) Aminoglycoside antibiotics and lectins cause irreversible increases in the stiffness of cochlear hair-cell stereocilia. "Mechanics of Hearing" proceedings, Eds: Wilson, J.P. and Kemp, D.T. (This volume)

Strelioff, D., Flock, Å. and Minser, K.E. (1985) Role of outer hair cells in mechanical frequency selectivity of the cochlea. Hearing Res. 18, 169-175.

Wersäll, J. and Flock, Å. (1964) Suppression and restoration of the microphonic output from the lateral line organ after local application of streptomycin. Life Sci. 3, 1151-1155.

Comments and Discussion

WIT

You showed that there is a strong mechanical coupling between hair cell bundle and cupula. This implies that different hair cells are mechanically coupled. The consequence could be that spontaneous activities of primary fibers coming from different hair cells are correlated. Do you know of any experiment that shows such a correlation.

VAN NETTEN AND KROESE

We don't know of any experiment that shows such a correlation in spontaneous activity. In the lateral line of the clawed frog (*Xenopus laevis*) it has been demonstrated (Harris and Milne, 1966) that the spontaneous afferent activity of the two fibres innervating a single neuromass is not correlated. Spontaneous afferent activity is defined as the activity under conditions where the cupula is not moving.

This activity is expected to be determined mainly by properties of the synapse.

Harris, G.T. and Milne, D.C. (1966) Input-output characteristics of the lateral-line sense organs of Xenopus laevis, JASA, 40, 32-42.

AMINOGLYCOSIDE ANTIBIOTICS AND LECTINS CAUSE IRREVERSIBLE INCREASES IN THE STIFFNESS OF COCHLEAR HAIR-CELL STEREOCILIA

G.P. Richardson, I.J. Russell, R. Wasserkort, and M. Hans

MRC Neurophysiology Group, School of Biological Sciences University of Sussex, Falmer, Brighton, BN1 9QG

Introduction

Aminoglycoside antibiotics such as neomycin and streptomycin are known to be both ototoxic and nephrotoxic. In the mammalian inner ear, chronic treatment with high doses of aminoglycosides causes an increase in auditory thresholds, impairment of tuning, the fusion of hair-cell stereocilia and the selective degeneration of hair cells (for reviews see Harpur 1987, Rybak 1986, Brown 1978, Hawkins 1976). The mechanisms underlying aminoglycoside induced ototoxicity are not properly understood. When applied directly to lower vertebrate hair cells, these drugs reversibly block the transducer channel in a manner that depends on both the voltage gradient across the membrane (Hudspeth and Kroese 1983) and the extracellular calcium concentration (Kroese and van den Bercken 1982). It has also been shown that aminoglycosides interact with phosphatidylinositol biphosphate and, therefore, may interfere with the phosphoinositide second messenger system (Schacht 1979). We have recently developed an organotypic culture system of the neonatal mouse cochlea (Russell, Richardson and Cody 1986, Russell and Richardson 1987), which can be used to directly investigate the effects that aminoglycosides have on the micromechanical and electrophysiological properties of mammalian cochlear hair cells.

Methods

PREPARATION OF CULTURES. Cultures were prepared from the cochleas of 1-2 day postnatal mice. The cartilaginous capsule, stria vascularis, Reissner's membrane and the immature mesenchymal internal spiral lamina were removed by dissection in HEPES-buffered (10mM, pH 7.2) Hanks balanced salt solution (HBSS), leaving the organ of Corti, greater epithelial ridge and attached spiral ganglion as one unit. These tissue pieces were then explanted onto collagen-coated round glass coverslips, fed with 50ul of complete medium (8 parts Eagle's minimum essential medium with Earle's salts, 1 part heat-inactivated horse serum, 1 part mouse embryo extract, buffered with 10mM HEPES pH 7.2) and maintained in Maximow slide assemblies in the lying drop position at 37°C for 1-3 days.

LECTIN HISTOCHEMISTRY. Three day old cultures were washed extensively with HBSS to remove medium, fixed for 1 hour in 3.7% formaldehyde buffered with 0.1 M sodium phosphate buffer pH 7.2 and then rinsed with Tris-HCl (10mM, pH 7.2) buffered saline (TBS). Non-specific protein binding sites were blocked by incubating the cultures in 3% w/v bovine serum albumin in TBS for 1 hour and the cultures were subsequently labelled with fluorescein isothiocyanate (FITC) conjugated lectins (Vector laboratories) for 1 hour at concentrations of either 50µg/ml or 5ug/ml. Cultures were then rinsed extensively with TBS, mounted in Tris-HCl(100mM, pH 8.4):glycerol (1:9) containing 0.1% w/v p- phenylenediamine and photographed on Kodak Tri-X rated at 1600 ASA.

MICROELECTRODE RECORDING. Microelectrodes were bent 0.2-0.5mm from their tips and filled with 3 M KCl (resistances 150-300 MOhm). Microelectrodes were positioned with the aid of Huxley micromanipulators (Goodfellow Metals, Cambridge). Recordings were made with a DC amplifier and records were stored on magnetic tape on an FM tape recorder (Racal 4DS) for future off-line analysis with a DEC PDP-1103 computer.

MECHANICAL STIMULATION. The sensory hair bundles were displaced by sinusoidal movements of the tip of a glass probe which was attached with insect wax to a piezoelectric bimorph (Vernitron PZT-5B) and was driven by a sinusoidal voltage. The probe tip was stepped in 5dB increments from about 2-100nm.

STIFFNESS MEASUREMENTS. The stiffness of the hair cell bundles was measured along the presumed axis of greatest sensitivity, ie., towards and away from the kinocilium (Fig. 1a) by measuring the bending at the tip of a silica probe that was attached to the tallest row of stereocilia, when the base of the probe was displaced by a known amount. Probes had diameters of 0.5-1.5 µm and the stiffness was determined by measuring the displacement of the tip in response to loading with acrylic beads of known mass using a horizontally mounted microscope (Howard and Ashmore 1985). The probes had stiffnesses of approximately 200pN/um and were glued to glass stubs which were then mounted on short lengths of piezoelectric bimorph. The resonant frequency of the bimorph driver was about 4 kHz and, in order to prevent excitation at this resonance, the driving voltage was low pass filtered with a cut off frequency of 1 kHz.

The displacement of the probe tip was monitored according to a method described by Crawford and Fettiplace (1985) in which the focussed and magnified (1000 x) image of the tip of the probe is projected onto a pair of photodiodes (Centronics LD 2-5). The photocurrents from each photodiode were converted to a voltage and the differential voltage was proportional to the position of the fibre over a distance equal to the optical diameter of the fibre. The displacement sensor was calibrated either by moving the silica probe a known distance using the piezoelectric driver or by moving the headstage several microns which, due to the optical magnification (1000 x), corresponds to a displacement of the probe of several nanometers.

The force delivered by a fibre can be calculated from the product of its known stiffness, Kf and the difference between steady state displacements of the fibre when it is just above and not in contact with the stereocilia (y1, off, Fig.1B) and when it is attached to the tips of the tallest rows of stereocilia (y2, on, Fig. 1b).

The bundle stiffness, Kb, is given by Kb = Kf((y1-y2)/y2). Steady state displacement measurements were made from averages of 10-32 records of the differential voltage output of the displacement sensor 80ms after the beginning of the displacement step.

Results

i) Steady state stereocilia stiffness. In Fig. 1c the stiffness of the stereocilia of an outer hair cell (OHC) located in the outermost row of the organ of Corti is plotted for displacements in the 0 to 60nm range. The stiffness is linear over this range and the cells are symmetrically stiff in both the excitatory and inhibitory directions; i.e., the stiffness is the same when the stereocilia are displaced either towards or away from the kinocilium. At any point along the length of the cochlea, the stereocilia of OHCs in the outermost row are stiffer than the stereocilia of adjacent inner hair cells (IHCs) by a factor of 1.5. The mean stiffness of IHC

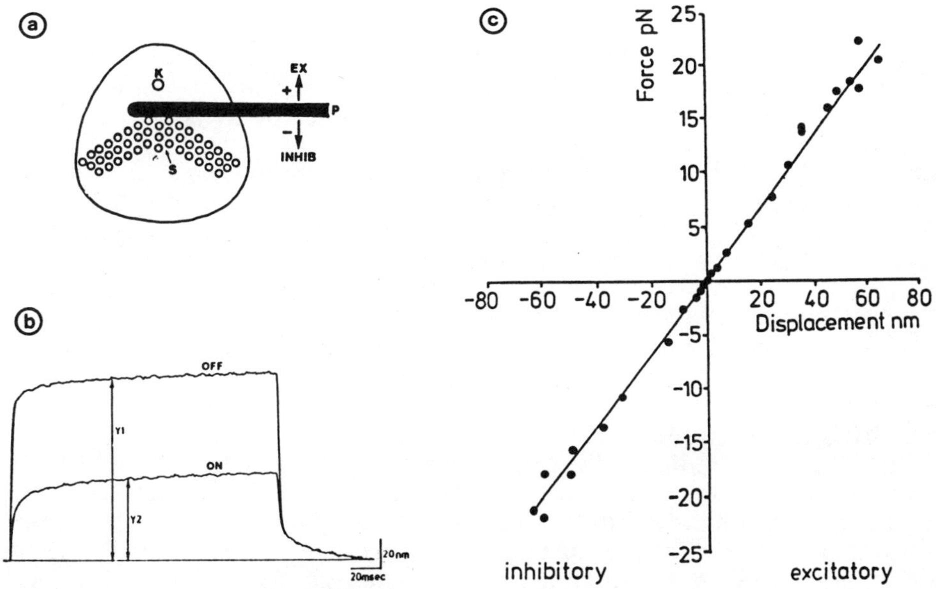

FIGURE 1. a) Schematic diagram illustrating the apical surface of a hair cell as viewed from above. The stiffness of stereocilia (S) was measured along the presumed axis of greatest sensitivity, i.e., towards (+ EX) and away (- INHIB) from the kinocilium (K) with a silica probe (P) attached to the tallest row of stereocilia.

b) The displacement of the tip of the probe was monitored according to a method described by Crawford and Fettiplace (1985). The force delivered by the fibre can be calculated from its known stiffness, Kf, and the difference between steady state displacements y1 (off the stereocilia) and y2 (on the stereocilia): the bundle stiffness, Kb, is given by Kb = Kf(y1-y2/y2).

c) The relationship between force versus displacement of the stereocilia for a single outer hair cell from the outermost row was made from averaged records similar to those in Fig.1b. The line is a regression line (r = 0.96) and the slope gives a bundle stiffness of 310 pN/µm. Unless stated all measurements were made in HEPES buffered (10mM, pH 7.2) Hanks balanced salt solution (HBSS) at room temperature.

stereocilia is 1040±390 pN/µm (n = 116) and of OHC stereocilia bundles is 1690±540 pN/µm (n = 130). OHC stereocilia in the apex of the cochlea are approximately 1.6 times less stiff than OHC stereocilia in the base of the cochlea.

ii) The effects of neomycin. Extracellular receptor potentials were recorded from IHCs and outer row OHCs in cultures bathed in HBSS in response to sinusoidal displacements of their stereocilia. The extracellular voltage responses are largest when recorded close to the tips of the stereocilia and are negative going when the stereocilia are displaced towards the kinocilium; an indication that the receptor current flows inwards near this point on the apical surface when the stereocilia are displaced in the excitatory direction. The relationship between the extracellular voltage response and displacement for an outer row OHC is shown in figure 2a. These voltage responses disappear within ten minutes when the culture is perfused with HBSS containing 50µM neomycin and similar amplitude responses return 20 minutes after the onset of washout with HBSS. Immediately after making each set of extracellular voltage recordings the mean stiffness of 10 adjacent outer row OHCs was determined for 40nm displacements of their stereocilia bundles. Ten to twenty minutes after the onset of perfusion with HBSS containing neomycin (50µM) the stereocilia stiffness increases from 1.6-2.0 fold. During washout with HBSS, transduction is restored (Figs. 2 a & inset) but the stereocilia stiffness remains elevated and does not return to control levels (Fig. 2b). Although transduction may be fully restored, return to pre-exposure stiffness levels has not been observed even after washout times of up to two hours. Similar results have been obtained with dihydrostreptomycin (50µM). Neomycin induced stiffness increases cannot be reversed by increasing the calcium concentration of the HBSS washout to 10 mM (Fig. 2b). Varying the calcium concentration of the HBSS in the range from 20 µM to 10 mM has no apparent effect on the steady state stiffness of stereocilia.

iii) Lectin binding. FITC-conjugated lectins have been used to examine the distribution of lectin binding sites on the apical surfaces of the hair cells. Lectins from Concanavalia ensiformis (Con A), Triticum vulgaris (WGA), Glycine max (SBA), Arachis hypogaea (PNA) and succinylated Con A all stain stereocilia, whereas binding sites for lectins from Dolichos biflorus (DBA) and Ulex europaeus (UEA 1) cannot be detected (Figs. 3 a-g).

iv) The effects of lectins. The effects of lectins on stereocilia stiffness was determined by first measuring the forces generated by the stereocilia in response to fixed 40nm displacements of the silica probe in 10 outer row OHCs when the culture was bathed in HBSS. The mean stiffness from these cells was then compared with the stiffness obtained in a further 10 adjacent OHCs about ten minutes after a lectin had been added to the bathing solution. All the FITC- conjugated lectins that bind to stereocilia, except succinylated Con A, cause an increase in stiffness (Fig.3h). The FITC-conjugated lectins for which binding sites on stereocilia cannot be detected by fluorescence microscopy (UEA 1 and DBA) do not increase stiffness. Saturating concentrations (see below) of native Con A (20 µg protein/ml) can cause up to 4 fold increases in stereocilia stiffness (Fig. 3h). At the same concentration succinylated native Con A causes no increase in stereocilia stiffness (Fig. 3h). Examination of both neomycin and Con A treated cultures by scanning and transmission electron microscopy indicates that the observed increases in stiffness caused by these agents are not associated with any obvious fusion of the stereocilia (not shown).

Recordings made from OHCs prior to and after the addition of WGA to the perfusion chamber at a concentration of 4 µg/ml (100nM) indicate that WGA does not block transduction (Figs. 4 a & inset), although there is an irreversible increase in stereocilia stiffness (Fig. 4b). Con A also does not block transduction. Dose response data (see Fig. 4c) indicate that half maximal stiffness increases are obtained with 8 nM Con A and 2 uM neomycin. The maximum stiffness increases obtained with saturating concentrations of WGA and Con A are 2 times greater than the increases obtained with saturating levels of neomycin. A comparison of the dose response curves for the effects of neomycin on the stiffness of inner (filled circles, Fig. 4c) and outer (open circles Fig. 4c) hair-cell stereocilia

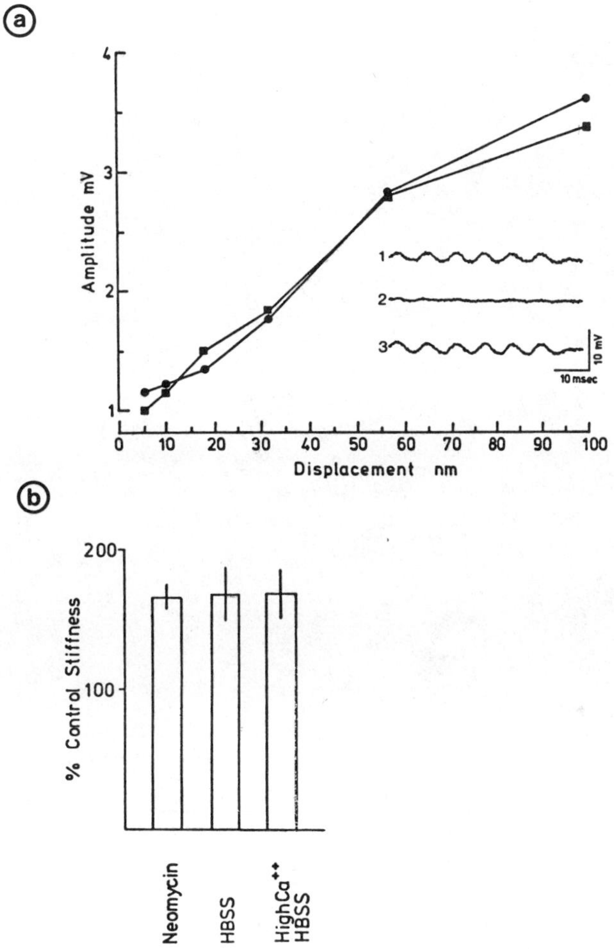

FIGURE 2. a) The relationship between the peak-to-peak amplitudes of receptor potentials recorded extracellularly from an outer row outer hair cell to sinusoidal peak-to-peak displacements of the stereocilia at 113 Hz in a cochlear culture during perfusion with HBSS (●) prior to treatment with neomycin and after washout of neomycin with HBSS (■). Insets are single traces of the voltage responses of the outer hair cell to 56nm displacements in HBSS (1), HBSS containing neomycin (2) and following washout of neomycin with HBSS (3).

b) The stiffness of outer hair cell stereocilia during perfusion of cochlear cultures with HBSS containing 50μM neomycin (when transduction was blocked) and during subsequent washout with HBSS (when transduction was restored), and during washout with HBSS containing 10 mM CaCl2, expressed as a percentage of the pre-exposure stiffness. Stereocilia stiffness was measured for 10 cells prior to the addition of neomycin, for 10 cells 10 mins after the onset of neomycin perfusion, for 10 cells 30 mins after the onset of washout and for 10 cells 30 mins after the onset of high Ca++ HBSS perfusion. Bars are the s.d.m. These measurements were made concurrently with those in Fig.2a.

indicate that both cell types have a similar sensitivity to neomycin. This effect of neomycin on stereocilia stiffness cannot therefore account directly for why OHCs are the first cells in the cochlea to be affected during aminoglycoside induced ototoxicity in vivo. The apparent differential sensitivity of OHCs to aminoglycoside ototoxicity may be a

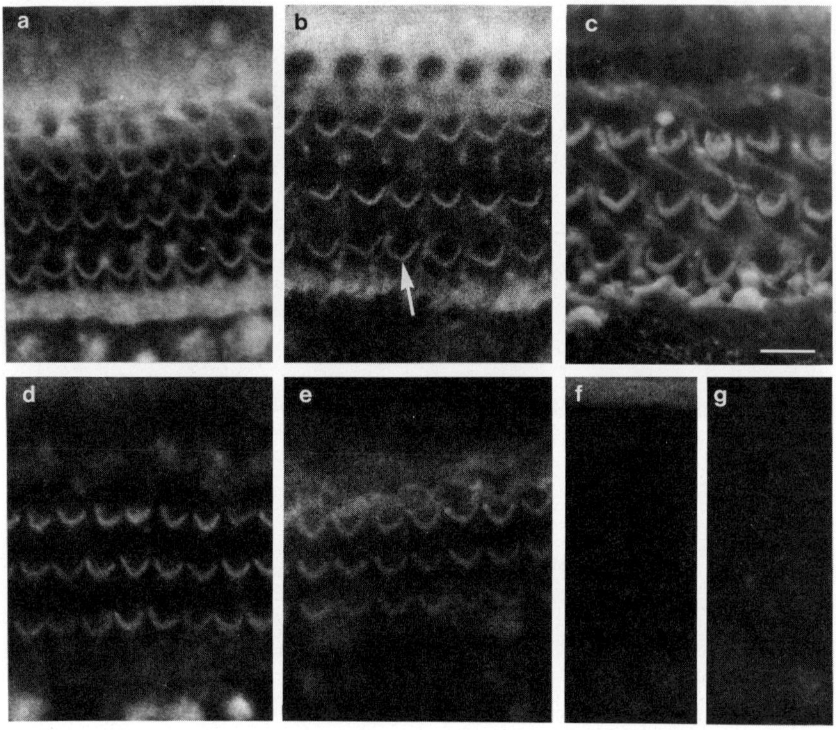

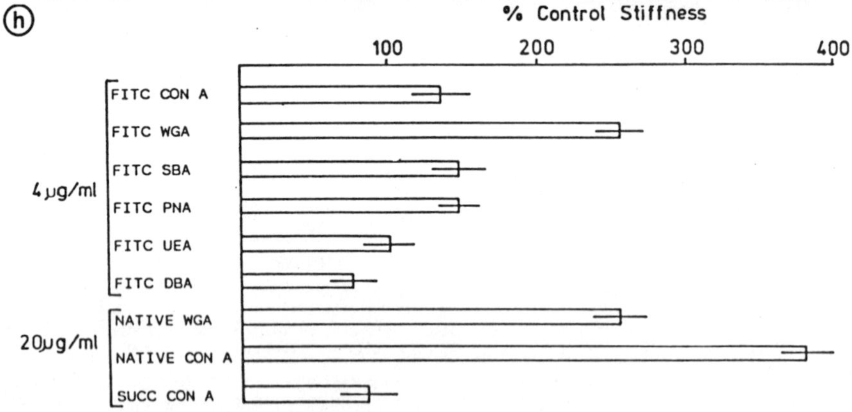

FIGURE 3. a-g) Three day old cultures stained with FITC-conjugated lectins. a) Con A, b) succinylated Con A, c) WGA, d) SBA, e) PNA, f) DBA, g) UEA I. Magnification = X 1280, bar = 10 µm. Arrow in b points to the stereocilia bundle of an outer hair cell in the outermost row. Inner hair cell stereocilia are partially obscured by the tectorial membrane and lie in a different plane of focus.

h) Effects of lectins on stereocilia stiffness. The forces generated by the stereocilia of 10 OHCs in response to a fixed 40nm displacement were measured in HBSS and then a lectin was added to the bathing solution. The forces generated in response to the same displacement were measured starting 10 minutes later for another sample of 10 cells in the same region of the culture over a period of 10 mins. Results are expressed as a percentage of the pre-exposure stiffness. Bars are the s.d.m. The FITC- conjugated lectins Con A, WGA, SBA and PNA all cause an increase in stereocilia stiffness. The lectins that do not bind to stereocilia, DBA and UEA I, and succinylated derivatives of Con A, do not cause an increase in stereocilia stiffness. FITC-conjugated lectins were tested at a concentration of 5µg/ml. Native forms of Con A, WGA and succinylated Con A were tested at a concentration of 20 µg/ml.

secondary effect related to, for example, either the metabolic activity of the OHCs or to their relationship with the tectorial membrane, another structure that may be affected by aminoglycosides.

The effects of Con A and neomycin are non-additive (Figs. 4 d & e). Sequential perfusion of cultures with HBSS containing Con A (5µg/ml, 50 nM) followed by HBSS and then by HBSS containing neomycin (50 µM) indicates that the subsequent addition of neomycin causes no further increase in stiffness over the initial increase caused by the lectin (Fig 4d). The reverse experiment, sequential perfusion with HBSS containing neomycin (50µM), followed by HBSS and then by HBSS containing Con A (5 µg/ml, 50 nM) indicates that neomycin prevents any subsequent effects of Con A (Fig. 4e), although similar concentrations of Con A would normally cause at least a 2- 3 fold increase in stiffness (Fig. 4c). Similar results have also been obtained with WGA. Succinylated Con A (25 µg/ml, 250 nM), which itself causes no increase in stiffness, prevents saturating concentrations of neomycin (50 µM) from causing any increase in stiffness (Fig. 4f), providing further evidence that lectins and aminoglycosides are interacting competitively for the same site.

Discussion

These results indicate that aminoglycoside antibiotics have two independent effects on early postnatal mammalian cochlear hair cells *in vitro*. One effect is to block transduction and this effect is reversible. The other effect is to cause an irreversible increase in stereocilia stiffness. An irreversible increase in stereocilia stiffness but of greater magnitude can also be caused by plant lectins, proteins that bind to carbohydrate residues and can agglutinate cells. The effects of lectins and aminoglycosides are non-additive. Native lectin from Canavalia ensiformis (Con A) can cause 2.5-4 fold increases in stereocilia stiffness but does not block transduction. Succinylated Con A, a modified form of Con A that retains binding but not agglutinating activity, does not increase stereocilia stiffness, suggesting that with lectins both binding and cross- linking are involved in causing increases in stereocilia stiffness.

A multistep hypothesis has been recently suggested to account for aminoglycoside induced ototoxicity (Schacht and Weiner 1986). In this model the first step is a reversible, Ca^{++} competitive, interaction of the drug with negatively charged components of the cell surface. This is followed by an energy dependent uptake of the drug and the subsequent, irreversible interference with a number of intracellular reactions, including inhibition of the phosphoinositide second messenger system. The results of this present study suggest that aminoglycosides may interact in two different ways with the hair cell surface.A previous study (Kroese and van den Bercken 1980, 1982) has described a dual action of aminoglycosides on lower vertebrate hair cells, a blockade of transduction and an increase in the phase lag of the response. However both of these effects were reversible and Ca^{++} competitive. The effect of neomycin that we have observed on stereocilia stiffness appears to be neither reversible nor Ca^{++} competitive and may contribute partially to the ototoxic effects that this drug is known to have *in vivo*.

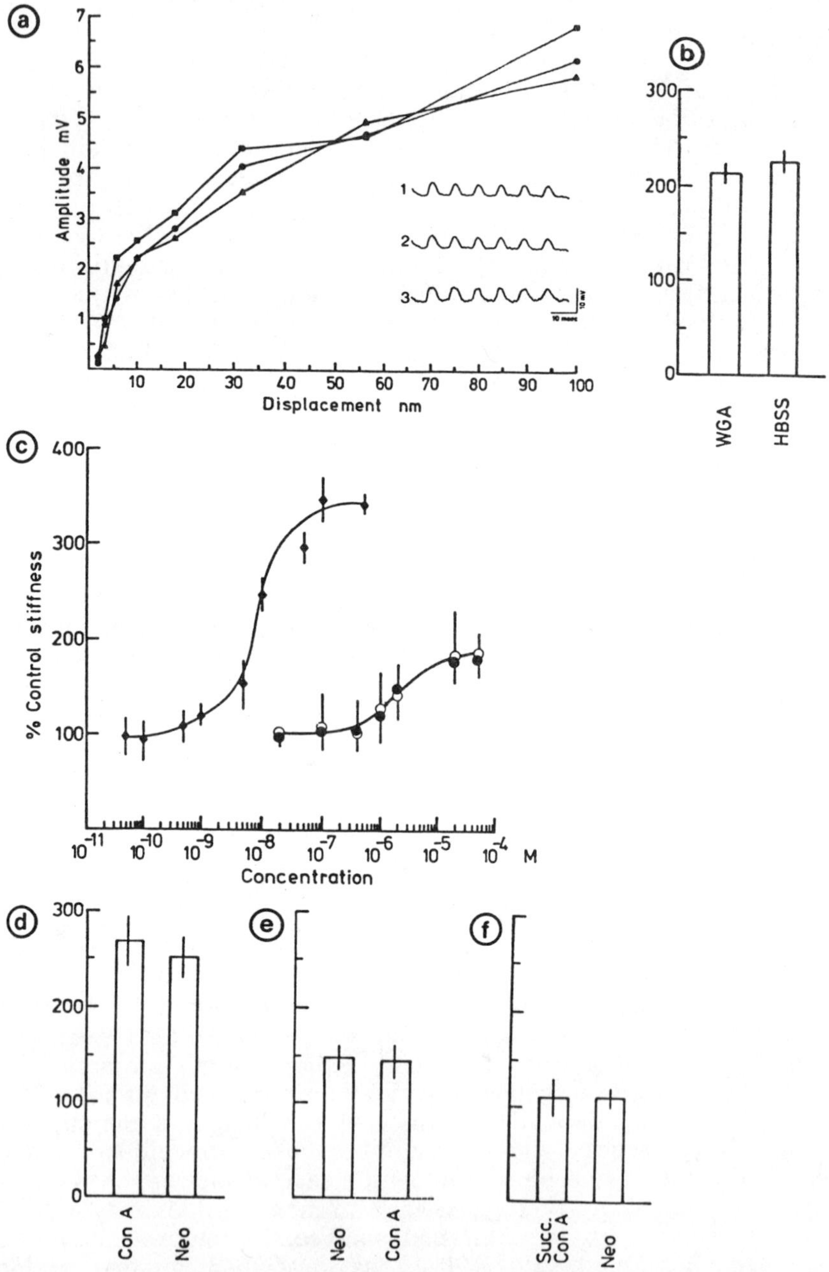

FIGURE 4. a) The relationship between the peak-to-peak amplitudes of receptor potentials recorded intracellularly from outer hair cells to sinusoidal peak-to-peak displacements of the stereocilia at 113 Hz in a cochlear culture which was successively perfused with HBSS (●), HBSS containing 4 µg/ml (100 nM) WGA (▲), and HBSS (■). Insets are the voltage responses of outer hair cells to 56nm displacements during perfusion with HBSS (1), HBSS containing WGA (2), and HBSS (3).

FIGURE 4.

b) The mean stiffness of outer hair cell stereocilia during perfusion with HBSS containing 4 µg/ml (100 nM) WGA and following subsequent washout with HBSS expressed as a percentage of pre-exposure stiffness. Bars = s.d.m., n = 10.

c) Dose response curves for the effects of Con A on outer hair cell stereocilia stiffness (closed diamonds) and neomycin on inner (filled circles) and outer (open circles) hair cell stereocilia stiffness. Half maximal stiffness increases are obtained with approximately 8 nM WGA and 2 uM neomycin. Concentrations of Con A and WGA have been calculated using molecular masses of 104 kDa and 36 kDa respectively. Bars = s.d.m., n = 10. d - f) The stiffness of outer hair cell stereocilia during perfusion of cultures with saturating concentrations of d) Con A (5 µg/ml, 50 nM) followed by neomycin (50 µM), e) neomycin (50 µM) followed by Con A (5 µg/ml, 50 nM) and f) succinylated Con A (25 µg/ml, 250 nM) followed by neomycin (50 µM) expressed as a percentage of the pre-exposure values for each experiment. Bar = s.d.m., n = 10.

Acknowledgements

We thank Elizabeth Cowley and Jim Hartly for excellent technical assistance and Ann Brown and Alan Cody for their comments on the manuscript. The work was supported by a grant from the MRC.

References

Brown, R.D. and Feldman, A.M. (1978) Pharmacology of hearing and ototoxicity. Ann. Rev. Pharmacol. Toxicol. 18, 233-252.

Crawford, C.F. and Fettiplace, R.J. (1985) The mechanical properties of ciliary bundles of turtle cochlear hair cells. J. Physiol. 364, 359-380.

Harpur, E.S. (1987) The pathophysiology of hearing. Brit. Med. Bulletin 43, 871-886.

Hawkins, J.E. (1976) Drug ototoxicity. In: Handbook of Sensory Physiology (Eds Keidel, S.D. and Neff, W.D.) Springer-Verlag, New York. pp. 707-748.

Howard, J. and Ashmore, J.A. (1986) Stiffness of sensory bundles in the sacculus of the frog. Hearing Res. 22, 93- 104.

Hudspeth, A.J. and Kroese, A.B.A. (1983) Voltage-dependent interaction of dihydrostreptomycin with the transduction channels in bullfrog sensory hair cells. J. Physiol., Lond. 345, 66P.

Kroese, A.B.A. and van den Bercken, J. (1980) Dual action of ototoxic antibiotics on sensory hair cells. Nature 283, 395-397.

Kroese, A.B.A. and van den Bercken, J. (1982) Effects of ototoxic antibiotics on sensory hair cell functioning. Hearing Res. 6, 183-197.

Russell, I.J., Richardson, G.P. and Cody, A.R. (1986) Mechanosensitivity of mammalian auditory cells in vitro. Nature 321, 517-519.

Russell, I.J. and Richardson, G.P. (1987) The Morphology and physiology of hair cells in organotypic cultures of the mouse cochlea. Hearing Res. 31, 9-24.

Rybak, L.P. (1986) Ototoxic mechanisms. In: Neurobiology of Hearing: The Cochlea. (Eds. Altschuler, R.A., Hoffman, D.W. & Bobbin, R.P.) Raven Press, New York, pp. 441-454.

Schacht, J. (1979) Isolation of an aminoglycoside receptor from guinea pig inner ear tissues and kidney. Arch Otorhinolaryngol. 224, 129-134.

Schacht, J. and Weiner, N. (1986) Aminoglycoside-induced hearing loss: A molecular hypothesis. Otorhinolaryngol. 48, 116-123.

MECHANICAL ANALYSIS OF HAIR CELL MICROSTRUCTURE AND MOTILITY

C.R. Steele and D. H. Jen*

Division of Applied Mechanics, Durand Building
Stanford University, Stanford CA 94305, USA
**General Products Division*
IBM, San Jose CA , USA

Introduction

In the past few years, a number of important discoveries have been made which deal with the microstructure of the cochlea and the possible relation with the active process in the normal function. The purpose of this paper is to summarize some considerations on the mechanical interpretation of these discoveries. Specifically, the implications of the tip and lateral fibers connecting the cilia on the inner and outer hair cells, and the motility of the outer hair cells is treated.

Stiffness of Components

Progress has been made on relating various measurements to the basic elastic properties of the tissue.

BASILAR MEMBRANE

Miller (1985) measured the static stiffness of the basilar membrane in guinea pig under a point load. From the fiber dimensions, the elastic modulus was computed to be E = 1.78 GPa, which is reasonably close to the value of keratin of E = 4 GPa given by Wainwright, *et al.* (1976). It is of interest that Raftenberg (1985), not aware of Miller's work, concluded from alternate sources that the basilar membrane fibers were in the keratin class of protein with a value E = 1.6 GPa. With this value established, it is possible to compute the significant part of the cochlear partition volume compliance if the anatomy is known, *i.e.*, the number and size of the transverse fibers of the basilar membrane, which is, perhaps, more easily obtained than direct stiffness measurements.

HAIR CELL CILIA

We have formulated a mechanical model for the cilia and the connecting upward tip fibers and the connecting lateral fibers. The conclusion is that the behavior suggested by Pickles, *et al.* (1984) and described by Flock and Strelioff (1986) is remarkably consistent with this model. Raftenberg (1985), from measurements of Yoshina and co-workers, computed the elastic modulus of F-actin filaments to be

$$\begin{aligned} E &= 30 \text{ MPa} \quad \text{without} \quad Ca^{+2} \\ &= 50 \text{ MPa} \quad \text{with} \quad Ca^{+2} \end{aligned}$$

The stiffness for a cilium with a load F and displacement d at the tip and clamped at the cuticular plate may be computed from the geometry and the assumption that E is constant everywhere in the cilium. On the point 10 mm from the stapes in the guinea pig, we take the length to be 4.5 μm, the diameter to be 0.3, and the tapered root region to have the length 0.3 and minimum diameter of 0.1 μm. The result for the stiffness, using the value of E without Ca is

$$\begin{aligned} F/d &= 0.15 \times 10^{-3} \text{ N/m} \quad \text{(cilium without lateral or tip fiber)} \\ &= 2.3 \times 10^{-3} \text{ N/m} \quad \text{(bundle of 15 cilia)} \end{aligned}$$

The measurements of Flock and Strelioff (1986) and Strelioff and Flock (1986) at this point for a group of fibers, 7-12 in the tall row but possibly three times that number because of the tip and lateral connections, are

$$F/d = 2 - 10 \times 10^{-3} \text{ N/m} \quad \text{(measurement, bundle of 7 - 21 cilia)}$$

which must be considered as remarkable agreement. Of interest is that the stiffness can be increased by 70% by the presence of the calcium ions.

Pickles, *et al.* (1984), suggest that the tip fibers will be in tension for a displacement of the tips of the long cilia in the excitory direction and will buckle for displacement in the opposite direction. In our calculation of this, the diameter of tip fibers found by TEM by Furness, *et al.* (1986), of 2-3 nm with a length of 300 nm was used. The conclusion is that buckling can occur at a very small tip displacement :

$$d_{cr} = 0.03 \text{ nm} \times (E_f / E_r) \qquad \text{(onset of tip fiber buckling)}$$

where E_f and E_r are the elastic moduli of the tip fiber and the ciliary root region, respectively. Thus if the fiber modulus is of the same order of magnitude or less than that of the cilia, then a very significant mechanical nonlinearity occurs at threshold levels. The displacement amplitude in the measurements of Flock and Strelioff was 1μm, greatly in excess of that required for the tip fiber buckling. Thus their result that the stiffness for displacement in the excitatory direction is higher than that in the opposite direction (by the ratio of 1.85 for IHC, 2.45 for OHC) is easily explained. In the first case the load is transferred to all three rows, while in the second case, the tip fibers buckle and only the tall row carries the load, which gives a factor of three difference. However some load is transferred by the lateral connecting fibers. From the geometry supplied by Furness and Hackney (1985) and Furness, *et al.* (1986), and the observation of Flock and Strelioff (1986) that the lateral connecting material causes a displacement of 2-4 of the tall cilia on each side of the probe, the modulus of the lateral fibers is computed to have the low value:

$$E = 60 \times 10^3 \text{ Pa}$$

Because of the hexagonal arrangement of the lateral fibers, a high modulus material is not required.

A consequence of the mechanical model is that the dependence on size of the forces can be computed. Table 1 shows results for the force acting between the tip fibers of the second and third rows of cilia. The proportions of the IHC are such that the fiber forces are noticeable larger than for the OHC at the base, middle and apex of the cochlea. This may well be related to the observation of Pickles, *et al.* (1987) that the first acoustic trauma occurs in the IHC tip fiber, separating the tallest row. The computation indicates that greater forces occur in the fibers between the second and third rows, however, the actual arrangement in this region is apparently not as regular as we have assumed in the model.

The conclusion is that the behavior suggested by Pickles, *et al.* (1984), correlated with the measurements of Flock and Strelioff (1986), holds up well under scrutiny by mechanical analysis. We now have the long-sought, strong mechanical nonlinearity at threshold levels, a means for chemical mediation of stiffness, and the first explanation for the site of acoustic trauma. This fits well with the model for hair cell transduction of Holmes and Bell (1985).

TABLE 1 Relative forces in tip fibers: F2, between cilia of the tallest and second row; F3, between cilia of the second and third rows. The lengths of the three rows L1, L2, L3 are for the chinchilla, scaled from the drawings of Lim (1980). The highest force occurs between the IHC cilia. Pickles, *et al.* (1987) report this to be the first region of acoustic trauma.

Location		L1	L2	L3	F2	F3
Base	IHC	2.5	1.2	0.4	1.39	2.0
	OHC1	1.5	1.2	0.8	0.83	0.63
	OHC2	1.7	1.1	1.0	1.0	0.57
	OHC3	1.8	1.5	1.0	0.8	0.6
Middle	IHC	3.2	1.4	0.4	1.52	2.67
	OHC1	2.0	1.5	0.9	0.89	0.74
	OHC2	3.9	2.1	1.8	1.24	0.72
	OHC3	5.2	2.8	2.1	1.24	0.83
Apex	IHC	4.7	1.8	1.0	1.74	1.57
	OHC1	3.2	2.3	1.3	0.93	0.82
	OHC2	4.8	2.6	1.7	1.23	0.94
	OHC3	5.8	3.0	1.3	1.29	1.49

CONNECT-DISCONNECT EXCITATION

Crane (1982) and in a recent, more comprehensive manuscript, considers the generation of difference and combination tones, which have many features which are inconsistent with any generating mechanism involving a polynomial nonlinearity. He shows that a connect-disconnect mechanism does produce the proper behavior of the known combination tones, as well as many others. Impact of the IHC cilia against the tectorial membrane is suggested for the actual physical source of the connect-disconnect activity. However, preliminary calculation of the interaction of the cilia and the fluid of the sub-tectorial membrane region indicates that the behavior at threshold levels will not have a sufficiently sharp impact, but will be linear. In contrast, the tip fiber on the cilia, according to our calculations, will undergo buckling at threshold levels of displacement and appears to provide exactly the connect-disconnect excitation needed. From a comparison with neural measurements, Crane finds that the mechanism should have a decay time of about 1.5 ms. Our first calculation of the response time of a cilium, based upon the root stiffness and the flow of fluid around the cilium was 1.3 ms. Subsequent analysis shows this to be, in fact, rather sensitive to the assumptions on the passages for the fluid flow between the cilia. Nevertheless, the decay time for the cilia is of the correct order of magnitude.

Cell Motility

The likely source of the direct feedback mechanism is the electrically induced displacement of the outer hair cells, which is found in the experiments of Brownell and Kacher (1985), Ashmore (1987), Ashmore and Brownell (1986), Holley and Ashmore (1988), and Zenner, *et al.* (1987). The process in the cell remains unknown. Nevertheless, some conclusions can be reached on the basis of the available experimental results.

ELECTROPHORESIS

Following the suggestion by Brownell, we have developed hair cell models in which the mechanical aspects are straightforward. The cell wall is assumed to be a homogeneous, isotropic material, and the intracellular and extracellular spaces are filled with viscous fluids. The interaction with the electrical field is considered to be due to either (1) charged particles in the intracellular fluid, or (2) charged particles imbedded in the cell wall. The calculations for the charged particles in the fluid yields interesting flow of the fluid but a rather weak distortion of the cell wall. In contrast the charged particles fixed to the wall yield good results. As reported by Jen and Steele (1987), "reasonable" values of the parameters yield a model response similar to that reported by Brownell and Karcher (1985) at 5 Hz.

A specific concern was whether or not the fluid viscosity would absorb the energy at high frequency. The "reasonable" parameters indicate this to occur for frequencies above 20 kHz. Subsequent measurements of Ashmore and Brownell (1986) of motility at 8 kHz, and Zenner (1987) at 1 kHz confirm that the effect is not restricted to low frequency. Ashmore (1987) provides a curve of cell elongation as a function of frequency which is similar to that calculated by Jen and Steele (1987), except that the rolloff occurs at a lower frequency. The details of the model and the experiment, however, do not agree at all. Charged particles in the wall under a uniform external electric field have a uniform axial body force which causes a parabolic variation in the axial displacement. Holly and Ashmore (1988) show a linear distribution of displacement due to an intracellular potential change.

CELL WALL ORTHOTROPY

The observation by Ashmore (1987) that the outer hair cell contracts in the axial direction due to internal pressure means that the cell cannot be of isotropic construction, as assumed by Jen and Steele (1987). Furthermore, an isotropic shell with a single layer of charged particles in the lateral wall will undergo a volume contraction or expansion due to intercellular potential change. If the shell is filled with an incompressible fluid, the total volume must be unchanged. This necessitates a pressure change in the fluid. Holley and Ashmore (1988) report no change in pressure during electrical stimulation of the OHC. The conclusion is that the cell wall is not isotropic.

Adding axial or circumferential stiffeners to the shell wall does not produce axial contraction with internal pressure. However, a wall construction consisting of fibers at an angle with the axis has such a behavior. As shown in Figure 1, for fiber angles less than about 55 degrees, the shell with internal pressure will undergo an increase in diameter and a decrease in the axial length.

Does the OHC wall have stiffness in preferred directions? The observations of Holley and Ashmore (1988, Figure 10) certainly indicate that a dominant stiffness of the wall is supplied by the lateral cisternae. The drawing of the outer hair cell by Lim (1986) shows the fenestrated cisternae. With a little imagination, it is possible to see that there may be a pattern to the shape and orientation of the perforations, which leaves bands of unperforated material making an angle of around 45 degrees with the axis. So it appears possible that the lateral cisternae could have a stiffness similar to a fiber reinforced composite. Flock, *et al.* (1986) find short pillars connecting the cisternae to the plasma membrane, which supports the notion that the composite wall, consisting of the cell membrane, the subplasma membrane, and the cisternae, has significant stiffness along with some special function.

The special function is to convert the electrical field into a mechanical force. A single layer of charged particles will cause a force on the wall which is radial for an intercellular potential change. In Figure 2, the effect of such a radial force is shown. The diameter and axial expansions are of opposite sign for all fiber angles. Of interest is that the volume expansion is zero for the angle of 55 degrees.

Another possibility mentioned by Terakawa (1985) is that the cell wall has an electrostrictive behavior. This could be represented by a bilayer of charge. A voltage gradient would cause a stress in the wall tending to expand or contract the wall thickness. The resulting mechanical behavior is shown in Figure 3. The measurements of Terakawa (1985) on the squid giant axon indicate that both the diameter and volume expand with depolarization.

The conclusion is that the cell wall has stiffness equivalent to a fiber reinforced shell. Either the single layer of charge or a bilayer could be consistent with the experiments on the squid axon and the outer hair cell for certain fiber angles. These angles may be consistent with the pattern of perforations in the lateral cisternae of the hair cell.

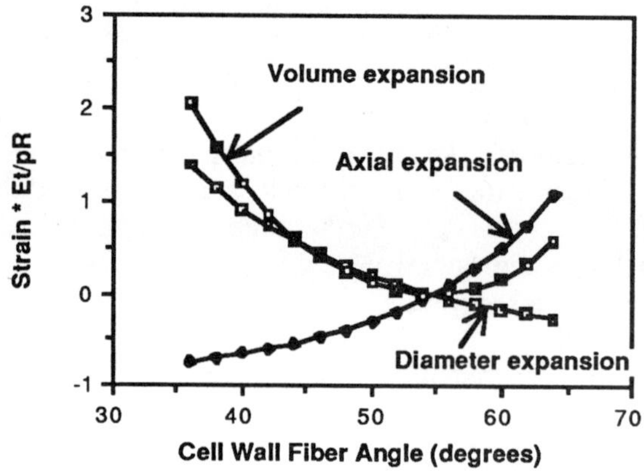

FIGURE 1 Behavior of an orthotropic cylindrical shell with internal pressure. When the cell wall fiber angle is less than about 55 degrees, the diameter increases while the axial length decreases, as observed by Ashmore (1987) in the OHC.

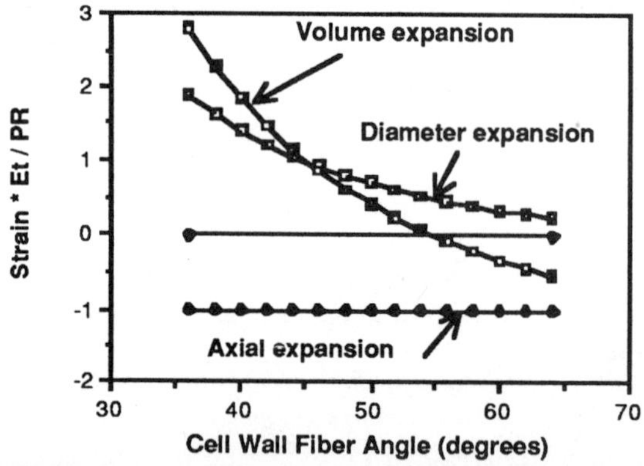

FIGURE 2 Behavior of an orthotropic cylindrical shell with a radial force on the lateral wall, which could simulate the behavior of charged particles in the wall with an intercellular potential. For wall fiber angles less than 55 degrees, both the diameter and the volume expand, as in the squid giant axon under electrical stimulation measured by Terakawa (1985). For the shell filled with an incompressible fluid, a pressure must be added to preserve volume. However, at 55 degrees the diameter increases, the length decreases, while the total volume change is zero, which means that the pressure is zero. This is similar to the response measured by Ashmore (1987) in the OHC under electrical stimulation.

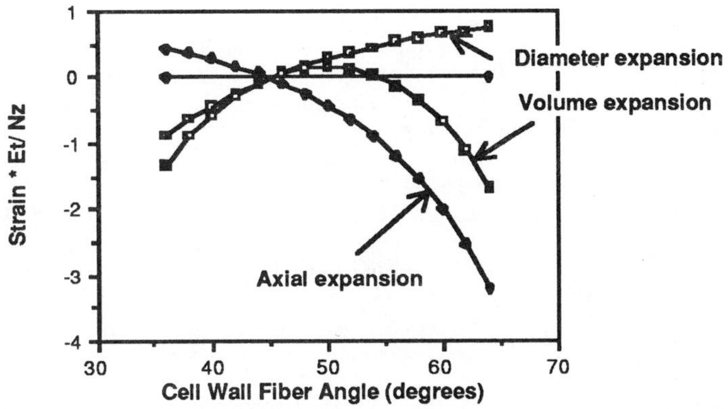

FIGURE 3 Behavior of an orthotropic cylindrical shell with the wall thickness expanded by the stress Nz, which could simulate the effect of electrostriction. For wall fiber angles between 45 and 55 degrees, both the diameter and the volume expand. At 55 degrees the diameter increases, the length decreases, while the total volume change is zero, which means that the pressure is zero.

Acknowledgment

This work was supported by Grant 2R01-NS12086 from the National Institute of Neurological and Communicational Disorders and strokes.

References

Ashmore, J.F. (1987) A fast motile response in guinea-pig outer hair cells: the cellular basis of the cochlear amplifier. J. Physiol., 388, 323-347.

Ashmore, J.F., and Brownell, W.E. (1986) Kilohertz movements induced by electrical stimulation in outer hair cells isolated from the guinea pig cochlea. J. Physiol., P41.

Brownell, W.E., and Kacher, B. (1985) Outer hair cell motility: a possible electrokinetic mechanism. In: Peripheral Auditory Mechanisms (Eds: Allen, J.B., Hubbard, A.E., Neely, S.T. and Tubis, A.) Springer, Berlin, pp. 369-376.

Crane, H.D. (1982) IHC-TM connect-disconnect and efferent control V. J. Acoust. Soc. Am. 72, 93-101.

Flock, Å, Flock, B., and Ulfendahl, M. (1986) Mechanisms of movement in outer hair cells and a possible structural basis. Arch. Oto-Rhino-Laryngol., 242, 83-90.

Flock, A. (1986) Mechanical properties of hair cells. Hearing Research 22, 80.

Flock, A. and Strelioff, D. (1986) Studies on hair cells in isolated coils from the guinea pig cochlea. Hearing Research 15, 11-18.

Furness, D.N., and Hackney, C.M. (1985) Cross-links between stereocilia in the guinea pig cochlea. Hearing Research 18, 177-188.

Furness, D.N., Hackney, C.M., and Evans, E.F. (1986) The ultrastructure of stereociliary cross-links. Hearing Research 22, 79.

Holley, M.C., and Ashmore, J.F., (1988) On the mechanism of a high-frequency force generator in outer hair cells isolated from the guinea pig cochlea. Proc. R. Soc. Lond. B 232, 413-429.

Holmes, M.H., and Bell, J. (1985) A model for transduction in hair cells involving strain-activated conductance. In: Peripheral Auditory Mechanisms (Eds: Allen, J.B., Hubbard, A.E., Neely, S.T. and Tubis, A.) Springer, Berlin, pp. 385-393.

Jen, D.H., and Steele, C. R. (1987) Electrokinetic model of cochlear hair cell motility. J. Acoust. Soc. Am. 82, 1667-1678.

Lim, D.J. (1980) Cochlear anatomy related to cochlear micromechanics. A review. J. Acoust. Soc. Am. 67, 1686-1695.

Lim, D.J. (1986) Functional structure of the organ of Corti: a review. Hearing Research 22, 117-146.

Miller, C.E. (1985) Structural implications of basilar membrane compliance measurements. J. Acoust. Soc. Am. 77, 1465-1474.

Pickles, J.O., Comis, S.D., and Osborne, M.P. (1984) Cross-links between stereocilia in the guinea pig organ of Corti, and their possible relation to sensory transduction. Hearing Research 15, 103-112.

Pickles, J.O., Osborne, M.P., and Comis, S.D. (1987) Vulnerability of tip links between stereocilia to acoustic trauma in the guinea pig. Hearing Research 25, 173-183.

Raftenberg, M.N. (1985) A model for cochlear micromechanics. Ph.D. Thesis, Johns Hopkins University.

Strelioff, D. and Flock, A. (1986) Stiffness of sensory-cell hair bundles in the isolated guinea pig cochlea. Hearing Research 15, 19-28.

Terakawa, S., (1985) Potential-dependent variations of the intracellular pressure in the intracellularly perfused squid giant axon. J.Physiol., Lond. 369, 229-248.

Wainwright, S.A., Biggs, W.D., Currey, J.D., and Gosline, J.M. (1976) Mechanical Designs in Organisms (John Wiley, New York).

Zenner, H.P., Zimmermann, U., and Gitter, A.H., (1987) Fast motility of isolated auditory sensory cells. Biochem. and Biophysic. Res. Comm. 149, 304-308.

Comments and Discussion

PICKLES

1. Transducer channels are about 20 - 30% open at rest, and if tip links are indeed involved in transduction (Pickles et al., 1984, and this volume), there should be a resting tension on the links. So it should be possible to produce small deflections in the inhibitory direction without any buckling of the links. This would be in accordance with the relatively constant stiffness measurements of Howard and Ashmore (1986), obtained for small deflections in the excitatory and inhibitory directions. However, I agree that there could be an asymmetry for larger deflections.

2. I think it is very dangerous to measure the geometry of hair bundles from electron micrographs prepared by standard techniques. Bundles are subject to substantial distortion, such as separation of the rows, and stretch or compression of the links, during the preparation process. I suggest therefore that the figures in Table 1 of the paper should be viewed with caution. Possibly the only way the correct information on geometry could be obtained is from high-resolution images obtained by Nomarski light microscopy, in living hair cells known to be in good physiological condition. However, the resolution would be inadequate for the level of detail required for the calculations.

Howard, J. and Ashmore, J.F. (1986) Stiffness of sensory hair bundles in the sacculus of the frog. Hearing Res. 23, 93-104.

A MODEL FOR BIDIRECTIONAL TRANSDUCTION IN OUTER HAIR CELLS

S. T. Neely

Boys Town National Institute
555 North 30th Street
Omaha, Nebraska 68131, USA

Introduction

There is considerable evidence for the existence of a cochlear amplifier which serves to increase the sensitivity and frequency selectivity of the cochlea to low intensity sounds (Davis, 1983). Earlier models of traveling-wave amplification in the cochlea used negative damping components to supply the additional energy used to power the cochlear amplifier (Kim, *et al.*, 1980; de Boer, 1983; Koshigoe and Tubis, 1983). The negative damping models are now being replaced by more realistic feedback force models in which the fast motile response of the outer hair cell is implicated as the driving force for the cochlear amplifier (Geisler, 1986; Zwicker, 1986; Neely and Kim, 1987).

Outer Hair Cell Motility

Cochlear outer hair cells (OHC) vary the length of their cell body in response to electrical stimulation (Brownell *et al.*, 1985). The motile property of OHCs is apparently linked to the presence of laminated cisternae adjacent to the plasma membrane. Because the OHCs are securely attached to Dieter's cells at their base and to the reticular lamina at their apex, a change in OHC length will change the separation between the reticular lamina and the basilar membrane (Brownell and Kachar, 1986).

In vitro studies of guinea pig OHCs indicate that length change is graded over a range of 1-2 μm (approximately 4% of the length) with a sensitivity of about 20 nm/mV of membrane polarization (Ashmore, 1987). Hyperpolarizing currents cause the cell to elongate and depolarizing currents cause the cell to contract. Although the sensitivity of the motile response decreases with frequency of sinusoidal electrical stimulation, length change has been observed at frequencies as high as 30 kHz (Gitter and Zenner, 1988).

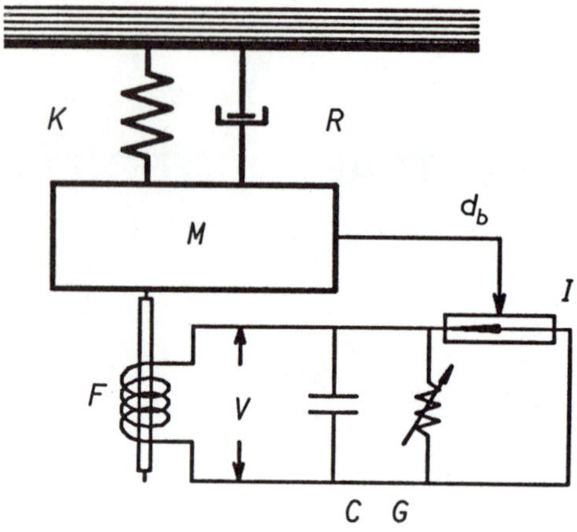

FIGURE 1 Schematic diagram of a model for an oscillating outer hair cell. The electrical components and transducers represent the motile outer hair cell and the mechanical components represent an isolated point on the basilar membrane. The transducer current I is assumed to be proportional to basilar membrane displacement d_b and the motile force F proportional to membrane potential V. The model is nonlinear since the transducer current saturates for large displacements.

It is becoming increasingly clear that bidirectional transduction in OHCs involves separate and distinct transducers for *mechanical-to-electrical* and *electrical-to-mechanical* transduction. The site of *mechanical-to-electrical* transduction is at the hair bundle (HB) at the apex of the cell where electrical current entering the cell (possibly through the tips of the stereocilia) is modulated by displacement of the HB (Hudspeth and Corey, 1977). The mechanical-to-electrical transducer is essentially the same for inner hair cells (IHC) as it is for OHCs. (One difference between IHCs and OHCs, however, is that the tips of the stereocilia are imbedded in the tectorial membrane for OHCs and not for IHCs.)

The site of *electrical-to-mechanical* transduction is at the plasma membrane of the OHC along the sides of the cell body (Ashmore, 1987). This motile response is not due to actin-myosin interaction (since it occurs in the absence of ATP) and is most likely driven by transmembrane voltage along the sides of the OHC (Ashmore, 1988). It is possible that the elongation of the OHC is due to constrictive forces along the sides of the cell with no net change in cell volume.

Oscillating Outer Hair Cell

Spontaneous otoacoustic emissions (SOAE) are low intensity narrow-band sounds which are present in about 25% of normal human ears. They are thought to be the result of continuous oscillations within the cochlea driven by one or more motile OHCs.

Fig. 1 shows a diagram of a simple model of an OHC coupled to an isolated place on the basilar membrane (BM). The mass, spring, and dashpot (M, K, and R) represent the mechanical properties of the cochlear partition. The current source I is controlled by displacement of the BM and represents mechanical-to-electrical transduction at the OHC. The capacitor and resistor (C and G) represent the electrical properties of the OHC membrane. Finally, the forcing function F acting on the mass of the BM represents electrical-to-mechanical transduction. This motile force is modeled as being proportional to the transmembrane voltage V.

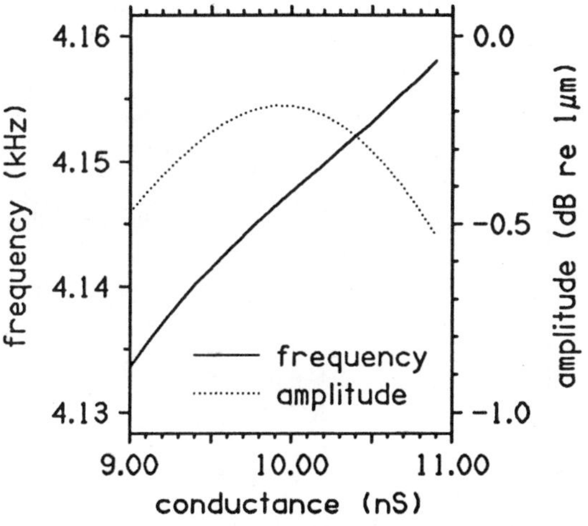

FIGURE 2 Amplitude and frequency of oscillation in the OHC model as a function of membrane conductance G. The curves indicate the results from numerical solution of eqs. (1) and (2) with the following parameter values:
K = 62.5 dyn/cm
R = 2.5 dyn·s/cm
M = 0.1 gm
G = 9-11 nS
C = 5 pF
I_o = 1 nA
d_o = 1 μm
α = -10 dyn/V
These parameter values provide a mechanical resonance of 3.98 kHz and an electrical time constant of 0.5 ms.

If the d_b, v_b, and a_b represent the displacement, velocity and acceleration of the basilar membrane, then the equations of motion can be written as

$$F = \alpha V = Ma_b + Rv_b + Kd_b \tag{1}$$

$$I = I_o \tanh(d_b/d_o) = C\,dV/dt + GV \tag{2}$$

where α, I_o, and d_o are transduction parameters. The mechanical-to-electrical transduction in eq. (2) is nearly linear for small displacements and saturates for large displacements (Hudspeth and Corey, 1977). The electrical-to-mechanical transduction in eq. (1) is modeled as a linear process, but has been observed to saturate for larger signals in a manner similar to the mechanical-to-electrical transduction (Ashmore, 1987).

If appropriate values are chosen for the parameters (see Fig. 2 caption), the OHC model becomes an oscillator. Numerical solutions to the equations show nearly sinusoidal oscillations with displacement amplitudes determined by the saturating nonlinearity of the mechanical-to-electrical transducer. The frequency of oscillation is determined primarily by the mechanical components and is slightly above the natural resonant frequency = $(K/M)^{1/2}$. Thus, the model suggests that SOAEs do not require the OHC to possess any intrinsic tuning (beyond the low-pass response of the cell membrane) as long as the electrical energy available to the OHC is bidirectionally coupled to the BM.

Another interesting observation with this oscillating OHC model is the effect of efferent stimulation on the frequency of oscillation. Efferent synapses at the base of the outer hair cells are thought to enhance the membrane conductance to ions when activated (Desmedt and Robertson, 1975). Fig. 2 shows that when the conductance in the OHC model is increased, the frequency of oscillation increases and the amplitude does not change significantly.

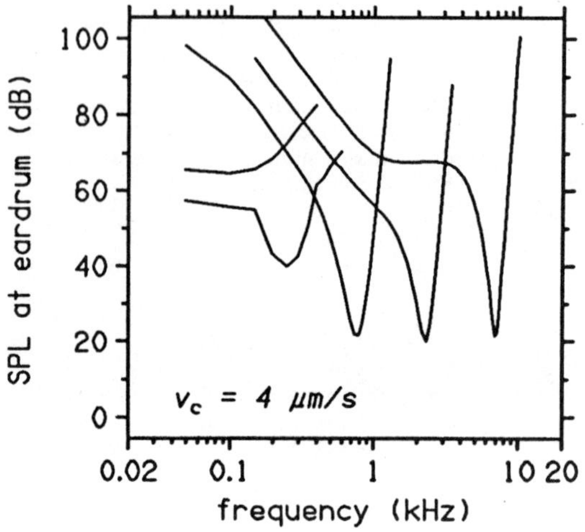

FIGURE 3 Isovelocity tuning curves for the active cochlear model without the transduction nonlinearity. The curves represent the sound pressure at the eardrum necessary to produce v_c = 4 μm/s in the model at 5 places along the cochlear partition. The frequency to place map is similar to that of a human cochlea. The following model parameter values (cgs units) were used:

$K_b = 4\cdot10^8\ e^{-3x}$
$R_b = 960\ e^{-1.4x}$
$M_b = 0.004$
$K_t = 2\cdot10^8\ e^{-3.2x}$
$R_t = 2000\ e^{-1.4x}$
$M_t = 0.037$
$K_c = 2.25\cdot10^8\ e^{-3.2x}$
$R_c = 0$
$K_a = 4.5\cdot10^8\ e^{-3.1x}$

The frequency of the SOAE has been observed to increase in human subjects when an external tone one-half octave lower in frequency than the SOAE is presented to the opposite ear (Mott *et al.*, 1988). The contralateral acoustic stimulation is thought to stimulate efferents to the OHCs via the uncrossed olivocochlear bundle (Warr and Guinan, 1979).

Active Nonlinear Cochlear Model

In this section, a representation of outer hair cell motility similar to the one presented in the previous section, will be used as the active element in a complete model of cochlear mechanics.

As before, let d_b, v_b, and a_b represent the displacement, velocity and acceleration of the basilar membrane (BM) perpendicular to its resting plane. Let d_t, v_t, and a_t represent the radial displacement, velocity and acceleration of the tectorial membrane (TM). The relevant stimulus to the HBs of the IHC and OHC will be $d_c = gd_b - d_t$ and $v_c = gv_b - v_t$, where g is the lever ratio which describes the radial motion of the reticular lamina (RL) due to basilar membrane displacement.

Let P_d be the fluid pressure difference across the BM and let P_a represent the additional force on the basilar membrane due to OHC motility (the active element). The equations of motion can be written as

$$M_b a_b + R_b v_b + K_b d_b + (R_c v_c + K_c d_c)/g = P_d - P_a \qquad (3)$$

$$M_t a_t + R_t v_t + K_t d_t - R_c v_c - K_c d_c = 0 \qquad (4)$$

The active pressure P_a is controlled by d_c in the following way:

$$P_a = -K_a d_c\ , \text{ for } d_c > 0$$
$$= 0\ , \quad \text{for } d_c < 0 \qquad (5)$$

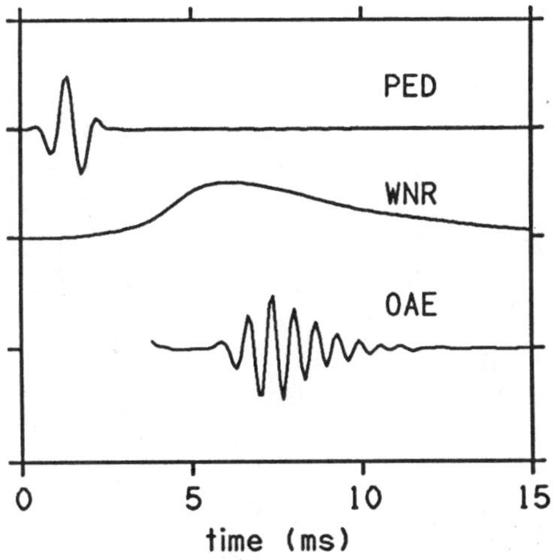

FIGURE 4 Transient response of the active, nonlinear cochlear model to a 1 kHz tone-burst stimulus. The model parameter values were the same as in Fig. 3. PED is the pressure at the eardrum showing the tone-burst stimulus. WNR is a measure of whole-nerve response computed by summing a rectified, low-pass filtered version of ν_c over the entire length of the cochlear partition. OAE is the same as PED except magnified to show the presence of an evoked otoacoustic emission.

The active element represented by eq. (5) is equivalent to the OHC model of the previous section except that the hyperbolic tangent is replaced by a rectifier function and the membrane capacitance is neglected. In terms of previous parameters, if $C = 0$, then $K_a = \alpha I_o/(d_o G)$. Any delay in the motile response (Ashmore, 1987) is also neglected in this model.

There are only two mechanical degrees of freedom represented by eqs. (3) and (4). Since the OHC are oriented perpendicular to the radial displacement of the TM, the active force P_a is applied only to the BM in eq. (3).

Isovelocity tuning curves for a linearized version of the model are shown in Fig. 3 to demonstrate the amount of sharpening and increased sensitivity provided by the active elements. The shape of these tuning curves is similar to that of neural tuning curves in a cat (e.g., Kiang and Moxon, 1972).

The response of the model (with the nonlinearity) to a 1 kHz tone-burst is shown in Fig 4. Because of the nonlinearity, the latency of the whole nerve response (WNR), shown in the second trace in Fig 4, varies with intensity in a manner similar to the variation observed in human auditory brainstem responses (Neely, 1988). The evoked otoacoustic emission (EOAE), shown in the third trace in Fig 4, is not present in the linear version of the model.

Discussion

Recent studies of OHC motility suggest that the OHC is capable of playing the role of the cochlear amplifier. The model of an oscillating OHC described above fits well with both the observations of SOAEs and the properties of OHCs. The dependence of the force F on membrane potential introduces a -90° phase shift (lag) at high frequencies relative to displacement d_b due to the membrane capacitance C. This makes the feedback force the equivalent of a *negative-damping* force.

In the complete (active, nonlinear) cochlear model, the fact that the nonlinearity facilitates the generation of the EOAE and makes the WNR dependent on stimulus intensity is encouraging. However, the fact that the membrane capacitance of the OHC was neglected to produce these results is contrary to the oscillating OHC model. If membrane capacitance were included (without altering the remainder of the model) then the effect of the active elements is substantially reduced for all but the lowest frequencies. It may be that the motile mechanism in the OHC is more sensitive to transducer current than membrane potential at high frequencies (Ashmore, 1987).

In the cochlear model the -90° phase shift is provided by the TM-HB resonance at $((K_t+K_c)/M_t)^{1/2}$ and, therefore, restricted to a narrow range of frequencies. Below this frequency the active force will add stiffness to the BM and above this frequency it will remove stiffness from the BM. The tuning of the *negative-damping* force in the cochlear model creates the separation between the *tip* and *tail* of the tuning curve.

References

Allen, J.B. (1980). Cochlear micromechanics -- A physical model of transduction. J. Acoust. Soc. Am. 68, 1660-1679.

Ashmore, J.F. (1987). A fast motile response in guinea-pig outer hair cells: The cellular basis of the cochlear amplifier. J. Physiol. 388, 323-347.

Ashmore, J.F. (1988). What is the stimulus for outer hair cell motility? In: Basic Issues in Hearing (Eds: Duifhuis, H., Hoorst, J.W., and Wit H.P.), Academic Press, London.

de Boer, E. (1983). No Sharpening? A challenge for cochlear mechanics. J. Acoust. Soc. Am. 73, 567-573.

Desmedt, J.E. and Robertson, D. (1975). Ionic mechanism of the efferent olivo-cochlear inhibition studied by perfusion in the cat. J. Physiol. 247, 407-428.

Brownell, W.E., Bader, C.E., Bertrand, D., and de Ribaupierre, Y. (1985). Evoked mechanical responses of isolated cochlear outer hair cells. Science 227, 194-196.

Brownell, W.E., and Kachar, B. Outer hair cell motility: A possible electro-kinetic mechanism. In: Peripheral Auditory Mechanisms (Eds: Allen, J.B., Hall, J.L., Hubbard, A., Neely, S.T., and Tubis, A.) Springer-Verlag, Munich, pp.369-376.

Davis, H. (1983). An active process in cochlear mechanics, Hearing Res. 9, 1-49.

Geisler, C.D. (1986). A model of the effect of outer hair cell motility on cochlear vibrations. Hearing Res. 24, 125-132.

Gitter, A.H., and Zenner, H-P. (1988). Auditory transduction steps in single inner and outer hair cells. In: Basic Issues in Hearing (Eds: Duifhuis, H., Hoorst, J.W., and Wit H.P.), Academic Press, London.

Hudspeth, A.J., and Corey, D.P. (1977). Sensitivity, polarity, and conductance change in the response of vertebrate hair cells to controlled mechanical stimuli. Proceedings of the National Academy of Science, (USA) 74, 2407-2411.

Kiang, N.Y.S., and Moxon, E.C. (1972). Physiological considerations in artificial stimulation of the inner ear. Ann. Otol. Rhinol. Laryngol. 81, 714-730.

Kim, D.O., Neely, S.T., Molnar, C.E., and Matthews, J.W. (1980). An active cochlear model with negative damping in the cochlear partition: Comparison with Rhode's ante- and post-mortem results. In: Psychological, Physiological and Behavioral Studies in Hearing (Eds: van den Brink, G., and Bilsen, F.A.), University Press, Delft, The Netherlands, pp. 7-14.

Koshigoe, S. and Tubis, A. (1983). Frequency-domain investigations of cochlear stability in the presence of active elements. J. Acoust. Soc. Am. 73, 1244-1248.

Mott, J.B., Norton, S.J., Neely, S.T., and Warr, S.T. (1988). Changes in spontaneous otoacoustic emissions produced by acoustic stimulation of the contralateral ear. (In preparation.)

Neely, S.T. (1988). Transient responses in an active, nonlinear model of cochlear mechanics. In: Basic Issues in Hearing (Eds: Duifhuis, H., Hoorst, J.W., and Wit H.P.), Academic Press, London.

Neely, S.T., and Kim, D.O. (1987) A model for active elements in cochlear biomechanics. J. Acoust. Soc. Am. 79, 1472-1480.

Warr, W.B. and Guinan, J.J. (1979). Efferent innervation of the organ of Corti: two separate systems. Brain Res. 173, 152-155.
Weiss, T.F. (1982). Bidirectional transduction in vertebrate hair cells: A mechanism for coupling mechanical and electrical processes. Hearing Res. 7, 353-360.
Zwicker, E. (1986). A hardware cochlear nonlinear preprocessing model with active feedback. J. Acoust. 80, 146-153.

Comments and Discussion

NEELY

If a component of a cochlear model adds energy to the mechanical system, we call it an *active element*. The influence of the active element on the mechanical system we call an *active process*. If this active process works on a "cycle-by-cycle" basis at acoustic frequencies and increases cochlear sensitivity, we call it a *cochlear amplifier*. In the Neely and Kim (1986) model, the cochlear amplifier adds acoustic energy to the cochlear (amplifier) and, thereby, acts as a *traveling-wave amplifer.*.

KOLSTON, VIERGEVER and DIEPENDAAL

This paper attempts to integrate several aspects of cochlear function into one cochlear model. The basic ideas are interesting and it is worthwhile to pursue them further. However, two points should be noted.

1. The results presented do not relate to a single cochlear model. Figs. 3 and 4 actually show calculations from two quite different models. The nonlinear model produces otoacoustic emissions (Fig. 4), whilst the linear model produces realistic neural tuning (Fig. 3). The nonlinearity saturates at a very low level (dm = 1nm) and so the nonlinear model will not exhibit realistic tuning. Furthermore, the fact that the linear model does not produce emissions is remarkable.

2. In Fig. 3 the cilia velocity is presented. 2-DOF cochlear models can easily produce this type of cilia motion, but usually do not succeed in coupling back the sharp tuning to the BM. It would have been interesting, therefore, if BM velocity (V_b) had been presented as well.

NEELY

Your points are well taken and I would caution the reader not to infer too much from the model results presented in this paper. I've attempted here only to present some ideas about the influence of OHCs on cochlear mechanics. I am still working on resolving the inconsistencies between the OHC model and the cochlear model.

WIT

If SOAE's in human ears and in frog ears are generated by the same mechanism, then the model for an oscillating outer hair cell presented in Fig. 1 in the paper by Neely should also describe frog SOAE's.

The consequence is that the model has to account for a more than 20% change of SOAE frequency, caused by a 10°C change of body temperature (Whitehead et al., 1986).

Furthermore, the model has to explain equally large frequency changes caused by direct current through the frogs' inner ear as shown in

Fig. 1. These frequency changes are much larger than the 0.6% change in Neely's Fig. 2.

The frequency spectra in Fig. 1 of a frog SOAE were recorded during DC flow between a wire electrode in the inner ear and a skin needle electrode. The permanent inner ear electrode was placed to record electrical correlates of SOAE's (Wit et al., this volume).

Whitehead, M.L., Wilson, J.P. and Baker, R.J. (1986). The effects of temperature on otoacoustic emission tuning properties. In: Auditory Frequency Selectivity (Eds. Moore, B.C.J. and Patterson, R.D.), Plenum, New York, pp 39-46.

WILSON

I would like to point out that OAEs, with the appropriate long delay, have been obtained in a linear model without recourse to a reverse travelling wave. Such a model would appear to be adaptable to explaining OAEs in frogs.

Sutton, G.J and Wilson, J.P. (1983) Modelling cochlear echoes: the influence of irregularities in frequency mapping on summed cochlear activity. In: Mechanics of Hearing, Eds: E. de Boer and M.A. Viergever, Delft Univ. Press, Delft, pp. 83-90.

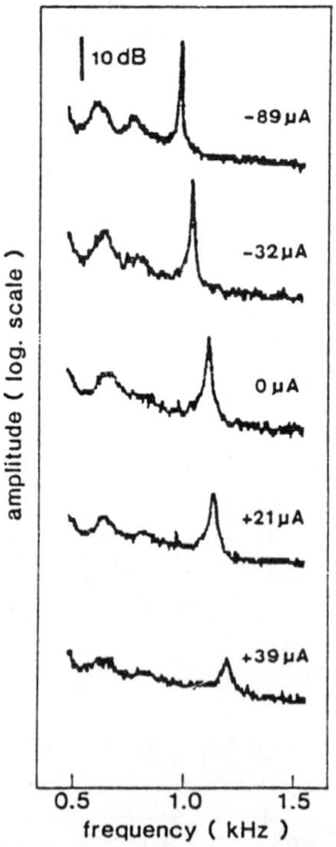

Figure 1. Frequency spectra of a frog SOAE for different values of DC through the inner ear. (Current is positive if the inner ear electrode is positive with respect to the skin electrode.)

A THREE-DEGREE-OF-FREEDOM ACTIVE MICROMECHANICAL MODEL OF THE COCHLEAR PARTITION

K.L. Jones and D.O. Kim

Div. Otolaryngology/Surgery; Neuroscience Program
University of Connecticut Health Center
Farmington, CT 06032, U.S.A.

Introduction

The earliest cochlear models were passive and macromechanical (e.g., Peterson and Bogert, 1950; Ranke, 1950; Zwislocki, 1950). In these models, the properties of the cochlear partition were lumped and represented by a single value of mass, stiffness, and damping for each location on the partition. Hence, we refer to these models as single degree-of-freedom (1-DOF) models. The results of calculations based on these models were in good agreement with the only measurements available at the time, those of von Békésy (1960), who worked with cochleas taken from cadavers.

Tuning of auditory nerve fibers (e.g., Kiang et al., 1965) was found to be much sharper than the cochlear partition tuning reported by von Bekesy. This contrast between the sharp tuning of auditory nerve fibers and the broad tuning of the cochlear partition motivated some researchers to hypothesize the existence of a "second filter" that would transform broad cochlear partition tuning into sharp neural tuning (e.g., Evans and Wilson, 1973; Zwislocki, 1974). Subsequent measurements of inner hair cell potential indicated that its tuning was similar to neural tuning (Russell and Sellick, 1978). The second-filter hypothesis led to the formulation of passive, micromechanical models (Zwislocki and Kletsky, 1980; Allen, 1980). These models represented the cochlear partition as two masses (the mass of the organ of Corti and the mass of the tectorial membrane) connected by a linear spring and dashpot (the stereocilia of the outer hair cells). The 2-DOF system thus created produced sharp inner hair cell tuning and broad cochlear partition tuning.

However, other researchers emphasized the view that the response properties of the cochlear partition (including the frequency selectivity) were significantly affected by the physiological condition of the cochlea (e.g., Kim and Molnar, 1975; Kemp, 1978). Recent direct measurements of cochlear partition motion paid more careful attention to the issue of physiological vulnerability and were able, by using refined measurement techniques that minimized disruption of normal cochlear function, to observe cochlear partition tuning that was much sharper than previously observed (Sellick et al., 1982; Khanna and Leonard, 1982; Robles et al.,

1984). This posed a problem for passive 1- and 2-DOF models of cochlear mechanics. It seemed impossible to get the required sharpness of tuning and sufficient sensitivity (at the threshold of hearing the amplitude of cochlear partition motion is estimated to be on the order of 0.1-10 angstroms; Sellick et al., 1982; Khanna and Leonard, 1982; Bialek, 1983) in these passive models while maintaining an acceptably small group delay (Neely, 1986).

With the discovery of otoacoustic emissions (Kemp, 1978), the idea that the cochlea might contain an active mechanism, first proposed by Gold (Gold, 1948), was given more serious consideration (e.g., Kemp, 1979; Kim et al., 1980; de Boer, 1983). More recent measurements of certain statistical properties of spontaneous otoacoustic emissions (Bialek and Witt, 1984) have lent support to this hypothesis. Support for the hypothesis that the outer hair cell is the likely source of otoacoustic emissions (and thus the site of the active generator) comes from the experimental observation that outer hair cells isolated from the cochlea expand and contract in response to electrical and chemical stimulation (e.g., Brownell et al., 1985; Zenner et al., 1985; Art et al., 1986; Ashmore, 1987). In the cochlea, such electrical stimuli could arise from a modulation of the electrical potential and/or current created by an electromotive force generator thought to be located in the stria vascularis.

Studies of active models of the cochlea have been pursued by many investigators in recent years (e.g., Koshigoe and Tubis, 1983; Mountain et al., 1983; Neely and Kim, 1983; Geisler, 1986; Zwicker, 1986). The model of Neely and Kim exhibits sharp tuning and a reasonable value for the magnitude of basilar membrane motion at threshold, while maintaining a reasonable group delay. The models of Zwicker, and Koshigoe and Tubis simulate the otoacoustic emissions found in many normal ears.

These active models have represented the cochlear partition as a 1- or 2-DOF system. We present, in this paper, the hypothesis that a micromechanical model of the cochlear partition must have a minimum of three DOF if it is to account for the following: (1) the active processes (thought to be due to the observed motility of outer hair cells) needed to explain the tuning, group delay, and threshold characteristics of the cochlea; (2) the stiffness of the stereocilia (Strelioff and Flock, 1984; Crawford and Fettiplace, 1985; Howard and Ashmore, 1986); and (3) the flexibility of the tectorial membrane.

The Model

A schematic drawing of the cochlear partition is given in Fig. 1a. Figs. 1b-d represent three possible models of the partition. Each model has a different number of DOF and incorporates a different combination of the three features referred to above. Fig. 1b shows a 1-DOF model of the cochlear partition. The tectorial membrane and organ of Corti are both rigid and are connected by a rigid hair bundle of an outer hair cell. Note that the hair bundles of the three rows of outer hair cells are represented by a single hair bundle. A 1-DOF model can embody neither a flexible tectorial membrane nor the time-varying change in length of the outer hair cell body that has been observed experimentally.

A 2-DOF model of the cochlear partition is depicted in Fig. 1c. This model is identical to the 1-DOF model shown in Fig. 1b, except that the reticular lamina is now allowed to move relative to the lower part of the organ of Corti as the bodies of the outer hair cells lengthen and shorten, permitting them to act as active force generators.

Incorporating flexibility of the tectorial membrane into the model adds another DOF, resulting in a 3-DOF model (see Fig. 1d). This model of the cochlear partition was implemented on PDP-11/23 and IBM PC/AT microcomputers. The model simulated an isolated single site on the cochlear partition. A brief discussion of the model follows (a more complete presentation will be given elsewhere).

The components of the model (organ of Corti, reticular lamina, and hair bundle) were modelled as rigid bodies, with the state of the system represented by the angular displacements and velocities of these components. The equations governing the time-evolution of the system were formulated using rigid-body dynamics.

The location of the modelled cochlear partition site was chosen to be at the approximate midpoint between the base and the apex of the cochlea with estimates of the various physical dimensions taken from Rhode and Geisler (1967), Lim (1980), and Spoendlin (1972). Estimates of the effective masses and moments of inertia (including the effects of fluid boundary layers) of each component were made, and the values of the various spring and damping constants were chosen to produce desired response characteristics.

The organ of Corti was modelled as a rigid body that was allowed to rotate about a fixed point located at the junction of the basilar membrane and the spiral lamina. Thus, a single differential equation could be written to describe the dynamics of the organ of Corti. This equation equated the time rate of change of the angular momentum of the organ of Corti to the sum of torques about the point of rotation. These torques were associated with the force the basal end of the outer-hair-cell body exerted on the Deiters' cells, the force the reticular lamina exerted on the pillar cells, and a driving force. The driving force was applied vertically at a point on the basilar membrane midway between the spiral lamina and the spiral ligament. The organ of Corti extended from the spiral lamina to this midway point and the basilar membrane was excluded from the model, its effect on the dynamics of the system being simulated by a rotary spring and dashpot located at the point where the organ of Corti joined the spiral lamina.

The reticular lamina was modelled to rotate about a point (the apex of the pillar cells) that was accelerating relative to an inertial frame of reference, and hence we could not simply equate the sum of torques about the center of rotation to the time rate of change of angular momentum. For this structure, three equations had to be solved simultaneously. Similarly, three equations were required to describe the motion of the hair bundle, which rotated about its point of attachment to the cuticular plate. By observing that the spatial configuration of the system could be represented by only three angles, we concluded that four of these seven equations could be eliminated. The three remaining equations included the effects of a rotary dashpot and spring placed at

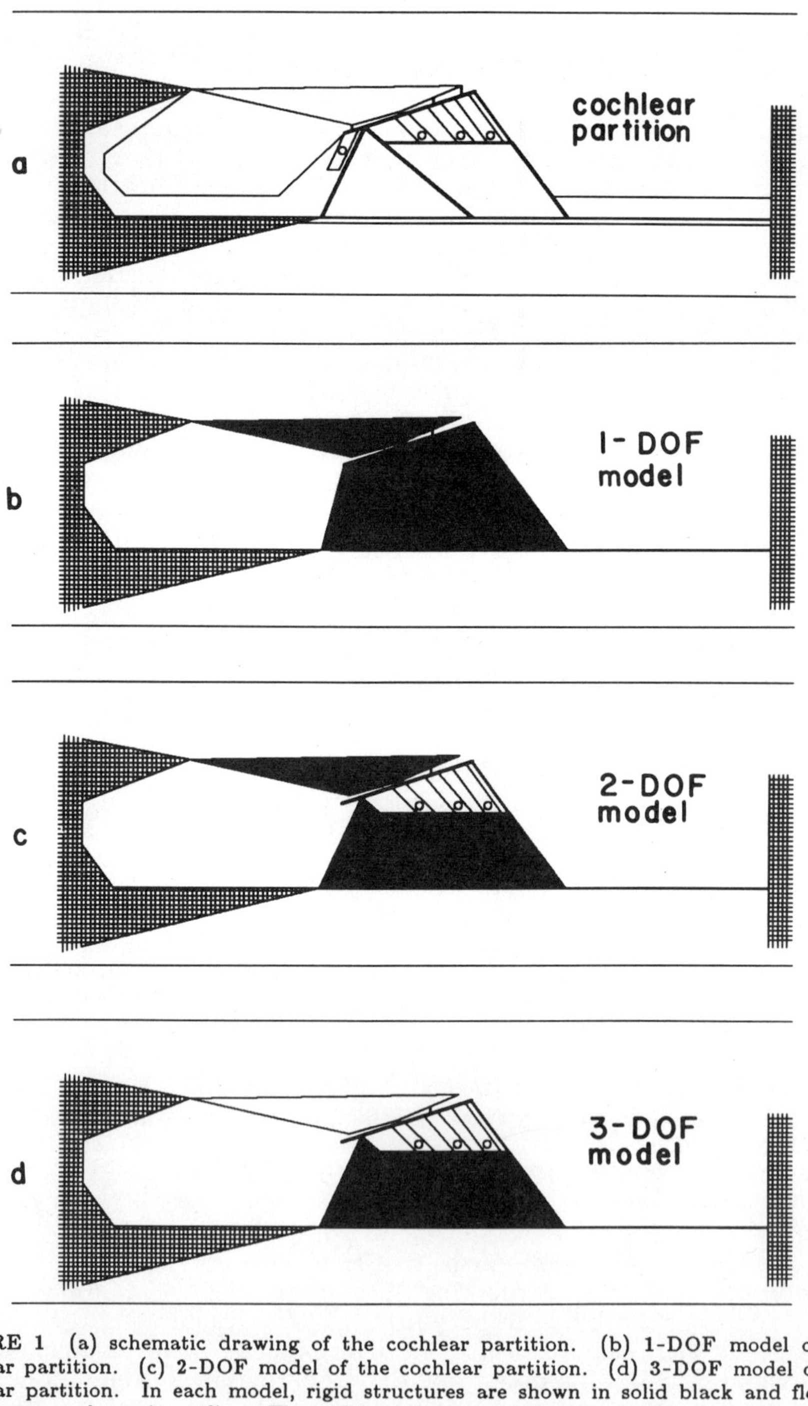

FIGURE 1 (a) schematic drawing of the cochlear partition. (b) 1-DOF model of the cochlear partition. (c) 2-DOF model of the cochlear partition. (d) 3-DOF model of the cochlear partition. In each model, rigid structures are shown in solid black and flexible structures are shown in outline. The width of the base of the organ of Corti is 124 microns and the length of the outer-hair-cell hair bundle is 3.8 microns.

the base of the hair bundle to represent the viscous damping force generated by the motion of the hair bundle through the surrounding fluid and the stiffness of the connection between the stereocilia and the cuticular plate.

The outer-hair-cell body was modelled as a spring in parallel with a dashpot. The spring not only represented the stiffness of the body of the outer hair cell, but also the stiffness of the other structures that connected the reticular lamina and the lower part of the organ of Corti. Part of the resistance represented the passive dissipative losses associated with rotation of the reticular lamina. Another element of the resistance modelled the active force generated by the body of the outer hair cell. This resistance was negative and, by combining with the positive resistance representing dissipative losses, acted to reduce the net resistance in the model of the outer-hair-cell body.

The tectorial membrane was represented by a point impedance (chosen to be anisotropic to reflect the experimental findings of von Bekesy (Bekesy, 1960)) and its inclusion in the model did not require an additional DOF. The forces exerted by the tectorial membrane on the hair bundle were eliminated by using the equations that specified the point impedance of the tectorial membrane. Thus, we obtained three equations in three unknowns driven by two forces: (1) the force exerted on the organ of Corti by the driving force; and (2) the active force generated by the extension and contraction of the outer hair cell bodies.

Results

The output of the model for three different values of outer-hair-cell-body mechanical resistance is shown graphically in Fig. 2. The upper and lower plots show the frequency response (FFT of the impulse response) of the angle of rotation of the organ of Corti and hair bundle, respectively. Both the organ of Corti and hair bundle have similar frequency selectivity, agreeing with the experimental observation that basilar membrane motion and inner hair cell potential show similar tuning. The effect of lowering the net outer-hair-cell-body mechanical resistance (by increasing negative damping) is to sharpen the tuning of both organ-of- Corti and hair-bundle motions. If the value of the outer-hair- cell-body mechanical resistance is given a large enough negative value, oscillation results (this case is not shown in Fig. 2). Since the present model contains no nonlinearity, the oscillation grows without bound over time, but the inclusion of nonlinearity should allow the attainment of a stable steady- state limit cycle oscillation, simulating spontaneous otoacoustic emissions.

Conclusions

Although most micromechanical models have, in the past, had either one or two DOF, we propose that it is necessary to have three DOF if one is to incorporate certain hypothesized aspects of cochlear mechanics, i.e., a mechanism whereby the body of the outer hair cell lengthens and shortens in a manner that releases energy into the micromechanical system, an outer-hair-cell hair bundle that acts as a rigid rod that pivots

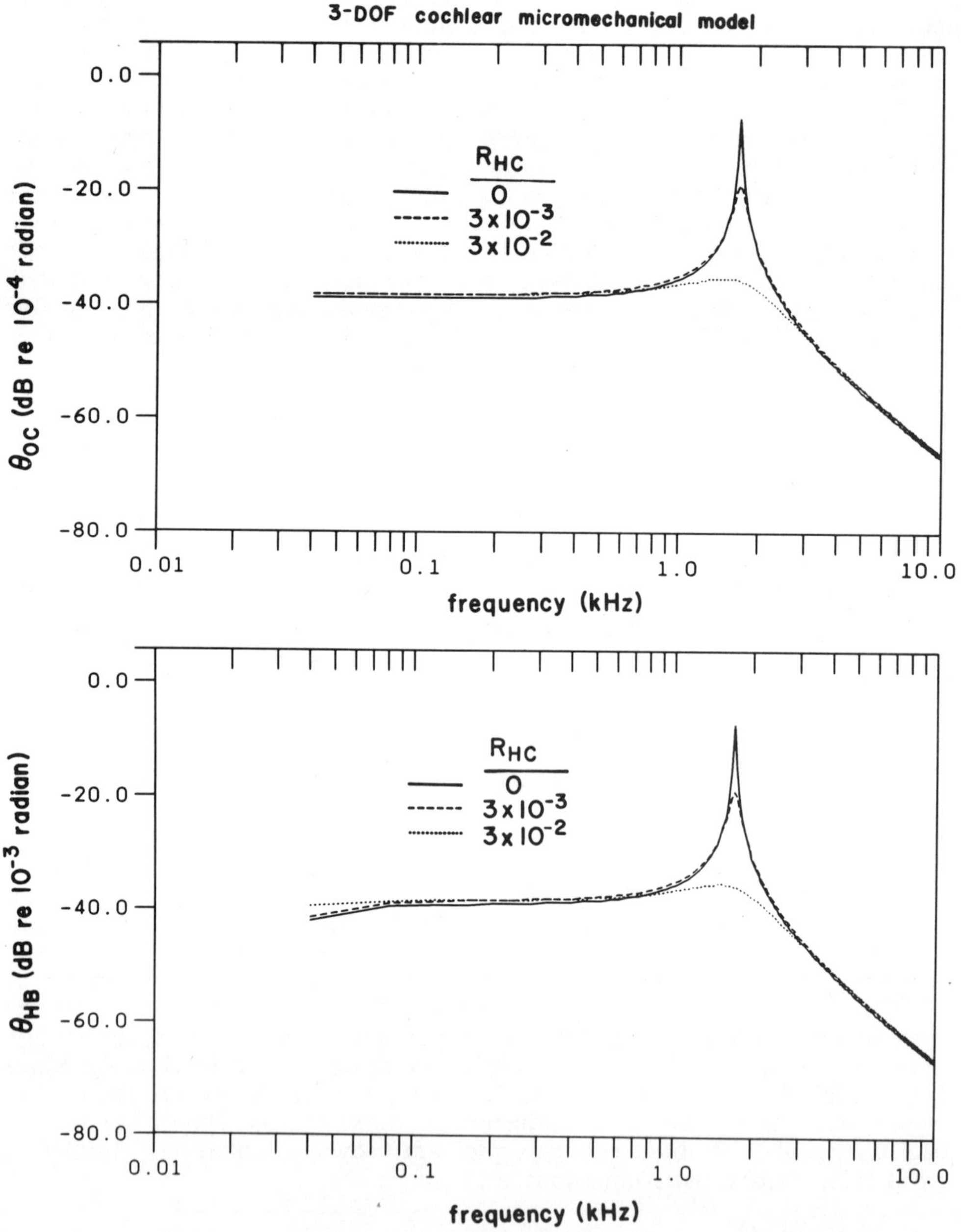

FIGURE 2 Output of a 3-DOF micromechanical model of a cross section of the cochlear partition. The FFT of the impulse response is shown for the angle of rotation of the organ of Corti (upper panel) and for the angle of rotation of the outer-hair-cell hair bundle (lower panel). R_{HC} is the mechanical resistance (in dyne x sec x cm^{-1}) of the outer-hair-cell body. Parameter values: time step = 12.5 microsec; driving impulse = 10^{-14} dyne x sec.

at its point of attachment to the cuticular plate, and a flexible tectorial membrane. The output of the model suggests that the outer hair cell can, by a negative damping mechanism, act to enhance the tuning and sensitivity of the cochlear partition. We believe that the insight gained from the analysis of the micromechanics of a cross section of the cochlear partition presented in this paper should be helpful in future extensions of the 3-DOF cochlear micromechanical model from one cross section to the full length of the cochlea.

Acknowledgements

This study was supported by a grant (NS23693) from US-NIH and grants from the University of Connecticut Health Center. We thank H.H. Nguyen and J.G. Sirianni for their assistance in computer programming and in other laboratory activities, and Dr. G. Leonard for helping us to acquire the equipment used in this study.

References

Allen, J.B. (1980) Cochlear micromechanics - A physical model of transduction. J. Acoust. Soc. Am. 68, 1660-1670.

Art, J.J., Crawford, A.C., and Fettiplace, R. (1986) Electrical resonance and membrane currents in turtle cochlear hair cells. Hearing Research 22, 31-36.

Ashmore, J.F. (1987) A fast motile response in guinea-pig outer hair cells: The cellular basis of the cochlear amplifier. J. Physiol. 388, 323-347.

Bekesy, G. von (1960) Experiments in Hearing, McGraw Hill, New York.

Bialek, W. (1983) Thermal and quantum noise in the ear. In: Mechanics of Hearing (Eds: de Boer, E. and Viergever, M.A.) Martinus Nijhoff Publishers, The Hague, pp. 185-192.

Bialek, W. and Witt, H. (1984) Quantum limits to oscillator stability: theory and experiments on acoustic emissions from the human ear. Phys. Lett. 10A, 173-177.

Brownell, W.E., Bader, C.R., Bertrand, D., and de Ribaupierre, Y. (1985) Evoked mechanical responses of isolated cochlear outer hair cells. Science 227, 194-196.

Crawford, A.C. and Fettiplace, R. (1985) The mechanical properties of ciliary bundles of turtle hair cells. J. Physiol. 364, 359-380.

de Boer, E. (1983) Power amplification in an active model of the cochlea - short- wave case. J. Acoust. Soc. Am. 73, 577-579.

Evans, E.F. and Wilson, J.P. (1973) The frequency selectivity of the cochlea. In: Basic Mechanisms in Hearing (Ed: Moller, A.R.) Academic Press, New York.

Geisler, C.D. (1986) A model of the effect of outer hair cell motility on cochlear vibrations. Hearing Research 24, 125-131.

Gold, T. (1948) Hearing II. The physical basis of action in the cochlea. Proceedings of the Royal Society of London B 135, 492-498.

Howard, J., and Ashmore, J.F. (1986) The stiffness of hair bundles of the frog sacculus. Hearing Research 23, 93-104.

Kemp, D.T. (1978) Stimulated acoustic emissions from within the human auditory system. J. Acoust. Soc. Am. 64, 1386-1391.

Kemp, D.T. (1979) Evidence of mechanical nonlinearity and frequency selective wave amplification in the cochlea. Arch. Otohinolar. 224, 37-45.

Khanna, S.M. and Leonard, D.G.B. (1982) Basilar membrane tuning in the cat cochlea. Science 215, 305-306.

Kiang, N.Y.S., Watanabe, T., Thomas, E.C., and Clark, L.F. (1965) Discharge patterns of single fibres in the cat's auditory nerve. In: Res. Monogr. M.I.T. 35, M.I.T. Press, Cambridge, MA.

Kim, D.O. and Molnar, C.E. (1975) Cochlear Mechanics: Measurements and Models. In: The Nervous System, Vol. 3: Human Communication and Its Disorders (Editor-in-Chief: Tower, D.B.) Raven Press, New York

Kim, D.O., Neely, S.T., Molnar, C.E., and Matthews, J.W. (1980) An active cochlear model with negative damping in the partition: Comparison with Rhode's ante- and post-mortem observations. In: Psychophysical, Physiological and Behavioural Studies in Hearing (Eds: van den Brink, G. and Bilsen, F.A.) Delft University Press, The Netherlands

Koshigoe, S. and Tubis, A. (1983) A non-linear feedback model for outer-hair-cell stereocilia and its implications for the response of the auditory periphery. In: Mechanics of Hearing (Eds: de Boer, E. and Viergever, M.A.) Martinus Nijhoff Publishers, The Hague, pp. 127-134.

Lim, D.J. (1980) Cochlear anatomy related to cochlear micromechanics, A review. J. Acoust. Soc. Am. 67, 1686-1695.

Mountain, D.C., Hubbard, A.E., and McMullen T.A. (1983) Electromechanical processes in the cochlea. In: Mechanics of Hearing (Eds: de Boer, E. and Viergever, M.A.) Martinus Nijhoff Publishers, The Hague, pp. 119-126.

Neely, S.T. (1986) Micromechanics of the cochlear partition. In: Peripheral Auditory Mechanisms (Eds: Allen, J.B., Hall, J.L., Hubbard, A., Neely, S.T., and Tubis, A.) Springer-Verlag, New York, pp. 137-146.

Neely, S.T. and Kim, D.O. (1983) An active cochlear model showing sharp tuning and high sensitivity. Hearing Research 9, 123-130.

Peterson, L.C. and Bogert B.P. (1950) A dynamical theory of the cochlea. J. Acoust. Soc. Am. 22, 369-381.

Ranke, O.F. (1950) Theory of operation of the cochlea: A contribution to the hydrodynamics of the cochlea. J. Acoust. Soc. Am. 22, 772-777.

Rhode, W.S. and Geisler, C.D. (1967) Model of the displacement between opposing points on the tectorial membrane and reticular lamina. J. Acoust. Soc. Am. 42, 185-190.

Robles, L., Ruggero, M., and Rich, N.C. (1984) Mossbauer measurements of basilar membrane tuning curves in the chinchilla. J. Acoust. Soc. Am. 76, S35.

Russell, I.J. and Sellick, P.M. (1978) Intracellular studies of hair cells in the mammalian cochlea. J. Physiol. 284, 261-290.

Sellick, P.M., Patuzzi, R., and Johnstone, B.M. (1982) Measurement of basilar membrane motion in the guinea pig using the Mossbauer technique. J. Acoust. Soc. Am. 72, 131-141.

Spoendlin, H. (1972) Innervation densities of the cochlea. Acta Otolar. 73, 235-248.

Strelioff, D. and Flock. A. (1984) Stiffness of sensory-cell hair bundles in the isolated guinea-pig cochlea. Hearing Research 15, 19-28.

Zenner, H.P., Zimmerman, U., and Schmitt, U. (1985) Reversible contraction of isolated mammalian cochlear hair cells. Hearing Research 18, 127-133.

Zwicker, E. (1986) A hardware cochlear nonlinear preprocessing model with active feedback. J. Acoust. Soc. Am. 80, 146-153.

Zwislocki, J. (1950) Theory of the acoustical action of the cochlea. J. Acoust. Soc. Am. 22, 778-784.

Zwislocki, J.J. (1974) A possible neuro-mechanical sound analysis in the cochlea. Acustica 31, 354-359.

Zwislocki, J.J. and Kletsky, E.J. (1980) Micromechanics in the theory of cochlear mechanics. Hearing Research 2, 505-512.

Comments and Discussion

VIERGEVER, KOLSTON, DIEPENDAAL

1. You present (on p. 2 of your paper) the hypothesis that a micromechanical model of the cochlear partition must have a minimum of three DOF if it is to account for (i) OHC motility, (ii) stiffness of the stereocilia, (iii) flexibility of the TM. However, you require implicitly that the model can account for rotation of the organ of Corti as well.

Since stiffness of the stereocilia does not represent a mechanical degree of freedom, your statement is not a hypothetical one but a trivial one.

2. The only numerical results of your study, shown in Fig. 2, do not support the need for three DOF. The depicted curves do not differ from responses of a 1-DOF (mass/spring/dashpot) system.

JONES AND KIM

We agree that a more logical presentation of our thoughts would have been as follows:

1) The rotation of the organ of Corti requires a degree of freedom;

2) an active mechanism due to changes in the lengths of outer-hair-cell bodies requires an additional degree of freedom; and

3) a flexibile tectorial membrane and rod-like outer-hair-cell hair bundle require a third degree of freedom in an active micromechanical model.

In light of the fact that previous *active* cochlear models have had 1 or 2 DOF, we wanted to emphasize that a minimum of 3 DOF are needed to incorporate these properties. We feel that the time has come to construct a model that allows the utilization of the increasing amount of experimental measurements of mechanical properties of cochlear partition elements. This was difficult to do in previous models because of the approximations and lumping of parameters made in these models.

Indeed, it is impossible in principle to model all aspects of the behaviour of a 3-DOF system with a 2- or 1-DOF system. We feel that previous models have yielded profound insights into the operation of the cochlea; in fact they have provided insights that may be obscured by the complexity of more realistic models. Simplicity has its virtues, but recent experiments have provided data that can be used by modellers to build the more sophisticated models needed to attempt to answer some of the most intriguing questions in cochlear modelling, e.g., is it possible for an active mechanism based on dynamic length changes of the outer-hair-cell body to produce sufficient power at high enough frequencies to significantly affect the dynamics of the cochlear partition? This is one of the long term goals of our modelling studies. The price that must be paid for such realism is the longer runtime and larger parameter space required by the inclusion of a third degree of freedom and the faithful adherence to Newton's laws of motion.

The results shown in Fig. 2 of our paper are preliminary and somewhat misleading. With a single cross section of the cochlear partition, we cannot, for theoretical reasons, design the model with the frequency response characteristics we desire. We believe that longitudinal coupling (energy transfer) is utilized by the cochlea to sharpen tuning. The model of Neely and Kim (1986) uses such a mechanism. An isolated cross-section of the cochlea exhibiting such tuning would be unstable because another section of the cochlear partition must be present to absorb and dissipate the energy released into the cochlear fluid. Although it would be possible to couple the fluid to a damped tuned circuit to dissipate this energy, this added complexity would not allow us to determine the frequency response needed for a cross-section embedded in a model of the entire cochlea. Hence, we chose to simply demonstrate that it was possible to attain sharper tuning and highest sensitivity by increasing the negative resistance component of the outer-hair-cell body impedance.

The tuning curves shown in Fig. 2 of our paper are not representative of the frequency response we will try to achieve for single sections of the model of the full cochlea. In fact, to simplify the task of choosing parameters, a large low-frequency peak was created by moving a resonance to such a low frequency that the middle-ear transfer function and the shunting action of the helicotrema would prevent its excitation. This resonance is of too low a frequency to appear on the frequency response curves shown in Fig. 2.

GEISLER

It is perhaps worth clarifying the point that results similar to those shown in their Fig. 1 can be obtained with models of less than 3 degrees of freedom (DOF). For example, my recent model, referred to in their paper, has 2 DOF, the essential variables being the angle of the basilar membrane at the inner-pillar rotation point and the angle of the reticular lamina around an outer-pillar rotation point, relative to their rest positions. This model produces a net impedance to the acoustic pressure wave that is composed of stiffness, mass and damping terms, the latter being a composite of viscous damping and an anti-viscous term contributed by the active OHCs. Such an impedance yields results similar to those shown in their Fig. 1. Similar results can also be achieved with a 1-DOF model, if one is not concerned with how the necessary small values of the damping term are achieved. This does not imply that a model's DOF do not matter, for they do. The more DOF a model has, the more flexible it is.

OUTER HAIR CELLS POSSESS ACETYLCHOLINE RECEPTORS AND PRODUCE MOTILE RESPONSES IN THE ORGAN OF CORTI

H.P. Zenner, G. Reuter, P.K. Plinkert, U. Zimmermann and A.H. Gitter

Department of Otolaryngology
University of Würzburg
D-8700 Würzburg, W.Germany

Introduction

Active mechanical processes in the mammalian cochlea are considered to be new general mechanisms in hearing that differ from the classical description of the passive travelling wave of the basilar membrane. Located in outer hair cells (OHCs) they are thought to contribute to sensitivity and frequency selectivity or to control the basilar membrane (BM) location and the operating point of the stereocilia. Reversible slow (Zenner et al., 1985; Zenner, 1986) and fast (Brownell et al., 1985; Zenner et al., 1987; Ashmore, 1987) active longitudinal movements of the cylindrical body of isolated OHCs that have been demonstrated in vitro support this notion. Furthermore, we could show, that the cuticular plate (CP) of OHCs is capable of slow and fast motile responses that displace the stereociliary bundle (Zenner, 1986, 1988; Zenner et al., 1988). Biochemical analyses revealed that an interaction of actin and myosin is the molecular basis of Ca^{2+}/ATP-dependend slow motile responses of OHCs (Zenner, 1988). A direct extrapolation, however, from these in vitro results to the conditions in the organ of Corti (OC) is rather dubious. Furthermore, the control mechanisms of OHC motility have not been finally elucidated. Control could be achieved e.g. by the efferent nerves as well as by a.c. and d.c. mo dulations of the OHC membrane potential.

However, neurotransmitter receptors, which are required for an efferent control, had not been identified in OHCs. Using monoclonal antibodies against internal and external epitopes of acetylcholine-receptors (AcChRs) we can now demonstrate the presence of AcChRs in the outer cell membrane of OHCs. To answer the question, whether the results obtained with isolated OHCs and IHCs can be applied to the in situ condition, we can show fast electrogenic motile responses of OHCs in the OC of guinea pigs. In addition OHC depolarizations in situ in the presence of increased perilymphatic K^+-concentrations induced slow shortenings of the three rows of OHCs in the OC.

Methods

Specific details of the preparation of isolated OHCs and of related techniques (patch clamping, chemical and electrical stimulation, cell culture, immunocytochemistry, photo-diode-technique, video-enhancement, digital image analyses) can be found in Gitter et al. (1986), and Zenner et al. (1988).

Results and Discussion

BIPHASIC SLOW MOTILE RESPONSES IN VITRO

Under cell culture conditions using patch-clamp techniques isolated OHCs had immediately stable membrane potentials (+ 2mV) of -45+ 16 mV (mean +SD, n = 17) with a minimum value of -69 mV for at least 5 min (Gitter et al., 1986). Similar results were obtained with microelectrode impalements (Gitter et al., 1987; Gitter and Zenner, 1988). A slow depolarization of OHCs in the presence of 25 - 125 mM K^+ was accompanied by a slow biphasic motile response of the cell body and the CP displacing the stereociliary bundle. Single frame recordings using digital image subtractions allowed to differentiate the two phases. (i) During the first 0.5 - 5 sec OHCs shorten and move their CP. (ii) A longer exposure to elevated K^+-concentrations results in an additional in crease of the cell volume, which is accompanied by a further length change of the cell. The experiments suggest two separate underlying mechanisms: (i) an early phase and possibly voltage dependent electro-mechanical process and (ii) a late phase volume regulatory mechanism of OHCs.

A depolarization of hair cells is thought to be associated with an increase of the intra intracellular Ca^{2+}-level. Recently, we were able to show biochemically that an increase of the intracellular calcium level activated the actomyosin- skeleton of isolated OHCs (Zenner, 1988). This resulted in slow contractions of the cell body and the CP with a velocity of 3-24 nm . msec-1 during a first phase of 50-200 msec. Longer stimulations induced an additional longer second phase of the motile response with time constants in the sec.- to min.-range. Results in the min.-range were also obtained by Flock et al. (1986). Exact mechanisms underlying a depolarization-induced rise of the intracellular Ca^{2+}-level remain unknown. Our own results suggest, that the increased Ca^{2+}-level can induce an actomyosin-activation and thus mechanical response of the OHC.

INOSITOL TRISPHOSPHATE AS A SECOND MESSENGER

Recently we could show,that the intracellular Ca^{2+}-level of OHCs is also controlled by inositol- trisphosphate ($InsP_3$) acting as a second messenger in hair cells (Schacht and Zenner, 1988). Thin-layer-chromatography revealed, that OHCs contain a cascade of phosphoinositides, and thus the biochemical maschinery to produce $InsP_3$ in their outer cell membranes. An experimental increase of intracellular $InsP_3$ in isolated OHCs induced motile responses during 50-200 msec. Thus $InsP_3$ can act as a second messenger to elicit a motile response, the molecular basis of which is thought to be the rise of the intracellular Ca^{2+}-level and the subsequent activation of actomyosin. However, in this proposed biochemical sequence of events resulting in hair cell contraction the adequate stimulus remained unknown.

ACETYLCHOLINE RECEPTORS IN OHC

A direct involvement of $InsP_3$ in the electro- mechanical process seems unlikely, as in other cell species the release of InsP3 is mostly a separate agonist-receptor operated process. However, no receptor in the outer cell membrane of OHCs has been identified, though the presence of a mixed AcChR or of GABA-receptors has been postulated (Klinke, 1986). Monoclonal antibodies against internal and external epitopes of the AcChR from torpedo allowed us a direct visualization of AcChRs in whole cell preparations from OHCs. AcChRs could be found exclusively in the basal and basolateral membrane parts of OHCs. Sometimes, they were arranged like a cup at the basal end of the sensory cell (Fig.1). Further more, the monoclonal antibodies showed patching of AcChRs suggesting a possible lateral diffusion of AcChRs in the membrane plane of OHCs. Moreover, labelling by the antibodies of AcChRs was found on both sides of the outer cell membrane, indicating the presence of a pleiotropic, transmembrane-protein. Thus, our results suggest with the presence of AcChR at the synaptic end of OHCs.

We hypothesize, that via AcCh efferent nerves activate these newly found AcChRs. This could result in an agonist-receptor operated release of $InsP_3$ from the membrane-bound phosphoinositide PIP_2 into the cytoplasma, thus generating a Ca^{2+} controlled response. In a separate model we suggest, that AcChR-operated ionic channels could generate a Na^+-influx into the cytoplasm, resulting in a depolarizing current. This could interfere with voltage dependent electro-mechanical events in OHCs.

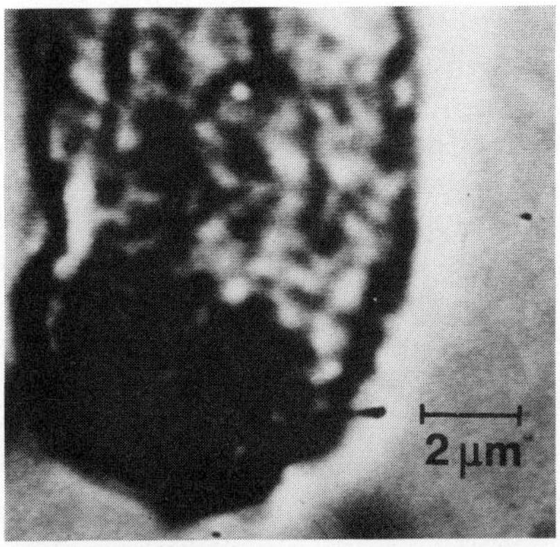

FIGURE 1: Visualization of AcChRs at the synapatic end of an isolated OHC (immune peroxydase staining using monoclonal anti-AcChR-anti-bodies and digital image contrast enhancement).

SLOW OHC-MOTILITY IN SITU

The question whether the concept of slow OHC movements can be applied to the in vivo condition could not be answered by these results. Recent joint investigations, however, with C.Fermin (Fermin et al, in preparation) demonstrated, that a perilymphatic perfusion with elevated K^+-concentrations induced a shortening of the OHCs. Histological controls revealed a reduced distance between BM and RL. Thus, the depolarization by K^+ of OHCs in situ is accompanied by motile OHC events in the OC.

FAST OHC-MOTILITY IN SITU

In addition to the slow longitudinal motility (Zenner et al., 1985; Zenner, 1986; Flock et al., 1986) the OHC body has been reported to oscillate in the presence of electrical stimuli (Brownell et al., 1985; Zenner et al. 1987; , Ashmore, 1987) up to at least 30 kHz (Gitter and Zenner, 1988). However, whether similar length changes and the dynamic tilting of the CP observed in isolated OHCs also occur in the OC remained unclear. Stiff ness changes of OHCs in situ without shape changes could not be excluded. Thus, viable half turns from guinea pig cochleae were cultured under con ditions, which had allowed isolated IHCs and OHCs to produce physiological cell potentials. Then the OC were exposed to a.c. fields ($E \approx 1$ kV/m) produced between Ag/AgCl-bath electrodes. A double photo-diode technique allowed to measure motile responses of the three rows of OHCs up to 15 kHz. Responses of IHCs and supporting cells were much smaller (Fig. 2) and were abolished following a mechanical decoupling from the OHCs. Thus, active electrogenic motile responses were restricted to the OHCs. Videostroboscopy (up to 500 Hz) and digital substractions of subsequent images allowed more precise observations of the in situ motility of OHCs. The experiments revealed oscillatory shortenings and elongations of the OHC-bodies, which were accompanied by oscillatory lateral shear motions of RL, CP and hair bundles in toto.

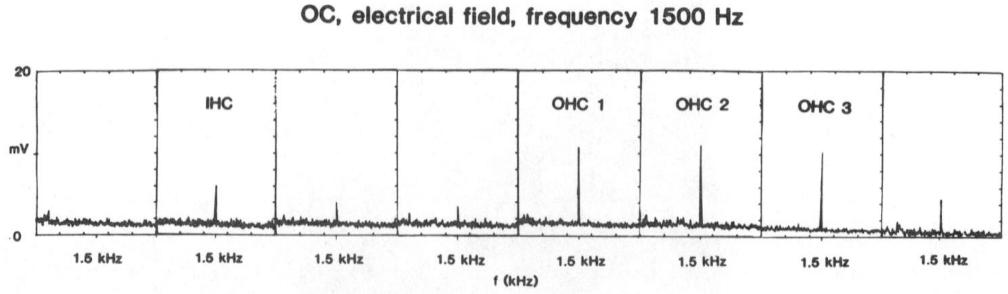

FIGURE 2: Electrogenic motile responses of 1,5 kHz at different locations in an OC. Measurements are from IHCs and OHCs where indicated. All other traces are from supporting cells. Note the high amplitudes produced in the three rows of OHCs and the reduced responses in other areas (power density spectra).

IMPLICATIONS

The present demonstration of slow and fast motile responses of OHCs in situ enhances the physiological significance of OHC motility as a possible common contribution of OHCs to the hearing process. Furthermore, OHCs possess AcChRs, which may modulate OHC motility.

The slow longitudinal and shear movements might directly influence the RL and BM motion and thus the operating conditions of the OC. They could control homeostasis of the location of the hair bundles and the BM and set the bias position of the cochlear partition. Under physiological conditions, a bias of the RL/BM location and of the operation point of the hair bundles induced by controlled, slow OHC movements could also contri bute to adaptation processes (automatic gain control) or TTS (Zenner 1986, 1988). Thus, by the Ca^{2+}-dependent actomyosin-driven motility of CP and cell body, OHCs could compress BM and hair bundle displacements during high SPLs. LePage (1987) speculated that the spatial dependence of such a long-term control of the BM-bias might define the tuning curve as a function of tone level. However, the "muscle-like" OHCs could also follow the sound stimulus cycle-by-cycle for fre quencies less than ca 1 kHz. A similar mechanical phase-locking has been proposed for low frequency coding, making possible the velocity response and phase-locking in neural period histograms (LePage, 1988). For sound frequencies above 1 kHz on the basis of models (Zwicker, 1979) and our own bio chemical results, we have suggested that the acto myosin skeleton might significantly help amplify the travelling wave by intermittent stimulations (Zenner, 1986; Zenner et al., 1988). Moreover, LePage (1988) proposed mechanical summations due to muscular OHC contractions which could dominate for high-frequency detection.

Furthermore, there is now some likelihood that the evoked fast motile mechanism could boost the local vibratory motion of the cochlear partition and/or the fluid-/TM-coupling to the IHCs. If present in vivo, it could have a significance for frequency selectivity, negative damping (cochlear amplifier) or oto-acoustic emissions.

References

Ashmore, J.F., (1987) A fast motile response in guinea-pig outer hair cells: The cellular basis of the cochlear amplifier. J. Physiol. 388, 323-347

Brownell,W.E. (1986) Outer hair cell motility and cochlear frequency selectivity. In : Auditory frequency selectivity (Eds: Moore ,B. C. and Patterson,R.D.) Plenum Press, New York and London, 109-120

Brownell W.E., Bader, C.R., Bertrand, D. and de Ribaupierre Y. (1985) Evoked mechanical responses of isolated cochlear outer hair cells. Science 227, 194-196

Flock,A., Flock, B. and Ulfendahl, M. (1986) Mechanisms of movement in outer hair cells and a possible structural basis. Arch.Otorhinolaryngol. 243, 83-90

Gitter, A.H., Zenner, H.P. and Frmter, E. (1986) Membrane potential and ion channels in isolated outer hair cells of the guinea pig cochlea. ORL. J. Otorhinolaryngol. Relat. Spec. 48,68-75

Gitter,A.H., Tietz,F. and Zenner, H.P. (1987) Inner ear outer hair cells viewed through microelectrodes. Pflgers Arch. 408, R 71

Gitter, A.H. and Zenner, H.P. (1988) Auditory transduction steps in single inner and outer hair cells. 8th Intl. Symp. Hear., University Press Groningen, in press.

Klinke,R. (1986) Neurotransmission in the inner ear. Hearing Re. 22, 235-243
LePage, E.L.(1987) A spatial template for the shape of tuning curves in the mammalian cochlea. J. Acoust. Soc. Am. 82, 155-164
LePage, E.L.(1988) Motility of outer hair cells and tuning in the mammalian cochlea. In: Ass.Res. ORL, Midw. Res. Meet. (Ed:Lim D.J.) Clearwater, pp.29-30
Schacht,J. and Zenner,H.P. (1988) Evidence that phosphoinositides mediate motility in cochlear outer hair cells. Hearing Res 31, 155-160
Zenner, H.P. (1986) Motile responses in outer hair cells.Hearing Res 22, 83-90
Zenner, H.P. (1988) Motility of outer hair cells as an active, actin-mediated process. Acta Otolaryngol. (Stockh.) 105, 39-44
Zenner, H.P., Zimmermann, U. and Schmitt, U. (1985) Reversible contraction of isolated mammalian cochlear hair cells. Hearing Res. 18, 127-133
Zenner,H.P., Zimmermann, U. and Gitter, A.H.(1987) Fast motility of isolated mammalian auditory sensory cells. Biochem. Biophys.Res.Commun. 49, 304-308
Zenner,H.P., Zimmermann,R. and Gitter,A.H. (1988) Active movements of the cuticular plate induce sensory hair motion in mammalian auditory hair cells. Hearing Res, in press
Zwicker, E. (1979) A model describing non- linearities in hearingby active processes with saturation at 40 dB. Biol. Cybern. 35, 243-250

MECHANO-ELECTRICAL TRANSDUCTION IN TURTLE HAIR CELLS

R. Fettiplace and A.C. Crawford

Physiological Laboratory
University of Cambridge
Cambridge CB2 3EG, UK

Introduction

The initial step in hair cell transduction involves coordinated flexion of an array of microvilli, the hair bundle, which gates a membrane conductance enabling a transducer current to flow into the cell (Hudspeth & Corey, 1977; Ohmori, 1985). Although the ionic selectivity of the transducer conductance is known (Corey & Hudspeth, 1979; Ohmori, 1985), the events leading to activation of the channel are not fully understood, and there is no consensus even on the precise form of relationship between bundle displacement and transducer current. Here we present some observations on the transduction process in turtle hair cells measured both directly in isolated cells under voltage clamp and indirectly from receptor potentials in the intact ear.

Methods

Experiments were performed on cochlear hair cells from the turtle *Pseudemys scripta elegans*. The first set of results was derived from intracellular recordings in an isolated half-head preparation employing procedures already documented (Crawford & Fettiplace, 1980). Sound stimuli, generated with a Beyer DT48 earphone, were delivered through a coupler to the tympanum and the sound pressure was measured with a condenser microphone. The scala tympani was filled with artificial perilymph whose normal composition was (in mM): NaCl, 130; KCl, 4; $CaCl_2$, 2.8; $MgCl_2$, 2.2; glucose, 8; NaHEPES, 5, pH 7.6. Tetraethylammonium bromide (TEA, 15 mM) was added by substitution for an equimolar amount of NaCl.

The techniques for dissociating and recording currents under whole cell voltage-clamp from solitary hair cells were similar to those described previously (Art & Fettiplace, 1987). Isolated cells were bathed in artificial perilymph and immobilised on

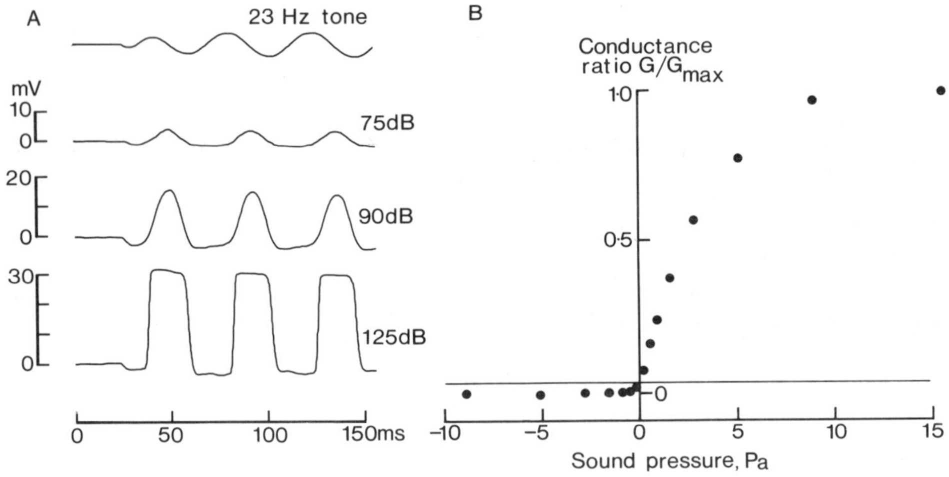

FIGURE 1. Mechano-electrical transduction in the intact ear. Fig 1A shows intracellular receptor potentials, relative to the resting potential (-44 mV) evoked by a 23 Hz tone burst (top trace) at the sound pressures (dB re 20 μPa) indicated by each trace. 15 mM TEA was added to the perilymph. In Fig 1B, peak depolarisations and hyperpolarisations have been converted to conductances according to eqn 1. The conductance relative to the maximum transducer conductance (25 nS) is plotted against peak sound pressure (Pascals). Note the pronounced asymmetry of the curve around zero pressure. Temp=23°C.

the floor of a recording chamber which had been coated with polylysine or concanavalin A. The chamber was mounted on a cooling stage (Crawford & Fettiplace, 1987) fitted to a Zeiss IM 35 inverted microscope. Patch electrodes were filled with a solution of composition (in mM): KCl, 125; $MgCl_2$, 2.8; K_2EGTA, 5; KHEPES, 5, pH 7.2. To elicit a transducer current, the tallest rank of cilia, about 6 μm in height, was deflected with a glass stylus attached to a piezoelectric bimorph. The driving voltage to the bimorph was low-pass filtered, so when a step input was delivered, the tip of the stylus settled in about 50 to 70 μs. The motion of the stylus was monitored using a dual photodiode detection system (Crawford & Fettiplace, 1985) with a bandwidth of more than 50 kHz.

Results

THE TRANSDUCER CONDUCTANCE IN THE INTACT EAR

Owing to the presence of voltage-sensitive conductances in turtle hair cells, it is difficult to relate the receptor potentials to the performance of the mechano-electrical transduction process. When the major voltage-dependent channels are blocked with TEA (Crawford & Fettiplace, 1981; Art & Fettiplace, 1987), thus rendering the cell's current-voltage relationship ohmic, the receptor potentials should accurately reflect the transducer current. Examples of receptor potentials obtained under these conditions are shown in Fig. 1A. The perilymph contained 15 mM TEA, and the ear was stimulated with tone bursts at 23 Hz, a frequency well below the corner frequency (160 Hz) imposed by the cell's time constant (1 ms). The receptor potentials swing asymmetrically around the resting potential, and at the highest sound levels, the cell depolarises by 32 mV on one phase of the stimulus but hyperpolarises by only about 5 mV on the other phase. The receptor potentials could be reversed by injecting steady currents which depolarised the cell by about 45 mV; the reversal potential of close to 0 mV is similar to values reported previously (Crawford & Fettiplace, 1981).

To extract the transducer conductance, the peak amplitudes of the depolarisations and hyperpolarisations from the resting potential were measured as a function of sound pressure, and then corrected for the instantaneous changes in driving force on ion movements (Crawford & Fettiplace, 1981) as follows:

$$G_t = G_{in} (V_r - V)/(V - E_{rev}) \quad (1)$$

where G_{in} and G_t are the input conductance and the change in transducer conductance respectively, V is the membrane potential on the peaks or dips of the receptor potential, V_r is the resting potential (-44mV) and V_{rev} is the transducer reversal potential. A plot of the transducer conductance scaled to its maximum value as a function of sound pressure is shown in Fig. 1B. A notable feature of the plot is the pronounced asymmetry, the steepest slope (and hence the largest sensitivity) occurring around the resting potential where only about 5% of the conductance is activated.

An absolute value for the transducer conductance can be obtained using the cell's input conductance inferred from current-injection experiments. The input conductance was 10 nS, the maximum transducer conductance therefore being estimated as 25 nS. This value is somewhat larger than those previously reported (Crawford & Fettiplace, 1981; Holton & Hudspeth, 1986), and reflects the large size of the receptor potential, on the peaks of which the membrane potential approaches the reversal potential. The calculation relies upon the value for the input conductance derived from bridge-balance measurements, but it seems unlikely that this would be out by more than a factor of two.

TRANSDUCER CONDUCTANCE IN ISOLATED HAIR CELLS

Measurements were performed on isolated cells whose bodies were firmly attached to the floor of the recording chamber, and transducer currents were evoked by displacing the hair bundle along its axis of bilateral symmetry. Clean glass probes normally adhered to the bundle, the resting position of which was adjusted to achieve a maximum current sensitivity for small deflexions. Currents were recorded under voltage-clamp at a holding potential of -70 mV where the voltage-dependent currents would be turned off.

Step displacements of the hair bundle produced a maintained transducer current that was graded with the size of the step (Art, Crawford & Fettiplace, 1986). Displacements of up to 1 μm towards the kinocilium led to an increase in inward current, whereas reverse displacements caused a smaller decrease (Fig. 3A), the current amplitude saturating for the largest movements in either direction. Fig. 2 shows an example of the steady-state relationship between current and displacement, which is an S-shaped function asymmetric about the resting position of the bundle (Holton & Hudspeth, 1986; Ohmori, 1986). All cells displayed some degree of asymmetry, though never as pronounced as that seen in the intact ear, and the peak sensitivity occurred when between 10 and 25 % of the total conductance was activated. At room temperature, response amplitudes of 200-300 pA were observed, corresponding to a maximum transducer conductance of about 4 nS.

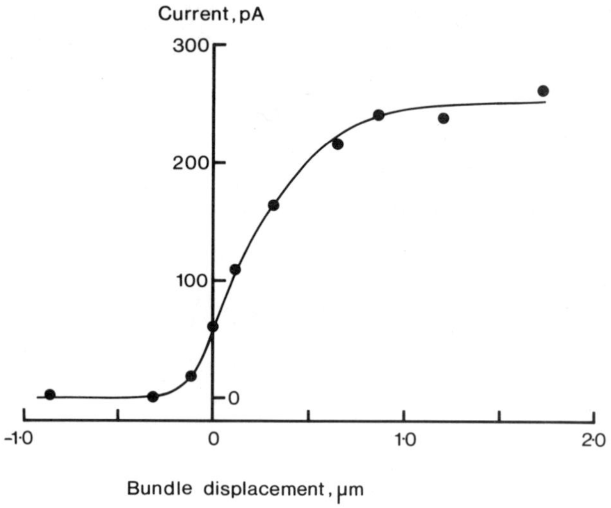

FIGURE 2 The relationship between steady-state transducer current and hair bundle displacement from an isolated cell under voltage-clamp. Movements towards kinocilium displayed positive; currents (pA) are inward. Holding potential -70 mV, temp. 23°C, same cell as Fig. 3A. Note the asymmetry of the curve around zero displacement.

Comparison of the scales on the abscissae in Fig. 1B and Fig. 2 enables one to calculate the transformation of sound pressure at the tympanum to hair bundle deflexion. The maximum conductance is attained for about 1 μm of bundle displacement and 10 Pascals of sound pressure, the conversion ratio therefore being 100 nm/Pa. This number is comparable to our previous estimate of 60 nm/Pa for the sound-evoked motion of the turtle basilar membrane (Crawford & Fettiplace, 1983), which suggests that, in the turtle, the tips of the hair bundles are displaced by approximately the same amount as the basilar membrane.

KINETICS OF TRANSDUCER CURRENTS

Fig. 3 shows examples of the onset of the current for step displacements of the hair bundle from the resting position. The records are taken from two different cells, one at room temperature (23°C) and the other at 3°C. In both cases, the current starts after a small delay and then develops with a single time constant that speeds up for larger displacements. The results are easier to interpret at the lower temperature, where the onset of the current is about five times slower and is clearly distinguishable from the rise time of the probe motion and the time constant of the voltage clamp, both about 50 μs.

To characterise the kinetics, the currents, I(t), have been fitted with a pair of time constants (τ_1, τ_2) using an equation of the form:

$$I(t) = I_{max} (1 - (\tau_2 \exp(-t/\tau_2) - \tau_1 \exp(-t/\tau_1))/(\tau_2 - \tau_1)) \quad (2)$$

where I_{max} is the steady-state current. At the lower temperature, one of the time constants is about 150 μs and independent of displacement, whereas the other decreases from 1.24 ms at the resting position of the bundle to 240 μs for the largest displacement. The fits are qualitatively similar at room temperature, with a level-invariant component

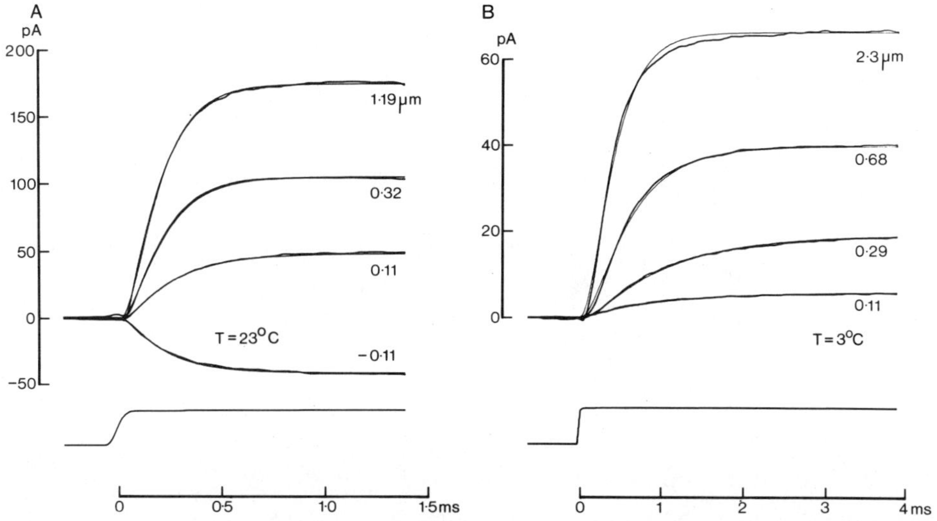

FIGURE 3 The onset of the transducer current when the hair bundle is stepped towards or away from the kinocilium. Increases in inward current are displayed as positive and displacement in µm shown beside each trace. Time course of probe motion is given below the records, which are from different cells: A, 23oC; B, 3oC. Note that the time scales differ between A and B, onsets slower in the cold. A line calculated from eqn. 2 has been superimposed on each current trace. For both cells holding potential -70 mV.

of 60 µs and a slower component decreasing with stimulus amplitude from 240 to 100 µs. In the latter case, however, it seems possible that the time course is limited, particularly at the highest levels by the time constants of the stimulation and recording systems. Assuming this is not the case for the smallest displacements, we estimate that the transduction mechanism has a Q_{10} of about 2.3, which is similar to the value reported by Corey & Hudspeth (1983).

We have no direct evidence about the nature of the kinetic processes involved. It may be that some part of the time course is dictated by mechanical relaxations within the bundle. However, the dependence of the slower time constant on stimulus level (Fig. 4) suggests that it may be determined by the gating properties of the transducer channel. Fig. 4 shows that this time constant (at 3oC) declines roughly in proportion to the fraction of current activated. A relationship of this form would arise if the transducer channel had two states, closed and open, and if the main effect of bundle displacement were to modulate the opening rate constant.

Discussion

The transducer conductance derived for a hair cell in the intact basilar papilla is larger and has a more asymmetric dependence on the mechanical stimulus than in solitary cells. The difference in magnitude might be due in part at least to the different ionic compositions of the solutions bathing the hair bundles: the isolated cells are completely surrounded by perilymph, whereas the bundles in the intact organ face a high K^+, low Ca^{2+} endolymph. The low Ca^{2+} in particular might be expected to augment the conductance (Corey & Hudspeth, 1983). With regard to the asymmetry, it seems

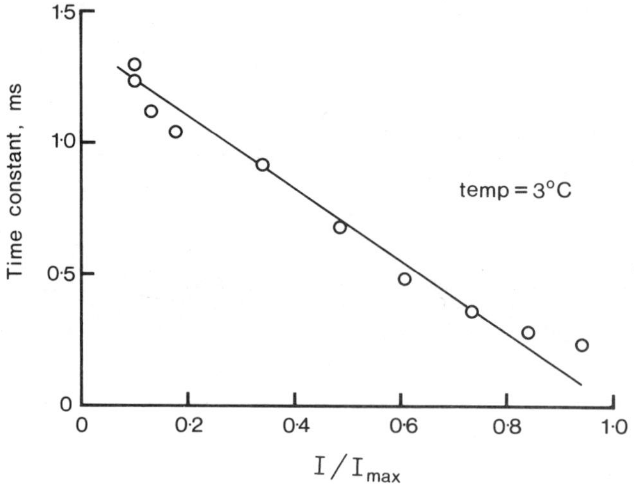

FIGURE 4 The slow time constant of the onset of the transducer current is plotted against the fraction of the steady-state current activated by bundle displacement (I/I_{max}). All measurements for movements towards the kinocilium. Same cell as Fig. 3B, temp. 3°C, I_{max} 80 pA. Line drawn through points by eye.

unlikely that the symmetrical sound pressure variations resulted in a rectified motion of the basilar or tectorial membranes. The measurements were performed in the presence of TEA, which if it were to produce a voltage-dependent block of the transducer channel at membrane potentials around the resting potential, might have distorted the conductance-stimulus relationship and accentuated the asymmetry. However no such blocking action of TEA has previously been reported (Corey & Hudspeth, 1979; Ohmori, 1985). Since significant asymmetry is still apparent in isolated cells, it seems most reasonable to conclude that it is an inherent property of the bundle mechanics or channel gating and that it is more pronounced in the intact papilla. It is worth noting that an asymmetry of the type observed is a requirement for maximum transducer sensitivity around the resting position coupled with the ability to generate sustained summating potentials at high frequencies. An asymmetrical transducer relationship has been deduced from voltage recordings in hair cells of the mammalian cochlea (Russell, Cody & Richardson, 1986) where this property is of clear importance.

Our observations on the kinetics of the transducer current are in general agreement with those of Corey & Hudspeth (1983), though it should be pointed out that in their experiments, the mechanical stimuli were administered indirectly to the otolithic membrane, and the cells were not properly voltage-clamped. To decide whether all or only part of the time course is determined by the behaviour of the transducer channel, it will be necessary to make more refined measurements of the motion of the hair bundle in response to mechanical stimuli. The kinetics of the transducer current at room temperature are more rapid than those of the voltage-dependent currents in turtle hair cells (Art & Fettiplace, 1987), and therefore transduction is never the limiting process. If however the time constants are extrapolated to 38°C on the basis of a Q_{10} of 2.3, the current would turn on in about 65 μs for small deflexions of the bundle. This time constant corresponds to a corner frequency of only 2.5 kHz, which does not seem compatible with the operation of mammalian cochlear hair cells at high frequencies.

One conclusion might be that either the channel properties or the bundle mechanics have been redesigned in mammals to enable the hair cells to generate periodic transducer currents up to frequencies of tens of kilohertz.

Acknowledgments

This research was supported by grants from the Medical Research Council and the Howe Fund of the Royal Society.

References

Art, J.J. & Fettiplace, R. (1987) Variation of membrane properties in hair cells isolated from the turtle cochlea. J. Physiol. 385, 207-242.

Art, J.J., Crawford, A.C. & Fettiplace, R. (1986) Ionic currents in solitary turtle hair cells. In: Auditory frequency selectivity (Eds: Moore, B.C.J. & Patterson, R.D.) Plenum Press, New York, pp. 81-88.

Corey, D.P. & Hudspeth, A.J. (1979) Ionic basis of the receptor potential in a vertebrate hair cell. Nature 281, 675-677.

Corey, D.P. & Hudspeth, A.J. (1983) Kinetics of the receptor current in bullfrog saccular hair cells. J. Neurosci. 3, 962-976.

Crawford, A.C. & Fettiplace, R. (1980) The frequency selectivity of auditory nerve fibres and hair cells in the cochlea of the turtle. J. Physiol. 306, 79-125.

Crawford, A.C. & Fettiplace, R. (1981) Non-linearities in the responses of turtle cochlear hair cells. J. Physiol. 315, 317-338.

Crawford, A.C. & Fettiplace, R. (1983) Auditory nerve responses to imposed displacements of the turtle basilar membrane. Hearing Res. 12, 199-208.

Crawford, A.C. & Fettiplace, R. (1985) The mechanical properties of ciliary bundles of turtle cochlear hair cells. J. Physiol. 364, 359-379.

Crawford, A.C. & Fettiplace, R. (1987) A substage cooling attachment for Zeiss IM microscopes. J. Physiol. 396, 13P.

Holton, T. & Hudspeth, A.J. (1986) The transduction channel of hair cells from bull-frog characterized by noise analysis. J. Physiol. 375, 195-227.

Hudspeth, A.J. & Corey, D.P. (1977) Sensitivity, polarity and conductance change in the response of vertebrate hair cells to controlled mechanical stimuli. Proc. Nat. Acad. Sci. U.S.A. 74, 2407-2411.

Ohmori, H. (1985) Mechano-electrical transduction currents in isolated vestibular hair cells. J.Physiol. 359, 189-217.

Ohmori, H. (1986) Gating properties of the mechano-electrical transducer channel in the dissociated vestibular hair cell of the chick. J. Physiol. 387, 589-609.

Russell, I.J., Cody, A.R. & Richardson, G.P. (1986) The responses of inner and outer hair cells in the basal turn of the guinea pig cochlea and in the mouse cochlea grown in vitro. Hearing Res. 22, 199-216.

TRANSDUCER MOTOR COUPLING IN COCHLEAR OUTER HAIR CELLS

J.F.Ashmore

Department of Physiology
Medical School
University Walk
Bristol BS8 1TD, UK

Introduction

Although many lines of evidence point to the outer hair cell as the element which controls basilar membrane mechanics, the precise nature of the interaction within the cochlear partition remains obscure. A minimum requirement of several theoretical models is that any work done by the outer hair cells on the basilar membrane has to occur synchronously with the movement of the membrane (e.g. Neely & Kim, 1986; Giesler, 1986). If so, outer hair cells must generate forces at acoustic rates. Isolated outer hair cells do indeed possess a high frequency motility (Ashmore 1987a), indicating that force is generated at rates too high to involve enzymatic intermediates, but probably based on simple physico-chemical mechanisms. If outer hair cells do function to oppose the basilar membrane fluid damping such dynamic forces need to be about three orders of magnitude less than the static deflection forces of the basilar membrane.

The questions addressed here are: 1) how large are the forces produced by the outer hair cells; 2) what activates these forces; and 3) what structures within outer hair cells might be responsible for force generation?

Methods

The experiments used tight-seal whole-cell recording to study the electrical properties of outer hair cells (OHC) isolated from the guinea pig organ of Corti and placed in short term culture. Isolation, optical and electrical recording techniques have been described elsewhere, (Ashmore, 1987a). Cells 60-80 μm in length from the apical portions of the organ of

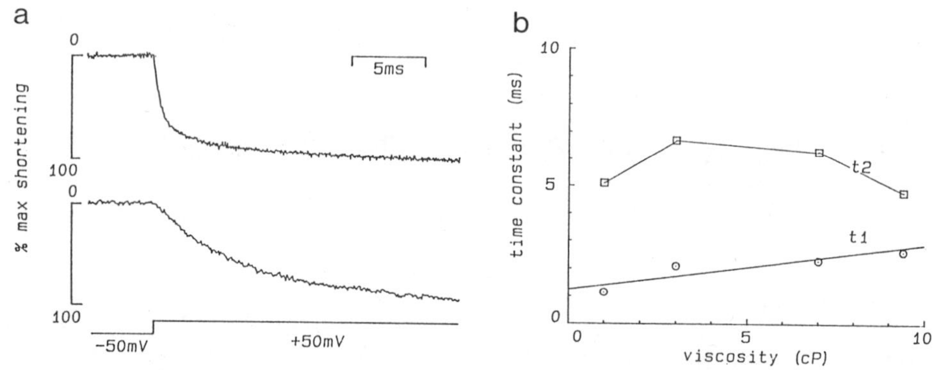

FIGURE 1 The effects of external viscosity on shortening of an OHC. a) Two cells in media of viscosity 1cP (above) and 9.5cP (below). b) Exponential time constants, t1, t2, obtained by 'pealing' length relaxations of 4 cells in different viscous L-15 media. Initial delay, typically 100us, has been ignored. Linear fit to t1 data, slope 0.115 ms/cP. Cells held at -50mV, +100mV depolarizing command steps. There was no significant difference in the steady state outward currents which settled within 3ms. Pipettes contained (mM): K (140), BAPTA (10). Signal averages, 100x.

Corti were used. It was estimated that the cells could be space-clamped essentially within 100μs. Data was sampled at rates of either 62.5kHz or 30.3kHz at repetition rates of 4Hz. The viscosities of the bathing solution, (L-15, GIBCO, 1x) were changed using methyl cellulose (concentrations not exceeding 1%), and viscosity was measured by capillary flow relative to water, (η=1cP). No significant increase in solution osmolality was detected. For solution viscosities above 20cP the cells could not be optically visualized and took an excessively long time to settle.

Results

FORCES PRODUCED BY OUTER HAIR CELLS

By placing cells in solutions of different viscosity, a measure of the force was obtained (Figure 1). From the rate of maximum length change (2mm/s), measured by a photosensor in standard extracellular solution, the maximum force under isokinetic constraints can be estimated to be about 200pN (Ashmore 1987a). This suggests that the passive stiffness of the cell would be of about the same magnitude, 100pN-1nN/μm

Fitting the initial length change by exponential time constants, it was found that the smallest time constant, representing the maximum velocity of increase, varied by a factor of only about 2.5 over a decade change of external viscosity. Modelling viscous forces as two dashpots in parallel, the data suggest that viscous damping from internal sources is about 10x that of the viscous damping in normal external media, (cf. Jen & Steele, 1987). Thus, under more nearly isometric conditions of force generation occurring in the intact cochlea, forces in excess of 1nN may be achieved, comparable to theoretical basilar membrane damping forces.

COUPLING OF FORCES TO THE APICAL TRANSDUCTION SITE

Patch clamp experiments indicate that OHC motility is driven by membrane potential (Ashmore, 1987a). Deflection of the stereocilia of OHC using a probe employing viscous coupling to the prcesses produced an inward current in the cell. This current was maximally 40pA at a trans-apical membrane potential of 160mV (Ashmore 1987b). Such currents correspond to a receptor potential of about 5mV, similar to that described in the intact cochlea (Dallos, 1985.).

The receptor current in isolated hair cells showed saturation with stimulus displacement. It also summated during repetitive stimulation, with a time course that followed the fluid movement. Assuming that mechanical gating of the apical transducer generates the length changes, an upper bound to the power available to drive OHC motility would be about 10^{-14}W for an input cell conductance of 20nS.

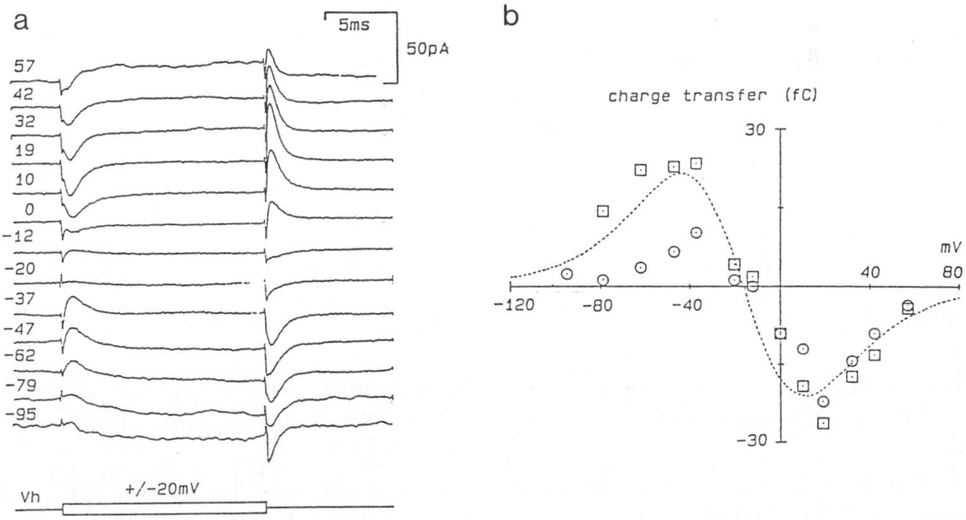

FIGURE 2 Asymmetrical current flow at early times. a) Cell voltage clamped at potentials shown. 20mV steps applied as an alternating sequence. Average of 250 pairs shown at each potential. Patch pipette contained (mM): CsCl (140), HEPES (5), pH 7.3; external solution, L-15 with 30mM Cs replacing equivalent Na. b) Integrated charge at ON (circles) and at OFF (squares) vs holding potential OFF charge reversed in sign. Continuous curve is Eqn (2) with K=25mV, V_0=-20mV and Q_{tot}=350fC.

ASYMMETRICAL CHARGE MOVEMENTS IN OUTER HAIR CELLS

Asymmetric movement of charge across the membrane was observed (Figure 2) using the experimental protocols used to study gating currents in axonal and muscle membranes (Keynes, 1983; Chandler et al, 1976). In this procedure equal and opposite pulses are summed to measure the departure from a simple RC cell membrane.

The maximum charge displaced by 20mV pulses was 30fC, i.e. about 5% of the total charge moved across the membrane when charging the cell capacitance. Currents reversed between -50 and -20mV. The simple exponential relaxation of these currents suggest that they arise from the difference between two first order current relaxations. Although some residual ionic currents contribute, it seems probable that currents arise from a voltage-dependent capacitance of the OHC membrane. No such asymmetry currents were observed with the pipette in the bath alone, or with the pipette recording whole cell from a control cell (an outer pillar cell).

The gating charge can be fitted by a simple two-state Boltzmann model for the probability distribution of a particle in a potential V:

$$f(V) = 1/(1 + \exp(-(V-V_0)/K) \qquad (1)$$

where K=RT/zbF, b is the fraction of the membrane potential in which the particle moves, z its valence, and V_0 the potential at equi-distribution of the particle (Adrian & Almers, 1976)

Using summation of equal and opposite pulses of magnitude ΔV, the asymmetrical charge transfer can be fitted approximately by

$$\Delta Q = Q_{tot}\, d^2F/dV^2.(\Delta V)^2 \qquad (2)$$

where Q_{tot} is the maximum charge that can be transferred

A fit is shown in Figure 2b, with K=25mV. This suggests that the apparent valence of the particle is 1. In muscle, the apparent valence is 2 (Adrian & Almers, 1976), and in neurones it is 3-6 (Kostyuk, et al, 1981). These systems also show more complex inactivation kinetics. However, like these gating currents, OHC asymmetry currents could be reduced by cell dialysis with isotonic fluoride. The currents were also blocked by bath application of La^{3+} (3mM) which was sufficient to prevent motile responses in the cell. In the absence of such ions cells immobilised on the bottom of the chamber still had measurable ionic currents and charge movements associated with them.

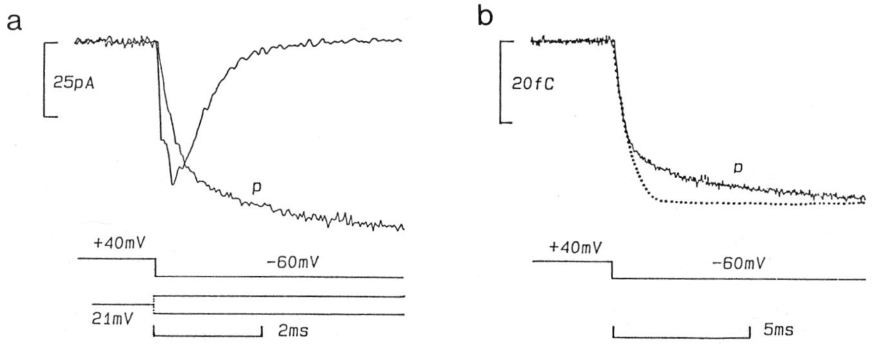

FIGURE 3 Comparison between asymmetry currents and cell length changes. a) Asymmetry current at pulse onset, (holding potential, +21mV) vs. cell shortening, (-100mV step from +40mV). b) Charge transfer, (integral of current in (a), dotted line) vs. cell shortening, normalized to same asymptote. Holding potentials chosen to overlapping command potentials. Photosensor responses labelled p, signal averaged 100x. Pipette contained (mM): CsCl (140), HEPES (5), pH 7.3.

CHARGE TRANSFER AND OUTER HAIR CELL MOTILITY

The charge movement has a latency too short to be measured with the present techniques (Figure 3a). The exponential time constant of its decay (1-2mS), although clearly voltage dependent below -90mV and above +50mV, is comparable to that of the cell length change. The integrated response matched the cell length change quite well (Figure 3b). This suggests that the charge movement may precede cell length changes, and might be the event generating the longitudinal forces.

Discussion

A SIMPLE MODEL FOR OUTER HAIR CELL FORCE PRODUCTION

The simplest model to account for the results is one where structures associated with the plasma membrane produce forces (Ashmore, 1987a; Holley and Ashmore, 1988). Changes in the tension of the plasma membrane are coupled hydrostatically to produce the observed length changes in the OHC. This model can also be represented by a passive longitudinal spring compressed by a voltage-dependent spring. It is proposed that this latter element is controlled by the mechanoelectric transducer.

The results can be interpreted as the transfer of a maximum of about 0.35pC or $2x10^6$ elementary charges across the cell membrane when the cell is polarized, i.e about 5% of the membrane capacitance is potential sensitive. One possibility is that redistributed charge alters the

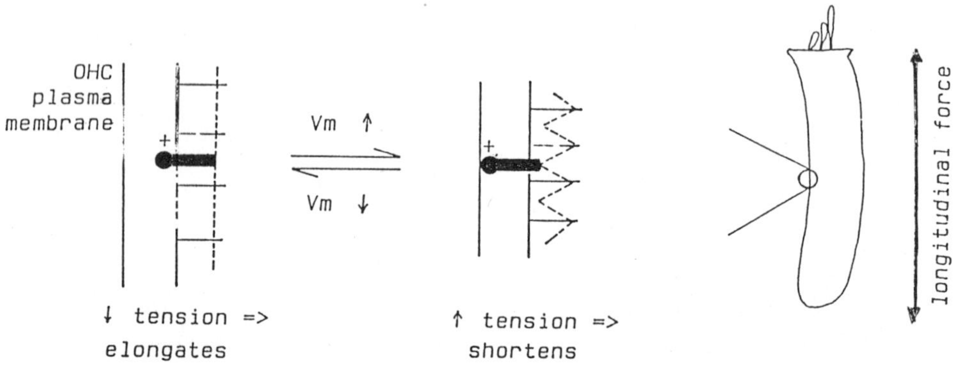

Figure 4 A model for charge movements in the OHC basolateral membrane. Depolarization moves positive charge outward. A linkage is shown which couples charge displacement to forces within the plane of the plasmalemma. The restoring forces are not shown.

membrane surface tension and gives rise to an intracellular pressure change. However, it is tempting to associate such charge displacement with the specialized network of filaments and pillar structures associated with the OHC plasmalemma (Flock et al., 1986; Bannister, 1988). This network has a lattice unit of 30nmx50nm and there would be about 10^6 such units ceach containing a pillar linking the subsurface cisternae with the membrane in an apical OHC 70μm long.

Figure 4 shows a hypothetical scneme which would couple the charge displacement to force generation by supposing that the movement distorts the network. In this scheme, a passive, element, possibly associated with the elastic properties of the network is required to lengthen the cell after shortening. It has been pointed out that there are similarities between the OHC pillars and elements responsible for excitation-contraction coupling between the T-tubule system and the sarcoplasmic reticulum of skeletal muscle (Flock et al, 1986). The higher valency of the associated charge movement found in muscle suggests the parallel is not complete. Nevertheless, the presence of a positive charge in the membrane which is linked to cell forces could explain a number of the actions of exogenously applied as well as intracellularly released cations on the cell which are reported to induce (irreversible) cell shortening.

The high frequency gain of the proposed coupling between mechano-electric transduction and forces in the cell is reduced by the RC time constant associated with membrane potential filtering. At low frequencies the potential generated by mechano-electric transduction would not be attenuated. If there is an additional series resistance between the capacitance formed by the membrane bilayer and the axis core, possibly associated with the space subjacent to the plasmalemma, then the charge which generates the observed asymmetry current could sense an unfiltered membrane potential. In this case high frequency gain would increase. In addition, the nonlinear membrane capacitance will also enhance gain slightly at high frequencies. It should be noted that the mechanism described is linear for small potential changes, but any nonlinearity of the OHC mechano-electric transducer would appear as a saturation of the forces at large vibration amplitudes of the cochlear partition.

Acknowledgements

This work was supported by the Medical Research Council. I thank Drs Matthew Holley and Bob Meech for discussion and critical comments.

References

Adrian, R. H. & Almers, W. (1976) Charge movement in the membrane of striated muscle. J.Physiol. 254,339-360.

Ashmore, J. F. (1987a) A fast motile response in guinea pig outer hair cells: the cellular basis of the cochlear amplifier. J.Physiol. 388,323-347.

Ashmore, J. F. (1987b) A mechanically evoked current in outer hair cells isolated from the guinea pig cochlea. J.Physiol. 392,37P

Bannister, L. (1988) The cortical lattice: a highly ordered system of subsurface filaments in guinea pig cochlear outer hair cells. Prog. Br. Res.74.

Chandler, W. K., Rakowski, R.F.,& Schneider, M.F. (1976) A non-linear voltage-dependent charge movement in frog skeletal muscle. J.Physiol. 254,245-284.

Dallos, P. (1985) Response characteristics of mammalian cochlear hair cells. J.Neurosci. 5,1591-1608.

Flock, A.,Flock. B and Uhlfendahl, M.(1986) Mechanisms of movement in outer hair cells and a possible structural basis. Arch Otorhinolaryngol. 243,83-90.

Geisler, D. (1986) A model of the effect of outer hair cell motility on cochlear vibrations. Hearing Res. 24,125-132.

Holley, M. C. & Ashmore, J. F. (1988) On the mechanism of a high frequency force generator in outer hair cells isolated from the guinea pig cochlea. Proc Roy. Soc. Lond. B. 232,413-429.

Jen, D. H. & Steele, C. R. (1987) Electrokinetic model of hair cell motility. J. Acoust. Soc. Am. 82,1667-1678.

Keynes, R.D. (1983) Voltage-gated ion channels in membranes. Proc Roy Soc,. Lond. B. 220,1-30.

Kostyuk, P.G., Krishtal, O.A. & Pidoplichko, V.I. (1981) Calcium inward current and and related charge movements in in the membrane of snail neurones. J.Physiol. 310,402-422.

Neely, S.T. & Kim, D.O.(1986) A model for active elements in cochlear biomechanics. J.Acoust. Soc. Am. 79,1472-1480.

Comment and Discussion

MOUNTAIN

Your results suggest that it is highly unlikely that the rapid length changes observed in isolated cells could act to reduce the damping in the intact cochlea. A simple interpretation of the data in your fig. 1 would be that the slow (5 msec) time constant represents the time it takes for the force to develop and the short time constant represents the mechanical load. In the intact cochlea the force generation would need to act on a cycle-by-cycle basis at frequencies perhaps as high as 100 to 200 kHz in some species. Electromechanical responses measured in intact cochleas have a rate limiting time constant of 35 usec or less (Mountain, 1986). Even if we assume that the force which gives rise to the length change develops instantaneously, then your results suggest that rate of contraction is limited by the cells own viscous damping. It seems unlikely that if the cell is incapable of overcoming its own damping at low frequencies that it could serve to reduce the damping of the basilar membrane at high frequencies.

Mountain, D.C. (1986) Electromechanical properties of hair cells. In: Neurobiology of Hearing. The Cochlea. (Eds. Altschuler, R.A., Bobbin, R.P. and Hoffnan, D.W.), Raven Press, New York, pp. 77-90.

ASHMORE

The internal viscous drag becomes critical for OHC when they change length at acoustic frequencies - for most cells it probably does not matter. It seems possible that outer hair cells have in fact minimized their internal viscosity by placing the nucleus at the basal end while concentrating organelles around the cortex. Even so, my estimates for internal viscosity may be underestimates because cells were recorded with whole cell dialysis using a saline solution and any additional material in the bath would also have tended to increase the external viscous drag. However, shorter cells from the basal end would be expected to have a smaller internal viscosity, and thus would work better in the acoustic frequency range. This matches a trend seen in Fig 6 of Mountain's reference where the cut-off frequency for electric acoustic emissions is higher in the basal turns.

The point raised seems to be a difficulty for models of outer hair cell function involving longitudinal force generation. More needs to be clarified about critical loads within the cochlear partition. Nevertheless, an alternative suggestion, that OHC action is mediated by changes in stereocilial pivotal stiffness, appears currently to have little direct experimental support. The dependence of longitudinal OHC forces on membrane potential produces forces of the correct phase to oppose basilar membrane damping forces at acoustic frequencies, but it is clearly necessary to make direct measurements of OHC forces.

PATUZZI

What is the possibility that some of the "gating charges" you observe are not actually due to transient, and possibly nonlinear, changes in the total membrane capacitance of the motile cell, which must undergo a complicated shape change during movement?

ASHMORE

I agree that cell deformation could, in principle, produce a gating current if the membrane curvature or thickness changed and thereby redistributed charge. This contribution is probably small for two reasons: firstly, the asymmetry currents could also be observed in cells effectively immobilized by high viscosity media, or stuck down to the bottom of the chamber; and secondly, such a contribution should reverse when the effective potential across the membrane bilayer is 0mV. There was no evidence for this reversal on the curves for the total charge transferred, which followed the Boltzmann function.

This comment was presented as a poster during the meeting.

STRUCTURE OF THE CORTICAL CYTOSKELETON OUTER HAIR CELLS FROM THE GUINEA PIG ORGAN OF CORTI

M.C. Holley and J.F. Ashmore

Department of Physiology, The Medical School, University Walk, Bristol. BS8 1TD

The mechanism of the length changes observed in outer hair cells isolated from the guinea pig (Brownell et al. 1985; Ashmore, 1987) is probably closely associated with the full length of the lateral plasma membrane (Holley and Ashmore, 1988). The structure of this region was studied in isolated cells which were extracted with 0.5% Triton X-100 in the presence of a buffer designed to stabilise cytoskeletal components (Fey et al., 1984). Triton-extraction removed the plasma membrane, lateral cisternae and 60-70% of the total cellular protein. Remaining structures included the cuticular plate, with its bundle of stereocilia and cytoplasmic processes, and the nucleus; these structures were connected by a self-supporting cytoskeletal sleeve which accurately outlined the original cell-shape. The sleeve possessed sufficient elasticity to restore its shape following small mechanical displacements with a micropipette.

Electron microscopy revealed that the sleeve was composed of circumferential filaments, 5-8nm in diameter and 40-50nm apart, which were pitched at a mean angle of 15° to the transverse axis of the cell. Circumferential filaments were cross-linked at 12-25nm intervals by thinner filaments 2-3nm in diameter. The sleeve was located between the plasma membrane and the lateral cisternae of the normal cell, in the region referred to as the sub-plasma membrane (Lim, 1986). Previous evidence suggests that the pillars described from the same region (Saito, 1983; Flock et al., 1986) are interconnected by fine filaments (Bannister et al., 1988). The spatial pattern of the pillars corresponds to that of the circumferential filaments, and images from extracted cells suggest that the pillars are attached to the circumferential filaments, projecting outward towards the plasma membrane.

We have modelled the cytoskeletal sleeve as a helical spring in which adjacent coils are cross-linked. The sleeve must confer significant passive elastic properties on the outer hair cell *in vivo*, and may be an important component of the force-generating mechanism which underlies cell length changes.

This work was supported by the M.R.C.

References

Ashmore, J.F. (1987) A fast motile response in guinea pig outer hair cells: The cellular basis of the cochlear amplifier. J. Physiol. 388, 323-347.

Bannister, L.H., Dodson, H.C., Astbury, A.F. and Douek, E.E. (1988) The cortical lattice: A highly ordered system of subsurface filaments in guinea pig cochlear outer hair cells. Prog. Brain Res. 74. (In press)

Brownell, W.E., Bader, C.R., Bertrand, D. and de Ribaupierre, I. (1985) Evoked mechanical responses of isolated cochlear outer hair cells. Science 227, 194-196.

Fey, E.G., Wan, K. and Penman, S. (1984) .... J. Cell Biol. 98, 1973-1984.

Flock, A., Flock, B. and Ulfendahl, M. (1986) Mechanisms of movement in outer hair cells and a possible structural basis. Archiv. Otorhinolaryngol. 243, 83-90.

Holley, M.C. and Ashmore, J.F. (1988) On the mechanism of a high frequency force-generator in outer hair cells isolated from the guinea pig cochlea. Proc. Roy. Soc. B232, 413-429.

Lim, D.J. (1986) Functional structure of the organ of Corti: A Review. Hearing Res. 22, 117-146.

Saito, K. (1983) Fine structure of the sensory epithelium of guinea pig organ of Corti: Subsurface cisterna and lamellar bodies in the outer hair cells. Cell Tissue Res. 229, 467-481.

GATING COMPLIANCE, A REDUCTION IN HAIR-BUNDLE STIFFNESS ASSOCIATED WITH THE GATING OF TRANSDUCTION CHANNELS IN HAIR CELLS FROM THE BULLFROG'S SACCULUS

A. J. Hudspeth, W. M. Roberts, and J. Howard

Department of Physiology
University of California School of Medicine
San Francisco, California 94143-0444, USA

Introduction

The electrical response of any organ of the internal ear or lateral-line system depends upon the hair cell's sensitivity to mechanical stimulation. This mechanosensitivity resides in the hair bundle, a cluster of 20-300 stereocilia that extends from the apical surface of the cell. Sound, acceleration, or water motion causes movement of an accessory structure such as a tectorial membrane, otolithic membrane, or cupula, which in turn deflects the hair bundle's tip. By opening transduction channels, excitatory deflection then produces a depolarizing receptor potential which modulates the cell's release of synaptic transmitter and hence the activity in eighth-nerve fibers.

Our earlier experiments on the kinetics of transduction suggested that stimulation opens channels by increasing the tension in elastic elements attached to the channels' molecular gates (Corey and Hudspeth, 1983; Howard *et al.*, 1988). If hair-bundle motion is indeed communicated directly to channels *via* such gating springs, it should be possible to detect in the bundle mechanical changes that correspond to the opening and closing of the channels. When a hair bundle's tip is displaced, the stimulus performs work against elastic elements in the bundle; some portion of that work is presumably done on the gating springs themselves. If this is so, it can be shown from thermodynamic principles that the opening and closing of transduction channels will affect the bundle's stiffness. More specifically, the mechanical give contributed by movement of the channels' gates should make the hair bundle less stiff over the range of displacements in which channels are opening and closing.

Methods

THEORY

Figure 1 shows the essential features of the gating-spring model for regulation of a mechanoreceptive channel (Corey and Hudspeth, 1983; Hudspeth, 1985a; Howard and

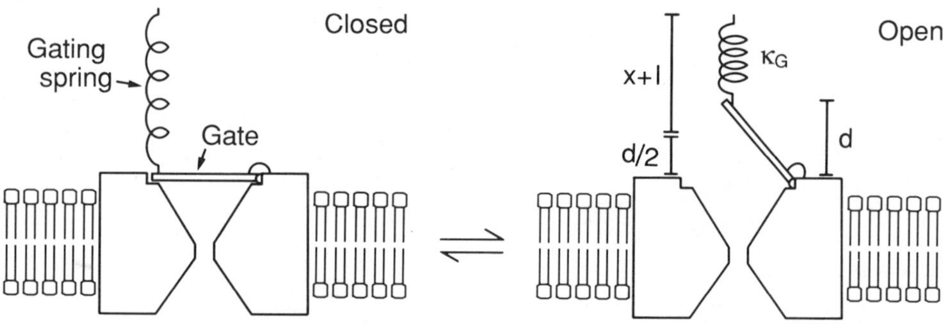

FIGURE 1 Schematic model of a transduction element in a hair bundle. Each element comprises an ion channel and an elastic element of stiffness κ_G, the gating spring, which is attached to the channel's molecular gate. With the gate in its open position, the spring is extended a distance $x - d/2$ beyond its natural length, l; closing of the channel farther lengthens the spring by a distance d.

Hudspeth, 1988; Howard *et al.*, 1988). For simplicity, it is assumed that the transduction channel can exist in either of only two conformations, closed or open. The channel is connected to an elastic gating spring, which is tensed by displacement of the hair bundle in the positive direction. If x_r is the spring's resting extension when the bundle is undisturbed, the extension of each gating spring, x, is

$$x = \gamma X + x_r$$

when the bundle's tip is displaced a distance X and when the gate is midway between its open and closed positions. The geometrical gain, γ, is determined by the arrangement of the gating springs within the hair bundle. If, for example, each stereociliary tip link (Pickles *et al.*, 1984) is a gating spring, then γ is approximately equal to the ratio of the spacing between stereocilia to the height at which the displacement, X, is measured. Because the mean stereociliary spacing along the axis of stimulation is 0.95 µm and the height of the kinociliary bulb at which forces are applied is 6.7 µm, γ is about 0.14 in the bullfrog's sacculus (Howard *et al.*, 1988).

Let each gating spring's stiffness be κ_G and let the difference in the spring's length between the open and closed states, the swing of the channel's gate, be d. For a transduction element comprising the spring and channel, the energy content when the channel is closed is

$$g_c^0 = \kappa_G(x + d/2)^2/2 + \mu_c^0.$$

Here μ_c^0 is the molecular free energy of the closed channel with no tension in the spring. The corresponding energy of the transduction element's open state is

$$g_o^0 = \kappa_G(x - d/2)^2/2 + \mu_o^0;$$

μ_o^0 is the molecular free energy of the open channel with a relaxed spring. The difference in energy when the channel opens is therefore

$$\Delta g^0 = g_o{}^0 - g_c{}^0 = -\kappa_G dx + \mu_o{}^0 - \mu_c{}^0.$$

By Boltzmann's law, the probability (p) of finding the channel in the open state when the system is in equilibrium is

$$p = [1 + \exp(\Delta g^0/kT)]^{-1},$$

in which k is the Boltzmann constant and T is the absolute temperature. From the equations above, the probability of a channel's being open in the steady state satisfies a Boltzmann relation,

$$p = \{1 + \exp[-z(X - X_0)/kT]\}^{-1}.$$

The single-channel gating force, z, which indicates the transducer's sensitivity to displacement, is equivalent to $\kappa_G d\gamma$ (Corey and Hudspeth, 1983; Hudspeth, 1985b; Holton and Hudspeth, 1986); X_0 is the bundle displacement at which $p = 1/2$. If the transduction elements are identical, then the steady-state transduction current is proportional to p and has a sigmoidal dependence on bundle displacement.

The mean free energy per transduction element, g, comprises an enthalpic component, h, and an entropic contribution, s. Because the volume change of the transduction element as the channel opens and closes is expected to be very small, the pressume-volume work can be ignored. The enthalpy is then the element's mean potential energy,

$$h = pg_o{}^0 + (1 - p)g_c{}^0 = g_c{}^0 + p\Delta g^0.$$

The free energy of a transduction element is thus

$$g = h - Ts = \kappa_G(x + d/2)^2/2 + \mu_c{}^0 + (\mu_o{}^0 - \mu_c{}^0)p - \kappa_G dxp + kT[p\cdot\ln(p) + (1 - p)\cdot\ln(1 - p)].$$

The force that each transduction element exerts on its insertions, f, is the derivative of the free energy with respect to displacement;

$$f = \kappa_G(x + d/2) - \kappa_G dp.$$

The stiffness of each transduction element, which would be measured by pulling directly on one end of the gating spring, is obtained by a further differentiation as

$$\kappa_{TE} = \kappa_G - \kappa_G{}^2 d^2 p(1 - p)/kT.$$

Because of the lever ratio, γ, between spring elongation and bundle displacement, the contribution of each transduction element to the stiffness of the entire hair bundle, as measured by deflection of the bundle's tip, is

$$K_{TE} = \kappa_G\gamma^2 - \kappa_G{}^2 d^2\gamma^2 p(1 - p)/kT = \kappa_G\gamma^2 - z^2 p(1 - p)/kT.$$

The expected total stiffness for a bundle with N gating springs, K_B, is therefore

$$K_B = K_S + N\kappa_G\gamma^2 - Nz^2 p(1 - p)/kT.$$

K_S is the stiffness of elastic components in parallel with the transduction elements, such as the basal tapers about which the stereocilia pivot (Crawford and Fettiplace, 1985; Howard and Ashmore, 1986).

The calculations indicate that, when the probability of the transduction channels' being open is very low ($p \sim 0$) or very high ($p \sim 1$), the bundle's stiffness reaches an asymptotic value that reflects the elastic properties of the stereociliary pivots (K_S) and the gating springs ($N\kappa_G\gamma^2$). These values for p correspond to extensive bundle deflections in respectively the negative or the positive direction. Over an intermediate range of bundle positions, the bundle should be less stiff, or more compliant; the stiffness is at a minimum when half of the channels are open, whereupon the bundle's stiffness is $Nz^2/4kT$ below its asymptotic value. A similar result is obtained by calculation of the bundle's stiffness from the average force exerted by each transduction element (Howard and Hudspeth, 1988; Howard *et al.*, 1988).

EXPERIMENTAL PROCEDURE

Experiments were conducted on macular epithelia, dissected from the sacculi of adult male and female bullfrogs (*Rana catesbeiana*), that were maintained and observed as described previously (Hudspeth and Corey, 1977; Howard and Hudspeth, 1987a, 1987b). The preparations were generally immersed in a saline solution consisting of 110 mM Na^+, 2 mM K^+, 4 mM Ca^{2+}, 118 mM Cl^-, 3 mM D-glucose, and 5 mM HEPES at pH 7.25; some maculæ were kept in a similar medium containing only 1 mM Ca^{2+}. Experiments were conducted at a temperature of approximately 21°C in a mechanically stabilized chamber on bedrock. Recordings of receptor potentials were obtained by conventional techniques with single microelectrodes, about 200 MΩ in tip resistance, filled with 3 M KCl buffered to a pH of 8.5 with 10 mM glycylglycine.

We determined the stiffness of each hair bundle by attaching to the kinociliary bulb, near the bundle's tip, a flexible glass fiber (Flock and Strelioff, 1984; Crawford and Fettiplace, 1985; Howard and Ashmore, 1986; Howard and Hudspeth, 1987a, 1987b, 1988). The fiber, typically about 100 μm in length and 0.5 μm in diameter, was short enough to permit measurements within 250 μs after a step stimulus. When a fiber's base was moved with a piezoelectrical micromanipulator (Corey and Hudspeth, 1980), the fiber flexed as it deflected the bundle's tip. The flexion of the fiber was measured to a precision of ±0.2 nm with a photodiode detector. From the fiber's calibrated stiffness and its measured deflection, we could then determine the bundle's stiffness at any time during a response.

Results

Our experiments demonstrate the predicted gating compliance. When a bundle was deflected extensively, more than 100 nm in either the excitatory or the inhibitory direction, its stiffness was approximately 650 $\mu N \cdot m^{-1}$ (Figure 2A). Near its resting position, however, the bundle was less stiff, or more compliant, by about 300 $\mu N \cdot m^{-1}$. In a sample of 34 hair cells, the mean stiffness for large displacements was 930 $\mu N \cdot m^{-1}$, while the minimal stiffness, measured with the bundle displaced an average of 22 nm positive to its resting position, was approximately 540 $\mu N \cdot m^{-1}$.

Simultaneous recordings of receptor potentials indicated that the range of bundle displacements over which the compliance increased corresponded to the range in which transduction channels opened and closed (Figure 2C). From the fit of a Boltzmann relation to the record shown, the receptor-potential data indicate a value for the single-channel gating force, z, of 248 fN. When fitted by the expression for hair-bundle stiffness, the corresponding data from the mechanical experiment (Figure 2B) yield a

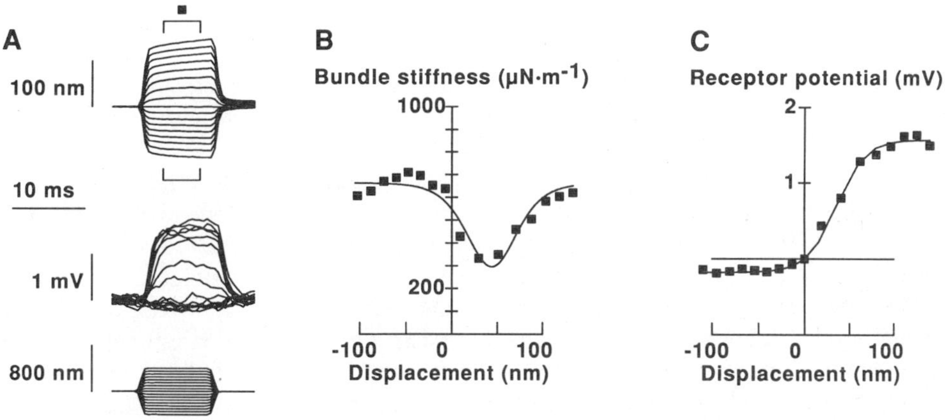

FIGURE 2 Demonstration of the gating compliance and its relation to mechanoelectrical transduction. *A)* Movements of the base of a flexible glass fiber (bottom set of traces) imposed force pulses on a hair bundle at the height of the kinociliary bulb. The displacements of the bundle's tip (top traces) elicited receptor potentials (middle traces) from a hair cell bathed in saline solution containing 1 mM Ca^{2+}. *B)* Plot of the bundle's stiffness determined from measurements in the bracketed region of the top set of traces in *A*. Although the bundle's stiffness was about 650 $\mu N \cdot m^{-1}$ for large displacements, the stiffness declined by roughly 300 $\mu N \cdot m^{-1}$ near the bundle's resting position. The continuous curve is a plot of K_B from the final equation of the Theory section. *C)* Plot of the displacement-response relation for the same hair cell. The transducer's sensitivity, as measured by averaging each response in the bracketed portion of the record, peaked at the same bundle displacement for which the bundle's stiffness reached a minimum. The range of bundle displacements in which the compliance increased also corresponded to the range over which the electrical reponse changed. The continuous curve represents a Boltzmann function, the theoretical displacement-response relation.

value for *z* of 218 fN. In a sample of 22 cells, the mean value for the single-channel gating force derived from mechanical measurements (290 fN) exceeded that from the simultaneously recorded electrical responses (180 fN). Although this systematic difference might indicate that the transduction channel is more complex than is portrayed in the two-state model presented above, it also remains possible that the mechanically and electrically derived values for *z* would coincide more closely if receptor currents, rather than receptor potentials, were used in the analysis.

Hair cells of the bullfrog's sacculus adapt to protracted stimulation (Eatock *et al.*, 1987). When the mechanosensitive range shifts during adaptation to prolonged stimuli, the gating compliance shifts to a similar extent (Howard and Hudspeth, 1988). A final indication that the increase in hair-bundle compliance is associated with transduction is that, like the receptor potential, the compliance increase is blocked by the ototoxic antibiotic, gentamicin.

Discussion

The demonstration of the gating compliance supports the hypothesis that the opening and closing of transduction channels in hair cells is controlled by tension in elastic gating springs. The gating of these channels operates in a manner formally similar to that of channels of other types (Howard *et al.*, 1988). The gating compliance of mechanosensitive channels is analogous, for example, to the gating capacitance contributed by voltage-sensitive channels, whose opening and closing involves the movement of charge within the transmembrane electrical field (Armstrong and Bezanilla, 1974).

The magnitude and spatial distribution of the gating compliance permit estimation of the values of several interesting features of transduction (Howard and Hudspeth, 1988). The force required to open a channel is approximately 290 fN; this value is plausible when compared with the forces thought to be exerted by molecular mechanical motors, such as myosin in muscle (Huxley and Simmons, 1971). The swing of the channel's gate is about 4 nm, a value again consistent with the motion estimated to occur during the force-producing steps of molecular motors. The results indicate that there are roughly 85 transduction channels per hair cell in the bullfrog's sacculus. Because such cells possess about 60 stereocilia apiece, there may be one channel per stereocilium. In that case, each channel may be attached to one of the morphologically demonstrable tip link between adjacent stereocilia (Pickles *et al.*, 1984). The stiffness of a gating spring, approximately 500 $\mu N \cdot m^{-1}$, is consistent with the hypothesis that each consists of a single molecular fiber of an elastic protein.

The mechanical changes in the hair bundle associated with adaptation of the receptor current (Howard and Hudspeth, 1987a, 1987b) also support the hypothesis that the gating of transduction channels depends upon tension in elastic elements. The measurements indicate that the elastic elements of the bundle undergo a rearrangement during adaptation. As the electrical response to a sustained stimulus declines with a time constant near 30 ms, the bundle's stiffness decreases at an identical rate to a steady-state value about 400 $\mu N \cdot m^{-1}$ less than the initial stiffness. Relaxation of the bundle occurs only for stimuli directed along a hair cell's axis of mechanosensitivity. The results suggest that the relaxation of gating springs results simultaneously in a reduction of the bundle's stiffness and in adaptation.

This study was motivated by our desire to understand the energetics of mechanoelectrical transduction. Deflection of a hair bundle of constant stiffness K_B through a distance X from its resting position would increase the bundle's potential energy by $K_B X^2/2$. Our naive expectation was that a fraction of this energy would be absorbed by the channels to alter their configuration (Guharay and Sachs, 1984; Hudspeth, 1985b). This line of reasoning leads to a contradiction: very small displacements would appear to increase the bundle's potential energy, which depends on the square of the displacement, by less than the resulting difference in energy between the open and closed states (zX), which depends linearly on displacement. For hair cells of the bullfrog's sacculus, this apparent paradox would arise for bundle displacements from the resting position of less than 1 nm. The difficulty is resolved by appreciating that the free energy of a transduction element includes an entropic as well as an enthalpic term. Thermodynamic analysis indicates why the force on the bundle and its derivative, the bundle's stiffness, depend on displacement: both the enthalpy and the entropy of the hair bundle depend on the configuration of the transduction channels.

Acknowledgements

The authors thank Mr. R. A. Jacobs for the construction of outstanding apparatus and preparation of figures and acknowledge the support of National Institutes of Health grant NS20429.

References

Armstrong, C. M. and Bezanilla, F. (1974) Charge movement associated with the opening and closing of the activation gates of the Na channels. J. Gen. Physiol. 63, 533-552.

Corey, D. P. and Hudspeth, A. J. (1980) Mechanical stimulation and micromanipulation with piezoelectric bimorph elements. J. Neurosci. Meth. 3, 183-202.

Corey, D. P. and Hudspeth, A. J. (1983) Kinetics of the receptor current in bullfrog saccular hair cells. J. Neurosci. 3, 962-976.

Crawford, A. C. and Fettiplace, R. (1985) The mechanical properties of ciliary bundles of turtle cochlear hair cells. J. Physiol. 364, 359-379.

Eatock, R. A., Corey, D. P., and Hudspeth, A. J. (1987) Adaptation of mechanoelectrical transduction in hair cells of the bullfrog's sacculus. J. Neurosci. 7, 2821-2836.

Flock, Å. and Strelioff, D. (1984) Sensory hairs in the mammalian hearing organ have graded and nonlinear mechanical properties. Nature 310, 597-599.

Guharay, F. and Sachs, F. (1984) Stretch-activated single ion channel currents in tissue-cultured embryonic chick skeletal muscle. J. Physiol. 352:685-701.

Holton, T. and Hudspeth, A. J. (1986) The transduction channel of hair cells from the bull-frog characterized by noise analysis. J. Physiol. 375, 195-227.

Howard, J. and Ashmore, J. F. (1986) Stiffness of sensory hair bundles in the sacculus of the frog. Hearing Res. 23, 93-104.

Howard, J. and Hudspeth, A. J. (1987a) Mechanical relaxation of the hair bundle mediates adaptation in mechanoelectrical transduction by the bullfrog's saccular hair cell. Proc. Natl. Acad. Sci. U.S.A. 84, 3064-3068.

Howard, J. and A. J. Hudspeth (1987b) Adaptation of mechanoelectrical transduction in hair cells. In: Sensory Transduction (Eds.: Hudspeth, A. J., MacLeish, P. R., Margolis, F. L., and Wiesel, T. N.) Report of the 1987 FESN Study Group; Discussions in Neurosciences, Volume IV, Number 3; *Fondation pour l'Etude du Système Nerveux Central et Périphérique*, Geneva, pp. 138-145.

Howard, J. and Hudspeth, A. J. (1988) Compliance of the hair bundle associated with gating of mechanoelectrical transduction channels in the bullfrog's saccular hair cell. Neuron 1, in press.

Howard, J., Roberts, W. M., and Hudspeth, A. J. (1988) Mechanoelectrical transduction by hair cells. Ann. Rev. Biophys. Biophys. Chem. 17, in press.

Hudspeth, A. J. (1985a) The cellular basis of hearing: the biophysics of hair cells. Science 230, 745-752.

Hudspeth, A. J. (1985b) Models for mechanoelectrical transduction by hair cells. In: Contemporary Sensory Neurobiology (Eds.: Correia, M. J. and Perachio, A. A.) Alan R. Liss, New York, pp. 193-205.

Hudspeth, A. J. and Corey, D. P. (1977) Sensitivity, polarity, and conductance change in the response of vertebrate hair cells to controlled mechanical stimuli. Proc. Natl. Acad. Sci. U.S.A. 74, 2407-2411.

Huxley, A. F. and Simmons, R. M. (1971) Proposed mechanism of force generation in striated muscle. Nature 233, 533-538.

Pickles, J. O., Comis, S. D., and Osborne, M. P. (1984) Cross-links between stereocilia in the guinea pig organ of Corti, and their possible relation to sensory transduction. Hearing Res. 15, 103-112.

SIMULTANEOUS RECORDING OF FLUCTUATIONS OF HAIR-BUNDLE DEFLECTION AND INTRA-CELLULAR VOLTAGE IN SACCULAR HAIR CELLS

Winfried Denk and Watt W. Webb

School of Applied and Engineering Physics
and Department of Physics
Cornell University, Ithaca, NY, 14853, USA

Introduction

The detection threshold of a sensory system depends on three factors: the coupling of the external stimulus such as sound pressure or acceleration to the input of the sensory cell, the transduction efficiency of the sensory cell, the transmission characteristics of the signal to the brain, and the noise associated with each stage. In this paper we describe experiments performed to elucidate the performance of sensory hair cells which are the site of mechano-electrical transduction in the inner ear of vertebrates. Mechanical deflection of the hair bundle protruding from these cells modulates the transmembrane resistance and consequently the transmembrane current and the intracellular potential. The magnitude of hair-bundle deflection necessary to obtain a significant receptor potential is determined by the size of the mechano-electrical transduction coefficient and by the amount of intracellular voltage noise.

Brownian motion of the hair bundle is expected to activate the mechano-electrical transduction mechanism, as does any mechanical stimulus, if no threshold exists for the modulation of membrane resistance by bundle deflection. The intracellular voltage noise should therefore contain a component due to the transduction of inevitable Brownian motion as well as components due to other noise soures. Transduced Brownian motion would be the sole component of the intracellular voltage noise for an ideal transducer.

Simultaneous observation of spontaneous bundle deflections (x) and intracellular voltage noise (V) provides information about the noise sources and about the transduction and tuning properties of hair cells. In the absence of electro-mechanical (reverse) transduction the fraction of the total intracellular noise spectral density due to transduced Brownian motion can be calculated from those data according to the following relation:

$$C_{xV}(f) = \frac{|X_{xV}(f)|^2}{P_x(f) \cdot P_V(f)} ,$$

where $X_{xV}(f)$ is the cross-correlation spectrum and $P_x(f)$ and $P_V(f)$ are the power spectra of the bundle position and the intracellular voltage fluctuations respectively. $C_{xV}(f)$ is also called the *coherence*; it is essentially the square of the absolute value of the correlation coefficient between the two signals as a function of frequency.

The same data permit the determination of the small signal transduction frequency response $(R_{xV}(f))$

$$R_{xV}(f) = \frac{X_{xV}(f)}{P_x(f)},$$

because the thermal motion can be viewed as a broadband noise source exciting the input of the "device under test", the hair cell. This relationship can be understood in the following way: The output noise(V_f) has one component $(R_{xV}(f) \cdot x_f)$ that is caused by transduction of the input (x_f) and another component that is independent of the mechanical input. The second component is uncorrelated with the input, therefore the sole contribution to the cross correlation $(X_{xV}(f))$ with a magnitude of $R_{xV}(f) \cdot \langle x_f^* x_f \rangle$ comes from transduced input fluctuations. By normalizing with the input power spectrum $(\langle x_f^* x_f \rangle = P_x(f))$ we obtain the above formula.

The mechano-electrical impulse response can be obtained by taking the Fourier transform of the frequency response.

Methods

Our experiments were performed on frogs of the species *Rana catesbeiana* and *Rana pipiens* using a preparation of the saccular sensory epithelium very similar to that described by Hudpeth and Corey (1977). The procedure was modified by including a 40 min enzymatic treatment in a mixture of collagenases I and II and subtilopeptidase (concentrations: 2 g·l^{-1}, 1 g·l^{-1}, and 50 mg·l^{-1}) to obtain an isolated sensory macula (A. J. Hudspeth, *personal commmunication*) which was then folded to allow the observation of hair bundles protruding horizontally from the bend. High resistance intracellular microelectrodes filled with $\approx$ 5 M potassium-acetate were used for electrical recordings. To measure the spontaneous motion of the hair bundle we developed an Optical Laser Differential Interferometer, capable of measuring the bundle displacements without attachment of a probe, over a wide bandwidth (100 kHz) with high sensitivity ($\approx 1\ pm/\sqrt{Hz}$, Denk *et al.*, 1986).

The output signals from the microelectrode amplifier and the interferometer were simultaneously filtered, digitized, recorded, and analyzed using a spectrum analyzer. Estimates of the power spectra for mechanical and electrical fluctuations and the cross correlation spectrum $(X_{xV}(f))$ between electrical and mechanical fluctuations were calculated according to the following formulas:

$$P_x(f) = \langle x_f^* x_f \rangle,$$

$$P_V(f) = \langle V_f^* V_f \rangle,$$

$$X_{xV}(f) = \langle x_f^* V_f \rangle,$$

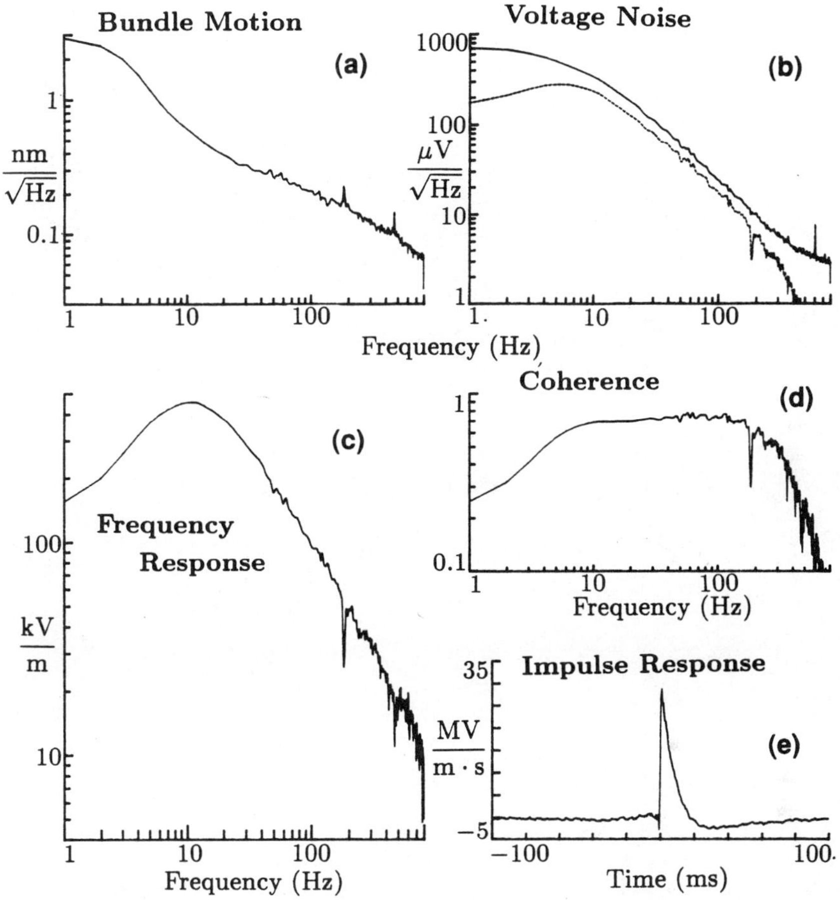

FIGURE 1: Results of a cross-correlation experiment; Power spectra of hair-bundle deflection fluctuations (a) and intracellular voltage noise (b, upper trace), transduced Brownian motion (b, lower trace), magnitude of the mechano-electrical frequency response (c) and coherence (d). Fourier transformation of the frequency response provided the impulse response (e) which shows no significant violation of causality in this case. The number of averages was 100. Peaks due to calibration motion and to line interference have been removed and the frequency domain traces have been smoothed by convolution with a Gaussian (width = 6 Hz).

where x_f and V_f are the Fourier transforms of time records of the mechanical and electrical signals. Complex conjugation is indicated by an asterisk (*). Angle brackets ($\langle\rangle$) denote averages.

For control experiments mechanical stimulation was performed by directing a pulsating jet of saline out of a micropipette (Inside diameter $\approx 5\ \mu$m) against the hair bundle. The pressure modulator driving the jet was fast enough to excite the bundle at frequencies up to several hundred Hertz. Microelectrodes filled with 0.5 M streptomycin sulfate were used to apply streptomycin iontophoretically to the hair bundles in order to block transduction (Hudspeth and Kroese, 1983).

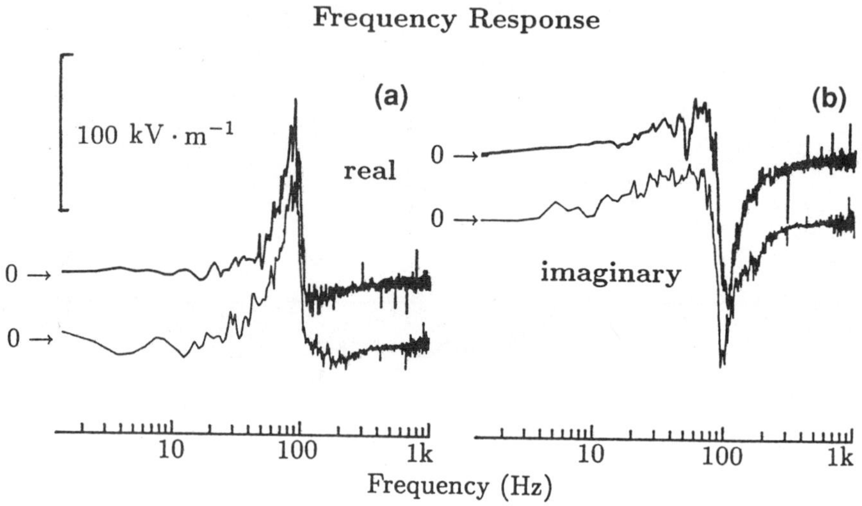

FIGURE 2: Comparison between real (a) and imaginary (b) parts of the mechano-electrical frequency response function obtained for the same cell by spontaneous noise correlation (upper traces) and stimulation with a fluid jet (lower traces). The traces have been separated vertically to eliminate overlap.

Results

As previously reported (Denk *et al.*, 1986) the spontaneous motion of saccular hair bundles shows root mean square (rms) amplitudes between 2 and 10 nm and roll off frequencies between 200 and 800 Hz. These results are consistent with the mechanical properties of these bundles as determined by direct force displacement measurements (Howard and Ashmore 1987).

The spontaneous bundle motion was frequently correlated with the intracellular electrical noise (Fig. 1). The strongest correlation usually occurred around the best frequency for electrically tuned cells (Lewis and Hudspeth, 1983). Of 41 cells, each of which had a peak coherence (maximum as a function of frequency) between mechanical and electrical signals of at least 5%, 10 cells showed peak coherences of more than 50% and 12 showed cells between 25% and 50%. In one cell (Fig. 1c) almost 75% of the intracellular noise in the range from 5 Hz to 150 Hz was correlated to bundle Brownian motion.

We also determined mechano-electrical transfer functions from the noise correlation experiments (Fig. 1d). Most peak transduction sensitivities ranged from 50 to 200 $kV{\cdot}m^{-1}$ with a few extreme cases at more than 400 $kV{\cdot}m^{-1}$. Frequency characteristics varied from a low-pass (knee frequencies 20-80 Hz) to a sharply tuned bandpass ($Q{\geq}10$, $50Hz \leq f \leq 150Hz$). Sometimes a reversible transition between these two types of frequency response could be caused by changing the membrane potential through direct current (DC) injection through the recording electrode. The shape of the electrical noise spectrum always resembled that of the transduction sensitivity. Noise-correlation was reversibly abolished by iontophoretic application

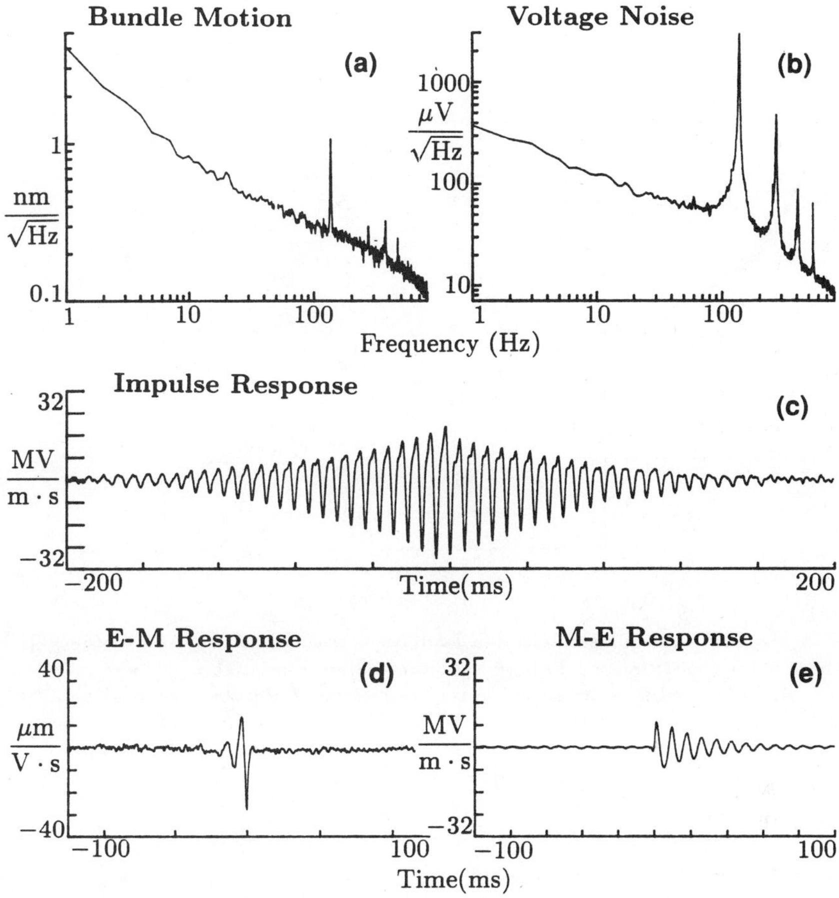

FIGURE 3: Tuned mechanical oscillation (f=136 Hz) of a hair bundle is visible as a peak in the displacement power spectrum (a) and coincides with the main peak in the electrical power spectrum (b). The calculated impulse response (c) violated causality, indicating the presence of a reverse transduction mechanism which was confirmed by broadband current injection and calculation of the electro-mechanical impulse response (d, inverted time axis). Mechanical stimulation confirmed that forward transduction was still causal (e). The ratio of the peak heights in (a) and (b) corresponds to a reverse transduction sensitivity of 366 nm/V. The reverse transduction sensitivity inferred from the current injection response is only about 178 nm/V (frequency trace not shown). The discrepancy is most likely due to an incomplete cancellation of the microelectrode series resistance leading to an overestimation of the intracellular voltage.

of streptomycin. Transfer functions agreed when measured by noise-correlation as well as by stimulating the same cell with a water jet. These results confirm that the observed correlation is indeed due to transduced Brownian motion.

The impulse response (FFT of R_{xV}) of most cells showed no significant deviations from zero along the negative part of the time axis, confirming physical causality of the mechano-electrical response of this system.

Causality was however violated by the "impulse response" of a subset of 10

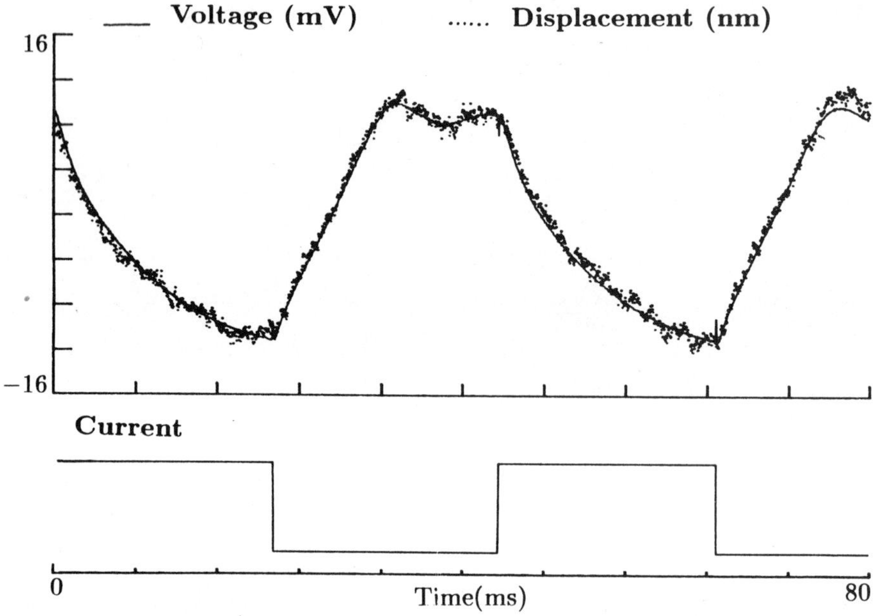

FIGURE 4: Square wave current injection leads to a mechanical response of the hair bundle (dots) whose shape closely follows the variation in membrane potential (solid line), rather than the current waveform (curve below, arbitrary units), with mechano-electrical response coefficient close to 1μm/V. A scaled version of the current waveform has been subtracted from the voltage trace to remove the remaining stimulus artifact. Curves are averages over 100 stimulus presentations.

cells, a result inconsistent with the existence of a forward transduction mechanism alone. These cells always showed sharply peaked electrical noise spectra often with harmonics at multiples of the main peak frequency. In one cell a peak in the displacement power spectrum was found coincident with the main peak in the electrical noise (Fig. 3). Peaks of the intracellular electrical noise and non-causality of the impulse response could be abolished by changing the membrane potential through current injection, whenever the attempt was made.

When injected with current in the form of broadband noise or square waves some cells showed a mechanical response with reverse transduction efficiencies of typically several hundred nm/V up to one μm/V (Fig. 4). This effect is large enough to account for the observed mechanical bundle oscillations (Fig. 3) as being reversly transduced voltage noise. It is unlikely that movements of the recording microelectrode are causing the bundle motion given our observation that the electrode can be moved by several microns laterally without interrupting the recording and without a discernible influence on bundle position and given that, as Fig. 4 shows, the movement follows the actual membrane potential of the cell. Mechanical responses to electrical stimulation have been found in cells with and without kinocilium. Current injection caused a mechanical response in all tested non-causal cells as well as in some causal cells.

The smallest detectable stimulus (for which the rms values of receptor potential and of intracellular noise are equal) has been found in some electrically tuned cells to be as much as 5 dB smaller than the rms bundle displacement due to Brownian motion.

Discussion

Our findings show that mechano-sensitive hair cells can perform close to the detection limit given by the thermal motion of the hair bundle and that some cells might even be able to detect stimuli at their best frequencies of an amplitude smaller than their total Brownian motion amplitude. The degree of correlation that we found between bundle displacement and voltage noise should probably be viewed as a lower limit because the trauma of dissection and impalement is likely to degrade transduction efficiency and increase intrinsic intracellular noise. To apply our analysis to the intact organ one has to assume that removing the otholitic membrane, to which the hair bundles are attached *in vivo*, does not change too drastically the bundle stiffness, and as a consequence the Brownian motion amplitude.

By demonstrating that the frequency response of mechano-electrical transduction can be determined purely by observing the spontaneous fluctuations of bundle position and intracellular potential without stimulation of the hair cells, we have shown that the transduction mechanism is activated by thermal motion, and therefore no displacement threshold exists for the opening of the putative transduction channels.

The appearent "non-causality" of the impulse response is most likely related to mechanical oscillation previously found in hair cells (Crawford and Fettiplace, 1985; Howard and Hudspeth, 1987). The existence of a reverse transduction mechanism driven by sharply tuned excess intracellular noise, which is sometimes observed in saccular hair cells, can account for those phenomena. The existence of reverse transduction by itself is not sufficient though for an obvious violation of causality because it was found in cells whose calculated impulse response showed no sign of causality violation. Without excess intracellular noise the degree of activation of the reverse tranduction mechanism seems to be too small to generate a significant effect.

The achievable round trip gain, viewing these hair cells as a closed loop in which mechanical input generates a electrical reaction leading to a mechanical action at the input again and using our peak values for forward and reverse transduction (400 $kV \cdot m^{-1}$ and 1 $\mu m \cdot V^{-1}$) is only 0.4, still smaller than unity, the minimum gain required for the generation of a genuine oscillation of the coupled system. It is more likely that the excess voltage noise is caused by the appearance of a negative dissipative part of the membrane impedance leading to oscillations of the membrane potential limited only by nonlinearities, a situation similar to the spontaneous firing of action potentials by neurons.

It was difficult to characterize the reverse transduction mechanism quantitatively because our electrical recordings were made with a single microelectrode. Our data nevertheless suggest that the reverse transduction mechanism depends on the membrane potential (Fig. 4) and has a frequency response faster than our recording bandwith (800 Hz). The size of the electro-mechanical transduction (less than $1\mu m \cdot V^{-1}$) is considerably smaller than the effect found in mammalian outer hair cells (Brownell, *et al.*, 1985; Ashmore, 1987) It is still unclear, as it is in the case of the mechanical contraction of nerve axons (Hill *et al.*, 1977), whether this reverse transduction mechanism has a biological function. Tuning in frog saccular hair cells does, different from the situation in the mammalian cochlea, not require a mechanical resonance (Lewis and Hudspeth, 1983).

Acknowledgements

This work was supported by grants from NIH (GM33028) and NSF (DMB8609084) and by an IBM graduate fellowship for W. D.. Furthermore we would like to mention the invaluable help from A. J. Hudspeth in the early stages of this work. We also thank R. Keolian and N. Gershenfeld for their comments on this manuscript.

References

Ashmore J. F., (1987), A fast motile response in the Guinea-pig outer hair cells: the cellular basis of the cochlear amplifier, J. Physiol. (London), 5, 323-347.

Brownell W. E., Bader C. E., Bertrand D., and Ribaupierre, (1985), Evoked Mechanical Responses of Isolated Cochlear Outer Hair Cells, Science, 5, 194-196.

Crawford A. C. and Fettiplace R., (1985), The mechanical properties of ciliary hair bundles of turtle cochlea hair cells, J. Physiol. (London), 5, 359-379.

Denk W., Hudspeth A. J., and Webb W. W., (1986), Optical Measurement of the Brownian Motion Spectrum of Hair Bundles in the Transducing Hair Cells of the Frog Auditory System, Biophys. J., 5, 21a.

Eatock R. A., Corey D. P., and Hudspeth A. J., (1987), Adaptation of Mechanoelectrical Transduction in Hair Cells of the Bullfrog's Sacculus, J. Neurosci., 5, 2821-2836.

Hill B. C., Schubert E. D., and Nokes M. A., (1977), Laser Interferometer Measurement of Changes in Crayfish Axon Diameter Concurrent with Action Potential, Science, 5, 426-428.

Howard J.and Ashmore J. F., (1986), Stiffness of sensory hairbundles in the sacculus of the frog, Hearing Res., 5, 93-104.

Howard J. and Hudspeth A. J., (1987), Mechanical relaxation of the hair bundle mediates adaptation in mechano-electrical transduction by the bullfrog's saccular hair cells, Proc. Natl. Acad. Sci. USA, 5, 3064-3068.

A.J. Hudspeth and A.B.A Kroese, (1983), Voltage dependent interaction of dihydrostreptomycin with the transduction channels in bullfrog sensory hair cells, J. Physiol. (London), 5, 66P.

Lewis E. R. and Hudspeth A. J., (1983), Voltage- and ion-dependent conductances in solitary hair cells, Nature, 5, 538-541.

Comments and Discussion

LEWIS

The presence of bidirectional transduction in bullfrog saccular hair cells, as shown by the data presented in this paper, opens the way for exchange of energy between the electrical resonances of neighbouring hair cells. Thus it is possible that the resonant system described by Lewis and Hudspeth (Lewis, 1985) is part of a filter with high-order dynamics, and could account for the high-order dynamics observed in the afferent axons from the intact sacculus.

Lewis, R.S. (1985) The Ionic Basis of Frequency Selectivity in Hair Cells of the Bullfrog's Sacculus. Ph.D. Dissertation, California Institute of Technology, Pasadena, California.

MICROMECHANICAL MOVEMENTS OF CHICK SENSORY HAIR BUNDLES TO SINUSOIDAL STIMULI

J.C. Saunders and Y.M. Szymko*

Department of Otorhinolaryngology and Human Communication
**Department of Bioengineering*
University of Pennsylvania, Philadelphia, PA 19104, U.S.A.

Introduction

Hair cell receptor potentials have been examined in both mammalian inner and outer hair cells (Russell, Cody, & Richardson, 1986; Dallos, Santos-Sacchi, & Flock, 1982; Russell & Sellick, 1978) and in hair cells from vestibular and cochlear organs of non-mammalian vertebrates (Crawford & Fettiplace, 1981; Harris, Frishkopf & Flock, 1970; Hudspeth and Corey, 1977). The outer hair cell may be a special case (Russell, Cody & Richardson, 1986), but in all other hair cells intracellular recordings of the receptor potential clearly reveal the presence of an asymmetric response, characterized as having a saturating non-linearity. This receptor potential in non-mammalian hair cells was partially attributed to a rectification property of the hair cell membrane (Crawford & Fettiplace, 1981, Hudspeth & Corey, 1977). In mammalian inner hair cells the receptor potential is non-linear (Russell & Sellick, 1978) as with other hair cells, but the membrane properties appeared more linear (Russell, 1983; Russell, Cody & Richardson, 1986).

The morphometry of the sensory hair bundle, which is decidedly asymmetric on all hair cells (Lim, 1980; Tilney & Saunders, 1983) suggests that this region may contribute to the non-linear receptor potential of the cell. Indeed, the "staircase" organization of the hair bundle suggests that its stiffness gradient for force applied against or away from the bundle may be quite different, thus providing a non-linearity at the mechanical input to the cell.

Attempts have been made to measure the mechanical stiffness of hair bundle deflections. Flock and Strelioff developed an in vitro preparation (1984b) to study the static stiffness of hair bundles from hair cells in the isolated guinea pig cochlea (Flock & Strelioff, 1984a). The stiffness was measured with a quartz fiber probe used to push the members of the tallest row of hairs. The force needed to achieve a criterion displacement of 1.0 micron was then derived. Results indicated that the stiffness of both inner- and outer-hair cell bundles was greater when the deflection was in the excitatory direction (the tallest hairs in the staircase were deflected away from the bundle) than in the inhibitory direction (the tallest hairs pushed toward the bundle).

The ratio of excitatory to inhibitory stiffness was different for outer and inner hair cells but together averaged 2.15 (Strelioff & Flock, 1984).

Hair bundle stiffness in the turtle cochlea (Crawford & Fettiplace, 1985) and the frog sacculus (Howard & Ashmore, 1986) however, appeared to be approximately the same for an excitatory or inhibitory deflection. In the turtle, the excitatory/inhibitory stiffness ratio was 0.91 and in the frog it was 1.1. These data were also based on static displacements of the hair bundle. In the case of the turtle the displacements were much smaller than 1 micron, while in the frog they were measured between + 1.5 microns. These data were different from those seen in the guinea pig and it is not clear if this was due to procedural variables or species differences. The hair bundles in the frog and turtle clump together and pushing on one hair moved them all. In the guinea pig, force applied to a single hair moved only a subpopulation of the total number of hairs (around 7 to 12, Strelioff & Flock, 1984).

The data described above report hair bundle stiffness for static or very low frequency stimuli. In the present study we will describe hair bundle motion in the excitatory and inhibitory direction for a sinusoidal stimulus. From this motion inferences can be made concerning the relative stiffness of the hair bundle by directly measuring its displacement patterns in response to a 300 Hz stimulus.

Methods

The temporal bones of chicks aged between 8 and 12 days were rapidly removed following decapitation. The oval and round windows were opened and the bones placed in culture medium at room temperature ($22^{o}C$). The culture medium (Leibovitz L-15, Gibco) partially simulated perilymph (K^{+} = 5.8 mM; Na^{+} = 138 mM; $Ca2^{+}$ = 1.26 mM). The papilla remained immersed in this medium throughout the dissection, transfer to the experimental microscope, and hair bundle testing. The surrounding bony capsule was dissected away to isolate and remove the membranous portion of the cochlea. The stump of the auditory nerve and much of the cochlear ganglion was then dissected free to permit an unobstructed light path through the basilar papilla. Further dissection cleared away the tegmentum vasculosum which revealed the tectorial membrane lying over the receptor epithelium. Darkfield illumination was essential for identifying the various cochlear structures in this unfixed tissue. Gentle prying at the proximal tip of the cochlea loosened the tectorial membrane. Grabbing the membrane at this point and pulling upward was about 80% effective in exposing large portions of the underlying sensory surface. In chicks aged younger than 7 days, the basilar papilla tended to lift off with the tectorial membrane, while in animals older than 13 days ossification of the temporal bone complicated access to the papilla.

The papilla was then mounted on a specially designed vise adapted from that described by Flock and Strelioff (1984b), and this was relocated to the experimental microscope (Zeiss ACM) equipped with DIC optics. At the microscope the tissue was immersed in a well containing culture medium (see Figure 1). The vise and stage

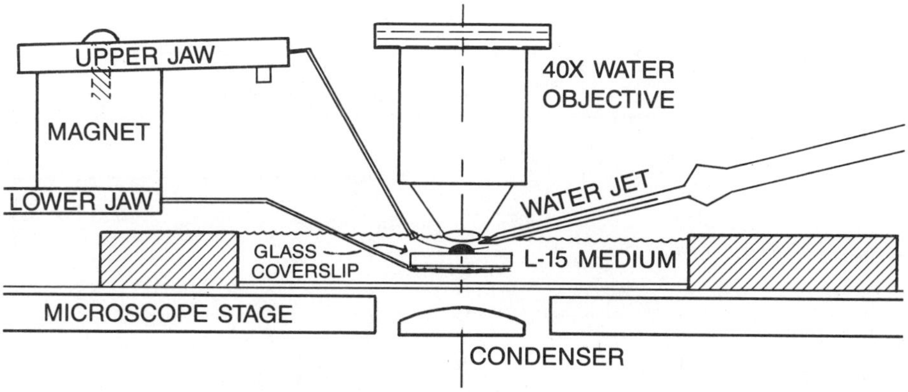

Figure 1. The illustration shows the vise assembly holding the basilar papilla to a piece of glass coverslip (part of the lower jaw) in the optical axis of the microscope.

assembly allowed the isolated cochlea to be tilted and rotated so that all hair cells on the papilla could be brought into the optical axis. The hair cell was viewed as seen from above, with the observer looking down on the tips of the hairs. A 40X water immersion objective (0.75 N.A. and 1.6 mm working distance) or a 63X objective (N.A. 1.2, 0.12 mm working distance) was used. Video imaging with analogue contrast enhancement permitted the hair bundles to be viewed on a TV monitor at magnifications between 4200X and 7500X.

A piezoelectric crystal (PZL-100, Burleigh) with a maximum peak-to-peak displacement of 100 microns (0.1 to 3.0 kHz) was used to drive (in an accordion like fashion) a small stainless steel bellows. The bellows was tightly clamped at one end and mated with a pressure fitting to accept a glass pipette. The arrangement of the water jet apparatus is seen in Figure 2A. The bellows was filled with water to which was added a few drops of photoflow (Kodak) to break the surface tension. Sonication assured the removal of all air bubbles. A glass pipette (15-30 microns tip diameter) filled with medium was mated to the bellows. When the far end of the bellows was sinusoidally driven by the crystal, the resulting pressure was conveyed through the fluid medium to the tip of the pipette, and produced an oscillating water jet stimulus.

The pressure field of the stimulus was complex, but within 10 to 15 microns of the tip there appeared to be a near-field in which a true oscillating pressure wave could be found. This was confirmed by observing the movements of glass micro beads. These 1 to 2 micron diameter beads were captured in the pressure field and their displacements measured. The peak-to-peak displacements of the beads at 300 Hz were sinusoidal and their response, measured over a 26-30 dB range was linear (Figure 2B).

The pipette was placed within 7 to 10 microns of the hair bundle and oriented so that it stimulated the bundle in its preferred axis of motion. The water jet effectively caused the hair bundle to move back and forth in the pressure field. In order to slow hair bundle motion,

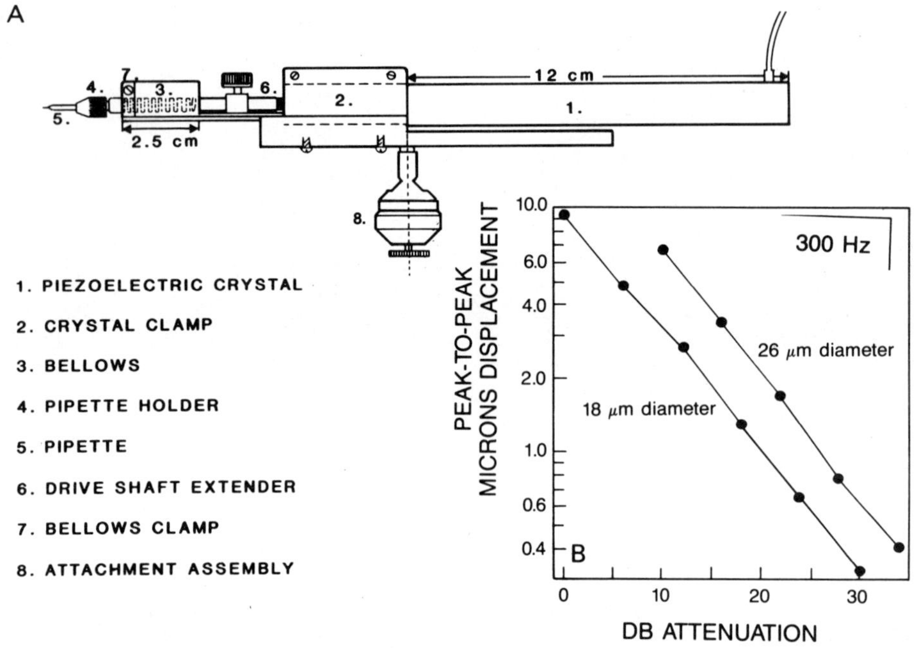

Figure 2. A. The apparatus used to produce the water jet stimulus is illustrated. B. The microns displacement of glass beads captured in the near-field of the water jet is indicated for two pipettes of different diameter. The linearity of the response at 300 Hz is apparent.

the microscope was illuminated with a 75-watt stroboscopic lamp which could be free-run, with the frequency slightly offset from the stimulus, or synchronized to specific phase angles of the stimulus. This caused the hairs to move back and forth a few times a second or to appear frozen at a fixed deflection.

In the present experiment, the strobe was synchronized to different stimulus phase angles, and then systematically "walked" through successive 45° steps of a single cycle. Hair bundle displacement from one step to the next was measured in two ways: either directly from the TV monitor, or from frame grabbed images stored on hard disk, in which length measures were calculated from the number of pixels traversed in the 45° step. All measures were based on the motion of the tallest row of hairs in the bundle and pixel resolution varied from 0.06 to 0.1 microns depending on the magnification.

Data were averaged for 12 cells, 8 of which were stimulated on the abneural side (toward the tallest hairs in the bundle) while 4 others were stimulated on the neural side (toward the staircase). The results from both were the same. In each cell hair bundle displacements were examined in 4 dB steps over a 20 dB range. Testing always proceeded from the lowest stimulus level to the most intense. Since stimulus levels varied due to pipette diameter and working distance (the space between the pipette tip and hair bundle), the 0 dB attenuation level was arbitrarily set to that intensity which produced an approximate 5 micron peak-to-peak hair bundle displacement. All the measured cells were located between 0.1 and 0.15 mm from the distal or low frequency end of the papilla. Exposure to the most intense stimuli was kept as short as possible to prevent a threshold shift in the mechanical response.

Results

A total of 42 cells were tested in the course of refining the procedures used in this study. The final 12 cells of this series are reported here where the dissection conditions, cochlear location, pipette diameter, and hair bundle imaging were all optimal. These data are from short hair cells located about 15 to 40 microns from the inferior edge of the cochlea. The thickness of the superior fibrocartilaginous plate made it difficult to to clearly image tall hair cells. As the procedures were developed, however, we occasionally identified a tall hair cell on which data could be collected. In the two instances where this was possible the data looked identical to that observed for the short hair cell bundles. These results must be considered preliminary at present.

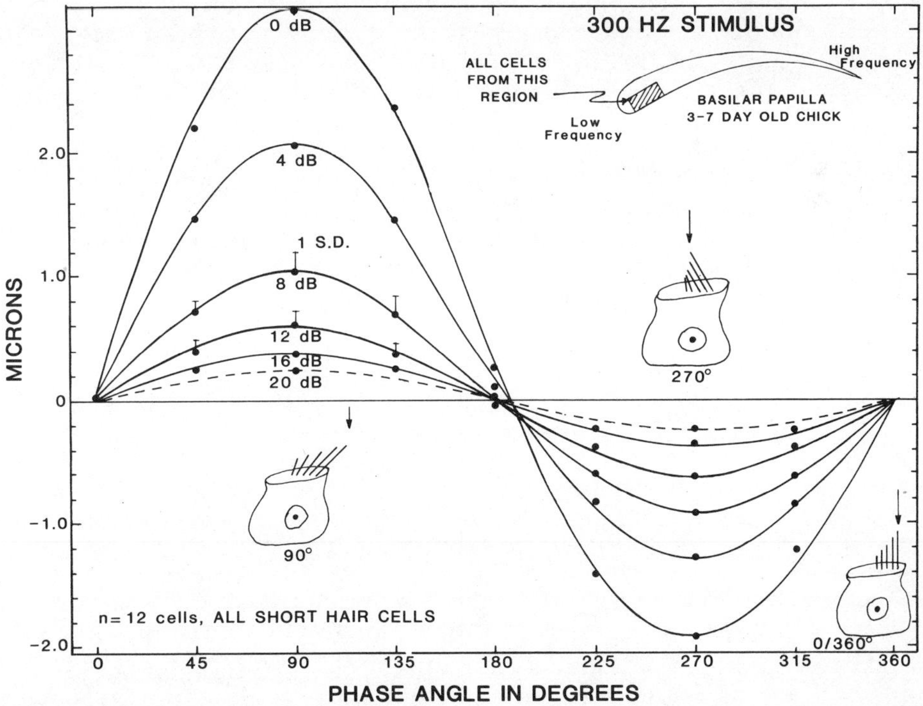

Figure 3. The waveform of the hair bundle response, measured at the tallest row of the bundle, is shown for six different stimulus levels. The curves are lines of best fit drawn by eye for the data. At stimulus levels between 8 and 20 dB attenuation the hair bundle response is nearly perfectly sinusoidal. The insert in the upper right corner shows the papilla surface and the location of the sampled hair cells.

In order to place some limits on testing, data were not collected longer than three hours from the time of sacrifice. This duration may seem conservative, but the hair cells up to that time had a normal appearance (Flock & Strelioff, 1984b). Given that it took about an hour or more to dissect and mount the papilla, and 30-40 minutes to obtain the data, only 2 to 3 cells could be studied in each ear. The results described below were obtained from five different basilar papillae.

The data presented in Figure 3 show the average waveform response for 12 cells. The positive deflections of the hair bundle are in the excitatory direction whereas the negative deflections are in the inhibitory direction. At the highest stimulus intensity (0 dB) the waveform was asymmetric with the excitatory deflection (3.19 microns) larger than the inhibitory deflection (1.96 microns). This indicates a relative difference in bundle stiffness being less in the excitatory direction than in the inhibitory direction. However, as stimulus intensity decreased the positive and negative peak deflections equaled one another. At 12, 16 and 20 dB attenuation the waveform closely approximated a sinusoid. Assuming that the normal operating range of a hair cell, as defined by the receptor potential, is something less than + 1.0 micron (Hudspeth & Corey, 1977; and others) than the data presented here suggest that the hair bundle is operating in a linear fashion within the physiologic range of hair cell operation.

The excitatory and inhibitory peak deflections have been plotted in Figure 4A, and the two values were nearly equal from 12 to 20 dB attenuation. From 0 to 8 dB attenuation the slope of the excitatory peak deflection curve increased while the slope of the inhibitory peak deflection decreased. Figure 4B illustrates that the peak-to-peak response was perfectly linear over the 20 dB range. Thus the increase in the excitatory peak was offset by the small deflection in the inhibitory direction. If we examined the peak-to-peak response (or the RMS value of the response) the non-linearity in the hair bundle would escape recognition. This is shown in Figure 4B.

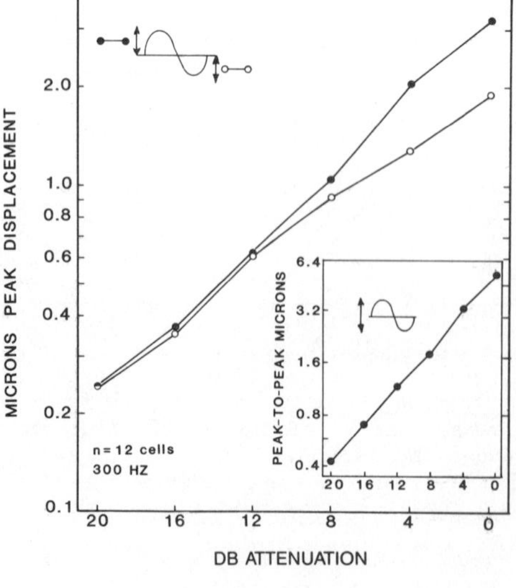

Figure 4. A. The excitatory and inhibitory peaks of the waveform are plotted as a function of stimulus attenuation. Between 12 and 20 dB the peak values are equal. B. (Inset) The peak-to-peak response of the waveforms are plotted as a function of stimulus intensity and appear linear over the entire test range.

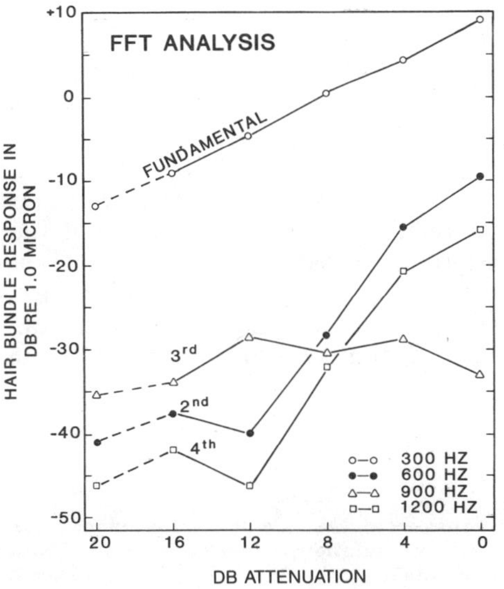

Figure 5. The results of an FFT analysis on the waveforms in Figure 3. At the highest stimulus intensities the amount of distortion product was greater than at lower intensities. The odd order harmonic remains relatively constant. The data at 20 dB are estimated, hence the dashed line.

Each of the waveforms in Figure 3 were further analyzed by subjecting them to an FFT analysis and the results are presented in Figure 5. Since only 8 data points were empirically measured in each waveform the analysis could not go beyond the fourth harmonic. The data are plotted as the hair bundle response in dB relative to a 1.0 micron displacement. The 300 Hz component of the waveform exhibits the linear slope demonstrated in the peak-to-peak representation of the data in Figure 4B. The second, third and fourth harmonic are also plotted. Between 20 and 12 dB attenuation, where the waveforms were most sinusoidal, the amount of distortion was minimal. Indeed we suspect the amount of distortion in this region is even less but was limited by the signal to noise ratio in our measurements. At attenuations lower than 12 dB the amount of energy in the second and fourth harmonics rose rapidly. This was the intensity region where the distortion in the hair bundle waveform became apparent (Figure 3).

Discussion

It is now possible to remove in an intact and healthy condition the basilar papilla from the inner ear of the chick. This papilla can be transferred to an experimental microscope where the hair bundles could be examined at high magnifications with video imaging. Moreover, the sensory hair could be stimulated at high frequencies with a water jet stimulus. Although the properties of the water jet are complicated and far from fully calibrated (a frequency response curve has yet to be constructed) it appears to be linear and sinusoidal over a considerable range of intensities. With stroboscopic illumination the bundle motion can be observed in slow motion or frozen at particular phase angles of the stimulus.

The waveform analysis of chick short hair cell bundle movements indicate nonsinusoidal behavior outside the physiological range of the hair cell response. However, within the physiologic range (less than +1 micron deflection) the hair bundle appeared to respond in a linear manner. One implication of these data is that the stiffness gradient is the same for deflections in the excitatory or inhibitory direction. This observation is in agreement with the data presented by Crawford and Fettiplace (1985) and Howard and Ashmore (1986). Moreover, it could be concluded from the present study that the asymmetric, non-linear receptor potential results from the transduction mechanism(s) in the hair cell, rather than an asymmetric input signal at the level of hair bundle mechanics. This conclusion needs to be further verified by directly relating hair bundle waveform, as in Figure 3 with intracellular measures of the receptor potential. Such experiments are underway.

Acknowledgements

This work was supported by research awards from the Pennsylvania Lions Hearing Research Foundation, the Deafness Research Foundation, The University Research Foundation, and BRSG funds to the School of Medicine. The assistance of Ms Diana Montgomery in preparing the manuscript is appreciated. Yvonne M. Szymko was supported by a General Electric Fellowship. The assistance of Dr. Roger Marsh is gratefully acknowledged.

References

Crawford, A.C. and Fettiplace, R. (1981) Non-linearities in the responses of turtle hair cells. J. Physiol. 315, 317-338.

Crawford, A.C. and Fettiplace, R. (1985) The mechanical properties of ciliary bundles of turtle cochlear hair cells. J. Physiol. 364, 359-379.

Dallos, P. Santos-Sacchi, J. and Flock A. (1982) Intracellular recordings from cochlear outer hair cells. Science 218, 582-584.

Flock, A. and Strelioff, D. (1984a) Graded and nonlinear mechanical properties of sensory hairs in the mammalian hearing organ. Nature 310, 597-598.

Flock, A. and Strelioff, D. (1984b) Studies on hair cells in isolated coils from the guinea pig cochlea. Hearing Res. 15, 11-18.

Harris, G.G., Frishkopf, L. S., and Flock, A. (1970) Receptor potentials from the lateral line. Science 167, 76-79.

Howard, J. and Ashmore, J.F. (1986) Stiffness of sensory hair bundles in the sacculus of the frog. Hearing Res. 23, 93-104.

Hudspeth, A. J. and Corey, D. P. (1977) Sensitivity, polarity, and conductance change in the response of vertebrate hair cells to controlled mechanical stimuli. Proc. Natl. Acad. Sci, (U.S.A.) 74, 2407-2411.

Lim, D. J. (1980) Cochlear anatomy related to cochlear micromechanics. A review. J. Acoust. Soc. Am. 67, 1686-1695.

Russell, I. J. (1983) Origin of the receptor potential in inner hair cells of the mammalian cochlea - evidence for Davis' theory. Nature 301, 334-336.

Russell, I. J. and Sellick, P. (1978) Intracellular studies of hair cells in the mammalian cochlea. J. Physiol. 284, 261-190.

Russell, I. J., Cody, A. R. and Richardson, G. P. (1986) The responses of inner and outer hair cells in the basal turn of the guinea-pig cochlea and in the mouse cochlea grown in vitro. Hearing Res. 22, 199-216.

Strelioff, D. and Flock, A. (1984) Stiffness of sensory-cell hair bundles in the isolated guinea pig cochlea. Hearing Res. 15, 19- 28.

Tilney, L.G. and Saunders, J.C. (1983) Actin filaments, stereocilia, and hair cells of the bird cochlea. I. Length, number, width, and distribution of stereocilia of each hair cell are related to the position of the hair cell on the cochlea. J. Cell Biol. 96, 807- 821.

MICROMECHANICAL BASIS OF HIGH-FREQUENCY TUNING IN THE BOBTAIL LIZARD

Geoffrey A. Manley, Christine Köppl and Graeme K. Yates*

Institut für Zoologie der Technischen Universität München
Lichtenbergstr. 4, 8046 Garching, FRG
**Department of Physiology, University of W. Australia*
Nedlands, W.A. 6009, Australia

Introduction

To date, a good understanding of the mechanisms of frequency selectivity has been achieved for the auditory papillae of the red-eared turtle (Crawford and Fettiplace, 1981), the alligator lizard (Weiss and Leong, 1985) and mammals (Khanna and Leonard, 1982; Russell and Sellick, 1978; Sellick et al., 1982). However, none of the three types of models proposed are directly applicable to the other cases. In the red-eared turtle, tuning seems to be mainly a function of the electrical properties of individual hair cells, whereas in the alligator lizard at least the high-frequency hair cells seem to be tuned by the resonance properties of individual hair-cell stereovillar bundles. Mammalian hair cells, however, show no indication of being electrically tuned and are covered by a thick tectorial membrane which, at least for outer hair cells, does not allow individual hair cell bundles to resonate independently. The mechanisms of frequency selectivity in vertebrate inner ears are obviously quite diverse (Manley, 1986), so that a comprehensive and comparative understanding of tuning mechanisms and their integration in the hearing organs of different vertebrate classes requires the detailed investigation of a greater variety of morphological types of inner ear.

We have previously described a more qualitative model of tuning in the basal area of the basilar papilla in the bobtail lizard Tiliqua rugosa (Manley et al., 1988a). The bobtail lizard is a large, common skink native to southern Australia. As a family, skinks possess a very well developed hearing organ. In the present paper, we briefly describe the measurements of basilar-membrane and neural tuning in the high-frequency area of this lizard which suggested a model for frequency sharpening. We then present quantitative morphological details which have permitted the calculation of absolute values for the frequency response of different locations on the papilla, using assumptions based on the previous model. A comprehensive description of the morphology is given in Köppl, 1988.

The measurements necessary for the model calculations described below were made using three different techniques. The tuning of the basilar membrane was measured using an optical technique (Yates, in preparation). The necessary surgical procedures, using a medial approach to the basilar membrane through the brain cavity, have been previously described (Manley et al., 1988a). The tuning of single auditory-nerve fibres emanating from those individual papillar regions for which basilar-membrane data were available (allowing a direct comparison of frequency selectivity) was measured using standard microelectrode techniques (Manley et al., 1988a). Quantitative data on the putative morphological substrate of the mechanical tuning proposed here were obtained on hearing organs investigated using both scanning-electron- and light-microscopy (Köppl, 1988).

Two tuning components in high-CF fibres of Tiliqua

The basilar papilla of the bobtail skink is an elongated, cylinder-shaped epithelium resting fully on the basilar membrane. It is more than 2 mm long and divided into a shorter apical segment and a long basal segment which occupies more than 80% of the length. Evidence from neurophysiological experiments not discussed here indicates that frequencies are tonotopically organized along the basal segment, between about 800 Hz and the upper limit of 4.5 kHz at the basal end. Due to the partial enclosure of the papilla by the limbus, only the basal two-thirds of this basal segment were accessible for basilar-membrane and neural tuning measurements. Using small, light-reflecting particles on the underside of the basilar membrane, we measured the displacement amplitudes of one or more locations to a broad range of frequencies in seven animals (Fig. 1). As can be seen, the basilar-membrane tuning is very broad; indeed, it is only slightly sharper than the tuning of the middle ear. It is also not place-dependent. Our estimates of the displacement amplitudes give values corresponding to those typical of the "tail" regions of basilar-membrane tuning curves of the basal turn of the mammalian cochlea (10nm at about 80 dB SPL). Sharply-tuned, sensitive regions of the basilar membrane were never found either with automatic or hand-swept tuning methods.

Primary auditory-nerve fibres in Tiliqua emanate from the basilar papilla in the immediate region of the hair cells they innervate. They then run in a gradually-narrowing fan-shaped bundle to the ganglion. It was possible to record from fibres adjacent to the papilla and, in the cases reported here, from fibres innervating hair cells over the basilar-membrane areas whose motion was previously investigated and where the reflecting objects were still in place. In contrast to basilar-membrane tuning, the tuning of the nerve fibres was very sharp, sensitive (Fig. 1), strictly tonotopically organized and indistinguishable from tuning curves measured in animals in which the inner ear was not opened. These neural data were collected subsequent to the basilar membrane measurements and indicate that the papilla was in very good condition. Over the accessible basal two-thirds of the basal segment of the papilla, the characteristic frequencies (CF) of nerve fibres varied systematically from 1.4 to 4.2 kHz, the latter being near the extreme basal end. A comparison of the tuning curves of many fibres indicated that they share common features. Each neural tuning curve shows a broad tuning at high SPL where the slopes of the low- and high-frequency flanks, respectively, are very similar for different fibres. The curves show their greatest individuality near

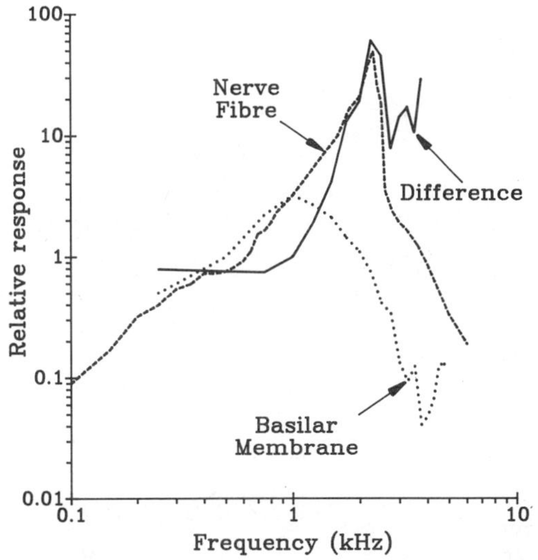

FIGURE 1. A comparison of the frequency selectivity of the basilar membrane (dotted line) and a single primary auditory-nerve fibre (dashed line) which innervated the same papillar location in the same individual bobtail skink. The two curves have been placed on the Y axis so that their low frequency flanks match up well. The difference between the two curves (solid line) strongly resembles a high-pass filter function.

their respective CFs, where a more sharply-tuned, relatively deep and sensitive "tip" region seems to be superimposed on the broad tuning (Fig. 2c).

It struck us that the tuning curves of the fibres appear to be the resultant of the concatenation of two components; a broad, insensitive tuning equivalent to the basilar-membrane tuning and a sharp, sensitive, individual and tonotopically-organized component with a different origin. A simple subtraction of the basilar-membrane tuning from the (inverted) neural tuning curve produced an interesting result: calculated for individual pairs of curves for specific measurement locations, the resultant difference curves each strongly resemble a simple high-pass filter function (Fig. 1). The subtraction of the common basilar-membrane tuning component from the neural curve thus revealed the characteristics of the second, individual and sharply-tuned component for each fibre. We suggested that this second component was the result of a mechanical resonance of local groups of hair cells and the attached portion of tectorial membrane (Manley et al., 1988a).

It is characteristic of this and some other lizard families, that the tectorial membrane of the high-frequency region is divided along its length into so-called sallets, which are individual masses of tectorial material connected to one another along the mid-line of the papilla. We modelled the tuning of different papillar locations as a set of simple resonant high-pass filters having graded corner frequencies and connected in series with the broad tuning of the basilar membrane. This procedure resulted in curves whose tip regions were too pointed and too shallow (Fig. 2a). A good match to the original neural tuning curves, with their deep, somewhat rounded tips, was only obtained when we assumed that the second component of tuning was the result of a pair of coupled simple high-pass filters (Fig. 2b,c). This strengthened our impression that the tectorial membrane, through its coupling of local groups of hair-cell stereovillar bundles (and thus of resonances),

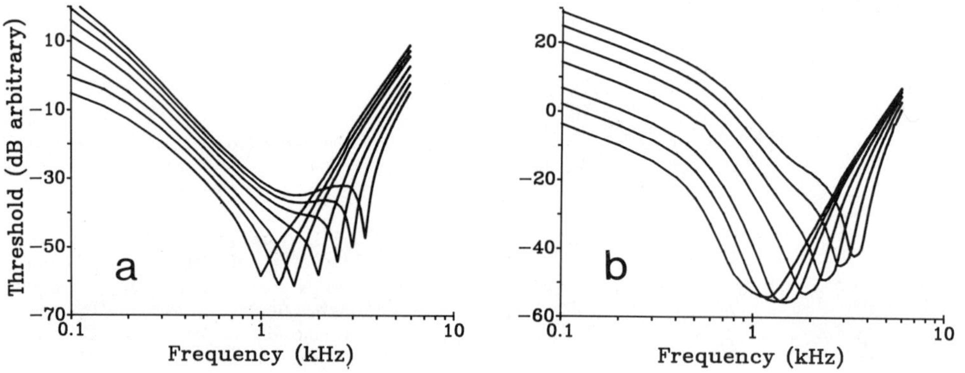

FIGURE 2 A comparison of families of modelled tuning curves calculated by cascading for each curve an approximation to the basilar-membrane tuning curve with a: a two-pole filter function and b: a coupled pair of two-pole filters. c: A family of tuning curves from primary auditory neurones in one animal. Both the general shape and the depth of the sharply-tuned tip region of the neural tuning curves are better matched by the coupled resonances shown in b. The Q-factors of the filters (roughly equivalent to the Q_{3dB}) of the filters in a: ranged from 3.75 to 26.25 from low to high CF; in b: they ranged from 1.25 to 8.5.

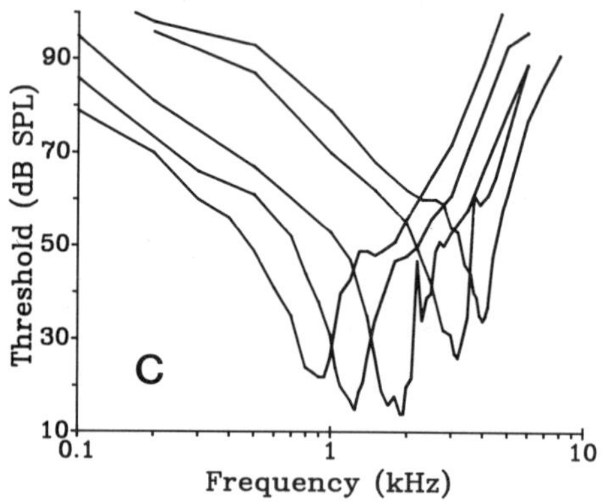

may be playing a critical role in determining the characteristics of local mechanical resonant groups. Rather than attempting to adjust the values of the assumed Q-values, etc., to achieve a perfect match, we returned to the morphological data to see if the assumption of a mechanical resonance of local hair-cell groups and their sallet could be tested on the basis of calculations of resonance frequencies using exact morphological data and reasonable assumptions of bundle stiffness and tectorial-structure mass.

Mechanical resonance frequencies - the morphological basis

In order to estimate resonance frequencies, it is necessary to have detailed information on the anatomical characteristics of the hair-cell stereovillar bundles and of the tectorial structures along the basal area of the papilla. We describe here briefly those features of the morphology of the papilla of Tiliqua relevant to the model. The values used in the model described below are based on averaged data for several specimens, whereby it should be noted that most features of the papillar morphology show considerable variation between individuals (Köppl, 1988).

The tectorial structure is a chain of 70-90 sallets which project (not necessarily symmetrically) from both sides of the connecting medial "rope" (Fig. 3a). We measured

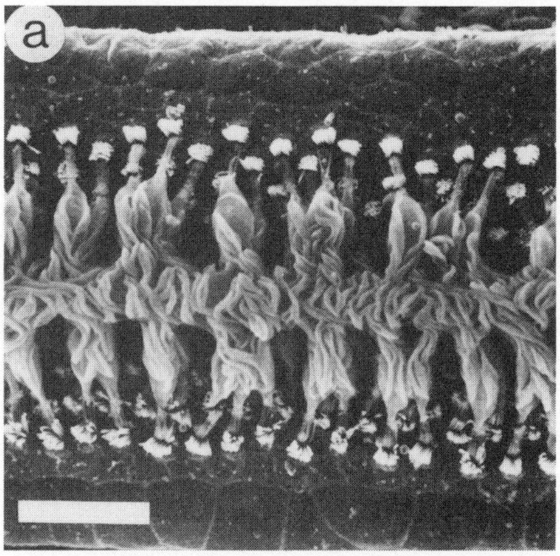

FIGURE 3 a: Scanning-electron micrograph of part of the surface of the basal segment of the basilar papilla of the bobtail lizard. Roughly 8 sallets can be seen extended to either side of a medial rope-like connection. Due to fixation and drying, the tectorial material is shrunken and pulled back to expose the hair-cell bundles on both sides of the papilla. b: Cross-sectional area of the sallets (compensated for shrinkage, see text) as a function of position from the apical end (0%) to basal end of the basal papillar segment. c: Number of hair cells connected to individual sallets as a function of the position along the basal segment. Calibration bar 25µm.

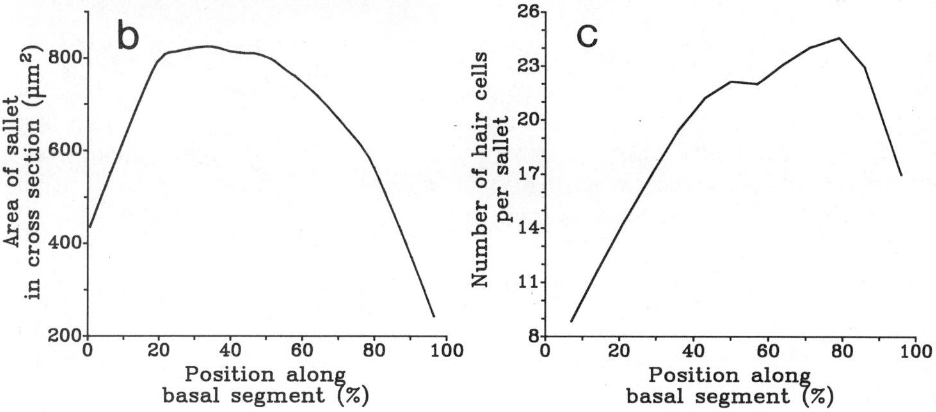

the dimensions of the different sallets in the fixed state from transverse sections of the papilla throughout the basal area and, because tectorial material always shrinks during the histological preparation (Köppl, 1988), assumed that this area is twice as large in the living state. For the same reason we assumed that their dimension along the length of the papilla is equivalent to the distance between their transverse axes as measured from SEM preparations. This distance is roughly 18 µm, being smaller only in the basal 20% (down to 10 µm). The cross-sectional area of the different sallets is smallest at the basal end and increases towards the apical area; it decreases again apically (Fig. 3). These data are necessary for estimating not only the mass of the sallets, but also, together with the known hair-cell density, how many hair cells are connected to each sallet (Fig. 3).

There are roughly 1650 hair cells along the basal segment and both neural and abneural orientations are seen at all locations. The hair-cell density increases from apical to basal; there are about 5 hair cells across the papilla apically and 9 basally. The hair-cell bundles are connected to the salletal chain only via the kinocilium, which, in turn, is

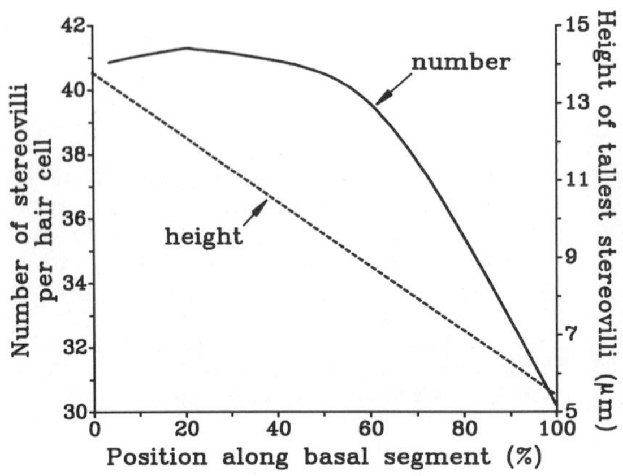

FIGURE 4. The number of stereovilli per hair cell (solid line, refer to left ordinate) as a function of position along the basal segment of the basilar papilla of the bobtail lizard. 100% is at the extreme basal end of the basal segment. The height of the tallest stereovilli within a bundle as a function of position along the basal segment is given as a simple linear regression line (dashed line, right ordinate).

connected to the tallest stereovilli. The salletal chain has no connections either to the limbus or to the surface of the basilar papilla. The hair-cell bundles vary systematically in a number of respects along the basal segment from apical (lower CF) to basal (higher CF; Fig. 4). The total number of stereovilli per hair cell is roughly constant over the apical two-thirds of the basal segment (41), but declines to 30 at the basal end. The height of the tallest stereovilli of a bundle varies from 13.75 µm apically to 5.4 µm basally.

Mechanical resonance frequencies - the calculation

We make the assumption that the local resonance frequency is dependent only on the mass of the sallet and the stiffness of all the stereovillar bundles connected to that sallet. Since tectorial gels are mostly water, the specific gravity of the sallets was assumed to be 1100 kg/m^3. The calculated mass of the sallets varies nonlinearly along the papilla (Fig. 5a). The stiffness depends on the number of hair cells connected to each sallet, on the number of villi in each bundle and on the height of the stereovillar bundle (Fig. 5a). We calculated the stiffness of each resonant unit according to the method of Crawford and Fettiplace (1985), whereby the stiffness of a single villus was assumed to be given by their measured value for the rotational stiffness of single hair-cell bundles in the red-eared turtle (2x10^{-14} N.m/rad) divided by the average number of villi in the turtle bundle (90). The calculated variation in stiffness is mainly due to the changing bundle height, rather than the number of stereovilli per hair cell or the number of hair cells per sallet. The stiffness gradient along the papilla is almost a mirror-image of the change in salletal mass (Fig. 5a). These inverse trends of mass and stiffness work together to produce the smooth gradient in resonance frequencies (Fig. 5b).

The absolute resonance frequency for each sallettal hair-cell unit is calculated as

$$1/(2\pi)\sqrt{(\text{stiffness}/\text{mass})}$$

and is shown in Fig. 5b. The calculated frequency ranges from 1080 Hz apically to 6808 Hz basally. The actual CF range estimated from neurophysiological experiments and

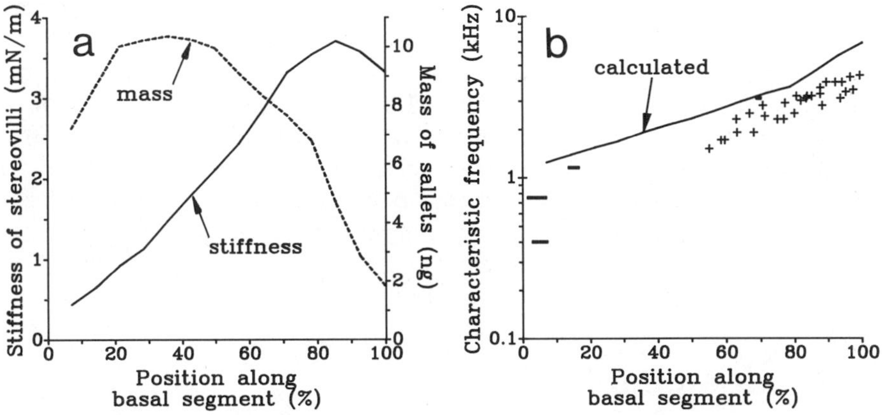

FIGURE 5 a: Change in the estimated mass of individual sallets (dotted line, right ordinate) and the total stiffness of all stereovilli connected to each sallet (solid line, left ordinate) as a function of position along the basal segment of the basilar papilla of Tiliqua. b: A comparison of the modelled CFs (solid line, for calculation, see text) and measured CFs as a function of position along the basal segment. The crosses represent the CF of individual primary fibres in four different animals as measured by recording with microelectrodes next to the papilla. There are four bars (one near the model line at 68%) which represent the position of single, cobalt-stained, physiologically-characterized primary fibres in three animals. The mean lowest CF of the basal segment as estimated from physiological data not discussed here is 850Hz.

measured for the basal end by recording from fibres next to the papilla is from 850 to 4500 Hz (Fig. 5b). Considering the uncertainty in the necessary assumptions and that some variables are not taken into account in the calculation (for example, that the slope of the heights of the villar rows in different bundles also varies systematically along the papilla), the agreement between the neural data and the calculated resonance frequencies is extremely good.

We thus propose that the tuning of the CF-region in high-frequency hair cells in Tiliqua is due to the mechanical resonance of local hair-cell groups and their sallet, superimposed on the broad basilar-membrane tuning. Frequency selectivity would be greatest if each resonant unit is only weakly coupled to adjacent units. We assume that the coupling is optimized by the sub-divided, salletal structure of the tectorial membrane of this basal region. This presumably enables the discrete units to resonate without substantially influencing the differently-tuned, more remote regions. The salletal structure could break up the basal area into maximally about 80 possible, independent "units", that is, about 30 per octave. This figure is, given the shape of the individual neural tuning curves, more than adequate to explain the frequency selectivity of the organ. This is also consistent with the assumption in our model of a degree of coupling of adjacent sallets to produce the characteristic tips of the tuning curves. In view of recent suggestions that the tectorial membrane of mammals is not stiff enough to act as a shearing partner for the hair cells but could act as a mass in a resonant circuit (Strelioff et al., 1985; Zwislocki et al., 1988), a model similar to ours could be applied to the mammalian organ of Corti.

The morphological characteristics of the apical segment of the basilar papilla are quite different from those of the basal segment discussed above. There is, for example, no obvious gradient in the height of stereovillar bundles. Also, the entire hair-cell area is covered with an enormous, undivided tectorial structure (Köppl, 1988). As in other reptiles and in birds, significantly less space is devoted to the low-frequency octaves in this apical area (200μm/octave) than to higher-frequency octaves (600μm/octave; Manley, 1986; Manley et al., 1988b). It seems to us likely that the frequency selectivity of hair cells in this apical segment is not primarily achieved through micromechanical factors, but by means of an electrical tuning mechanism such as that described for the red-eared turtle (Crawford and Fettiplace, 1981).

Acknowledgements

Supported by a travel fellowship to G.A.M. from the Stiftung Volkswagenwerk and to C.K from the Boehringer-Ingelheim Fond, a grant to B.M. Johnstone from the NH&MRC of Australia and a grant to G.A.M. from the Deutsche Forschungsgemeinschaft within the programme of the Sonderforschungsbereich 204 "Gehör". We thank B.M. Johnstone for support and encouragement.

References

Crawford, A.C. and Fettiplace, R. (1981) An electrical tuning mechanism in turtle cochlear hair cells. J. Physiol. 312, 377-412.

Crawford, A.C. and Fettiplace, R. (1985) The mechanical properties of ciliary bundles of turtle cochlear hair cells. J. Physiol. 364, 359-379.

Khanna, S.M. and Leonard, D. (1982) Basilar membrane tuning in the cat cochlea. Science 215, 305-306

Köppl, C. (1988) Morphology of the basilar papilla of the bobtail lizard Tiliqua rugosa. in press.

Manley, G.A. (1986) The evolution of the mechanisms of frequency selectivity in vertebrates. In: Auditory frequency selectivity (Eds: Moore, B.C.J. and Patterson, R.D.) Plenum press, New York, London, pp 63-72.

Manley, G.A., Yates, G. and Köppl, C. (1988a) Auditory peripheral tuning: evidence for a simple resonance phenomenon in the lizard Tiliqua. Hearing Res. 33, 181-190.

Manley G A, Brix J, Gleich O, Kaiser A, Köppl C, Yates G (1988b) New aspects of comparative peripheral auditory physiology. In: Syka J (ed) Auditory System - Structure and Function. Plenum Press, London, N.Y. in press.

Russell,1 I. and Sellick, P.M. (1978) Intracellular studies of hair cells in the mammalian cochlea. J. Physiol. 284, 261-290.

Sellick, P.M., Patuzzi, R. and Johnstone, B.M. (1982) Measurement of basilar membrane motion in the guinea pig using the Mössbauer technique. J. Acoust. Soc. Am. 72, 131-141.

Strelioff, D., Flock, A. and Minser, K.E. (1985) Role of inner and outer hair cells in mechanical frequency selectivity of the cochlea. Hearing Res. 18, 169-175.

Weiss, T.F. and Leong, R. (1985a) A model for signal transmission in an ear having hair cells with free-standing stereocilia. III. Micromechanical stage. Hearing Res. 20, 157-174.

Zwislocki, J.J., Slepecky, N.B. and Cefaratti, L.K. (1988) Tectorial-membrane stiffness and hair-cell stimulation. Abstr. 11th. Mtg. Assoc. Res. Otolaryngol. p.160.

Comments and Discussion

LEWIS

When their Q's are high, second order resonances are good for sorting signals with respect to frequency but poor for sorting them with respect to time. To do both well, a filter bank needs to employ high order dynamics in its channels. In that respect, the four-pole model you propose is better than the two-pole version. The fact that high-order dynamics are being discovered in so many vertebrate acoustic sensors implies to me that there is a compelling adaptive advantage in the ability to sort signals in both time and frequency. Perhaps we should think of the cochlea and other acoustic sensors not as mechanical or electromechanical frequency analyzers, but as analyzers of time and frequency.

MANLEY

It is not easy to know which selective pressures may have been operating at the time in which the basic structure of the basilar papilla of land vertebrates was being established. Although it may appear attractive to examine the responses in terms of modern filter theory, an explanation in non-biological terms will necessarily remain speculative. The bobtail lizard papilla (similar to other terrestrial vertebrates) only shows sharp tuning in the frequency domain at low levels and at higher CFs. The division into an apical region of low-CF cells which show good phase-locking and a basal region with poorer phase-locking but higher Qs may, for example, be an adequate compromise for coding time and frequency information.

MECHANICAL COUPLING BETWEEN INNER AND OUTER HAIR CELLS IN THE MAMMALIAN COCHLEA

D.C. Mountain and A.R. Cody*

Departments of Biomedical Engineering and Otolaryngology
Boston University
44 Cummington St.
Boston, MA 02215, U.S.A.
**M.R.C. Neurophysiology Group*
School of Biological Sciences
University of Sussex
Falmer, Brighton BN1 9QG. U.K.

Introduction

The mammalian cochlea is often described as a mechanical frequency analyzer in which the basilar membrane acts as a bank of mechanical filters tuned to different frequencies. The inner hair cells (IHC) in such descriptions passively respond to the displacement or velocity of the basilar membrane and pass the acoustic information on to the auditory nerve. The outer hair cells (OHC) are now believed to act as electromechanical amplifiers and serve to increase the movement of the basilar membrane over a limited frequency range. Mountain et al. (1983) proposed that the output of the mechanical-to-electrical transduction process in the OHC drives an electrical-to-mechanical transduction process which is, in turn, coupled back to the motion of the basilar and tectorial membranes. This feedback system is inherently nonlinear due to the limited dynamic range of the forward transduction process.

A careful examination of a variety of experimental data suggests that the IHC receptor potential can not be explained simply as a basilar membrane displacement or velocity response. Several authors have reported that for low-frequency acoustic stimulation, the IHC receptor potential appears to respond in phase to basilar membrane velocity towards scala vestibuli (Nuttall et. al., 1981, Sellick and Russell, 1980, Patuzzi and Yates, 1987). Sellick et al. (1982) and Ruggero and Rich (1983, 1987) however, found that the phase of excitation (inferred from spiral ganglion and afferent fiber recording) depends on stimulus level and cochlear location. Sellick et al. (1982) concluded that at low intensities the response was due to electrical excitation from extracellular OHC currents. Ruggero and Rich (1987) suggested that at low stimulus levels the IHC in the basal portion of the cochlea are mechanically excited in phase with displacement or velocity towards scala tympani. At higher stimulus levels the excitatory phase corresponds to basilar membrane velocity towards scala vestibuli. Ruggero and Rich (1983) also reported that at stimulus intensities corresponding to the phase transition the period histograms became quite distorted often exhibiting several peaks (peak splitting).

We have recently recorded basal turn IHC receptor potentials and input-resistance changes to low-frequency stimuli and conclude that peak splitting and the phase shifts with intensity reflect the mechanical stimulus to the IHC (Cody and Mountain, 1988). In addition, the analysis of a simple electrical model of the organ of Corti suggests that electrical interactions between the OHC and the IHC are minimal (Mountain, 1988).

A comparison of IHC and OHC responses measured in the same animal suggest that the mechanical input to the IHC is the difference between the basilar membrane motion and the motion of a second structure which is coupled to the basilar membrane via the OHC. The data further suggest that the coupling between the basilar membrane and the secondary element is proportional to OHC receptor current or receptor potential.

Methods

Pigmented guinea pigs (180-270g) were anaesthetized with sodium pentabarbitone (30 mg/kg). Sedation and analgesia were maintained throughout the experiment by an initial dose of Droleptan (droperidol, 5mg/kg) followed by regular injections of Operidine (phenoperidine hydrochloride, 1 mg/kg). The animals were given a muscle relaxant (Flaxidil, gallamine triethiodide, 5mg/kg) and artifically respirated.

Acoustic stimuli were delivered by an Oticon (type PP-055) earphone to the animal via a closed system. For this paper the stimulus frequencies used were 63, 115, and 125Hz which gives an upper limit for the third harmonic of 375Hz, well below the estimated cut-off frequencies of the hair cell and the recording system. The stimuli were monitored at the tympanum with a calibrated 1mm probe tube coupled to a Bruel and Kjaer 13mm condensor microphone (type 4134). The frequency and intensity of the acoustic stimuli were under computer control.

The right bulla was opened and a small hole made in the bone over scala tympani of the basal turn. Cochlear potentials were monitored at selected sites within the organ of Corti with glass micropippetes (100-120 MOhm, 3M KCl). The micropipette was also used to pass a dc hyperpolarizing current (-0.5 to -1.0nA) into the IHC using an active bridge circuit in order to measure the IHC input resistance. A silver wire electrode positioned on the round window was used to monitor the compound action potential and remote cochlear microphonic. All potentials were recorded with respect to an indifferent electrode in the neck. Potentials were recorded on magnetic tape and subsequently digitized for latter waveform analysis.

The IHC receptor potential was calculated by subtracting the potential recorded just outside the IHC from the IHC potential measured intracellularly. This subtraction significantly reduces the contamination of the IHC response by extracellular currents from the OHC (Cody and Mountain, 1988; Mountain, 1988) and more accurately reflects the presynaptic potential.

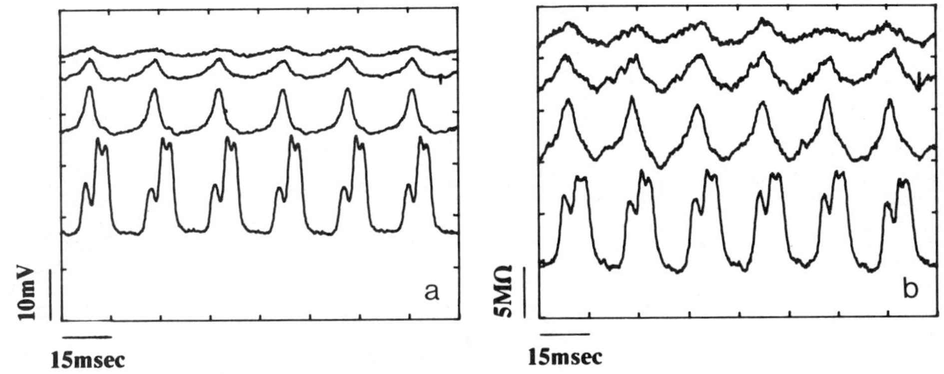

FIGURE 1. a. IHC receptor potentials in response to a 113Hz tone delivered at SPL's of 96, 105, 114 and 124dB respectively. b. IHC resistance change during acoustic stimulation shows a similar waveform to that seen in the receptor potential.

The technical difficulties associated with intracellular recording in OHCs were avoided by assuming that the extracellular potentials recorded in the organ of Corti are proportional to the local OHC receptor current (Cody and Mountain, 1988; Dallos et al, 1982; Russell and Sellick, 1983).

Results

Figure 1a illustrates the IHC receptor potential in response to a 113 Hz stimulus. The receptor potential exhibits a systematic change in waveshape as the sound pressure level (SPL) is increased. At very low stimulus levels the waveform is sinusoidal. As the level is increased the waveform becomes more distorted, often with two or more peaks per stimulus period. In some cells, at the highest levels, the response becomes more regular but assymetrical with the depolarizing phase being up to 5 times larger than the hyperpolarizing phase. The IHC responses illustrated in figures 1-3 are typical of the range of waveforms observed in this study. Fourteen out of 16 cells in this study showed at least a local minimum in the depolarizing phase of the response for one or more sound pressure levels. The complex distortion seen in the receptor potential at low stimulus frequencies is similar to the distortion observed in the input-resistance waveforms. Figure 1b illustrates input-resistance waveform measured at the same stimulus levels as in fig. 1a. In both cases multiple peaks per stimulus period can be seen.

The onset of the distortion in the IHC waveform occurs at sound pressure levels for which the OHC response begins to saturate. Figure 2 illustrates the magnitude of extracellular response in the organ of Corti at the acoustic frequency as a function of sound level. The inserts are the IHC waveform measured at the same SPL. As the OHC response begins to deviate significantly from the broken line (extrapolated linear response) the IHC response begins to become quite distorted.

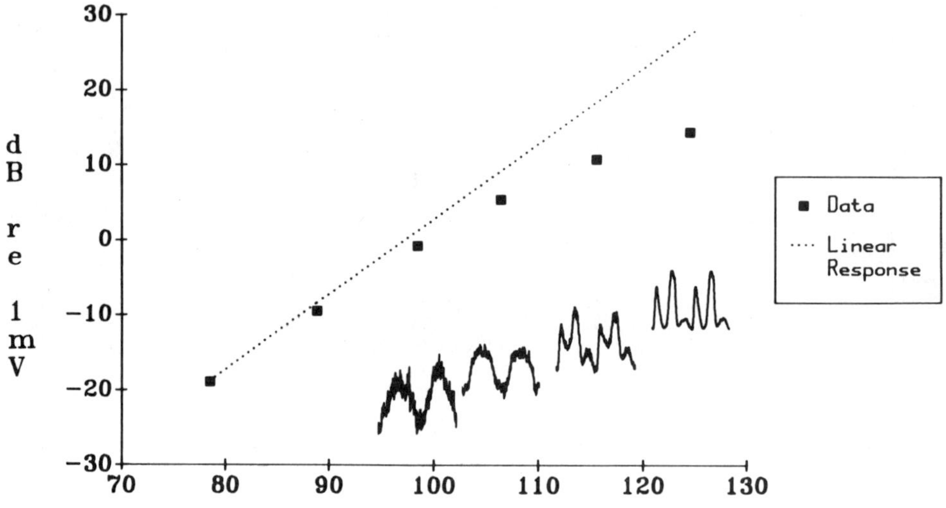

FIGURE 2 Growth of the cochlear microphonic recorded in the organ of Corti (■) and the corresponding IHC receptor potential (inserts) recorded at the same SPL's. The dotted line indicates an extrapolated linear growth. When the growth of the cochlear microphonic starts to deviate significantly from the linear response the IHC receptor potential demonstrates an increasingly distorted waveform. The IHC receptor potentials have been normalized so that they approximate the amplitude of the potential at the highest stimulus level.

In all cells, a phase shift of the fundamental Fourier component of the response with SPL was observed. In 10 out of 13 cells, the IHC phase showed an increased lead with increasing SPL. The average phase shift for these cells was 24° . One additional cell, not included in the above phase statistics showed a phase shift of approximately 180°. Figure 3 illustrates the phase shift in this cell along with the associated waveforms. The highly distorted waveforms coincide with the phase shift region.

Discussion

The similarity of the distortion in the IHC receptor potential and the input resistance waveforms supports the hypothesis that the distortion is present in the mechanical input to the IHC (Cody and Mountain, 1988, Mountain, 1988). If this is true then the stimulus to the IHC is not simply proportional to basilar membrane displacement or velocity because there is no evidence for this level of distortion in the basilar membrane motion.

Other investigators have discounted the distortion observed in basal turn IHC receptor potentials at low frequencies because of possible contamination of the IHC response by the extracellular currents from the OHC. We believe we have minimized this problem by calculating the differential potential across the IHC basolateral membrane.

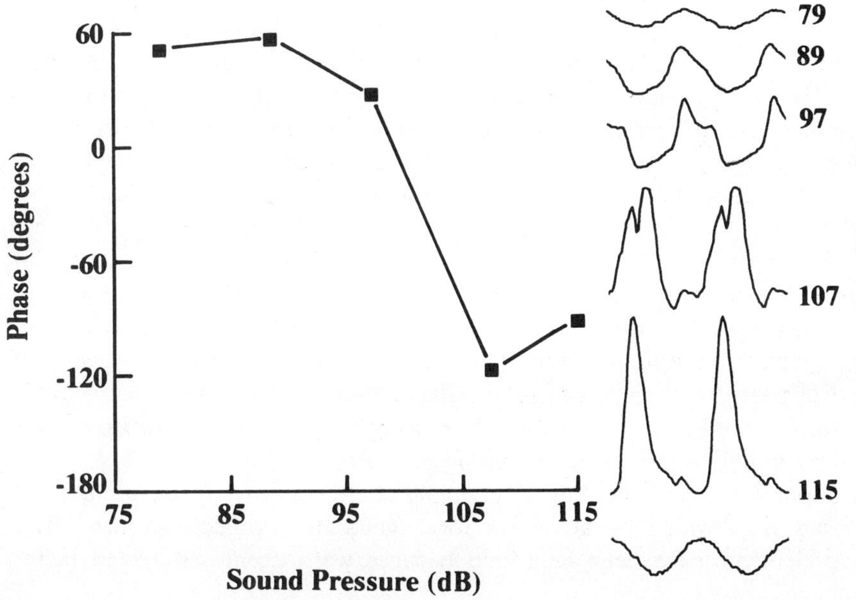

FIGURE 3. Phase of the fundamental of the IHC receptor potential to a 115Hz stimulus as a function of stimulus level. The phase is referenced to the SPL recorded at the tympanum. The inserts are the IHC receptor potentials recorded at the SPL's indicated. The lowermost insert is the sound pressure waveform with postive values corresponding to condensation. At stimulus intensities between 97 and 107dB there is a significant phase change in the fundamental component of the receptor potential.

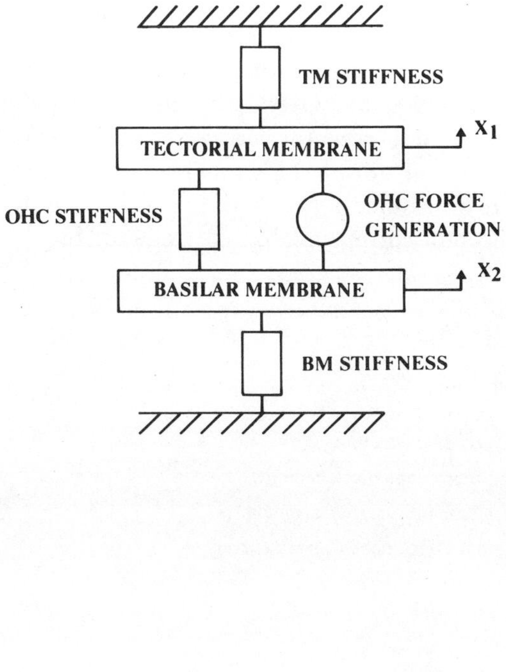

FIGURE 4. Simple mechanical model of the cochlear partition adapted from one originally proposed by Zwislocki (1986) where the nonlinear coupling between the basilar membrane and the tectorial membrane have been replaced by an active force located in the outer hair cells. The displacement of the tectorial membrane and the basilar membrane is indicated by X_1 and X_2 respectively. Sound is assumed to act directly only on the basilar membrane.

The stimulus frequencies and intensities used in the present study are outside the normal response area of basal turn IHCs. We are of the opinion, however, that the distortion observed imposes important constraints on any hypothesis of cochlear micromechanical function. Similar distortion has been observed as well by Dallos et al. (1986) in apical turn hair cells. In these cells stimulus frequencies much closer to the characteristic frequency of the cell can result in very distorted receptor potentials. An examination of the published apical turn data also suggests that the appearance of distorted IHC receptor potentials correlates with saturation of the OHC response.

The abrupt phase shifts in the IHC response with increasing sound level (Cody and Mountain, 1988; Sellick et al., 1982; Ruggero and Rich, 1983) can be produced by models in which the IHC respond to a combination of the movements of two structures. These are usually assumed to be the basilar membrane and a secondary structure, usually the tectorial membrane (Zwislocki, 1986). The tectorial membrane must be coupled to the basilar membrane via a nonlinear element and must excite the IHC out of phase with respect to the basilar membrane. One must also assume that the tectorial membrane is capable of moving in the radial direction. Figure 4 illustrates a modified model based on one proposed by Zwislocki (1986). The major modifications are that nonlinear coupling between the tectorial and basilar membranes is provided by an active force generation process in the OHC and damping elements have been neglected because we are only interested in the low frequency response.

Our data support the hypothesis that the nonlinear coupling is due to a force produced by the OHC which is proportional to the OHC receptor current or receptor potential. As the OHC mechanical-to-electrical transduction process saturates the coupling between the basilar membrane and the tectorial membrane is reduced. At low sound levels the tectorial membrane is assumed to be the dominant input to the IHC and at higher levels the basilar membrane is the dominant input and the phase of the IHC response abruptly changes.

The results of the nonlinear coupling can be illustrated with a very simple mathematical model. Assume that at very low frequencies that the tectorial membrane can be modeled as a spring and that the OHC exert a force on this structure which is directly proportional to the OHC receptor current. Further assume that the OHC receptor current is a function of the displacement between the basilar membrane and the tectorial membrane. If we assume a two-state channel model for the transduction process then the OHC receptor current can be approximated by:

$$I_{OHC} = \frac{I_{Max}}{1 + \exp(x_2 - x_1)}$$

where: I_{OHC} is the OHC receptor current
x_1 is the basilar membrane displacement
x_2 is the tectorial membrane displacement
I_{Max} is the maximum OHC peak to peak current

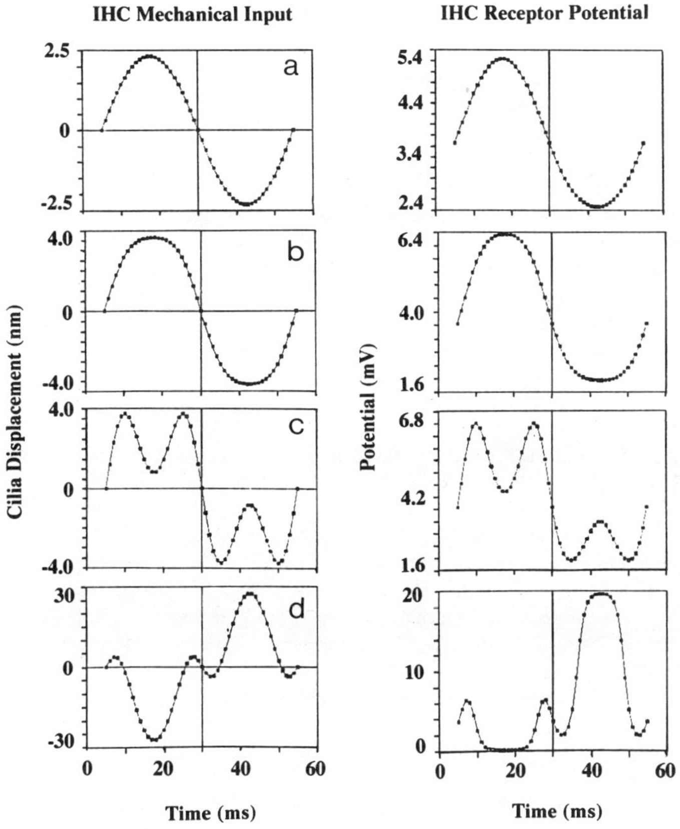

FIGURE 5. The mechanical input and the receptor potential of a simulated IHC to the simple mechanical model shown in figure 4. From the top to the bottom of the figure the sound pressure level is increasing in 6dB steps. Note that there is no increase in the peak-to-peak cillia displacement between panels B and C even though the stimulus level has increased 6 dB.

If the IHC are more sensitive to the displacement of the tectorial membrane than to the basilar membrane, then the transfer characteristic relating the mechanical input of the IHC to basilar membrane displacement may be nonmonotonic. Fig. 5 illustrates the response of a simulated IHC to such a mechanical system for low, moderate, and high sound pressure levels. At low sound levels (panel A) the tectorial membrane is the dominant input to the IHC. As the sound level is increased the fundamental components of the basilar and tectorial membrane movements cancel (panel C), but the harmonic components reinforce and a very distorted waveform results. At higher sound levels (panel D) the basilar membrane movement becomes the major input to the IHC. The cilia displacement waveform is further distorted by the rectification and saturation of the IHC transduction process as shown in fig. 5.

The exact waveshapes produced by such a model are very sensitive to small changes in model parameters such as the ratio of the passive stiffness of the OHC stereocilia to the sensitivity of the OHC force generator and the assymetry in the OHC mechanical-to-electrical transduction process. This sensitivity to small changes in mechanical properties may underlie the variablity observed in the experimentally obtained waveforms.

Acknowledgments

This work was supported in part by the MRC and NINCDS.

References

Cody, A.R. and Mountain, D.C. (1988). Low frequency inner hair cells: Evidence for a mechanical origin of peak splitting. Submitted for Publication.

Dallos, P., Santos-Sacchi, and Flock, A. (1982). Intracellular recordings from cochlear outer hair cells. Science 218, 582-584.

Dallos , P., Cheatham, M.A. and Oesterle, E. (1986). Harmonic components in hair cell responses. In: Auditory Frequency Selectivity (Eds: Moore, C.J. and Patterson, R..D.) Plenum, London, pp. 73-80.

Mountain, D.C. (1988). Measurement of low frequency receptor potentials in inner hair cells: A theoretical analysis. Submitted for Publication.

Mountain, D.C., Hubbard, A.E. and McMullen, T.A. (1983). Electromechanical processes in the cochlea. In:Mechanics of Hearing (Eds: deBoer, E. and Viergever, M.A.) Delft University Press, Delft, pp. 119-126.

Nuttall, A.L., Brown, M.C., Masta, R.I. and Lawrence, M. (1981). Inner hair cell responses to the velocity of basilar membrane motion in the guinea pig. Brain Res. 211, 171-174.

Patuzzi, R.B. and Yates, G.K. (1987). The low frequency response of inner hair cells in the guinea pig cochlea: Implications for fluid coupling and resonance of the stereocilia. Hearing Res. 30, 83-98.

Ruggero, M.A. and Rich, N.C. (1983). Chinchilla auditory-nerve responses to low-frequency tones. J. Acoust. Soc. Am. 73, 2096-2108.

Ruggero, M.A. and Rich, N.C. (1987). Timing of spike initiation in cochlear afferents: Dependance on site of innervation. J. Neurophys. 58, 379-403.

Russell, I.J. and Sellick, P.M. (1983). Low-frequency characteristics of intracellularly recorded receptor potentials in guinea pig cochlear hair cells. J. Physiol. 338, 179-206.

Sellick, P.M., Patuzzi, R. and Johnstone, B.M. (1982). Modulation of responses of spiral ganglion cells in the guinea pig cochlea by low frequency sound. Hearing Res. 7, 199-221.

Sellick, P.M. and Russell, I.J. (1980). The responses of inner hair cells to basilar membrane velocity during low frequency stimulation in the guinea pig cochlea. Hearing Res. 2, 439-445.

Zwislocki, J.J. (1986). Are nonlinearities observed in the firing rates of auditory-nerve afferents reflections of a nonlinear coupling between the tectorial membrane and the organ of Corti. Hearing Res. 22, 217-221.

Comments and Discussion

PATUZZI

We have observed responses from 52 IHCs responding to low frequency tones over the frequency range 20 Hz to 3200 Hz, and at levels that produce saturation of these cells. We have not observed "peak-splitting" under these conditions. It may be that the "peak splitting" you have observed is a correlate of the very high level complications in the neural histograms we have observed. If this is the case we must be careful in defining the different categories of "peak splitting".

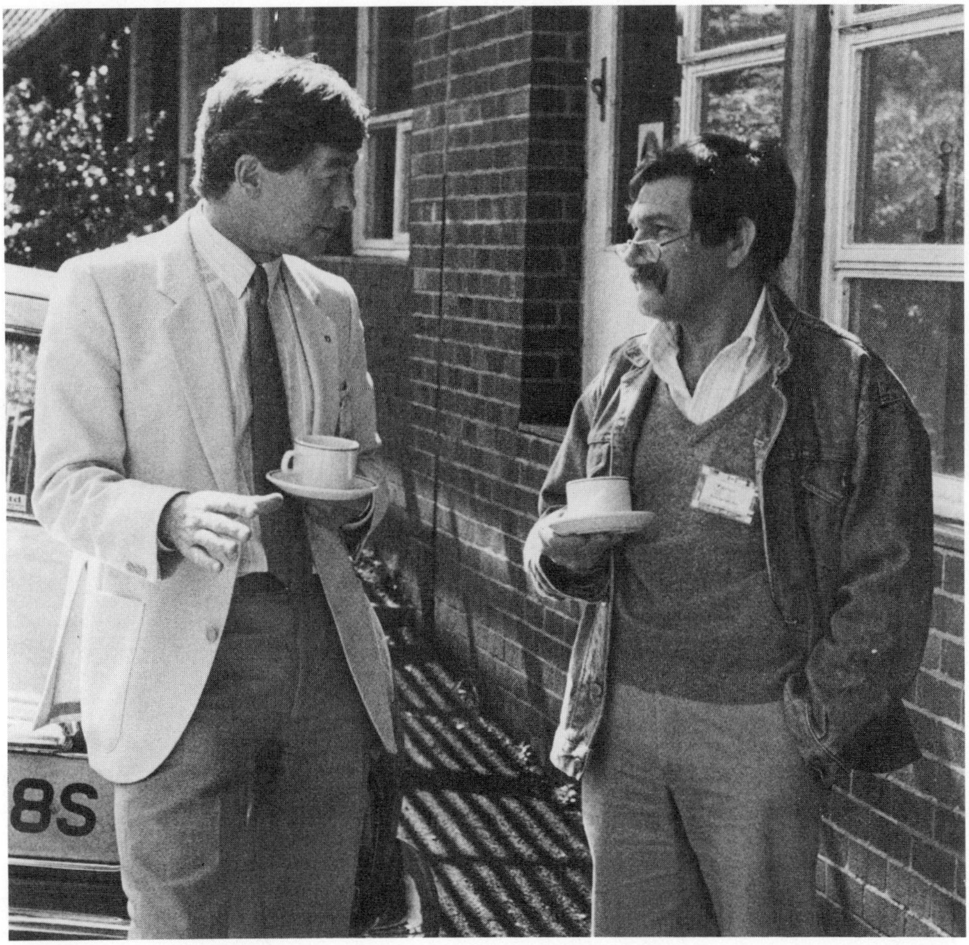

E.F. Evans and P. Dallos

3. ELECTROPHYSIOLOGICAL MEASUREMENTS

PHASE REVERSAL IN OHC RESPONSE AT HIGH SOUND INTENSITIES

J.J. Zwislocki and R.L. Smith
Institute for Sensory Research
Syracuse University, Syracuse, NY 13244, USA

Introduction

Kiang and his associates (e.g. Kiang, 1984) discovered an enigmatic phase shift of about 180° occurring in responses of auditory-nerve fibers at high sound intensities. One of us has demonstrated with the help of an electrical-network model that the phase shift can result from a nonlinear mechanical coupling between the tectorial membrane and the organ of Corti (Zwislocki, 1986). The associated distortion pattern produced by the model is essentially the same as found by Kiang's group.

If the phase shift does have a mechanical origin, it should also occur in the receptor potentials of the inner hair cells (IHCs) and, because of the mechanical coupling through the organ of Corti and the tectorial membrane, in those of the outer hair cells (OHCs) as well. To test this prediction, we recorded the alternating component of OHC receptor potentials directly, and also indirectly by determining Hensen-cell potentials and cochlear microphonics (CM).

Methods

The measurements were performed on Mongolian gerbils anesthetized with sodium pentobarbithal or dial in urethane. The surgical procedure was essentially the same as described by Schmiedt and Zwislocki (1977) for recording CM. In short, the animals were tracheotomized but not artificially respirated. The right pinna with the cartilagenous part of the ear canal as well as the soft tissues over the ventrolateral part of the right bulla were removed, and the bulla was opened between the tympanic ring and the vicinity of the trachea. The tympanic ring and the middle-ear ossicles were left intact. The opening revealed the entire ventrolateral aspect of the cochlea. A separate, small opening was made for a silver-wire round-window electrode used for measuring CAP (compound action potential) and also CM as gross indicators of the state of the cochlea. In preparations accepted for the experiments, the visual CAP threshold was around 20 dB SPL.

The sound was delivered to the ear by means of a miniature earphone with a flat transfer function within 6 dB in the frequency range between .5 and 12 kHZ. The sound pressure in the ear canal was monitored with a miniature electrette microphone with a flat transfer function in the same frequency range. Both transducers were coupled to the bony part of the ear canal by means of an insert especially developed for the purpose. The insert was sealed in the ear canal by means of a malleable plastic compound.

We recorded the cochlear potentials in the second turn (best frequency, BF, between 1.5 and 2 kHZ), using the approach of Dallos, Santos-Sacchi and Flock (1982) through scala media. However, only a small hole was drilled in the bony cochlear capsule, and the recording electrode was directed toward OHCs with the help of external landmarks rather than under visual observation. The small hole allowed us to maintain the endolymphatic potential at the high level of about 80 to 90 mV usually encountered in CM recordings. With proper electrodes, we were able to find Hensen's and outer hair cells without difficulty. The location of the electrode tip was monitored with the help of several indices — the distances from the bony capsule, the surface of stria vascularis and the surface of the organ of Corti, and the recorded direct and alternating potentials. The resting potentials of OHCs were between -60 and -85 mV, and those of Hensen's cells tended to be somewhat more negative, as described by Dallos et al. (1982). The alternating receptor potentials of OHCs were clearly larger than the alternating potentials recorded in intercellular space and in Hensen's cells. When the electrode penetrated the outermost Hensen cell, it could be guided through the rest of Hensen's cells up to the outer tunnel of Corti which was approximately at the 0 potential. Further advancement of the microelctrode by a few microns placed its tip at the outermost row of OHCs. The cells were penetrated with the help of capacitive ringing.

The intracellular microelectrodes were pulled on the Brown-Flaming puller P-77 and were filled with 3-M KCl. The most successful ones had resistances between 20 and 30 MOhms, as measured in the endolymph, after the penetration of the spiral ligament and stria vascularis. CM potentials were recorded either with the same electrodes or electrodes with tips broken to a diameter of 1 to 3 μm and filled with isotonic 0.15-M KCl.

The sound stimuli consisted of 5-sec bursts of sinusoids whose frequency was swept logarithmically from about 0.2 to about 12 kHz within each burst. The recorded potentials were amplified in a preamplifier with capacitance compensation and a lock-in amplifier with the filter bandwidth set to 3 or 10 Hz, depending on conditions. The lock-in amplifier improved the signal-to-noise ratio and limited the recordings to the fundamental frequency of the response wave forms. The frequency sweeps produced transfer functions that were displayed on a cathode-ray oscilloscope and photographed with a Polaroid camera. All the figures of this article represent such photographs. The transfer functions were displayed in terms of magnitude and the sine, y sin ($\omega\Delta t + \phi$), of the phase relative to the voltage at the earphone terminals. The displays had logarithmic frequency and linear amplitude scales.

Results

As a basis for subsequent comparisons, Fig. 1 shows the magnitude and sine-phase transfer functions of an OHC at a SPL of 30 dB. The best frequency is at approximately 1.7 kHz. Note the corresponding amplitude and phase perturbations below the best frequency. Their significance was discussed in preceding articles (Zwislocki, 1984, 1986 b,c) and will become more apparent in connection with the results that follow. A sine-phase function obtained on another OHC at 40 dB SPL is shown in Fig. 2 by

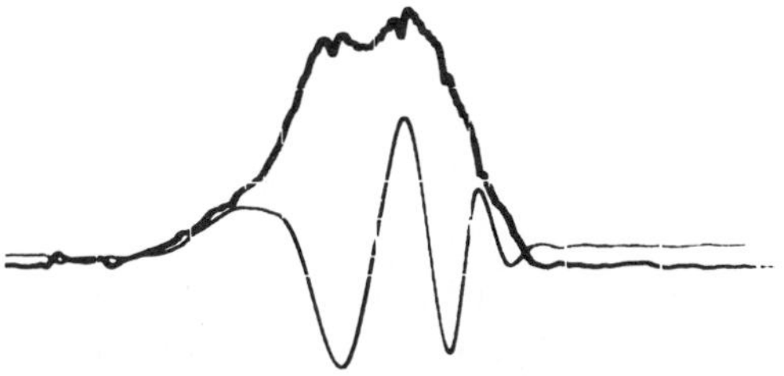

FIGURE 1 Intracellular magnitude and sine-phase (thin line, amplification reduced) transfer functions of a OHC. Frequency scale is log., amplitude scale is linear. The main peak (right) is at about 1.7 kHz; the second peak was caused by a strong peak in the middle-ear tranfer function. Note the phase perturbation (departure from sinusoid) at low sound frequencies resulting from the 180° phase shift. SPL at 30 dB. Animal: GZ-87.

the thin line. The thick line shows the transformation of this function at 100 dB (The amplification was decreased by a factor of 10). Note that the response phase is practically reversed in the neighborhood of low-SPL BF , and that the phase change decreases toward the low frequencies. The associated change in amplitude distribution can be ascribed in part to the known decreased frequency selectivity at high SPLs. Its analysis is beyond the scope of this article.

To demonstrate that the phase reversal of Fig. 2 is not due to an artifact caused by inserting a microelectrode into an OHC, we recorded corresponding phase characteristics in Hensen's cells and in the endolymphatic space. They are reproduced in Figs. 3 and 4, respectively. The recordings were made on the same preparation (GZ-133). Since the same phase reversal occurred at all three recording sites, the reversal found in the OHC potential could not have been produced by an electrode artifact. Similar results were obtained on other preparations, and the phase reversal at high SPLs proved to be a robust phenomenon. It persisted even after moderate cochlear deterioration.

Discussion

The phase reversal in the alternating OHC receptor potential at high SPLs can hardly be ascribed to the OHCs themselves since their response polarity is determined by their morphology. As a consequence, the reversal must take place in the mechanical stimulus that controls the deflection of the OHC stereocilia. How can this happen?

If we persist in accepting the classical shear-motion model of hair-cell stimulation, according to which the shear motion between the tectorial membrane and the reticular lamina is due solely to the geometry of the organ of Corti, no answer becomes readily apparent. If, on the other hand, we are ready to accept that the tectorial membrane is capable of resonance vibration in the radial cochlear direction and, in addition, that cochlear damping increases with sound intensity, an answer is provided almost automatically. That the damping increases with sound intensity is well established. How a tectorial-membrane resonance in the radial direction can occur has been explained on several occasions, and a substantial body of experimental evidence for such a resonance has been assembled (Zwislocki, 1980, 1982, 1983, 1985, 1986 b). It has been found that, in live Mongolian gerbils, the tectorial membrane is quite compliant in the radial

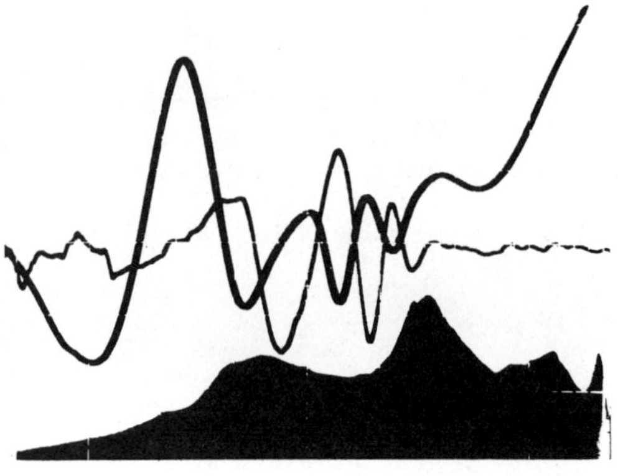

FIGURE 2 Intracellular sine-phase transfer functions of another OHC taken at two SPLs, 40 (thin line) and 100 dB. Note the phase reversal between the two curves and the lack of the low-frequency phase perturbation in the 100-dB curve. Black area at bottom indicates ear-canal sound pressure, but 0-coordinate is not shown. Animal: GZ-132.

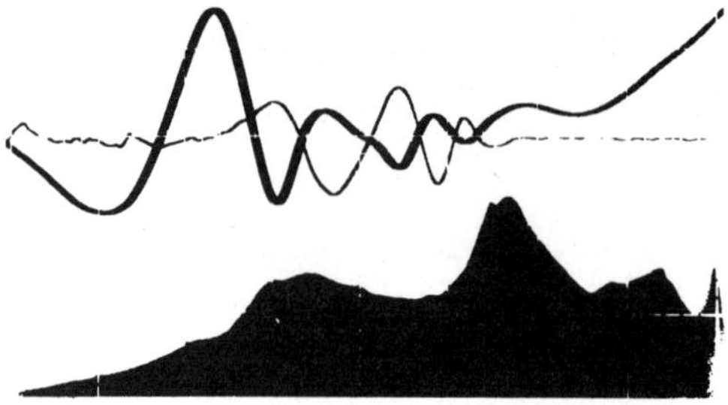

FIGURE 3 Same as Fig. 2, but for a Hensen's cell. Same animal.

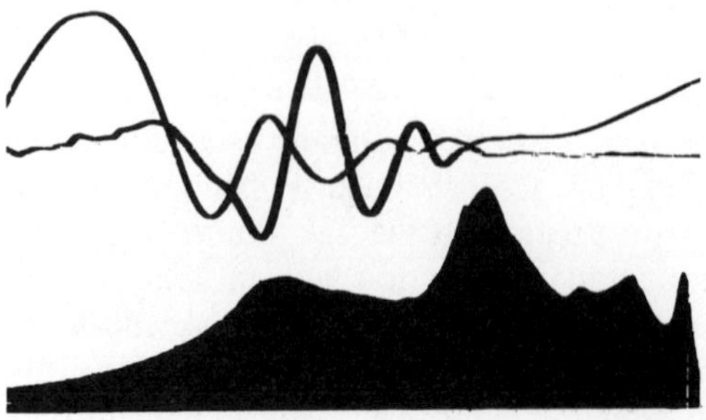

FIGURE 4 Same as Fig. 2, but for CM. However, thick line for 40 dB SPL. Note phase opposition between this figure and Figs. 2 and 3. Same animal.

cochlear direction, so that a strong radial vibration is possible. The measured compliance was greater by one order of magnitude than that of the corresponding aggregate of the OHC stereocilia (Zwislocki, 1988). This means that the tectorial membrane must act on the stereocilia as a mass load rather than a stiff anchor. According to the resonance model of the tectorial membrane, the resonance results from an interaction between the distributed mass of the tectorial membrane and the stiffness of the OHC stereocilia (Zwislocki, 1980). On the basis of their measurements of the stereocilia stiffness in guinea pigs and estimations of the effective mass of the tectorial membrane (Zwislocki, 1980), Strelioff, Flock and Minser (1985) calculated that the resonance frequency agrees approximately with cochlear BF for any given cochlear location.

In the classical model, the geometry of the organ of Corti demands that the radial component of the tectorial-membrane motion be always smaller than the radial component of the reticular-lamina motion (e.g. Zwislocki, 1986 b). Under such conditions, the hair-cell stereocilia are always deflected toward Hensen's cells and the OHC depolarized during basilar-membrane displacement toward scala vestibuli. On the other hand, the resonance model of the tectorial-membrane predicts that the radial vibration amplitude of the tectorial membrane substantially excedes the radial vibration amplitude of the reticular lamina in the broad vicinity of BF when the cochlear damping is small. According to the model, the stereocilia are deflected toward Hensen's cells during basilar-membrane displacement toward scala tympani in all frequency regions where the radial vibration of the tectorial membrane is roughly in phase with the radial component of the reticular-lamina vibration. Simple mathematical considerations and computer simulations show that this is true everywhere in the broad vicinity of the best frequency (e.g. Zwislocki, 1986 b). At high SPLs at which the cochlear damping becomes high, the effect of the tectorial-membrane resonance is practically abolished. As a consequence, the radial amplitude of the tectorial-membrane vibration becomes smaller than the radial amplitude of the reticular-lamina vibration, and the phase of the stereocilia deflection becomes the same as in the classical model. The same phase must hold for very low sound frequencies at which the effect of the tectorial-membrane mass is negligible. The model predicts the following phase patterns of OHC depolarization:

At low SPLs, depolarization during basilar-membrane displacement toward scala vestibuli at low sound frequencies but during its displacement in the opposite direction in the broad neighborhood of BF,with a phase shift of 180° between the two regions.

At high SPLs, depolarization during basilar-membrane displacement toward scala vestibuli at all sound frequencies (no phase shift between the low and high frequencies).

A phase reversal between the low- and high-SPLs in the broad vicinity of the best frequency; no such reversal in the low frequency region.

The phase shift between the low and high frequencies is evident in all the figures in the sine-phase curves obtained at 30 or 40 db SPL. No such phase shift is evident in the sine-phase curves recorded at 100 dB SPL. The phase reversal between the low- and high-SPL patterns in BF region is clearly documented in Figs. 2, 3 and 4. The phases converge toward the low-frequency end of the patterns.

Our findings have an important corollary for the use of CM as reference for cochlear measurements. Comparison between Figs. 2 and 4 shows no substantial difference in phase patterns between the OHC receptor potentials and scala-media CM, except for phase oppostion. This means that CM phase cannot be assumed to be always in the same relation to the phase of basilar-membrane displacement. The relation changes with sound frequency and SPL. The depolarizing phase of CM indicates basilar-membrane displacement toward scala vestibuli only at sound frequencies well below the best frequency, unless the sound pressure is very high.

Acknowledgements

Preliminary surgery was performed by L.K. Cefaratti. Work supported by NIH Javits Grant RO 1 NS 03950.

References

Dallos, P. , Santos-Sacchi, J. and Flock, Å. (1982) Intracellular recordings from cochlear outer hair cells. Science 218, 582-584.

Kiang, N.Y.S. (1984) Peripheral neural processing of auditory information. In: Handbook of Physiology, Sect. 1, Vol. 3 (Ed.: Darian-Smith, I.) American Physiological Society, Bethesda, Maryland, pp. 639-674.

Schmiedt, R. A. and Zwislocki, J. J. (1977) Comparison of sound-transmission and ccochlear-microphonic characteristics in Mongolian gerbil and guinea pig. J. Acoust. Soc. Am. 61, 133-149.

Strelioff, D., Flock, Å. and Minser, K. E. (1985). Role of inner and outer hair cells in mechanical frequency selectivity of the cochlea. Hearing Res. 18, 169-175.

Zwislocki, J. J. (1980) Five decades of research on cochlear mechanics. J. Acoust. Soc. Am. 67, 1679-1685.

Zwislocki, J. J. (1982) Micromechanics of the cochlea and possible changes caused by intense noise. In: New Perspectives on Noisc-Induced Hearing Loss (Eds: Hamernik, R. P., Henderson, D. and Salvi, R.) Raven Press, New York, pp. 209-224.

Zwislocki, J. J. (1983) Cochlear micromechanics—a model and some of its consequences. In: Mechanisms of Hearing (Eds: Webster, R. W. and Aitkin, L. M.) Monash University Press, Clayton, Victoria, Australia, pp. 21-26.

Zwislocki, J. J. (1984) How OHC lesions can lead to neural cochlear hypersensitivity. Acta Otolaryngol. 97, 529-534.

Zwislocki, J. J. (1985) Cochlear function—An analysis. Acta Otolaryngol. (Stockh) 100, 201-209.

Zwislocki, J. J. (1986a) Are nonlinearities observed in firing rates of auditory-nerve afferents reflections of a nonlinear coupling between the tectorial membrane and the organ of Corti? In: Procedings of Nobel Symposium 63: Cochlear Mechanisms in Hearing (Eds: Flock, Å. and Wersäll, J.) Elsevier, Amsterdam, pp. 217-221.

Zwislocki, J. J. (1986b) Analysis of cochlear mechanics. In: Proceedings of Nobel Symposium 63. Cellular Mechanisms in Hearing (Eds: Flock, Å. and Wersäll) Elsevier, Amsterdam, pp. 155-169.

Zwislocki, J. J. (1986c) Changes in cochlear frequency selectivity produced by tectorial-membrane manipulation. In: Auditory Frequency Selectivity (Eds: Moore, B.C.J. and Patterson, R. D.) Plenum, New York, pp. 3-11.

Zwislocki, J. J. (1988). Mechanical properties of the tectorial membrane in situ. Acta Otolaryngol. (Stockh) 105 (in press).

OUTER HAIR CELL RECEPTOR CURRENT AND ITS EFFECT ON COCHLEAR MECHANICS

R.B. Patuzzi, G.K. Yates and B.M. Johnstone

Department of Physiology
University of Western Australia
Nedlands, Western Australia 6009

Introduction

In 1948 Gold suggested that the vibration of the organ of Corti relied on active mechanical feedback to maintain its sensitivity and frequency selectivity. Since then mathematical models of its labile vibration (Khanna and Leonard, 1982; Sellick et al, 1982, 1983, 1984; Robles et al, 1986) agree with Gold's view that forces must be applied to the organ to partially cancel the inherent viscous forces (Neely and Kim, 1983,1986; de Boer, 1983). This force generation process within the cochlea has been termed the active process, while the forces themselves have been termed negative damping. More recently, it has been observed that isolated outer hair cells (OHCs) from the mammal contract in vitro in response to applied electric current (Brownell et al, 1983, 1985; Ashmore, 1987). These and other observations (see Patuzzi and Robertson, 1988) suggest that the OHCs are the negative damping elements in cochlear mechanics, and that their synchronous contraction is controlled by the AC receptor current that flows through them, or by voltages that these currents produce. This combination of mechano-electric (ME) transduction at the apex of the hair cells (Holton and Hudspeth, 1987) and electro-mechanical (EM) cellular contraction has been termed "bi-directional transduction" (Weiss, 1982).

On the basis of these findings, many forms of sensori-neural loss can be explained by disruption of at least one of the stages of bi-directional transduction, with a consequent loss of mechanical sensitivity. For example, under certain conditions of acoustic overstimulation dramatic threshold elevations near the characteristic frequency (CF) of a neuron can be accompanied by little or no threshold change on the low-frequency tail of the neural tuning curve (Cody and Johnstone, 1980). Similar changes are also seen after other traumatic manipulations of the cochlea (see Patuzzi and Robertson, 1988). This lack of change on the tail of the tuning curve indicates that after such trauma synaptic transmission and detection of organ of Corti vibration by the inner hair cells are normal. By exclusion, the changes in neural sensitivity near CF are probably due to changes in the vibration of the organ of Corti. Indeed, there is some direct experimental evidence in the case of acoustic trauma that this is the case (Sellick et al, 1982; Patuzzi et al, 1983).

Although a disruption of bi-directional transduction is consistent with these changes it is still not clear which of its ME or EM stages is impaired by any particular cochlear manipulation or trauma. The changes in the mechanical and electrical responses at CF following trauma provide little information about the site of the disruption since they are inextricably linked within a feedback loop. To determine which of the ME or EM processes is compromised in any particular lesion we would need to monitor at least one of them independently of the function of the overall feedback system.

As already noted, however, vibration of the organ of Corti at frequencies much below CF is relatively robust, presumably because the vibration at these frequencies is dominated by stiffness restoring forces that are much greater in magnitude than the negative damping forces. This ineffectiveness of the EM feedback process for frequencies much below CF does allow the integrity of the ME stage of transduction to be tested independently of the integrity of the entire bi-directional process. Any fall in the AC receptor currents through OHCs on the tail of the tuning curve following trauma is probably due to impairment of the ME transduction process at the apex of these cells, rather than to a change in the mechanical stimulus to their hair bundle. Consequently, the extent to which impairment of ME transduction contributes to the disruption of the bi-directional process may be estimated by measuring OHC transduction currents below CF and vibration of the organ of Corti at CF. Fortunately, we need not measure either of these responses directly. The low-frequency microphonic potential may be used as an assay of the integrity of the OHC ME transduction in the first turn of the guinea pig since it is well established that this potential is dominated by AC receptor currents through the OHCs of this region (see Cheatham and Dallos, 1982; Patuzzi et al, 1988a). Similarly, the gross eighth-nerve compound action potential (CAP) evoked by tone bursts may be used as an indicator of the vibration of the organ of Corti at CF (Sellick et al, 1982; Robles et al, 1986).

In this paper we present results from such experiments in which the low-frequency microphonic and neural sensitivity in the first turn in the guinea pig have been monitored before and after various manipulations of the cochlea, including acoustic overstimulation. Our results indicate that the most vulnerable step in bi-directional transduction is the ME transduction process at the apex of the outer hair cells. We also present in this and a subsequent paper (Yates et al, this volume) evidence that the nonlinearity of the ME transduction process is the major cause of the many nonlinear phenomena observed in cochlear mechanics.

Acoustic trauma and mechano-electrical transduction

As already mentioned, one of the simplest manipulations of the cochlea that produces elevation of neural threshold near the tip of the tuning curve, with little or no elevation on the tail, is acoustic trauma. We have measured the relationship between threshold elevation at CF and the integrity of the ME transduction process by exposing anaesthetized guinea-pigs repeatedly to a traumatizing pure tone stimulus (10kHz, 115dB SPL) for successive periods of 30s, 30s, 45s and 45s. The elevation of neural threshold in the first cochlear turn was estimated by averaging the neural threshold elevation after each exposure for frequencies of 10, 12, 14, 16, 18 and 20kHz. This average elevation was a reasonable estimate of the desensitization in the whole basal turn because the threshold elevation was approximately flat for frequencies above 10kHz. The reduction in the efficiency of the ME transduction process of the OHCs of the first turn was determined by measuring the amplitude of the low-frequency microphonic evoked at the round window by a 200Hz probe tone presented at 105dB SPL. The changes in the amplitude of the 200Hz microphonic and neural thresholds were determined 4 minutes after each exposure. This delay avoided the rapid partial recovery period immediately after exposure.

After each exposure the amplitude of the microphonic potential was reduced, and the neural thresholds were elevated for frequencies above 8kHz. The reductions in neural and microphonic sensitivities were highly correlated, as shown in figure 1a. Here the percentage reduction in microphonic amplitude is plotted against mean neural threshold elevation. The relationship between the microphonic amplitude, n, normalized to initial amplitude and the associated threshold elevation, HL, is given by the empirical relationship

$$HL = 55dB\ (1-n/(1+0.85(1-n))$$

The relatively constant shape of the distorted microphonic waveform (figure 1b) supports the view that the fall in microphonic amplitude was not due to a reduction in the mechanical stimulus to the OHC hair bundle. This is also consistent with the vertical, rather than horizontal, repositioning of the microphonic input-output function after trauma (figure 1c). These changes are consistent with a reduction in the number of operational ME transduction channels at the apex of the OHCs, without a change in the properties of the remaining channels. Potential measurements in scala media of the first turn support this view, and indicate that the reduction in channel numbers probably results from an inactivation of channels in a closed conformational state. This can be seen in figure 2. Following each exposure to the traumatic stimulus the endocochlear potential was unaltered for peak excursions of the organ of Corti towards scala tympani (the direction producing closure of the transduction channels), while the peak negative going excursions of the endocochlear potential became more positive for low-frequency displacements towards scala vestibuli (the direction producing opening of the transduction channels).

Regardless of the mechanism producing the reduction in the amplitude of the low-frequency microphonic, these results indicate an impairment of the ME transduction

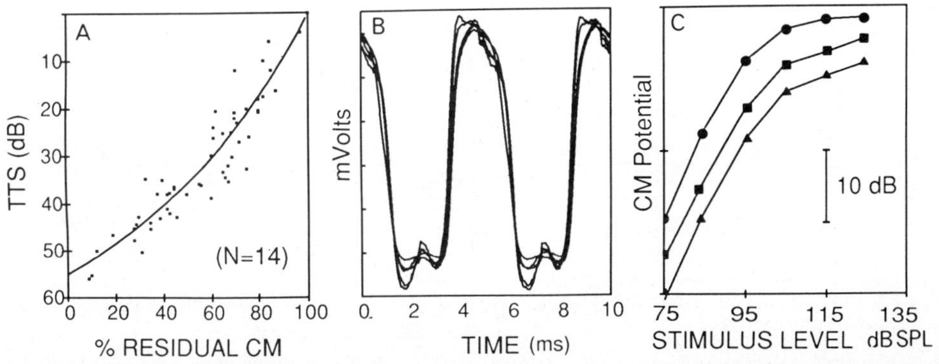

Figure 1: (a) The correlation between elevation of neural threshold and reduction of 200Hz microphonic in the first turn after acoustic trauma. The solid line is the empirical equation given in the text. (b) Normalized 200Hz microphonic waveforms in the tunnel of Corti before and after acoustic trauma. The waveshapes are very similar despite reduction of the amplitude to less than 20% of its initial value. (c) Input-output functions for the 200Hz round window microphonic before (●) and after cumulative exposures of 30s (■) and 60s (▲).

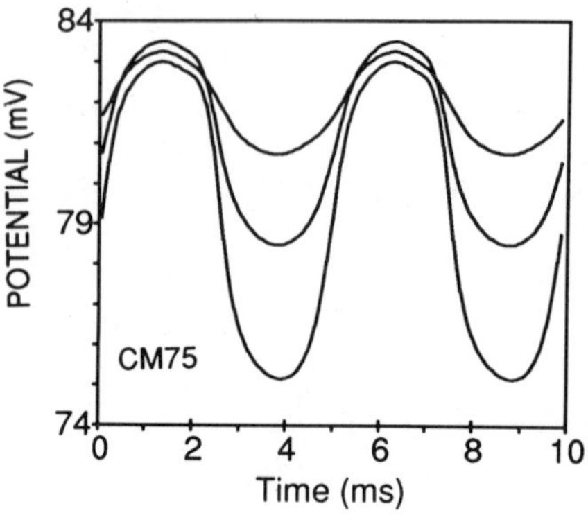

Figure 2: Averaged DC-coupled potential waveforms in scala media before and after cumulative exposures of 30s, 60s and 105s. Negative going potentials are produced by partition displacements towards scala vestibuli, and correspond to opening of OHC mechano-electric transduction channels. Positive going potentials occur during displacements towards scala tympani, and indicate closure of channels. Note that after acoustic trauma the potentials for displacements towards scala vestibuli are less negative indicating inactivation of transduction channels.

process at the apex of the OHCs in the first turn. At first appearance the fall in microphonic amplitude may appear insignificant when compared with the dramatic elevation in neural threshold. Such small changes are likely to be quite significant, however, as may be seen from a simple model of bi-directional transduction.

Negative damping and mechanical sensitivity

Only a relatively small reduction in the magnitude of the negative damping forces applied to the cochlear partition would be required to dramatically alter the mechanical sensitivity near CF. We can appreciate how important negative damping is to the mechanical sensitivity of the organ of Corti by considering a simple second order resonant system as shown in figure 3a. The sensitivity of such a system at its resonance frequency is proportional to the reciprocal of the net damping coefficient, R_{tot}, which relates the velocity of the organ of Corti, v, to the frictional forces that damp its movement by $F_{damp}=R_{tot}.v$. We can make three basic assumptions at the outset in our consideration of the active process. First, we can assume that the total damping coefficient is comprised of a passive component, R_{pass}, and an active component, R_{act}.

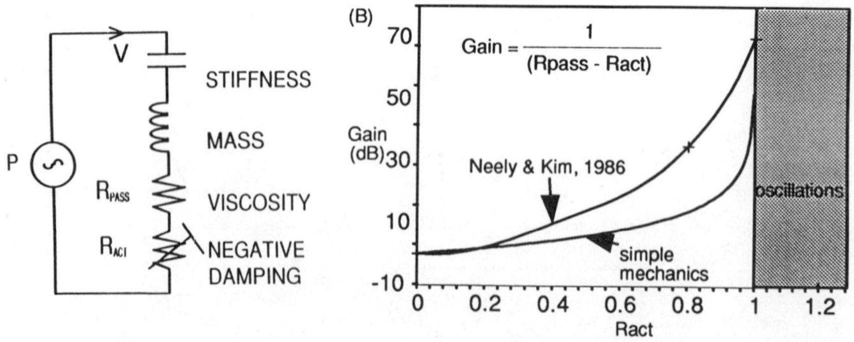

Figure 3: (a) A simple second order electrical analogue of bi-directional transduction. The total damping coefficient is Rtot=Rpass-Ract. The gain of the system at its resonance frequency is proportional to 1/Rtot. (b) The variation of system gain at the resonant frequency as a function of the negative damping component -Ract. Also shown for comparison are the model results of Neely and Kim (1986).

Second, we can assume that the active component of the damping coefficient is itself proportional to the product of the sensitivity of the ME transduction process at the apex of the OHCs (R_{me}) and the sensitivity of the EM feedback process (R_{em}). And third, we can assume that the active feedback forces simply subtract from the inherent viscous forces. The net damping coefficient is then given by the simple expression $R_{tot}=(R_{pass}-R_{act})=(R_{pass}-R_{me}.R_{em})$. As a consequence, the increase in sensitivity or gain, G, produced by the active process at the resonance frequency of the simple model is given by $1/(R_{pass}-R_{me}.R_{em})$.

This simple hyperbolic relationship between sensitivity at the resonance frequency and the magnitude of the negative damping component is shown in figure 3b for a negative damping coefficient, R_{act}, within the range 0 to R_{pass}. Neely and Kim (1986) have calculated analogous mechanical sensitivities for a number of values of the negative damping component in their more complex hydrodynamic model. The values they calculated are also shown in figure 3b for comparison. The point emphasized by this figure is that the mechanical sensitivity of a resonant system is extremely sensitive to the magnitude of the negative damping component when the negative and passive damping terms are nearly equal and sensitivity is high. This appears to be the case in the normal mammalian cochlea. As a consequence, the percentage reduction in the sensitivity of the ME transduction process, R_{me}, and the resulting fall in OHC receptor current following acoustic trauma is not insignificant. On the contrary, on the basis of the hydrodynamic model of Neely and Kim it would appear sufficient to explain the observed elevation in neural threshold.

Since the disruption of the ME stage of bi-directional transduction does seem sufficient to explain the threshold shift observed, the EM stage of transduction must be relatively robust. This is consistent with the fact that contraction of OHCs can be observed in vitro under decidedly abnormal conditions. Furthermore, if disruption of the ME transduction efficiency of the OHCs is sufficient to explain acoustic trauma under certain conditions, we may ask if a similar disruption is responsible for sensori-neural loss produced by other cochlear manipulations. We argue in the remainder of this paper that this is the case.

Disruption of ME transduction by other means

If the hearing loss produced by acoustic trauma is due to an inactivation of the ME transduction channels and a fall in the AC receptor currents that drive the active process, we might expect any cochlear manipulation that reduces these currents to cause a similar sensori-neural loss. There are many other means of impairing the efficiency of the ME transduction process at the apex of OHCs. Apart from acoustic trauma, the AC receptor currents through OHCs may be reduced by a fall in the endocochlear potential, as in asphyxia or furosemide intoxication, and by blockage of the transduction channels at the apex of these cells. This blockage can result from intoxication with ototoxic drugs such as streptomycin or 4-aminopyridine, or may be produced by driving the population of ME transduction channels into saturation. This may result when either an intense single tone stimulus is presented, or when a relatively low intensity stimulus is presented with a second relatively intense interfering tone. The interference tone may be either a very low-frequency bias tone (Patuzzi et al, 1984) or be presented at a frequency closer to the CF of a particular region of the cochlea. In each case the relative amplitude of the crucial AC receptor currents through the OHCs that drive the active process would be reduced.

In each of these manipulations there is, of course, the possibility of also impairing inner hair cell ME transduction and/or synaptic transmission. As a result, the elevation of neural threshold produced by any particular manipulation may be more than that predicted on the basis of the reduction of OHC receptor current and the mechanical desensitization observed after acoustic trauma (figure 1a). As with acoustic trauma, however, under certain conditions some of these manipulations can produce elevations of neural threshold for frequencies near CF without threshold elevation on the tail of the neural tuning curve. In such cases it is probably only OHC function that is impaired, and neural and mechanical desensitization at CF would be equal.

For example, elevation of neural sensitivity at CF without elevation on the tail of the tuning curve is observed in two tone suppression experiments in which a suppressor elevates the tip of the tuning curve without stimulating of the neuron directly (Sachs and Kiang, 1968). Similarly, neural sensitivity at CF can be elevated cyclically by an intense very-low-frequency suppressor (Sellick et al, 1982b; Patuzzi et al, 1984a). Peak threshold elevation is observed for peak displacements of the organ of Corti towards scala tympani and scala vestibuli, and at levels of the suppressor tone that do not stimulate the neuron when presented alone. We would expect that threshold elevation in such cases would be due to disruption of OHC receptor currents alone, and that the relationship between the efficiency of OHC ME transduction and threshold elevation at CF would be similar to that observed in acoustic trauma. Our experimental measurements support this view.

Figure 4 shows the relationship between neural threshold elevation and fall in OHC ME transduction efficiency as the intensity of a low-frequency suppressor tone was increased. As in the case of acoustic trauma the change in mechanical sensitivity at CF was estimated by averaging the elevation of CAP threshold for frequencies between 10 and 20kHz. The OHC ME transduction efficiency in the first turn was estimated by measuring the amplitude of the microphonic potential evoked by low-frequency probe tones presented at frequencies of 6, 7, 8 and 9kHz, and at an intensity of 70dB SPL. For each intensity of a 6.5kHz suppressor tone in the range 65 to 95dB SPL the mean threshold elevation was estimated, and the percentage reduction in the round window microphonic was averaged across probe frequency. Note that the relationship between disruption of the OHC receptor currents and the elevation of neural threshold observed in

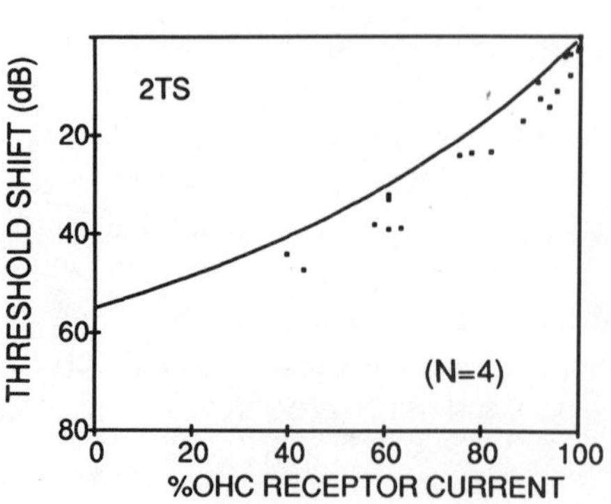

Figure 4: The correlation between elevation of neural threshold and reduction of low-frequency microphonic at the round window produced by a 6.5kHz suppressor tone at levels between 65 and 95dB SPL. The solid line is the empirical equation describing the data following acoustic trauma (figure 1a).

two-tone suppression is almost identical to that seen after acoustic trauma. Essentially Figure 4 is the link between two-tone interference in the gross microphonic and two-tone suppression in the neural response.

The neural threshold elevation produced by displacement of the organ of Corti from its rest position follows a similar pattern. If a 40Hz pure tone is presented at intensities above about 90dB SPL it cyclically reduces the efficiency of OHC ME transduction by driving the majority of transduction channels at the apex of the OHCs into either the open or closed states. Under these conditions they are unavailable to transduce any high-frequency mechanical stimulus presented at the same time. As a result, the amplitude of the high-frequency receptor currents through the OHCs are modulated in synchrony with the low-frequency displacement, and the EM feedback loop within the cochlea is broken cyclically. This cyclic reduction in the AC receptor currents through the OHCs is illustrated in figure 5a for 3 different levels of the 40Hz suppressor tone.

If we plot the percentage reduction in the efficiency of OHC ME transduction at peak low-frequency displacements towards scala tympani (indicated by the arrow in figure 5a) against the corresponding elevation of neural threshold at the same instant we obtain a relationship very similar to that obtained following acoustic trauma and during two-tone suppression (figures 1a and 4). In this case neural threshold elevation is monitored at only 18kHz, and a 7kHz probe tone is used to monitor OHC transduction efficiency.

In conclusion, the similarity between the correlations between neural threshold and low-frequency microphonic for acoustic trauma, two-tone suppression and low-frequency biasing, and the predictions based on the model of Neely and Kim, suggests that all three experimental manipulations produce a sensori-neural loss by the same mechanism: namely a reduction in the high-frequency OHC receptor currents that drive the active process and produce negative damping. Moreover, since the lack of threshold

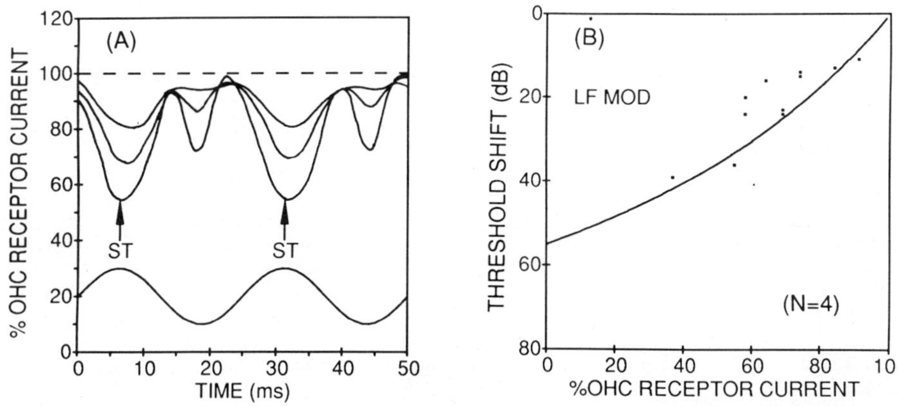

Figure 5: (a) The cyclic reduction of the 7kHz microphonic measured at the round window through two cycles of a 40Hz suppressor tone presented at levels of 115dB, 118dB and 120dB SPL. The depth of modulation increases with suppressor intensity. The low-frequency phase corresponding to maximum displacement towards scala tympani is indicated by the arrow. (b) The correlation between the percentage reduction in the 7kHz microphonic and the elevation of neural threshold at 18kHz at maximum displacement towards scala tympani. The solid line is the empirical equation describing the data following acoustic trauma (figure 1a).

elevation on the tail of the neural tuning curves indicates little disruption of inner hair cells and synaptic processes, this relationship probably represents a pure OHC hearing loss. In the case of acoustic trauma, desensitization of the ME stage of transduction is probably due to an inactivation of ME transduction channels at the apex of the OHCs into a closed state, while in the case of two-tone suppression and low-frequency biasing of the cochlear partition it is due to saturation of the channel population (Holton and Hudspeth, 1987). These results are consistent with the saturation-feedback model of Zwicker (1979), and with other forms of sensori-neural loss described in detail elsewhere (Patuzzi et al, 1988b).

Acknowledgements

This work was supported by grants from the Australian N.H. & M.R.C.

References

Ashmore, J.F. (1986) A fast motile response in guinea-pig outer hair cells. J. Physiol. 388, 323-347.
Ashmore, J.F. and Brownell, W.E. (1986) KiloHertz movements induced by electrical stimulation in outer hair cells from the guinea pig cochlea. J. Physiol. 377, 41P.
de Boer, E. (1983) No sharpening? A challenge for cochlear mechanics. J. Acoust. Soc. Am. 73, 567-573.
Cheatham, M.A. and Dallos, P. (1982) Two-tone interactions in the cochlear microphonic. Hearing Res. 8, 29-48.
Cody, A.R. and Johnstone, B.M. (1980) Single auditory neuron response during acute acoustic trauma. Hearing Res. 3, 3-16.
Gold, T. (1948) Hearing. II. The physical basis of the action of the cochlea. Proc. Roy. Soc. B. (Edinburgh) 135, 492-498.
Holton, and Hudspeth, A.J. (1987) The transduction channel of hair cells
Khanna, S.M. and Leonard, D.G.B. (1982) Basilar membrane tuning in the cat cochlea. Science, 215, 305-306.
Neely, S.T. and Kim, D.O. (1983) An active cochlear model showing sharp tuning and high sensitivity. Hearing Res. 9, 123-130.
Neely, S.T. and Kim, D.O. (1986) A model for active elements in cochlear micromechanics.
Patuzzi, R.B., Sellick, P.M. and Johnstone, B.M. (1984a) The modulation of the sensitivity of the mammalian cochlea by low-frequency tones: I. Primary afferent activity. Hearing Res. 13, 1-8.
Patuzzi, R.B., Johnstone, B.M. and Sellick, P.M. (1984b) The alteration of the vibration of the basilar membrane produced by loud sound. Hearing Res. 13, 99-100.
Patuzzi, R.B. and Robertson, D. (1988) Tuning in the mammalian cochlea. Physiological Reviews, (in press).
Patuzzi, R.B., Yates, G.K. and Johnstone, B.M. (1988a) The origin of low-frequency microphonic potentials measured in the first turn of the guinea pig cochlea. Hearing Res. (submitted).
Patuzzi, R.B. Yates, G.K. and Johnstone, B.M. (1988b) Outer hair cell receptor current and sensori-neural hearing loss. Hearing Res. (submitted).
Robles, L., Ruggero, M.A. and Rich, N.C. (1986) Basilar membrane mechanics at the base of the chinchilla cochlea. I. Input-output fucntions, tuning curves, and phase responses. J. Acoust. Soc. Am. 80: 1364-1374.
Sellick, P.M., Patuzzi, R.B. and Johnstone, B.M. (1982) Measurement of basilar membrane motion in the guinea pig using the Mossbauer technique. J. Acoust. Soc. Am. 72, 131-141.
Sellick, P.M., Patuzzi, R. and Johnstone, B.M. (1982) Modulation of responses of spiral ganglion cells in the guinea pig cochlea by low-frequency sound. Hearing Res. 7, 199-221.
Sachs, M.B. and Kiang,N.Y.S. (1968) Two-tone inhibition in auditory nerve fibers. J. Acoust. Soc. Am. 43, 1120-1128.
Weiss, T.F. (1982) Bidirectional transduction in vertebrate hair cells: a mechanism for coupling mechanical and electrical vibrations. Hearing Res. 7, 353-360.
Yates, G.K., Geisler, C.D., Patuzzi, R.B. and Johnstone, B.M. (1988) Saturation of receptor currents accounts for two-tone suppression. This volume.
Zwicker, E. (1979) A model describing nonlinearities in hearing by active processes with saturation at 40dB. Biol. Cybern. 35, 243-250.

SATURATION OF RECEPTOR CURRENTS ACCOUNTS FOR TWO-TONE SUPPRESSION

G.K. Yates, C.D. Geisler*, R.B. Patuzzi, and B.M. Johnstone

Department of Physiology, University of Western Australia, Nedlands 6009 Western Australia
**Departments of Neurophysiology and of Electrical & Computer Engineering, University of Wisconsin-Madison, Madison, Wisc. USA*

Introduction

In a preceding paper of this symposium (Patuzzi et al., this volume), evidence was given of an intimate connection between the electrical activity of the outer hair cells (OHCs) and the threshold sensitivities of primary fibers in the neighborhood of the OHCs. Small reductions in the responsiveness of the OHCs (as indicated by small reductions in the magnitudes of the locally recorded cochlear microphonic potentials) were used, through presumed high-gain active feedback processes, to account for large reductions observed in the neural thresholds near the characteristic frequencies (CFs) of the fibers. In this paper we will present evidence that the "two-tone rate suppression" (2TRS) which is observed in the response discharges of these primary fibers is a natural consequence of the limited dynamic range of the electrical drive to these same active processes: that is, a saturation of feedback (cf. Zwicker, 1979).

Methods

In the experiments reported here, extracellular recordings were made from the organ of Corti in anesthetized guinea pigs. A full account of the experimental procedure is given elsewhere (Geisler et al., 1988). Briefly, a small hole was scraped in the wall of scala tympani in the first turn of the cochlea, and a hyperfine micropipette (Z>100 Mohm) was inserted through the hole, under visual control, directly into the basilar membrane. Stimuli used were either pure tones, or combinations of two tones, presented in a closed acoustic system that had an approximately "flat" response (±3 dB) from 6-28 kHz (between 6 and 4 kHz, the intensity dropped by about 10 dB). The stimulus was usually gated on and off at a 23-Hz rate with a 1:1 on-off ratio. This gating signal was low enough in frequency that steady-state values of the various potentials were reached during each of the 21.7-msec "on" periods. A small silver wire was glued in place on the bone near the round window for measurement of compound action potentials (CAPs). Regular monitoring of the intensities needed to produce just detectable CAPs at various frequencies (the "CAP audiogram") provided a running measure of cochlear integrity.

After amplification, potentials from the microelectrode were led into a lock-in amplifier. Various synchronization signals to the lock-in were used to obtain different

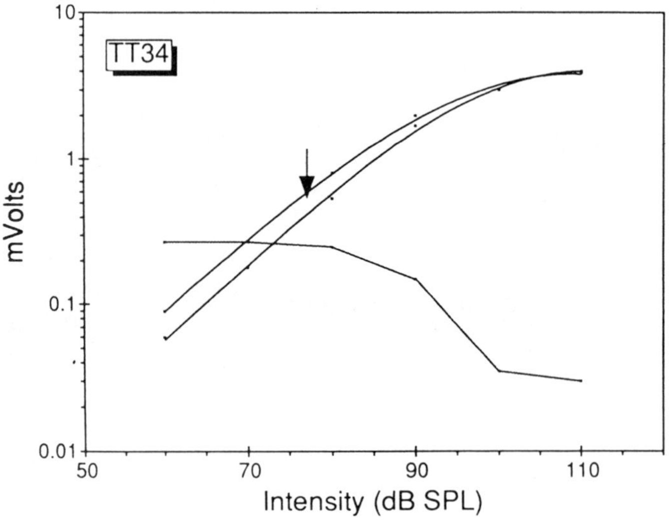

FIGURE 1 CM responses recorded from the basal-turn organ of Corti, illustrating interference. Each of the top two curves is a 2nd or 3rd order polynomial fitted to the data points obtained with single tones of 1.0 and 1.2-kHz frequency, respectively. The point on the 1.2-kHz curve at which the nonlinear terms equal 0.05 of the linear term is indicated by an arrow (at 78 dB SPL). The lower line connects response amplitudes produced by a constant-amplitude 1.0-kHz probe tone, as the intensity of a simultaneously presented 1.2-kHz suppressor is increased. Animal TT34 (the same electrode location also provided the data in Fig. 6).

components of the output. For a cochlear microphonic (CM) response, the desired frequency component of the stimulus was used as the synchronization signal. To obtain the summating potential (SP) response, the gating signal was used for synchronization. We will interpret these extracellular potentials to be direct reflections of intracellular receptor potentials of local hair cells. In the case of the CM potentials, there is a large body of evidence which indicates that they are principally a reflection of local OHC activity (e.g. Dallos et al., 1974; Cheatham and Dallos, 1982; Patuzzi et al., 1988). The SP potentials appear to reflect the DC receptor potentials of the local IHCs. This conclusion is supported by several observations, notably the close match which occurs between primary-fiber threshold frequency tuning curves and the threshold-level iso-amplitude curves of the SP potentials obtained from the same cochlear region (Geisler et al., 1988). There was no sign, on an oscilloscope monitor, of any CAP contamination of the SP responses.

Results

The principal process which we believe to be operative in 2TRS is illustrated by the data in Fig. 1, which are of the same type obtained many years ago by Engebretson and Eldredge (1968). First, single tones of 1.0 and 1.2 kHz were presented to the animal. As can be seen, the respective CM response curves grow linearly with intensity up to a level of approximately 80 dB SPL. With further increases in intensity, the responses enter a saturating region. The two tones were then presented simultaneously. The 1.0-kHz tone,

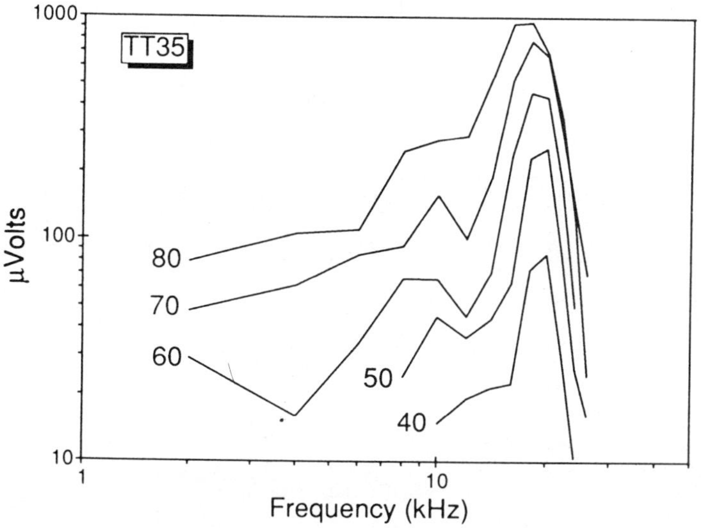

FIGURE 2 SP responses to single tones obtained from the basal-turn organ of Corti. Nominal SPL of the constant-attenuation sweep used to obtain each curve is indicated. The same electrode location in animal TT35 provided the data in Figs 2-5.

used as a probe tone, was presented at a constant intensity, while the 1.2-kHz tone was presented at a series of steadily increasing levels. It is apparent that the CM response to the probe tone was unaffected by the presence of the 1.2-kHz tone so long as the latter's intensity was less than about 80 dB SPL. Any increases in the amplitude of the higher frequency tone beyond that level, which marks the end of the linear response range, reduced the response to the probe tone proportionately.

Such "suppression" of the response to the probe tone is easily accounted for if, as already stated, we assume that the CM reflects the AC receptor potentials of the OHCs. These hair cells have been shown to have a saturating type of input-output curve (Russell et al., 1986), and a saturating curve has been shown to produce this same type of suppression (Engebretson and Eldredge, 1968). Basically, the AC receptor potential due to the suppressing tone carries, at its peak excursions, the voltage output of the cell into its saturating region, so that the superimposed components of the receptor voltage generated by the probe tone are smaller than would be produced by the probe tone acting alone.

The data in Fig. 1 were collected using frequencies so low that the active processes operating in the basal turn of the cochlea were believed to be unimportant. Let us assume that the same suppressing process illustrated there takes place no matter what the stimulating frequencies are. Imagine, therefore, the probe tone to be set at the CF of the recording site. A second tone is added. At high enough amplitudes it, like the 1.2-kHz tone of Fig. 1, will produce a reduction in the AC response to the probe tone. In this case, however, the OHC is presumed to be an element in a high-gain feedback loop (Patuzzi et al., this volume). Thus, if the output of the haircell drops by only a small amount (say 20%), the loop gain of this feedback path may be reduced by a large amount, perhaps an order of magnitude. Thus, at frequencies near CF, a relatively small reduction in the

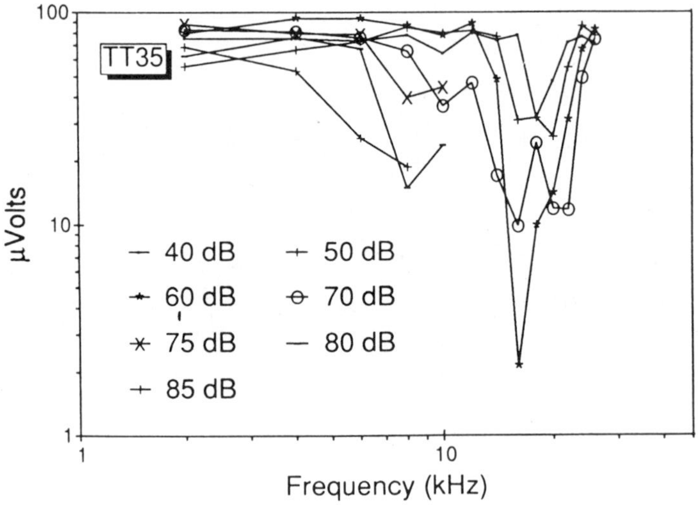

FIGURE 3 SP suppression curves. Each point shows the amplitude of the SP response evoked by a gated 18-kHz probe tone of 40 dB SPL, as a function of the (continuously presented) suppressor-tone frequency. Nominal SPL of the suppressor tone in each of its constant-attenuation sweeps is given. The amplitude of response to the probe tone alone was 74 µv

responsiveness of the OHCs is thought to cause a large reduction in the overall gain of the active process, and hence a large reduction in the sensitivity of the basilar- membrane complex. For different probe tones, the effects will vary. The more important the active processes are at a particular probe frequency and intensity, the more system suppression will be produced by OHC saturation.

One test of the hypothesis given above is to compare the intensity level at which a suppressing tone just begins to produce 2TRS with the level at which the OHC responses to the suppressing tone, given alone, just begin to saturate. We have made such a comparison, using indirect measures of the important variables: extracellular CM as a measure of OHC responses and the extracellular SP as a measure of neural responses. Ample evidence of the local origin of both of these extracellular responses exists (see Geisler et al., 1988).

A typical example of the extracellular SP responses obtained with pure tones is shown in Fig. 2. The data were collected by setting the attenuation of the system at a fixed level (producing nominally constant intensity) and varying the frequency in 2-kHz steps. At the lowest intensity level shown, 40 dB SPL, a clear response profile with a peak at 20 kHz is seen. This intensity is presumably close to the CF thresholds of single afferent fibers originating in the area, as the CAP threshold, shown in the guinea pig to be about 10 dB above the CF thresholds of local primary fibers (Johnstone et al., 1979), was 45 dB at 20 kHz in this animal. With further increases in intensity, the magnitudes of the SP responses grew and eventually saturated. A two-tone suppression paradigm was then instituted. A probe tone of 18-kHz frequency, presented at a constant intensity of 40 dB SPL, was gated on and off at the 23-Hz rate. A suppressor tone, not gated but left on continuously, was then added. The gating signal of the probe tone formed the synchronization signal applied to the lock-in amplifier. As only the probe tone was modulated by the gating signal, the

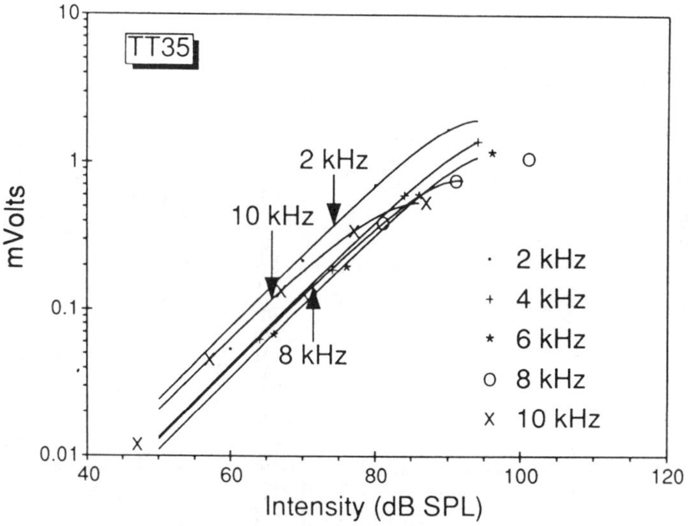

FIGURE 4 CM responses to single tones of 5 different frequencies. For each frequency, the solid curve shows a 2nd or 3rd-order polynomial fitted to its data points. For several curves, an arrow marks the "threshold of saturation" (the point at which the nonlinear terms equal 0.05 of the linear term).

amplifier's output registered only that part of the SP that was synchronised to the presence of the probe tone.

Figure 3 shows SP responses to the probe tone obtained with this paradigm using suppressor tones of different intensities. The results are very orderly. When the suppressing tone was at 18.0 kHz, it produced suppression at all intensity levels used, even at the same level as the probe tone itself. As the intensity of the suppressor tone was raised, the region of suppression expanded. At 85 dB SPL, the highest intensity used, suppression was produced at all frequencies above 2 kHz. Such data, while tracing out quite differently shaped suppression areas from those seen with neural 2TRS (Sachs and Kiang, 1968), are very similar to corresponding suppression data obtained from IHCs (Sellick and Russell, 1979). For purposes of testing our hypothesis, a "threshold of suppression", defined to be that intensity of the suppressor tone which produced a just noticeable decrease in the probe-tone response, was determined at each frequency.

Cochlear microphonic data were also obtained from the same electrode site that yielded the SP data in Figs. 2 and 3. Frequencies were restricted to the range below 10 kHz, where the extracellular CM responses are thought to be accurate representations of the AC receptor potentials of the local OHCs (cf. Cheatham and Dallos, 1982). The amplitude function at each of the 5 frequencies is shown in Fig. 4. Each curve grows linearly with intensity at the lower levels and then begins to enter a saturation region. For purposes of quantification, each of these amplitude functions was fitted with a 2nd-order polynominal (a 3rd order was used with the 10-kHz curve). The "threshold of saturation" for each curve was defined as that intensity for which the nonlinear terms just equalled 0.05 of the linear term. These saturation-threshold values, several marked by arrows in Fig. 4, are plotted in Fig. 5, along with the threshold curve for SP suppression derived from Fig. 3 and a constant-amplitude SP response curve derived from Fig. 2.

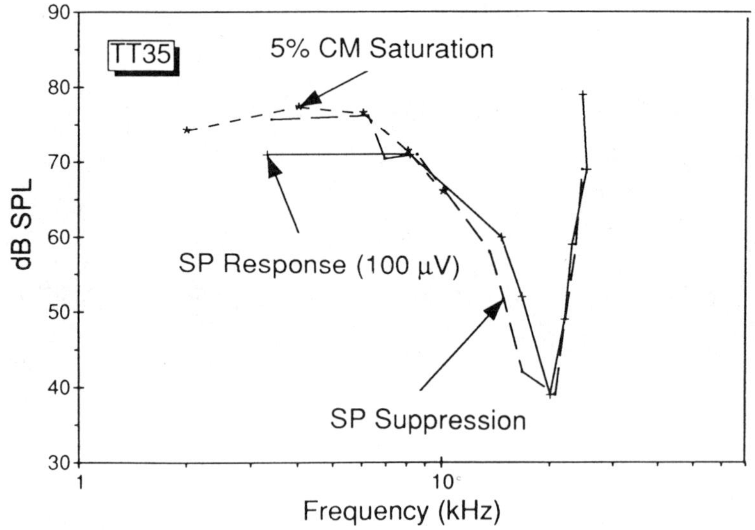

FIGURE 5 Comparison of "threshold" curves for SP probe-tone suppression (from Fig. 3, using a 57 μv criterion) and CM nonlinearity (from Fig. 4). Also shown is a constant-amplitude SP response curve (from Fig. 2, using a 100 μv criterion).

Several features of the data in Fig. 5 are important. Most significantly for purposes of this paper, is the key comparison between the threshold curves for CM saturation and SP suppression. These two curves are, in fact, very similar to one another, both in amplitude and shape, over the whole range of common existence. This agreement is predicted by the interference theory, which holds that suppression begins at the lowest intensity level at which the active processes involving the OHCs can no longer respond linearly to the stimulus waveform.

We have obtained close agreement between the CM saturation-threshold and SP suppression-threshold curves in all 4 of the animals in good condition from which we obtained the relevant data (cf. Geisler et al., 1988). We conclude, from the consistent agreement obtained, that, at least so far as the threshold levels are concerned, the suppression of the SP response to a probe tone by a second tone can be accounted for with the interference (saturation-feedback) theory.

The frequency-intensity patterns of classical 2TRS, however, differ markedly from those shown in Fig. 5, in that the neural data display two separate and distinct suppressive areas, one on either side of CF. It must be remembered, however, that the data in Fig. 5 represent the SP responses to the probe tone alone. Measuring the total SP response yields an entirely different picture. To obtain such measurements, we gated both the probe and suppressor tones on and off simultaneously at the 23-Hz rate and applied the gating signal as the synchronization signal to the lock-in amplifier. Results obtained from one of the two experiments in which this paradigm was systematically pursued are shown in Fig. 6. The familiar pattern seen in the neural data is observed: two suppressive areas separated by an area of excitation. The lower of the two suppressive areas in Fig. 6 coincides very closely with the low-frequency end of the suppression area for the probe tone alone (cf. Fig. 3).

In the middle range of frequencies, the combination of the two tones produces an increase in the SP response. Since this increase is coupled with a decrease in the response

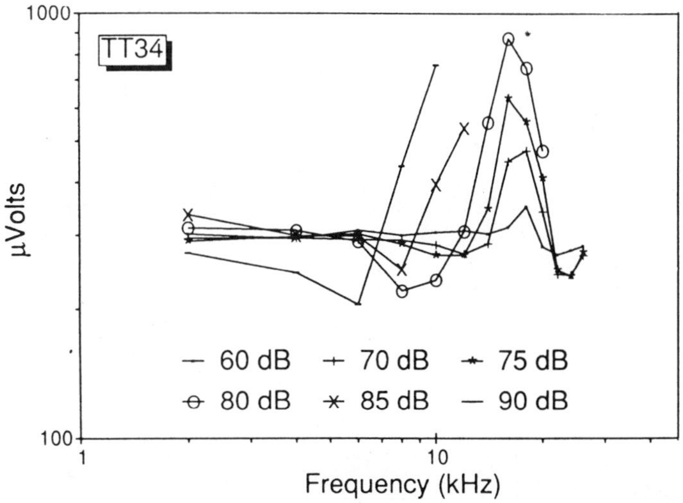

FIGURE 6 SP responses to a two-tone complex (both tones gated at 23 Hz), as a function of suppressor-tone frequency. The probe tone was an 18-kHz tone of 39-dB SPL. The nominal SPL of the suppressor tone in each of its constant-attenuation sweeps is given. Note that, to minimize cochlear damage due to overstimulation, suppressor tones having the higher intensities were limited to the lower frequency ranges. The amplitude of response to the probe tone alone was about 300 µv

component produced by the probe-tone (cf. Fig. 3), the suppressing tone must be causing an excitatory response of its own. We know, for the data in Fig. 2, that this is indeed the case. We thus have the remarkable situation that the suppressing tone simultaneously exerts both excitatory and suppressive effects. Such behavior is in fact predicted by the interference hypothesis: the excitation is due to the driving of IHC receptor potentials by the suppressor tone, while the suppression is due to the forcing of the OHC receptor potentials into their nonlinear regions and the subsequent reduction in the effectiveness of the active process. Strong evidence exists that just such a balance between excitation and suppression determines the net discharge rate of a primary fiber. Schmiedt (1982), for example, found that a fiber's 2TRS threshold contour overlapped, in some cases, the fiber's response area. In short, we believe that the interference theory also accounts for neural 2TRS.

Discussion

In addition to providing strong support for the interference (saturation-feedback) hypothesis of suppression origin, the data obtained in these experiments have other implications. For example, there is close agreement between the SP suppression-threshold data and the constant-amplitude SP response curve over the whole frequency range in Fig. 5. This was a general finding: there was always a criterion level that generated, from the SP response curves, an iso-amplitude response curve which closely matched the SP suppression-threshold curve. These close matches suggest, if one grants that the extracellular SP responses obtained near an IHC are a measure of local ciliary deflections and hence of local basilar membrane motion (cf. Geisler et al., 1988), that the threshold of suppression occurs at a particular amplitude of basilar-membrane vibration, regardless of the frequency of the probe tone. This conclusion is not only consistent with the interference hypothesis, it is interesting in its own right. It is also consistent with the relatively invariant boundaries of neural 2TRS found by Schmiedt (1982) using low-frequency suppressors.

The same processes that produced the SP suppression in Figs. 3 and 6, and presumably the 2TRS in primary-fiber discharges, would also be expected to produce "synchrony suppression" in the neural discharges of more apically located fibers (a loss there in amplitude of the probe tone's receptor potential, such as shown in Fig. 3, would surely be reflected in reduced synchronization to the probe-tone's frequency). Yet, because other cochlear processes, such as depletion of transmitter stores, have also been implicated as causes of synchrony suppression (e.g. Geisler and Greenberg, 1986), further experimentation is needed to unravel the contributions of the various candidate processes.

Acknowledgements

This work was supported by grants from the Australian N.H. & M.R.C. and by the United States N.I.H.

References

Cheatham, M.A. and Dallos, P. (1982) Two-tone interactions in the cochlear microphonic. Hearing.Res. 8, 29-48.

Dallos, P., Cheatham, M.A. and Ferraro,J.(1974) Cochlear mechanics, nonlinearities and cochlear potentials. J. Acoust. Soc. Am. 55, 597-605.

Engebretson, A.M. and Eldredge, D.H. (1968) Model for the nonlinear characteristics of cochlear potentials. J. Acoust. Soc. Am. 44, 548-554.

Geisler, C.D. and Greenberg, S.G. (1986) A two-stage nonlinear cochlear model possesses automatic gain control. J. Acoust. Soc. Am. 80, 1359-1363.

Geisler, C.D., Patuzzi, R.B., Yates, G.K. and Johnstone, B.M. (1988) Relationships between two-tone suppression and outer hair cell function. Hearing Res. (submitted).

Johnstone, J.R., Alder, V.A., Johnstone, B.M., Robertson, D. and Yates, G.K. (1979) Cochlear action potential threshold and single unit thresholds. J. Acoust. Soc. Am. 65, 254-257.

Patuzzi, R.B., Yates, G.K. and Johnstone, B.M. (1988) The origin of low-frequency microphonic potentials measured in the first turn of the guinea pig cochlea. Hearing Res. (submitted).

Patuzzi, R.B., Yates, G.K. and Johnstone, B.M. (1988) Outer hair cell receptor current and its effect on cochlear mechanics. This volume.

Russell, I.J., Cody, A.R. and Richardson, G.P. (1986) The responses of inner and outer hair cells in the basal turn of the guinea-pig cochlea and in the mouse cochlea grown in vitro. Hearing Res. 22, 199-216.

Sachs, M.B. and Kiang, N.Y.S. (1968) Two-tone inhibition in auditory nerve fibers. J. Acoust. Soc. Am. 43, 1120-1128.

Schmiedt, R.A. (1982) Boundaries of two-tone rate suppression of cochlear-nerve activity. Hearing Res. 7, 335-351.

Sellick, P.M. and Russell, I.J. (1979) Two-tone suppression in cochlear hair cells. Hearing Res. 1, 227-236.

Zwicker, E. (1979) A model describing nonlinearities in hearing by active processes with saturation at 40 dB. Biol Cybern. 35, 243-250.

Comments and Discussion

PICKLES

Q1. You suggest that the suppressor acts by reducing the active process that generates the peak and sharp tuning of the travelling wave to the *suppressed* tone. How does this theory account for the result of Robertson and Johnstone (1981), where by traumatising a localised region of the cochlea, it was possible to abolish two-tone suppression for suppressors above an auditory-nerve fibre's CF, without affecting the threshold or tuning at the suppressed-tone place?

Q2. In your model, how is it possible for the low-frequency two-tone suppression area to lie well below the excitatory tuning curve in threshold (e.g. by nearly 40 dB as in the data of Sachs and Kiang, 1968)? Surely, if the suppressor is only a little below the CF in frequency, it will begin to excite inner hair cells as soon as it begins to affect the outer hair cells.

Robertson, D. and Johnstone, B.M. (1980) Primary auditory neurons: nonlinear responses altered without changes in sharp tuning. J. Acoust. Soc. Am., 69, 1096-1098.
Sachs, M.B. and Kiang, N.Y.-S. (1968) Two-tone inhibition in auditory-nerve fibers. J. Acoust. Soc. Am., 43, 1120-1128.

GEISLER AND PATUZZI

A1. Before answering the question regarding the Robertson-Johnstone results, we must first describe how the feedback-saturation theory can account for rate suppression when the suppressor tone has a frequency higher than that of the probe tone. To do this requires the additional assumption that the OHC feedback processes which contribute to the sharp tuning at a particular place on the cochlear partition are located over an appreciable longitudinal band of the cochlea. This band is depicted in the sketch below, along with the resulting cochlear-partition vibration envelope. The response of the suppressing tone, which in many cases does not excite the probe-tone place (cf. Deng and Geisler, 1985), is also contributed to by a longitudinal band of OHCs, this band displaced somewhat basally from the probe-tone band but partially overlapping it (see sketch). If the suppressor tone were intense enough, the OHCs in the apical portion of the suppressor-tone band would be driven into the

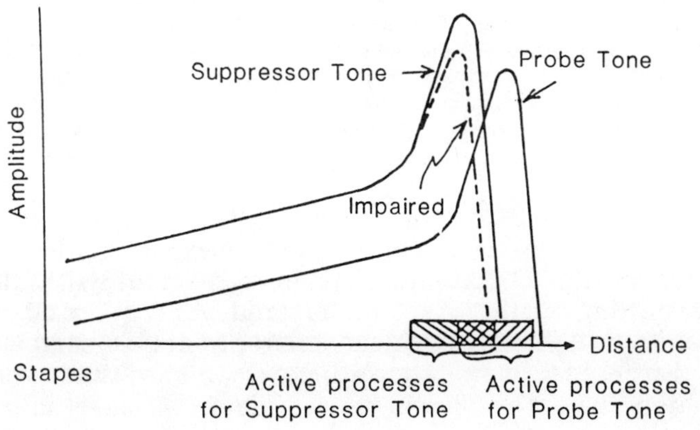

non-linear regions of their input-output curves. According to the theory, they would then no longer be able to contribute fully to the probe-tone response, to which they contribute. As a result, the amplitude of the probe-tone response would drop: suppression would have occurred.

To account for the Robertson-Johnstone results, we assume that the acoustic overstimulation they used would partially impair the electromechanical functioning of OHCs in the basal portion of the suppressor-tone band. This impairment in turn would cause the amplitude of the response to the suppressor tone to be reduced, as shown in the sketch by the dashed-line. This reduction in amplitude, which has been demonstrated experimentally (Geisler et al., 1988) would in turn cause a reduced suppression effect on the OHCs in the entire suppressor-tone band. Thus, the OHCs common to both bands would no longer be driven so far into their nonlinear regions and so suppression of the probe-tone response would be reduced. The probe-tone band of OHCs would have remained unimpaired and so normal frequency tuning of the probe-tone resonant point would be maintained.

A2. Central to the justification of the feedback-saturation theory are the data showing that the threshold-of-saturation versus frequency curve parallels the threshold-of-excitation curve at low frequencies (see Fig. 5). Schmiedt (1982) and Allen and Fahey (1983) have observed similar trends in auditory-nerve-fiber data. In the region of the tip of the probe tone's response, things are more complicated. Not only is that the region in which Sachs and Kiang observed the large difference between the thresholds of suppression and excitation, but near the tip, no suppression occurs at all (cf. our Fig. 6). The reason for this behaviour, we believe, is that both tones utilize the feedback contributions of the same group of OHCs (as in the sketch above). Thus, if suppression were instituted at the onset of a suppressor tone, the level of excitation of the common OHCs would drop as the probe-tone response was attenuated. But that in turn would drop the level of excitation by the suppressor tone also. Suppression of the suppressor would occur. It thus becomes quite difficult, without explicit models, to determine the magnitude of suppression in this area.

Allen, J.B. and Fahey, P.F. (1983) Nonlinear behaviour at threshold determined in the auditory canal and on the auditory nerve. In: Hearing - Physiological Bases and Psychoacoustics. Eds. R. Klinke and R. Hartmann, Springer-Verlag, New York, pp. 128-133.
Deng, L. and Geisler, C.D. (1985) Changes in the phase of excitor-tone responses in cat auditory-nerve fibers by suppressor tones and fatigue. J. Acoust. Soc. Am., 78, 1633-1643.
Geisler, C.D., Patuzzi, R.B., Yates, G.K. and Johnstone, B.M. (1988) Relationships between two-tone suppression and outer hair cell function. Hearing Res. (submitted).
Schmiedt, R.A. (1982) Boundaries of two-tone rate suppression of cochlear-nerve activity. Hearing Res., 7, 335-351.

ALLEN

Our published two-tone suppression measurements made in the auditory nerve of the cat seem to be in agreement with the hypothesis that you are putting forth. As I understand your proposal, you feel that the saturation point of the cochlear microphonic is correlated with the suppression threshold. In the figure below, we show that your hypothesis is approximately true for our measured data. I have taken the figure below from Fahey and Allen (1985), J. Acoust. Soc. Am. 77, pp. 599-612, Fig. 13. This figure shows the locus of suppressor level vs. frequency that is required to reduce the rate due to a probe tone at the best frequency, to its spontaneous rate. In all cases shown, the unit being tested does not respond (e.g., its rate is not changed) to the suppressor tone. These suppressor levels make a family of curves that approximately follow the middle ear transfer function. They also approximately correspond to the level where the CM becomes nonlinear (e.g., the point where it deviates by 1 dB from linear) as you have described in your paper. To show this, we have added to the figure (curve marked with the O symbols) a plot of the sound pressure level, as a function of frequency, where the CM becomes nonlinear. We define this point by where the CM deviates from linear by 1 dB. We have used the CM data published in Allen (1983), J. Acoust. Soc. Am. 73, pp. 2071-2092, Fig. 16a. The distortion threshold has the same shape as the rate suppression-to-threshold locus. The difference between the two curves will be affected by the fact that our CM data was recorded on the round window and not in scala media. This difference will be greatest at lower frequencies, where the travelling wave, and therefore the CM, is largest in the apex, and is not well represented by the round-window CM.

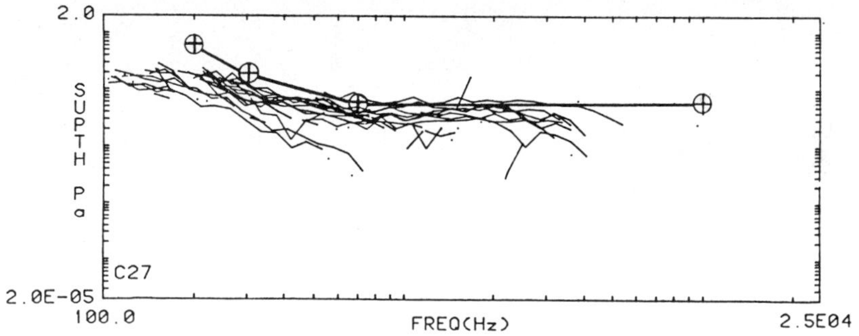

MOUNTAIN

I am pleased to see that your data supports the model that we presented at the 1983 Mechanics of Hearing Symposium (Mountain et al., 1983; see also Mountain, 1985; Mountain, 1986), but I am concerned that the data you present in your fig. 5 may be from a damaged cochlea. The tip-to-tail ratio of your SP tuning curve is only just over 30dB and your threshold for suppression coincides or is higher than the SP tuning curve for almost all frequencies.

Mountain, D.C., Hubbard, A.E., and McMuller, T.A. (1983) Electromechanical Processes in the Cochlea. In: Mechanics of Hearing (Eds: de Boer, E. and Viergever, M.A.), Delft University Press, Delft, pp. 119-126.

Mountain, D.C. (1985) Active filtering by hair cells. In: Peripheral Auditory Mechanisms (Eds: Allen, J.B., Hall, J.L., Hubbard, A., Neely, S.T., and Tubis, A.), pp. 179-188.

Mountain, D.C. (1986) Electromechanical Properties of Hair Cells. In: Neurobiology of Hearing. The Cochlea (Eds: Altschuler, R.A., Bobbins, R.P. and Hoffman, D.W.), Raven Press, New York, pp. 77-90.

GEISLER

Animal TT35, from which the data in Figs. 2-5 were obtained, had normal sensitivity. Its CAP threshold at 20 kHz was about 26 dB SPL, implying, on the basis of past correlations (Johnstone et al., 1979), a single-fiber threshold of about 15 dB SPL, which is normal. The "SP Response" curve of Fig. 5 is not intended to be a theshold curve, but was chosen from other supra-threshold curves as the one most easily compared with the "SP Suppression" curve. In fact, SP "threshold" (i.e. our noise level of about 10 uvolts) would have been about 20 dB SPL at 20 kHz. Concerning the SP tip-to-tail ration, values of 30-40 dB were obtained from animals with normal sensitivity. These values are less than those obtained in single-fiber experiments, probably due to the contributions of remote sites to the SP at stimulus frequencies much lower than CF.

COMPONENTS OF THE MEMBRANE CURRENT IN GUINEA-PIG INNER HAIR CELLS

C.J. Kros and A.C. Crawford

The Physiological Laboratory
Downing Street
Cambridge CB2 3EG, U.K.

Introduction

Movement of a hair cell's stereociliary bundle results in the generation of a receptor potential. The shape of this receptor potential is not only determined by the transducer current and the passive electrical properties of the cell (capacitance and input impedance) but also by time- and voltage-dependent currents if these are activated in the membrane potential range of the receptor potential. Such time- and voltage-dependent currents have been described in hair cells isolated from the bullfrog's sacculus (Lewis and Hudspeth, 1983) and amphibian papilla (Roberts, Robles and Hudspeth, 1986), the chick's vestibulum (Ohmori, 1984) and the turtle's cochlea (Art and Fettiplace, 1987).

We have recently provided evidence for the presence of similar currents in inner hair cells isolated from the cochlea of the guinea-pig (Kros and Crawford, 1988). Here we present a more detailed analysis of some of the underlying conductances.

Methods

Inner hair cells were isolated mechanically from the fourth and part of the third turn of cochleas of pigmented guinea-pigs, killed by cervical dislocation (weight 190 to 650 grams). The isolation procedure was similar to that reported by Lim and Flock (1985), but without any enzymatic treatment. Inner hair cells were mostly grouped in clusters of two to ten cells; truly isolated cells were only occasionally found.

In most experiments the cells were maintained on the stage of a heated compound microscope at 35-38 $^{\circ}$C for 4 to 8 hours and viewed using differential interference contrast optics with a x40 water immersion objective. They were superfused with extracellular medium at a flow rate which changed the bath volume every 5 minutes. The medium was not oxygenated.

The extracellular solution used was bicarbonate-free Hanks' MEM (Gibco), modified by the addition of 10 mM HEPES-NaOH, pH 7.3 at 38°C. The composition of the salts (in mM) was: 137 NaCl, 0.3 Na_2HPO_4, 5.4 KCl, 0.4 KH_2PO_4, 1.3 $CaCl_2$, 0.5

$MgCl_2$, 0.4 $MgSO_4$. In some experiments 25 mM tetraethylammonium-Cl (TEA-Cl) or 4-aminopyridine (4-AP) replaced an equal amount of NaCl. In other experiments a simple gravity-feed superfusion system was used to apply these modified solutions to local cell groups, using a glass pipette with a tip of 35-60 um internal diameter.

Membrane properties of the cells were studied using the patch-clamp technique (Hamill et al. 1981) in the whole-cell and cell-attached patch configurations. Both voltage clamp and current injection experiments could be performed on the same cells. In the whole-cell configuration it was possible to compensate part of the series resistance of the pipettes. In whole-cell experiments the pipettes were filled with (mM): 140 KCl, 5 EGTA-KOH, 0.3 $CaCl_2$, 5 $MgCl_2$, 2.5 Na_2ATP and 5 HEPES-KOH, pH 7.2. In some experiments 10 mM 4-AP replaced an equal amount of KCl. The series resistance after compensation was between 2.5 and 6.2 MOhm. The inner hair cell's capacitance was 9.2 ± 1.6 pF (mean ± S.D., n = 13). The time constant of the voltage clamp in the experiments presented here was 30-90 μs.

Cell-attached patches were studied at room temperature (20-21° C). In these experiments the pipettes were filled with (mM): 142 KCl, 0.9 MgCl, 1.3 CaCl, 10 HEPES-NaOH, pH 7.4. In some experiments 10 mM TEA-Cl replaced an equal amount of KCl.

Voltage and current signals were stored on a Racal Store 4 FM tape recorder, mostly using a bandwidth of 0-5 kHz. The tape recordings were digitized via a CED 502 interface at a 10 kHz sampling rate on a PDP 11-34 for later analysis.

Current fluctuations in whole-cell voltage clamp were studied using ensemble-variance analysis in a similar way as Fenwick, Marty and Neher (1982).

Results

MEMBRANE CURRENTS IN NORMAL MEDIA

The resting potentials were -67 ± 3 mV (mean ± S.D., n = 29). In voltage clamp the cells were held at a potential of -74 or -84 mV (at this potential all time- and voltage-dependent conductances were turned off). When the cells were depolarized for 40 ms large time- and voltage-dependent outward currents developed over the first 10 ms of the step. Most of the conductance turned on in the potential range of -50 to -30 mV. Hyperpolarizing steps of 10 to 40 mV from the same holding potential showed only a small instantaneous current consistent with an ohmic leakage conductance of 1-2.5 nS.

An example is shown in Fig. 1. The currents that developed on stepping the potential to the values indicated next to each trace are shown for the first 20 ms of the step. The onset of the currents became faster as the potential was stepped to more depolarized levels. The currents developed without an appreciable delay at a recording bandwidth of 5 kHz and the time course of the onset could not be described by a single exponential.

We have previously suggested that these outward currents are mainly carried by potassium ions and that they may be modulated by the concentration of intracellular free calcium ions (Kros and Crawford, 1988).

KINETICS OF THE CURRENTS

As can be seen in Fig. 1. the currents rise to their steady-state values with a fast and a slow component. The fast component is not much in evidence for small depolarizing steps but grows rapidly with further depolarization until it dominates the response at large depolarizations. The current records of this cell as well as a number of other cells could be fitted fairly well with a combination of two exponentials with time constants differing by about an order of magnitude. The fast time constant ranged from about 0.7 ms for small voltage steps to 0.15 ms for steps to an absolute potential of +20 mV. The slow time constant varied similarly from about 8 to about 1.2 ms.

The current relaxations at the end of the depolarizing steps could also be fitted with two exponentials whose time constants differed by about an order of magnitude. The time constants were independent of the membrane potential level of the depolarizing step and only determined by the level to which the membrane potential was returned.

The simplest explanation for this type of kinetic behaviour is the presence of two independent underlying conductances, one with fast and one with slow kinetics. Therefore an attempt was made to isolate these conductances by pharmacological means.

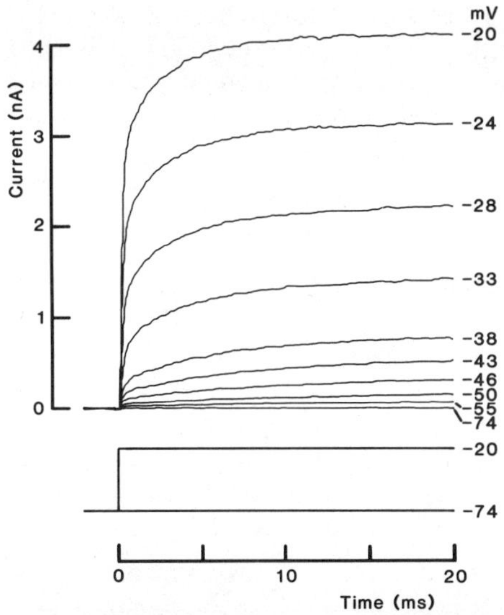

FIGURE 1 Membrane currents of an inner hair cell under voltage clamp with normal intra- and extracellular solutions. Lower part: schematic representation of voltage step protocol. Upper part: currents elicited by steps to absolute membrane potentials (corrected for 6.2 MOhm series resistance) shown by each trace (averaged from 12 repetitions). Leakage and capacity current subtracted. Temp. 38°C.

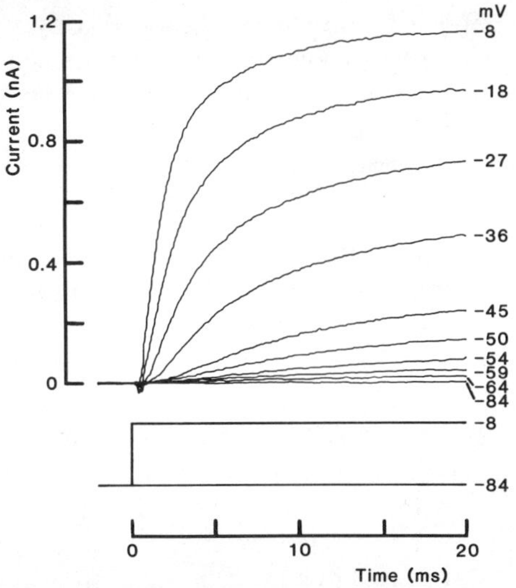

FIGURE 2 Membrane currents of an inner hair cell under voltage clamp with 25 mM TEA in the extracellular solution. Lower part: schematic representation of voltage step protocol. Upper part: currents elicited by steps to absolute membrane potentials (corrected for 3.5 MOhm series resistance) shown by each trace (averaged from 27 repetitions). Leakage and capacity current subtracted. Note different scale of ordinate from Fig.1. Temp. 36°C.

CURRENTS IN THE PRESENCE OF TETRAETHYLAMMONIUM IONS

When cells were superfused during voltage clamp with a solution in which 25 mM TEA, a blocker of a variety of potassium channels (Stanfield, 1983), replaced an equal amount of NaCl the currents were reversibly reduced in size and their kinetics changed dramatically. In some experiments 25 mM TEA was permanently present in the extracellular solution without deleterious effects on the cells, judging from morphological criteria. These cells had resting potentials similar to those in normal extracellular medium and showed the same changed kinetics as the cell which were only intermittently superfused with TEA.

An example is shown in Fig. 2. The voltage step protocol is similar to that in Fig. 1. The currents in response to depolarizing steps from the holding potential of -84 mV could be seen to develop with a delay, especially pronounced for small depolarizations, and to become faster with larger voltage steps. Most of the conductance turned on in the range -60 to -30 mV. A fast initial inward current which reached a maximum size of 20-50 pA at an absolute potential of about -20 mV was also found under these conditions. This component tended to decline more than the other currents with prolonged contact with a cell. This inward current may be carried by calcium ions but was not studied further.

The current relaxations after a 40 ms step were exponential. The time constants were similar to those of the slow component in normal extracellular solution. The current onsets could not be fitted very well either with a single exponential or with higher order exponentials, so that the conductance was not describable by a Hodgkin-Huxley scheme of any order (Hodgkin and Huxley, 1952). The size of the currents (note the different scales of the ordinates) is similar to that of the slow component in normal extracellular medium.

CURRENTS IN THE PRESENCE OF 4-AMINOPYRIDINE

When cells were superfused with a solution in which 25 mM 4-AP (4-aminopyridine, a blocker of some types of potassium channel, (Dubois, 1983)) replaced an equal amount of NaCl the slow component of the current was reversibly suppressed. Whereas the onset and washout of the effect of TEA developed within about ten seconds the effect of 4-AP developed very slowly over minutes and washout took even longer, making it impossible to achieve complete suppression and reversal. It has been suggested that 4-AP may be membrane permeant and act on the intracellular side of the cell membrane (Hermann and Gorman, 1981). Therefore, in some experiments 10 mM 4-AP was used to replace an equal amount of KC1 in the intracellular solution instead of using it extracellularly. In these cells the onset of the action of 4-AP was very rapid. In three cells the resting potentials were -54, -67 and -64 mV with 4-AP in the intracellular solution.

An example is shown in Fig. 3. The voltage step protocol was similar to that in the previous figures. The current onsets were fast without an appreciable delay. There is no evidence of a slow component. The currents became faster for larger depolarizing steps and could be fitted well with a single exponential. The time constant and size of the currents were similar to those of the fast component of cells in normal extracellular medium. Most of the conductance was activated in the range -60 to -20mV.

The current relaxations following a depolarizing step were exponential in form, the time constants of decay depending only on the level to which the potential was returned.

CURRENT FLUCTUATIONS AND SINGLE CHANNEL CURRENTS

Analysis of membrane current fluctuations can give useful information about underlying ionic channel conductances provided that not more than one species of ionic channels dominates these fluctuations. Current fluctuations were studied in experiments with TEA superfusion and in experiments with 4-AP in the intracellular medium. Examples of both experiments are shown in Fig. 4. The fluctuations were similar for both experiments at the holding potential of -84 mV, at which potential the ionic currents are largely not activated. When the cells were depolarized to a potential sufficient to generate a current of 1 nA, the current variance in both cases increased, though to a much greater extent in the 4-AP experiment where the slow current had been blocked. This may mean that TEA suppresses a current with a considerably larger underlying single channel conductance than 4-AP.

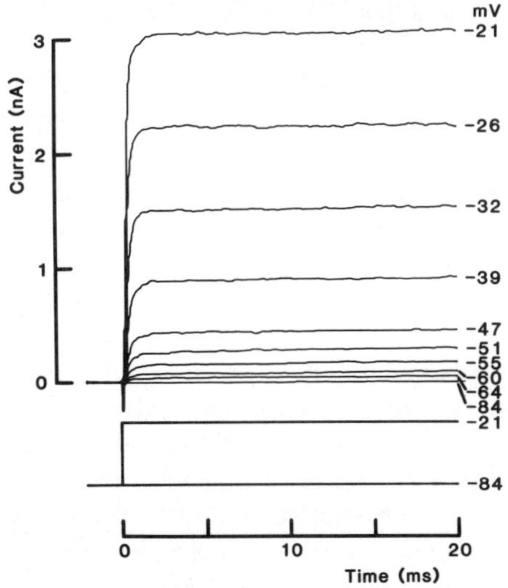

FIGURE 3 Membrane currents of an inner hair cell under voltage clamp with 10 mM 4-AP in the intracellular solution. Lower part: schematic representation of voltage step protocol. Upper part: currents elicited by steps to absolute membrane potentials (corrected for 5.5 MOhm series resistance) shown by each trace (averaged from 7 repetitions). Leakage and capacity current subtracted. Temp. 35°C.

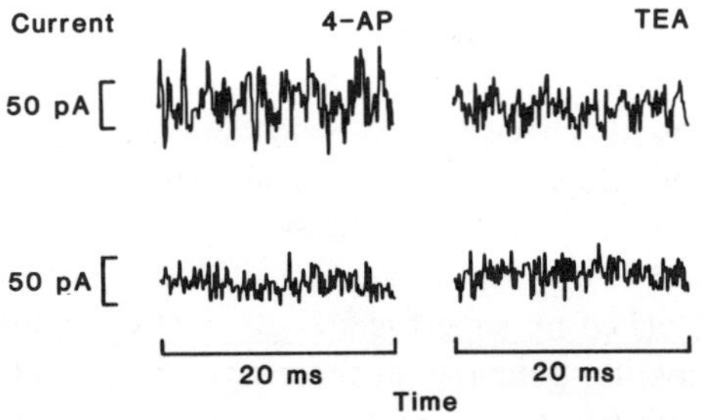

FIGURE 4 Membrane current fluctuations of two inner hair cells under voltage clamp with (left) 10 mM 4-AP in the intracellular solution and (right) 25 mM TEA in the extracellular solution. Lower traces: steady-state currents at a holding potential of -84 mV; Upper traces: current fluctuations at a mean steady-state current of (left) 0.9 nA and (right) 1.0 nA. Only the fluctuations around the mean current are shown. Temp. 35°C (left) and 36 °C (right).

Some preliminary experiments on cell-attached patches support this idea. In 4 cells in which the patch-pipette contained a high-potassium extracellular solution, all patches contained a well-resolved large-conductance channel (120 $\pm$ 14 pS, mean $\pm$ S.D.) with a reversal potential about 45 to 65 mV depolarized from the holding potential of the pipette (0 mV). This reversal potential range would be expected from a channel carrying mainly potassium ions. Patches also contained one or more smaller conductance channels of about 10-20 pS with a similar reversal potential. In 4 experiments in which 10 mM TEA replaced an equal amount of KC1 no large-conductance channels were found. It seems that the fast, TEA-sensitive current is carried by the large conductance channels.

Discussion

These results provide strong evidence for the presence of two distinct potassium conductances in isolated guinea-pig inner hair cells, both activated in the membrane potential range of the receptor potentials (Cody and Russell, 1987).

The current with fast kinetics, blocked by TEA, with a large underlying single-channel conductance is probably a calcium-dependent potassium conductance (Blatz and Magleby, 1987). Similar conductances have been described in hair cells of a variety of lower vertebrates (Lewis and Hudspeth, 1983; Ohmori, 1984; Art and Fettiplace, 1987). We have not been able to detect delays in the onset of the fast current, though the limited bandwidth of the voltage clamp means that delays less than 200 us would probably have been missed.

The current with slow kinetics, blocked by 4-AP, is also a potassium conductance. The reversible suppression of all currents evoked by depolarizing steps in cells superfused with 1 mM cadmium ion which we reported previously (Kros and Crawford, 1988) suggests that this current may also be calcium-dependent (Hagiwara and Byerly, 1981). However, calcium-dependent potassium conductances suppressed by 4-AP have not been described before. Further evidence from inside-out patches exposed to different concentrations of free calcium ions on their intracellular surface is needed to clarify this point. Superfusion of apamin, which is known to suppress small-conductance calcium-dependent potassium channels in a variety of other systems (Blatz and Magleby, 1987) had no effect on the slow current. This current is also different from the current suppressed by 4-AP in hair cells from the bullfrog's sacculus (Lewis and Hudspeth, 1983), since it does not inactivate in the range of potentials studied, is blocked by superfusion with 1 mM cadmium ions and is unaffected by the value of the holding potential in the range -84 to -44 mV. In normal extracellular solution, when both fast and slow currents are present, the delay in the slow current is obscured by the fast component. A small but consistent discrepancy with double exponential fits at small depolarizations shows that the delay is there, however, and not likely to result from some unusual change in the kinetics of the current due to external TEA.

In outer hair cells Ashmore and Meech (1986) and Gitter, Zenner and Frömter (1986) have described at least two populations of potassium channels, which may also be present in inner hair cells and underly the potassium currents described here. But the large conductance channel they describe has a somewhat larger unit conductance (about 200 pS) than the 120 pS channel found here.

One of the more remarkable aspects of the inner hair cell currents is the speed with which they develop. For instance in Fig. 3. the fast component is virtually completely turned on at all potentials in less than a millisecond. This is faster than previous reports of conductances in other hair cell preparations (see for instance Ashmore and Meech (1986), Lewis and Hudspeth (1983) and Art and Fettiplace (1987)), though the difference must in part arise from our use of 35-38° C rather than room temperature. Physiologically however, the speed of the currents may be very important since they must operate to modify the receptor potentials on a time scale as fast as a few kHz.

Acknowledgements

This work was suppported by the M.R.C. and Trinity College Cambridge. We are indebted to Professor H.B. Barlow for the loan of equipment and to Dr. R. Fettiplace for many helpful discussions throughout the course of this work.

References

Art, J.J. and Fettiplace, R. (1987), Variation of membrane properties in hair cells isolated from the turtle cochlea. J. Physiol. 385, 207-242.

Ashmore, J.F. and Meech, R.W. (1986). Ionic basis of membrane potential in outer hair cells of guinea pig cochlea. Nature 322, 361-371.

Blatz, A.L. and Magleby, K.L. (1987). Calcium-activated potassium channels. Trends in Neurosciences 10, 463-467.

Cody, A.R. and Russell, I.J. (1987). The responses of hair cells in the basal turn of the guinea-pig cochlea to tones. J. Physiol. 383, 551-569.

Dubois, J.M. (1983). Potassium currents in the frog node of Ranvier. Prog. Biophys. Mol. Biol. 42, 1-20.

Gitter, A.H., Zenner, H.P. and Frömter, E. (1986). Membrane potential and ion channels in isolated outer hair cells of guinea pig cochlea. ORL J. Otorhinolaryngol. Relat. Spec. 48, 68-75.

Hagiwara, S. and Byerly, L (1981). Calcium channel. Ann. Rev. Neurosci. 4, 69-125.

Hamill, O.P., Marty, A., Neher, E., Sakmann, B. and Sigworth, F.J. (1981). Improved patch-clamp techniques for high-resolution current recording from cells and cell-free membrane patches. Pflügers Arch. 391, 85-100.

Hermann, A. and Gorman, A.L.F. (1981). Effects of 4-aminopyridine on potassium currents in a molluscan neuron. J. Gen. Physiol. 78, 63-86.

Hodgkin, A.L. and Huxley, A.F. (1952). A quantitative description of membrane currents and its application to conduction and excitation in nerve. J. Physiol. 117, 500-544.

Kros, C.J. and Crawford, A.C. (1988). Non-linear electrical properties of guinea-pig inner hair cells: a patch-clamp study. In: Basic Issues in Hearing, (Eds: Duifhuis, H., Horst, J.W. and Wit, H.P.) Academic Press, London (in press).

Lewis, R.S. and Hudspeth, A.J. (1983). Voltage- and ion-dependent conductances in solitary vertebrate hair cells. Nature 304, 538-541.

Lim, D.J. and Flock, Å. (1985). Ultrastructural morphology of enzyme-dissociated cochlear sensory cells. Acta Otolaryngol. 99, 478-492.

Ohmori, H. (1984). Studies of ionic currents in the isolated vestibular hair cell of the chick. J. Physiol. 350, 561-581.

Roberts, W.M., Robles, L. and Hudspeth, A.J. (1986). Correlation between the kinetic properties of ionic channels and the frequency of membrane-potential resonance in hair cells of the bullfrog. In: Auditory Frequency Selectivity (Eds: Moore, B.C.J. and Patterson, R.D), pp. Plenum Press, New York, pp. 89-95.

Stanfield, P.R. (1983). Tetraethylammonium ions and the potassium permeability of excitable cells. Rev. Physiol. Biochem. Pharmacol. 97, 1-67.

COCHLEAR NONLINEARITIES REFLECTED IN INNER HAIR CELL RESPONSES

P. Dallos and M.A. Cheatham

Auditory Physiology Laboratory (Audiology) and Department of Neurobiology and Physiology
Northwestern University, Evanston, IL 60201 USA

Introduction

The growth pattern of spectral components in a system's output with increases in its input is revealing of its internal structure. Inferences about various properties of the peripheral auditory system from the harmonic structure of its various responses have been made since the days of Helmholtz. In contemporary work the focus has been on magnitude functions recorded for a variety of variables at differing peripheral sites. Thus basilar membrane displacement, gross cochlear potentials, inner and outer hair cell responses and discharge rates of auditory nerve fibers have all been considered. Here we study some properties of intracellular potentials recorded from inner hair cells of guinea pigs in the low frequency region of the cochlea.

Of interest is the relation between growth patterns of fundamental, dc, and lower harmonic components in inner hair cell responses to sinusoidal stimuli, chosen to be near the cell's characteristic frequency. Inner hair cell input-output functions for intracellular dc and ac components have been studied before (Russell and Sellick, 1978, 1983; Sellick et al., 1983; Patuzzi and Sellick, 1983; Goodman et al., 1982; Brown and Nuttall, 1984). All the cited experiments were performed on the high frequency, basal end of the cochlea, rendering quantitative comparisons between harmonic components difficult. We have provided some information about response growth in the low frequency region (Dallos, 1985, 1986).

Methods

All results presented here are obtained from inner hair cells (IHC) in the third turn of the guinea pig's cochlea. Hair cells were approached with microelectrodes using the lateral approach (Dallos et al., 1982). Experimental details are identical to those previously reported (Dallos, 1985). All data are at the stimulus frequency of 700 or 800 Hz; just below, or at the best frequency (BF) of these cells (800-1000 Hz). The information provided is based on averaged responses to tone bursts. Response magnitude and phase are computed from fast Fourier analysis of the averaged waveforms, and were obtained off line. Both amplitude and phase of the fundamental and lower harmonics as well as the dc component are obtained. Dc responses are also determined from actual waveforms as the difference between baseline and average of positive and negative excursions of the wave. This method is useful when the baseline is noisy or contains a low frequency component.

Results

The most commonly éncountered response pattern is shown in the various panels of **Figure 1a.** Here the fundamental component first rises linearly, then saturates and virtually flattens out by 80 dB SPL with modest further increases accompanying any additional rise in sound level. The corresponding dc pattern is similar; a rapid rise is followed by pronounced saturation. This IHC is a reasonably sensitive one, albeit it is not the very best that one may encounter. Thus this cell produces 1 mV-p ac response at 35 dB SPL, whereas the two best cells in our collection yield such a response at 5 and 10 dB SPL.

The phase of the fundamental component shows a smooth accumulation of lag with intensity, as seen before for stimulus frequencies below BF (Dallos, 1986). The combined ac and dc response characteristics exhibited by this IHC may be construed as a "simple" saturating pattern. In fact, this is the one most likely to be encountered, and this is the one characterized by most previous investigators of IHC responses (Patuzzi and Sellick, 1983; Russell and Sellick, 1978; Goodman et al., 1982).

Another informative depiction of the level-dependence of the ac response obtains when maximum depolarizing and hyperpolarizing responses are plotted as a function of peak magnitude and phase of the stimulus. Such response patterns have been published for a variety of hair cell types, such as the saccular hair cell of the frog (Hudspeth and Corey, 1977), cochlear hair cell of the terrapin (Crawford and Fettiplace, 1981), mammalian inner hair cell (Russell and Sellick, 1983; Dallos, 1986) and mammalian outer hair cell (Dallos, 1986; Russell et al., 1986). In **Figure 1b** a linear plot of peak depolarizing and peak hyperpolarizing responses (corresponding to the plot of **Fig. 1a**) are given as a function of peak sound level, covering +/- 10 Pa. In **Figure 1c** the same data are shown for a more limited range with the horizontal scale expanded over +/- 1 Pa. These plots clearly show the two most conspicuous features of the responses: saturation and asymmetry. In this case both depolarizing and hyperpolarizing phases of the response saturate smoothly but the magnitude of the positive phase is about eigth-times that of the negative half cycle. Restricting the input range to +/- 1 Pa (**Fig. 1c**) permits a quite satisfactory analytic fit to the data by two simple rectangular hyperbolae as has been proposed before (Lipetz, 1971; Russell and Sellick, 1983):

$$V_D = V_{D\text{-max}}/(p_D/p+1) \quad \text{for } p>0$$
$$V_H = V_{H\text{-max}}/(p_H/p-1) \quad \text{for } p<0$$

Where $V_{D\text{-max}}$ and $V_{H\text{-max}}$ are the saturated positive and negative response magnitudes and p_D and p_H are the pressure values at $V_{max}/2$. The fit provided by this formula is shown for comparison with the data in **Figure 1c.**

Finally, we include in **Figure 1a** plots of the second and third harmonic components in the response. The patterns shown here are characteristic of those commonly

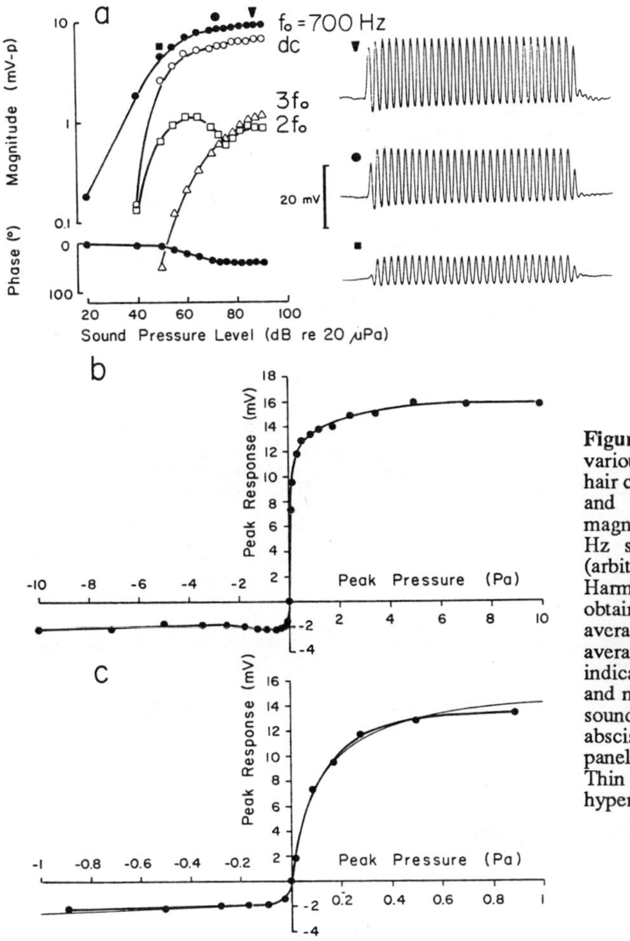

Figure 1. **a.** Responses to tone bursts at various intensities from a third turn inner hair cell. Fundamental (f_0), dc, second ($2f_0$) and third harmonic ($3f_0$) component magnitudes are shown in response to a 700 Hz stimulus. Phase of the fundamental (arbitrary phase reference) is also shown. Harmonic magnitudes and phases are obtained from Fourier transformation of averaged responses. Three inserts give averaged response waveforms at the levels indicated by matching symbols. **b.** Positive and negative response peaks plotted against sound pressure magnitude. Note linear abscissa from -10 to +10 Pa. **c.** Same as panel **b.** but abscissa is restricted to +/- 1 Pa. Thin line indicates fit by two rectangular hyperbolae (see text).

encountered. As reported before (Dallos et al., 1986), the second harmonic seen in IHCs almost invariably has two lobes in its magnitude function. A first maximum is reached between 50 and 70 dB SPL, followed by a notch of variable depth. At higher levels the response rises again, to reach a maximum within the range of levels tested (illustrated here) or to continue to rise. Even in the latter case, a maximum and eventual decline is surely reached (presumably at SPLs outside the test range), for complete saturation dictates the dominance of the response by odd harmonics. The third harmonic magnitude tends to rise monotonically, as shown here, in the majority of cases that we have encountered

Not all IHC responses may be characterized by the above described "simple" intensity dependence. In **Figure 2** we include another commonly encountered pattern (closed symbols). Here both ac and dc responses saturate and show a true maximum around 70 dB SPL. This cell is again a fairly sensitive one, producing 1 mV-p response at 30 dB SPL; 5 dB more sensitive than the cell shown in **Fig. 1.** Yet, the maximal response of the Figure 1 cell is about 2 dB greater within the test range, due to a lack of its complete saturation.

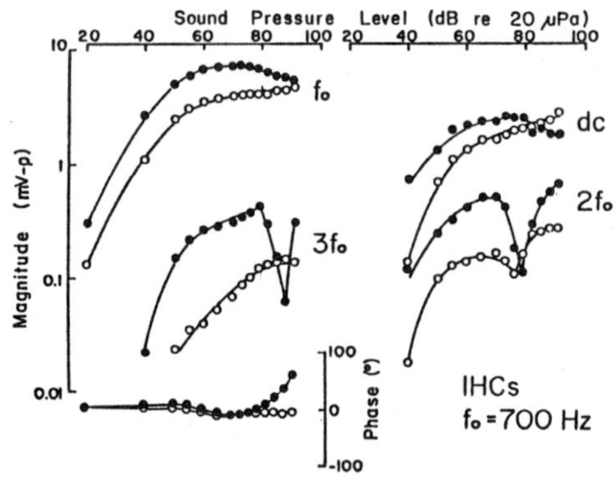

Figure 2. Response magnitudes from two inner hair cells in the same organ of Corti. Fundamental (f0), dc, second (2f0), and third harmonic (3f0) magnitudes are given as well as fundamental phase (arbitrary phase reference). All stimulus and recording conditions are identical for the two cells (shown with closed and open symbols respectively).

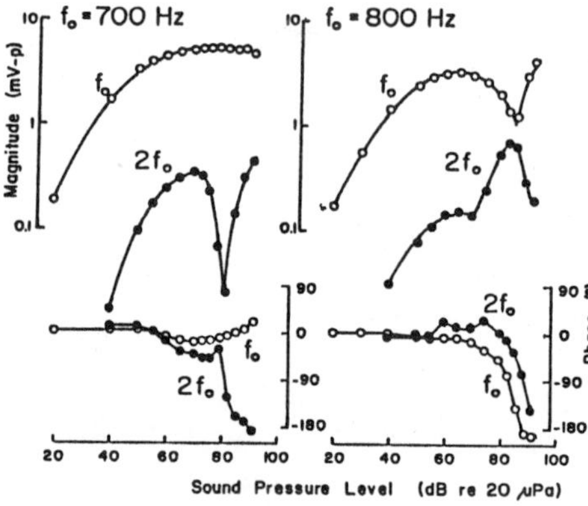

Figure 3. Magnitude and phase of fundamental (f0) and second harmonic (2f0) responses from two inner hair cells recorded from two different preparations. Phase reference is arbitrary.

The fundamental component's phase dependence appears to be similar to that seen before, at least for lower sound levels. In the declining portion of the input-output function the phase-change reverses direction with intensity and suggests rapid accumulation. (We will return to this pattern with a suggested explanation after considering other types of response patterns that one may encounter). The second harmonic of the ac response exhibits the already discussed common characteristics of this distortion component. It has a peak at 65 dB SPL and a pronounced notch at approximately 78 dB. The third harmonic produced by this cell is unusual in its nonmonotonicity. A pronounced notch is evident at 88 dB SPL.

To illustrate variations in IHC responsiveness, responses from another cell, recorded from the same guinea pig, are also included in **Fig. 2** (open symbols). The various harmonic *patterns* more closely resemble those seen in **Fig. 1** than the ones illustrated with closed symbols in **Fig. 2**, albeit the former was obtained from a different animal. Thus the fundamental and dc components rise monotonically throughout the intensity range tested, and so does the third harmonic. The second harmonic component possesses the now familiar notch at 76 dB. While the general patterns are similar, interesting quantitative differences exist in the nonlinear response properties of this cell and that shown in **Fig. 1**. First note that the sensitivities (dB SPL at 1 mV-p ac response) of the two cells are within three decibels. Yet, the maximum ac and dc responses of the **Fig. 1** cell are more than 6 dB greater. More impressive is that the 2nd and 3rd harmonic components are nearly 20 dB greater.

Visual comparison between response patterns in **Fig. 2** reveal different qualitative characteristics for all components, except the 2nd harmonic which has the expected two-lobed appearance. All components are different quantitatively. We should note that differences in these IHC responses are seen while the gross cochlear responses (measured in scala media and in the organ of Corti fluid space with the recording microelectrode) show essentially no change in repeated determinations bracketing the IHC measurements.

One interesting input-output pattern that can be seen occasionally in IHC responses is characterized by non-monotonic fundamental and dc response components. They both reach a local maximum at about 65 dB SPL, followed by a relatively deep notch showing minima for both components at the same sound level (~80 dB SPL). Beyond the notch both ac and dc responses rise with some hint of saturation within the test range of sound levels. The notch is accompanied by a phase reversal of the fundamental component. We illustrate this pattern in **Fig. 3** where fundamental and second harmonic responses are included for two cells. These are chosen for comparison because their sensitivities are essentially identical, ~35 dB SPL at 1 mV-p, as is their low-level second harmonic production. Yet, one cell exhibits "well behaved" growth pattern while the other a non monotonic one.

For cells showing notched fundamental the second harmonic maximum occurs at higher than usual SPL; in fact, the maximum coincides with the fundamental minimum. The example of **Fig. 3** represents a very interesting such situation in that there is an apparent buildup of the second harmonic coinciding with the drop in the fundamental.

Discussion

One advantage of our apical recording location is that various harmonic components in a cell's response to tones can be studied near the characteristic frequency. At the third turn recording location this is typically between 800 and 1,000 Hz. Low-pass filtering is expected due to the recording electrode (usual corner frequency ~1,500 Hz) and the cell membrane capacitance (typical corner frequency 470 Hz; Dallos 1984). In this paper all data are presented just below the best frequency, at 700 or 800 Hz. Thus, the fundamental is attenuated to a modest degree, maybe 3 dB, the second harmonic to a greater extent, possibly 9 dB, and the third harmonic component conceivably as much as 16 dB. Consequently, the actual harmonic content of the hair cell-input/transducer processes is greater than depicted in the present graphs, implying a more distorted waveform than represented in the cell's voltage response (**Fig. 1 inserts**).

The most commonly seen IHC response at best frequency is illustrated in **Fig. 1**. In agreement with virtually all intracellular data from hair cells, these responses contain a large dc component. Plotting peak responses against peak pressure (**Fig,1b, c**) reveals a pronounced asymmetry with $\mathbf{V_{D\text{-}max}/V_{H\text{-}max}}$ ratio of about eight. In harmony with other reports (Crawford and Fettiplace, 1981; Corey and Hudspeth, 1983; Russell and Sellick, 1983) the response saturation is much more pronounced in the hyperpolarizing direction. In fact, the degree of asymmetry seen here is most reminiscent of that manifested by terrapin hair cells in which the electrical membrane resonance was suppressed or absent (Crawford and Fettiplace, 1981). The saturation in the hyperpolarizing direction, as seen here, is much harder than presented for high frequency inner hair cells by Russell and Sellick (1983). The difference is easy to explain by the fact that our measurements are much nearer to the cell's best frequency than was possible for the basal turn inner hair cells. The peak response-versus-peak pressure characteristic curves are frequency-dependent, such that away from the best frequency the nonlinearity is milder and the response asymmetry is less.

The fits of these functions with two rectangular hyperbolae are better than what may be obtained by the hyperbolic tangent functions proposed by Weiss and Leong (1985). The curves seem not to possess continuous derivatives at the origin. To give an idea about the expected slope (gain) changes between depolarizing and hyperpolarizing directions, the derivatives to the fitted functions of **Fig. 1c** are evaluated at the origin, where they take on the values of $\mathbf{V_{D\text{-}max}/p_D}$ and $\mathbf{V_{H\text{-}max}/p_H}$. The slope in the depolarizing direction is obtained as 145 mV/Pa, while that in the hyperpolarizing direction as 262 mV/Pa, or a roughly two-fold difference.

The apparent discontinuity at the origin, seen to various degrees in all inner hair cells that we have evaluated, has implications about the character of the expected harmonic pattern in the response. Weiss and Leong (1985) showed that if a hyperbolic tangent-type transducer nonlinearity is incorporated in a simple electric circuit representing the hair cell, then it is possible to find notches in certain harmonic input-output functions, accompanied by 180° phase shift in that harmonic's phase. Thus they have shown that such notches do not necessarily imply (while do not rule out) the presence of two competing processes producing response cancellation. The model generated notches only for odd order harmonics. We have shown (Weigelt and Dallos, to be published) this conclusion to be true also when the hyperbolic tangent type transducer nonlinearity was introduced into the hair cell circuit model proposed by one of us (Dallos, 1983, 1984). Transducer functions with discontinuous derivatives, when incorporated into our circuit model, however, could yield input-output functions with notches for any harmonic component, including the fundamental.

It is thus possible to envision nonlinear transducer functions that produce notches in fundamental, dc, or harmonic magnitude functions (with attendant 180° phase shifts) without the need to propose cancellation between two response components. This is particularly interesting in relation to the fundamental where we have seen such notches and phase shifts, conceivably corresponding to those seen in single auditory nerve fiber rate-level functions (Kiang and Moxon, 1972). The latter are interpreted as the result of interaction between two response producing processes (Kiang et al., 1986). The nonlinearity responsible for these behaviors does not have to be the inner hair cell transducer function, it could reside in preceding mechanical properties. Zwislocki (1986) proposed that the notches are a consequence of the nonlinear coupling between tectorial membrane and organ of Corti. Notches have been seen in basilar membrane velocity responses in the guinea pig (Patuzzi et al., 1984). On the other hand, the peak intracellular response-versus-peak input pattern, obtained with direct mechanical input to the cilia in organ culture, is remarkably similar to that seen in the adult animal *in vivo* (Russell et al., 1986). It is thus possible that the character of the nonlinearities residing in cochlear micromechanics and IHC transduction have certain similarities and that they both contribute to the ultimate response. If outer hair cell (OHC) response characteristics are not dissimilar from those of IHCs, as seems to be the case in the apical cochlea (Dallos, 1985, 1986), and if OHCs are actuators in a mechanical feedback path, then similar response properties should be seen at differing loci of measurement. In other words, the OHC transducer nonlinearity [as represented in the *in vitro* responses seen by Russell at al. (1986)] should be manifested in basilar membrane motion (Patuzzi et al., 1984), in IHC responses (this report), and in nerve fiber discharges (Kiang and Moxon, 1972).

How prevalent are amplitude notches and related phase inversions in IHC responses? In much of our early work only course intensity steps (20 dB) were used to outline input-output functions. With such a raster the notches are usually missed. However, even using small steps does not assure the presence of a notch. In many cases these are definitely absent within our explored intensity range (20 to 91 dB SPL). It is possible to see notches in the input-output function from one IHC of a given organ of Corti but not in others. We have also seen the sound level where the notch is deepest move toward higher values during the course of recording from an IHC. It is conceivable that if higher sound levels were routinely explored with small steps, more amplitude notches would be found. For example, the decline of magnitude and change of phase of the response shown in **Fig. 2** intimate that a notch and 180° phase shift might be seen at higher levels than those examined.

It is not uncommon to record from IHCs in a given preparation that show different response properties, as illustrated in **Fig. 2**. Even if a change in the animal's condition may be ruled out by examinining gross potential recordings, IHC response properties do vary. It is probable that the principal determining factor of the nature of the response, all other variables being unchanged, is the quality of the electrode penetration into the cell. Thus, variations in membrane potential (due to interference with cell homeostasis by the electrode, or artificially controlled) can have significant effects on nonlinear response properties (Dallos and Cheatham, to be published). Of course, one cannot rule out certain inherent differences in transducer properties among inner hair cells.

Acknowledgment

Work supported by Grant NS08635 from the NINCDS, NIH

References

Brown, M.C. and Nuttall, A.L. (1984) Efferent control of cochlear inner hair cell responses in the guinea pig. J. Physiol. (London) 354, 625-646.

Corey, D.P. and Hudspeth, A.J. (1983) Kinetics of the receptor current in bullfrog saccular hair cells. J. Neurosci. 3, 962-976.

Crawford, A.C. and Fettiplace, R. (1981) Non-linearities in the responses of turtle hair cells. J. Physiol. (London) 315, 317-338.

Dallos, P. (1983) Some electrical circuit properties of the organ of Corti. I. Analysis without reactive elements. Hearing Res. 12, 89-119.

Dallos, P. (1984) Some electrical circuit properties of the organ of Corti. II. Analysis including reactive elements. Hearing Res. 14, 281-291.

Dallos, P. (1985) Response characteristics of mammalian cochlear hair cells. J. Neurosci. 5, 1591-1608.

Dallos, P. (1986) Neurobiology of cochlear inner and outer hair cells: intracellular recordings. Hearing. Res. 22, 185-198.

Dallos, P., Santos-Sacchi, J. and Flock, A. (1982) Intracellular recordings from cochlear outer hair cells. Science 218, 582-584.

Goodman, D.A., Smith, R.L. and Chamberlain, S.C. (1982) Intracellular and extracellular responses in the organ of Corti of the gerbil. Hearing Res. 7, 161-179.

Hudspeth, A.J. and Corey, D.P. (1977) Sensitivity, polarity, and conductance change in the response of vertebrate hair cells to controlled mechanical stimuli. Proc. Natl. Acad. Sci. U.S.A. 74, 2407-2411.

Kiang, N.Y.S. and Moxon, E.C. (1972) Physiological considerations in artificial stimulation of the inner ear. Ann. Otol. Rhinol. Laryngol. 81, 714-730.

Kiang, N.Y.S., Liberman, M.C., Sewell, W.F. and Guinan, J.J. (1986) Single unit clues to cochlear mechanisms. Hearing Res. 22, 171-184.

Lipetz, L.E. (1971) The relation of physiological and psychological aspects of sensory intensity. In: Handbook of Sensory Physiology. Vol. 1. Principles of Receptor Physiology. (Ed. Loewenstein, W.R.) Springer-Verlag, Berlin, pp. 191-225.

Patuzzi, R. and Sellick, P.M. (1983) A comparison between basilar membrane and inner hair cell receptor potential input-output functions in the guinea pig. J. Acoust. Soc. Amer. 74, 1734-1741.
Patuzzi, R., Johnstone, B.M. and Sellick, P.M. (1984) The alteration of the vibration of the basilar membrane produced by loud sound. Hearing Res. 13, 99-100.
Russell, I.J. and Sellick, P.M. (1978) Intracellular studies of hair cells in the guinea pig cochlea. J. Physiol. (London) 284, 261-290.
Russell, I.J. and Sellick, P.M. (1983) Low-frequency characteristics of intracellularly recorded receptor potentials in guinea-pig cochlear hair cells. J. Physiol. (London) 338, 179-206.
Russell, I.J., Cody, A.R. and Richardson, G.P. (1986) The responses of inner and outer hair cells in the basal turn of the guinea-pig cochlea and in the mouse cochlea grown in vitro. Hearing Res. 22, 199-216.
Sellick, P.M., Patuzzi, R. and Johnstone, B.M. (1983) Comparison between the tuning properties of inner hair cells and basilar membrane motion. Hearing Res. 10, 101-108.
Weiss, T.F. and Leong, R. (1985) A model for signal transmission in an ear having hair cells with free-standing stereocilia. IV. Mechanoelectric transduction stage. Hearing Res. 20, 175-195.
Zwislocki, J.J. (1986) Are nonlinearities observed in firing rates of auditory-nerve afferents reflections of a nonlinear coupling between the tectorial membrane and the organ of Corti? Hearing Res. 22, 217-221.

Precirculated comment/discussion

ASYMMETRIES IN MOTILE RESPONSES OF OUTER HAIR CELLS IN SIMULATED IN VIVO CONDITIONS

B.N. Evans, P. Dallos and R. Hallworth

Auditory Physiology Laboratory (Audiology)
Department of Neurobiology and Physiology
Northwestern University, Evanston, IL 60201 USA

It is now well known that electrical stimulation of isolated mammalian outer hair cells results in a motile response (Brownell, 1983; Ashmore, 1987; Zenner et al., 1987). The fast response component is apparently capable of following a sinusoidal current stimulus in the audio frequency range (Ashmore, 1987; Zenner et al., 1987). Fast motility is a robust response that has been shown under conditions that are distinctly non-physiological. In all experiments reported thus far, all cell surfaces were bathed in a high-sodium medium. Of course, under *in vivo* conditions only the basolateral cell membrane is exposed to perilymph (high Na^+) while the hair-bearing apical end is bathed in endolymph (high K^+). We demonstrate here that isolated cells show two kinds of rectification in their motility with sinusoidal current stimuli, that there are quantitative differences in the responses as a function of cell length, and that these phenomena persist when the apical and basolateral cell surfaces are exposed to their proper biochemical environment.

Outer hair cells were isolated from individual turns of guinea pig cochleas to assure proper correlations between their length and cochlear origin. The cells were maintained in a Liebovitz L-15 nutrient medium. Flame polished pipettes (tip dia. 4 um) were attached at the synaptic end to stabilize the cells and to pass current. Cell movement was measured by a calibrated photodiode/imaging system and averaged displacement responses were stored in a computer. Sinusoidal current bursts (100 Hz) of variable magnitude were the stimuli. Movement thresholds were obtained at approximately 2 pA.

It was observed that motile responses were asymmetrical. At low current levels the frequency-following response was superimposed on a DC response component toward cell contraction. With increasing stimulation this asymmetry first increased, then diminished, to be superseded by an asymmetry producing net cell extension. Both long (apical) and short (basal) cells exhibited this phenomenon, but the latter had thresholds and transition levels from 12-30 dB higher. Apical cells showed pronounced saturation at the highest current levels, while basal cells did not within the measured range. In **Figure 1 (left)** the DC response components are shown for one long and one short cell. These are similar for both cell types, albeit with a considerable difference in effective stimulus levels. For comparison, the DC receptor potential components recorded *in vivo* from an apical and a basal outer hair cell are given in **Figure 1 (right)**. The similarity of patterns in DC receptor potentials and motile responses is interesting and suggests the possibility of a common origin.

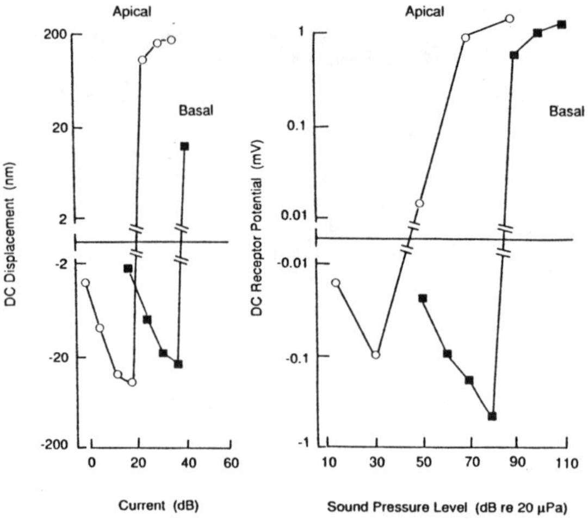

Figure 1. Left. DC motile response components to 100 Hz sinusoidal current bursts from long (apical) and short (basal) outer hair cells. Contraction is plotted below the baseline, elongation above. **Right.** DC receptor potential components recorded intracellularly from outer hair cells of apical (Dallos, unpublished data, 1983) and basal origin (Cody and Russell, 1987). Relation between stimulus and best frequencies of these cells is shown in octaves. Hyperpolarization is plotted below the baseline, depolarization above.

To test whether these phenomena, including the basic motile response, persist under more natural conditions, we adopted the methods of Baylor et al. (1979). Isolated outer hair cells were drawn into flame polished pipettes, synaptic end first, so that only the cuticular plate was exposed to the outside medium. The pipette was filled with standard high-Na^+ electrolyte and the bath was initially also a high-Na^+ medium. Cell motility was established under these conditions and then the bathing medium was changed to artificial endolymph. All outer hair cells remaining in the medium contracted while the cell within the pipette remained unchanged. Upon application of current, the cell exhibited fast motility and the above-described rectification. It may be concluded that outer hair cells do have the ability to show asymmetric fast motility under conditions that mimic those *in vivo*.

Work supported by grants from the NIH.

References

Ashmore, J.F. (1987) A fast motile response in guinea-pig outer hair cells: the cellular basis of the cochlear amplifier. J.Physiol. (London) 388, 323-347.
Baylor, D.A., Lamb, T.D. and Yau, K-w. (1979) The membrane current of single rod outer segments. J.Physiol. (London) 288, 589-611.
Brownell, W.E. (1983) Observations on a motile response in isolated outer hair cells. In: Mechanisms of Hearing (W.R. Webster and L.M. Aitkin, Edts.) Monash Univ. Press, Clayton, Australia, pp. 5-10.
Cody, A.R. and Russell, I.J. (1987) The responses of hair cells in the basal turn of the guinea-pig cochlea to tones. J.Physiol. (London) 383, 551-569
Zenner, H.P., Zimmerman, U. and Gitter, A.H. (1987) Fast motility of isolated auditory sensory cells. Biochem. and Biophys. Res. Com. 149, 304-308.

ROUND WINDOW COCHLEAR MICROPHONIC AND ATROPHY OF SHORT AND MIDDLE STEREOCILIA ON OUTER HAIR CELLS IN HYDROPIC COCHLEAS IN GUINEA PIGS

K.C. Horner, Y. Cazals and A. Guilhaume

Laboratoire d'Audiologie Expérimentale
INSERM U229, Hôpital Pellegrin, Université de Bordeaux II
Place Amélie Raba Léon, 33076 Bordeaux, France

Introduction

Endolymphatic hydrops of the inner ear in man is a major pathology but since the etiology is not known treatment of the disease remains obscure. Induction of endolymphatic hydrops in animals is an experimental manipulation which has been employed for the past 60 years (Portmann, 1927) with the aim of providing an animal model for the investigation of hydrops. Despite the fact that hydrops can be surgically induced (Kimura, 1967) with almost 100% success in the guinea pig, the model has, in general, failed to reveal any specific characteristics and indeed instead of providing an insight to the disease the model itself has remained poorly understood. Despite this rather disconcerting appraisal there has recently been a renewed wave of interest in the model. In the past couple of years a considerable amount of data on the histopathology of experimental hydrops has been published including outer hair cell loss (Kimura, 1967) as well as progressive loss of inner hair cells (Aran et al., 1984; Albers, et al, 1987) towards the apex which can account well for the elevation of thresholds. However the physiological basis for the most characteristic and intriguing symptom of the disease - that of fluctuant thresholds - is still at the stage of hypotheses which are discussed by us elsewhere (Horner et al., 1988). Clearly, whilst the thresholds remain fluctuant we can consider that the sensory hair cells are still present and functional to some degree at least intermittently. Indeed by employing chronically implanted guinea pigs (Horner and Cazals, 1987) it has been shown that the early stage in experimental hydrops is indeed associated with fluctuant thresholds and in particular for the lower frequencies. Whilst hair cell loss can account for sensitivity loss, fluctuant aggravation of the sensitivity loss can be more fully explained by a perturbation of the remaining hair cells. Indeed we have recently pin-pointed a specific stereocilia pathology which could represent a candidate to explain the physiological data.

We have described a selective atrophy of short and middle stereocilia of outer hair cells in the upper cochlear turns while the tall stereocilia appear to be conserved (Horner at al., 1988). These observations were indeed essentially novel, given that this particular pattern of atrophy had, to our knowledge, never before been described. In this paper we take the opportunity of describing in further detail this atrophy which becomes evident only after about four months of hydrops when the CAP audiogram is relatively flat. In addition we present the data on the round window cochlear microphonics and their harmonic distortion recorded at this period. In addition we have attempted to highlight the potential significance of this specific atrophy to stereocilia in normal and hydropic cochleas.

Methods

The electrophysiological methods employed here have for the most part been described in detail several times by us. In brief, the animals were chronically implanted with round window platinum ball electrodes. The AP audiogram changes were registered on awake animals, often over a period of four months. The present study investigated the input-output functions of the round window cochlear microphonics (RWCM). In addition spectrum analyses of the microphonics allowed us to note the amplitude of the harmonic distortion products of the microphonic.

The preparation of specimens for scanning electron microscopy was similar to that described by us recently. In order to expose all three rows of stereocilia on the hair cell bundles along the whole length of the cochlea, we have found that the most appropriate fixation procedure is intracochlear perfusion with osmium tetroxide (1%) in sodium cacodylate buffer (0.1M). The cochleas are left to bathe in this fixative for 1 h and then flushed with the same buffer solution before being dehydrated to 70% ethanol for dissection. The specimens were critical point dried in CO_2 before being coated with gold/palladium (Balzers SCD 030) and observed on a MEB Philips 505 scanning electron microscope.

Results

During early stages of hydrops when there is either a low frequency CAP sensitivity loss or a low and very high sensitivity loss the RWCMs were found to be little affected or not affected at all (Horner and Cazals, 1987, 1988). In this study we have chosen to present data from 10 animals which had been operated to induce hydrops 4 months earlier. The CAP audiograms from all hydropic ears four months after the surgical induction of endolymphatic hydrops are presented in figure 1. The hatched area represents the minimum and the maximum limits of audiograms taken from a group of 15 normal guinea pigs indicating that the sensitivity loss in hydropic ears was between 30 and 70 dB. Figures 1 also illustrates the amplitude of the RWCM as a function of stimulus frequency for the same hydropic ears and control ears. Two particular features are striking and will be dealt with separately. First, the amplitude of the microphonic responses in 7/10 hydropic ears appear to be less affected by hydrops than the neural CAP responses. It is clear that the microphonic amplitudes are reduced but the deterioration certainly does not extend to the same degree as that seen for the corresponding CAP. Second, in those 3 cases which have the highest CAP thresholds and smallest microphonic responses, it is the microphonic responses for the lower (1 kHz and 2kHz) which are more seriously reduced - in contrast to normal cochleas hatched area) where the RWCM increases towards lower frequencies.

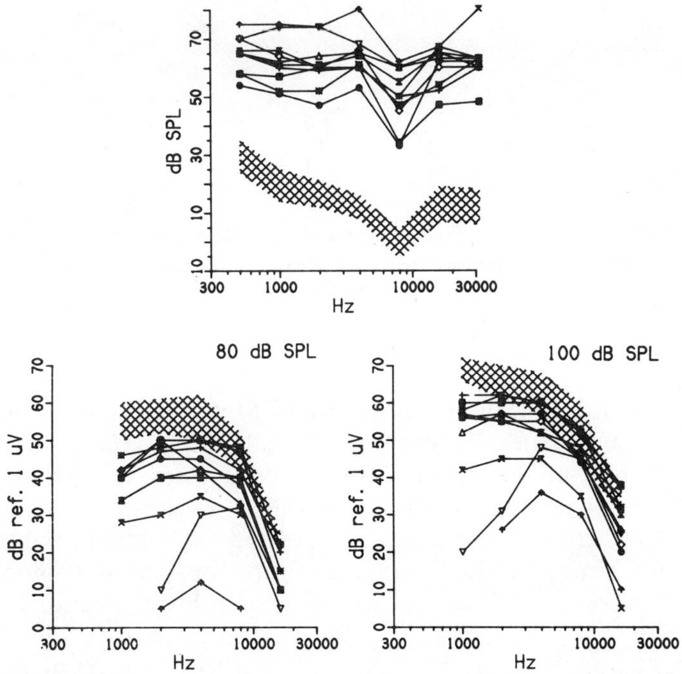

Figure 1. (Upper) CAP audiograms from 10 different hydropic guinea pig ears. The hatched area represents the maximum and minimum limits of the audiograms from a group of control ears. (Lower left) Amplitude of RWCM, at 80 dB SPL, as a function of stimulus frequency for 10 different hydropic ears. The hatched area is the maximum and minimum limits from a group of control ears. (Lower right) the same as for "Lower left" but for stimuli at 100 dB SPL

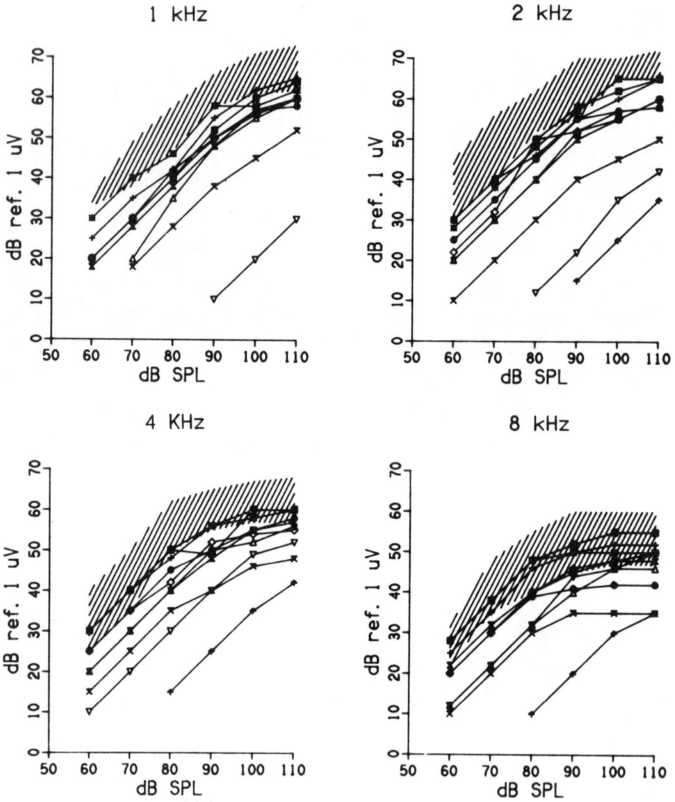

Figure 2. Input/output functions for RWCM for each of 10 hydropic ears. The hatched area represents the maximum and the minimum limits in a control group of animals.

The input/output functions for the RWCM are completely in keeping with that noted by us earlier (Horner and Cazals, 1987; Horner and Cazals, 1988). The input/output function for hydropic ears is shifted towards higher stimulus levels and the plateau level is reduced as illustrated in figure 2. In this study we were interested to know whether the microphonics were simply reduced in amplitude or whether there was an additional modification to the quality of microphonic responses. In order to probe this aspect we investigated the composition of the harmonic distortion by spectrum analyses. It is clear that while there is at least 20 dB difference in the amplitude of the fundamental RWCM at 100 dB SPL, between the control and hydropic ears (figure 3) the level of harmonic distortion of those microphonics is more similar to the controls at 100 dB SPL that the controls at 80 dB SPL. These findings are particularly evident for the lower frequencies (1kHz and 2kHz) where up to eight harmonics could be recorded even in hydropic cochleas.

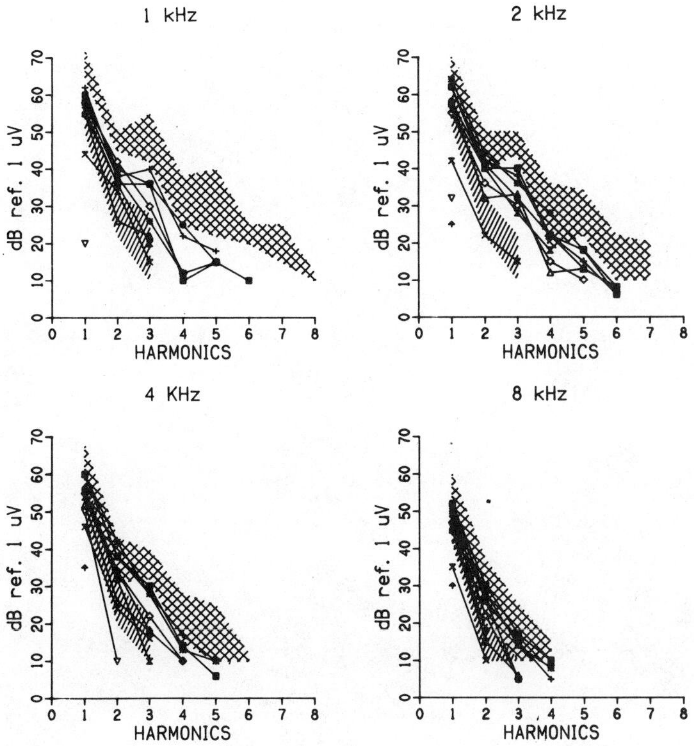

Figure 3. The maximum and minimum limits of the harmonic distortion of RWCM in control ears for pure tone stimuli presented at 100 dB SPL (crossed hatched) and at 80 dB SPL (simple hatched). The harmonic distortions for each of 10 hydropic ears for pure tone stimuli is presented at 100 dB SPL.

In short, four months after the experimental induction of hydrops there is an important sensitivity loss across the CAP audiogram whilst the input-output functions of RWCM appear to affected to a much lesser degree and they appear to be very rich in harmonic distortion. We would like to present some SEM observations from an hydropic ear of a guinea pig operated 6 months previously. We have recently described a most peculiar atrophy of the short and middle stereocilia from the outer hair cells (OHCs) - restricted to the upper 2/3 of the cochlea (Horner et al., 1988). SEM observations of the hydropic cochlea of GP660 (figure 4) showed that the pathology progresses from OHC row 1 where the atrophy is discrete, to row 2 where the two rows (short and middle) can be completely absent, to row 3 where there is often absence of cells. In fact before atrophy of the stereocilia becomes evident all three rows of stereocilia in a bundle adopt a swollen appearance and are glued together (figure 4a). Often the first stereocilia atrophy begins at the centre of the

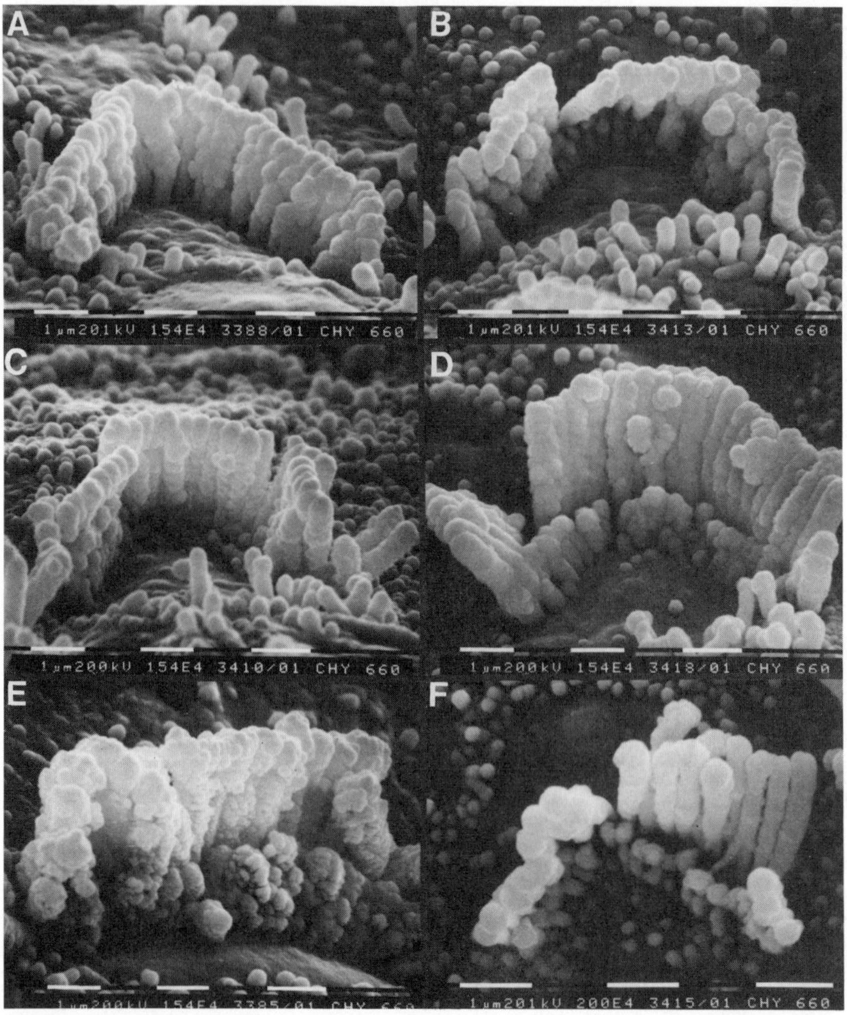

Fig. 4. Examples of hair cell stereocilia tufts from the hydropic cochlea of GP660. A first row OHC (A) and second row OHCs (B) (C) and (D) taken at a location around 2 kHz in the second cochlear turn. A second row OHC taken at a location around 500 Hz in the fourth cochlear turn (E). A third row IHC taken at a location around 4 kHz in the second cochlear turn.

hair cell stereocilia bundle and the lateral stereocilia are the last to atrophy (fig 4 b,c). Tall stereocilia can be seen bent slightly forward (fig 4b, c) before the complete atrophy of the short and middle stereocilia. On the other hand the tall stereocila can be seen to be upright after the complete atrophy of the short and middle stereocilia (fig 4d) and almost all the inter stereociliary bridges are broken (fig 4f). Whilst absence of stereocilia was not observed on the inner hair cell it was clearly evident that the stereocilia of the IHCs are swollen and give the impression that the three rows of stereocilia are glued together with a "cauliflower" appearance (fig 4e).

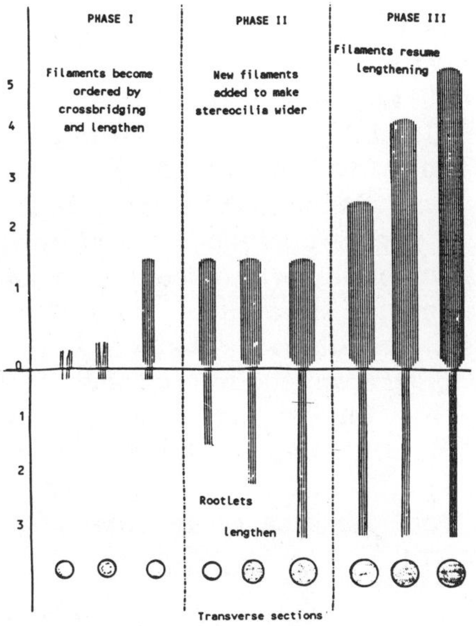

Figure 5. (With permission of Tilney and Tilney, 1986) Diagram illustrating the three phases of growth of the stereocilia and the rootlet and the gradual ordering of the bundle of actin filaments.

Discussion

Our observations from electrophysiology suggest that there are at least two simultaneous phenomena occurring in hydropic cochleas of the guinea pig. First we suggest on the bases of RWCMs that OHCs (towards the base of the cochlea) are partially functional, albeit with a reduced output, but the sensorineural function of the IHCs and OHCs along the length of the cochlea (as seen from the CAP audiograms) is impeded. We must therefore conclude, as we have done earlier (Horner and Cazals, 1988) that this discrepancy must be located at the level of the intimate coordination of function between OHCs and IHCs. Second it appears from the RWCM data that the low frequency response of the base of the cochlea is disturbed to a greater extent than that for higher frequencies in keeping with clinical observations on Menière's patients (Dauman et al., 1986). In addition we have earlier shown that the very first change seen after induction of hydrops is an elevation of the thresholds for the low/mid frequencies (below 6.4 kHz) (Horner and Cazals, 1987, 1988) - hence a disturbance of the low frequency response towards the apex of the cochlea. Indeed from CAP recordings we have shown that there is reduced excitation of the base of the cochlea by brief low frequency tones (Cazals and Horner 1988).

We propose that that the progressive atrophy of the short and middle stereocilia on OHCs together with "cauliflower-like" appearance of the other stereocilia in the upper 2/3 of the cochlea is the most likely bases for the pathophysiology in hydropic cochleas described by us. At this point we would like to draw attention to the striking resemblance between the pattern of *pathological atrophy* in hydropic cochleas and the pattern of *embryonic development* in chick cochleas (Tilney and Tilney, 1986). In brief, those authors have defined three phases of stereocilia growth : first, an elongation of the stereocilia throughout the length of the cochlea; second, the lengthening is brought to a halt and the stereocilia thicken except for the tall stereocilia which have already attained their mature diameter and finally a third phase begins where the stereocilia towards the upper 2/3 of the cochlea elongate once again (figure 5). Indeed the atrophy of stereocilia in hydropic cochleas might ressemble a form of counteraction of phase III (as seen for the chick) in the mature stereocilia . Tilney and Tilney suggest that the controlled growth of stereocilia is by the addition of subunits to the actin filaments at the tips of the stereocilia and that this growth process is critically controlled by the removal of certain impediments or "preferred end cappers" from the tips. In the same vain perhaps the loss of subunits from stereocilia tips in hydropic cochleas is due to the over-activity of "cappers" and understanding of the pathology might be achieved by biochemical investigations.

Acknowledgements

Kathleen Horner was supported by La Fondation de France during this research.

References

Aran, J-M, Rarey, K.E. and Hawkins, J.E. (1984) Functional and morphological changes in experimental endolymphatic hydrops. Acta Otolaryngol. 97, 547-557.

Albers, F.W.J., Veldman, J.E. and Huizing, E.H. (1987) Early hair cell loss in experimental hydrops. Ann Otol. Rhinol. Laryngol. 96, 282-285.

Cazals, Y. and K.C. Horner (1988) Abnormal two-sound interactions in hydropic cochleas of the guinea pig. In: 8th International Symposium on Hearing. Basic Issues in Hearing. (in press).

Dauman, R., Aran, J-M. and Portmann, M. (1986) Summating potential and water balance in menire's disease. Ann. Otol. Rhinol. Laryngol. 95, 389-395.

Horner, K.C. and Cazals, Y. (1987) Rapidly fluctuating thresholds at the onset of experimentally-induced hydrops in the guinea pig. Hearing Res. 26, 319-325.

Horner, K.C. and Cazals, Y. (1988) Evolution of recruitment at different frequencies during the development of endolymphatic hydrops in the guinea pig. Arch. Otorhinolaryngol. (in press).

Horner, K.C., Guilhaume, A. and Cazals, Y. (1988) Atrophy of middle and short stereocilia on outer hair cells of guinea pig cochleas with experimentally induced hydrops. Hearing Res. 32, 41-48.

Kimura, R.S. (1967) Experimental blockage of thebendolymphatic duct and sac and its effect on the inner ear of the guinea pig. A study on endolymphatic hydrops. Ann. Otol. Rhinol. Laryngol 76, 664-687.

Portmann, G. (1927) Surgical treatment by opening the saccus endolymphaticus. Arch. Otolaryngol. 6, 309-319.

Tilney, L.G. and Tilney, M.S. (1986) Functional organisation of the cytoskeleton. Hearing Res. 22, 55-77.

Comments and Discussion

PICKLES

Q1. Could it be that the loss of the shortest and middle stereocilia simply represents the earliest stage of a progressive loss of all three rows? In our own study of the effects of kanamycin, stereocilia were lost progressively, the middle ones next, and the tallest stereocilia least (Pickles et al., 1987). However, there was never such a clear distinction between the effects on the different rows as you have shown.

Q2. If tip links are indeed involved in transduction (Pickles et al., 1984, and this volume), and if the transducer channels are indeed situated at the lower end of the link (our preferred hypothesis), then the middle and short stereocilia, but not the tallest, carry the transducer current. Is it possible that this in some way is related to the relative protection of the tallest stereocilia during hydrops?

Q3. Is there any evidence that "over-activity of preferred-end cappers" can occur, as you suggest, and that this will lead to dissolution of the stereocilia from the tips? My understanding is that cappers would simply stabilise the apical end of the stereocilium. However, it could be that if the cappers did not allow any addition of actin monomers at the tips, the stereocilium would be progressively dissolved by the removal of monomers from the preferred end for *removal* of monomers, which is at the lower (hair-cell) end.

Pickles, J.O., Comis, and Osborne, M.P. (1984) Cross-links between stereocilia in the guinea pig organ of Corti, and their possible relation to sensory transduction. Hearing Res., 15, 103-112.

Pickles, J.O., Comis, and Osborne, M.P. (1987) The effect of chronic application of kanamycin on stereocilia and their tip links in hair cells of the guinea pig cochlea. Hearing Res., 29, 237-244.

HORNER

A1. From our observations, it does not seem that the 3rd row (tall) of stereocilia atrophy. There is complete atrophy of the short and middle stereocilia and the next stage seems to be loss of hair cell.

A2. Yes - we would also prefer that the transducer channels be associated with short and middle stereocilia tips - since this would fit with out hypothesis that rapid fluctuations are due to perturbation of interciliary bridges.

The tall stereocilia may be protected by the tectorial membrane.

In addition one might envisage some kind of overstimulation of transducer channels by some kind of abnormal forces on the bridges introduced by hydrops - which could be selectively toxic on those middle and short stereocilia.

A3. No - there is no evidence for overactivity of preferred end cappers. On the other hand, as I understand it there is not a preferred end for *removal* of monomers at the lower (hair cell end). Tilney & Tilney suggest that growth can occur from both ends but the tip is the preferred end. In the case of hydrops, as the tips disappear, I would not be surprised to find that the rootlets shorten also.

POSTNATAL DEVELOPMENT OF THE COCHLEA IN HORSESHOE BATS

M. Vater and R. Rübsamen

Zoologisches Institut, Luisenstr.14, 8 München 2 Lehrstuhl für Zoologie Ruhruniversität Bochum, Bochum FRG

Introduction

The mammalian cochlea exhibits immature features in early postnatal development. Physiological responses are restricted to the low frequency range, and structural maturation is proceeding from basal cochlear locations towards the apex (review: Romand, 1983). The development of the cochlear frequency representation is an intriguing problem, however there are few frequency mapping studies in mammals. Cochlear microphonic measurements in gerbils showed that in postnatal development a shift in frequency place map takes place for basal regions of the cochlea (Arjmand et al.,1988) which are tuned to frequencies about 1.5 octaves lower than in the adult. The hypothesis that a reorganization of the cochlear frequency mapping pattern occurs during development (Lippe and Rubel, 1983) is thus supported for locations responsive to high frequencies in adult mammals, although it does not apply for apical cochlear regions (Arjmand et al., 1988) and has been generelly questioned by a developmental study in birds (Manley et al., 1987).

This study lends further supporting evidence for developmental shifts in cochlear frequency representation in mammals by investigating cochlear development in young horseshoe bats (Rhinolophus rouxi) with combined physiological and anatomical techniques. In adult bats, the cochlea is exceptionally sharply tuned to a narrow frequency band encompassing the long constant frequency (CF) component of the echolocation signal, (review: Vater, 1987) which is mapped onto hydromechanically specialized regions of basilarmembrane (BM). Evoked potential studies in young horseshoebats (Rübsamen, 1987) demonstrated that similar to other mammals, the hearing range expands towards higher frequencies and the adult characteristics are gradually established within a period of three postnatal weeks. The experimental approach reported here comprises single unit recordings from cochlear nucleus (CN) and analysis of horseradish peroxidase (HRP) transport patterns to the cochlea, accompanied by studies of cochlear morphology.

We demonstrate a clear age-dependent shift in the frequency response characteristics of a given place in the cochlea of horseshoe bats, which in the adult is sharply tuned to the individuals CF-component.

Methods

The procedures used in this study generally follow previously published protocols (Feng and Vater, 1985, Vater et al., 1985). Young bats were caught in a large maternity colony in Sri lanka. Their age was assessed in measurements of forearm length (Rübsbsamen, 1987) and ranged from 8 to 22 days. In all experimental animals, the middle ear was airfilled and clear of fluid or mesenchym. Neurophysiological recordings and tracer injections in 8-17 day old bats were performed in a field laboratory in Sri lanka, experiments on 18-23 day old bats were performed in Munich. For CN-recordings, a dorsal stereotactic approach through the intact cerebellum was chosen. Fine tipped KCL-filled glasselectrodes or HRP-filled glasselectrodes (10% in acetate buffer, pH 7.2; tip diameter 5-8 um; impedance 8-10 MOhm) were used to record single and multi unit activity from CN. Best frequencies (BF: frequency of lowest threshold) and frequency threshold curves (FTC) were determined with audiovisual criteria. HRP was iontophoretically injected through the recording electrode (0.5-1 uA for 4-8 min) into the physiologically characterized region. Perfusion and histochemical procedures followed those given in previous reports (Feng and Vater, 1985; Vater et al., 1985). Electrode tracts, HRP-injection sites and transport patterns in the CN of young bats were reconstructed and compared with data from adult bats. The labeling pattern in the cochleae of young bats was compared with the adult cochlear frequency map obtained with identical techniques.

Results

COCHLEARMORPHOLOGY

Lightmicroscopical investigations of cochlear morphology (Vater, in press) are summarized briefly. There is no significant change in BM-length during postnatal development. At birth, the specialized BM-thickness and width profile is established in final dimension and the histological picture of the organ of Corti is more mature than in cat or rodents (review: Romand, 1983). Baso-apical gradients in maturation of cochlear morphology (tectorial membrane, pillar cells) are clearly seen in prenatal specimens. Postnatally, there are only subtle differences among different turns. The most pronounced deviation from the adult organ of Corti is the presence of a thick cell layer attached to the scala tympani side of the BM (tympanic cover layer, TCL) throughout the cochlea (Fig.2). This cell layer atrophies in the course of development evidenced by a decrease in cell size and a loss of cells. In the basal turn of 3 weeks old bats and adult bats, this layer has almost completely disappeared, while it persists in reduced form in apical turns. Surface preparations of the basal turn of young bats revealed that the TCL cells are spindle shaped with the long axis oriented parallel to the spiral course of the BM.

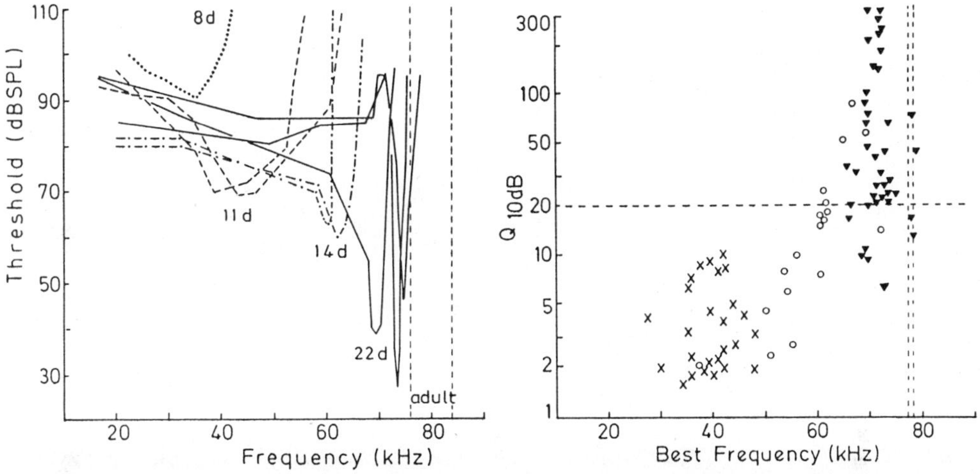

Fig.1 A: Representative tuning curves recorded in PVCN of young horseshoe bats. Numbers give postnatal age in days. Stippled lines border the range of BFs recorded in similar locations in adult female bats. With age, there is a concomittant change in tuning curve shapes and their BFs. B: Q 10dB values of single units recorded in PVCN of young horseshoe bats grouped according to different age (different symbols). Within age groups data are pooled across different individuals. Stippled lines indicate frequency range of maximal Q10dB in the adult.

TUNING CHARACTERISTICS IN COCHLEAR NUCLEUS

In young bats, single unit recordings were obtained mainly from dorsal parts of the posteroventral CN (PVCN), which in the adult (CF-frequency 78 kHz) process the frequencies above and including the echolocation signal (76-84 kHz). Reconstructions of electrode penetrations, localization of the HRP- injection sites and analysis of intranuclear transport patterns clearly show, that the frequency representation in CN is subjected to age dependent changes, while the wiring diagram remains stable.

Frequency threshold curves of single units recorded in PVCN of young bats are shown in Fig.1.

The oldest bat (female, 22 days) exhibited adultlike tuning features as evidenced by the exceedingly sharp FTC at 73.9 kHz, i.e. close to its echolocation call. The frequency range of sharp tuning is thus significantly lower than in adult females (78 kHz). Sharp tuning is not seen in bats up to 17 days old. In the youngest bat (8 days), only one acoustically driven single unit could be recorded in a penetration through PVCN and this was broadly tuned with a BF around 30 kHz and insensitive. In the 11 day old bat, sensitivity improved, but tuning characteristics were still broad to 42 kHz and both high and low frequency slopes of FTCs were shallow. In bats 14 days old, the high frequency slope of the FTCs steepened and tiny tip segments appeared tuned around 60 kHz.

Q10 dB values of single units recorded in young bats are plotted in Fig. 1B and grouped into three categories. Stage 1 (crosses) encompasses the

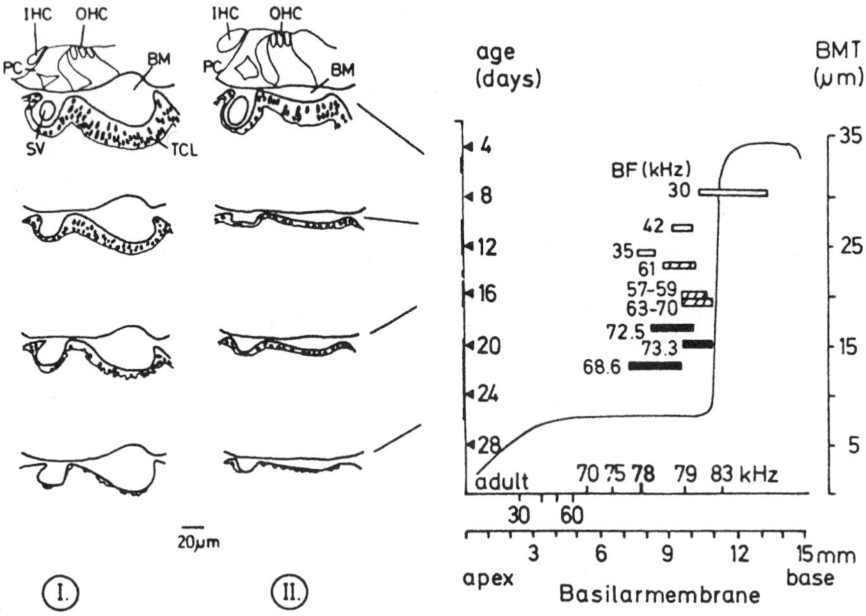

Fig.2 right: Comparison of location of HRP-labeled spiral ganglion cells (bars) in young bats (age given on left ordinate) with the cochlear frequency map of adult bats (female, CF-frequency 78 kHz) plotted on BM-scale (abscissas). Numbers next to bars give the BF or BF-range recorded at the HRP-injection site in PVCN. Open bars denote broad tuning characteristics, striped bars denote transition towards higher Q 10dB values and black bars denote sharp tuning characteristics, the injections at 72.5 kHz and 73.3. kHz were done in female bats, the injection at 68.6 kHz was done in a male (adult CF-frequency 74 kHz). Also plotted is the BM-thickness profile (thin line, BMT, right ordinate). Left: Crossections through the first and second half turn at different ages. BM, basilar membrane; IHC, inner hair cell, PC, pillar cells; SV, spiral vessel, OHC, outer hair cell.

postnatal days 8 to 13 and exhibits Q10dB values below 20. In stage 2 (14-18 days, open circles), a transition is seen towards higher Q10 dB values, the first Q10 values exceeding 50 are seen at frequencies around 65 kHz. Bats of stage 3 (19 to 22 days, filled triangles) possess the adult tuning sharpness (Q10dB up to 300) but at lower frequencies.

COCHLEAR FREQUENCY MAP

In adult bats, HRP-injections in the dorsal parts of PVCN label spiral ganglion cells within the second half turn and the upper basal half turn of the cochlea. Fig.2 compares the locations of labeled ganglion cells in young bats with the cochlear frequency map of adults plotted on the scale of BM- length. The extent of label is given by bars, and the numbers on the left side denote the BFs at the injection site. Open bars indicate broad tuning characteristics, striped bars indicate transitional stages with steep high frequency slopes and tip segments, filled bars denote sharp tuning characteristics. As expected from the locations of most injection sites, labeled ganglion cells were found in the second half turn apical to the decrease in BM- thickness (plotted as thin line, right ordinate). The injection in the youngest bat at a BF of 30 kHz was confined to most dorsal parts of PVCN, which processes the highest frequencies in the adult and receives input from most basal cochlear locations. The data clearly reveal, that in early postnatal development, the second half turn of the cochlea changed BF as well as tuning characteristics. Cross-sections through the first and second half turn of the cochlea of young bats are plotted on the left of Fig. 2. Corresponding to the time, were a transition of tuning characteristics is seen in young bats, the TCL is starting to atrophy. The TCL is nearly completely reduced in bats which are sharply tuned to lower frequencies than the adult.

Discussion

Our results demonstrate clear changes in frequency mapping and response characteristics of specialized high frequency regions of the horseshoe bat cochlea in early postnatal development. The development of sharply tuned FTCs in horseshoe bats is more complex than the hypothetical developmental scheme proposed for high frequency FTCs in the cat (Romand, 1983). In cats, development proceeds from broadly tuned reponses towards FTCs with clear tip and tail regions. "Virtual" BFs in early life correspond to the tail regions of FTCs in the adult. During the period of improving sensitivity of the tip region, no clear shifts in BF take place. In the horseshoe bat, development also starts with broadly tuned responses. Once a sharply tuned tip with steep high and low frequency slopes is formed, its BF is shifting upwards in frequency towards the adult range.

Morphological analysis of cochlear development in horseshoe bats reveals that postnatal growth in cochlear dimensions is not a critical factor, similar to other mammals (Harris and Dallos, 1984). In cats and rodents, immaturity of receptor cell innervation, in particular the efferent supply of outer hair cells has been proposed to represent a critical factor (Romand, 1983). We can exclude this possibility, since the horseshoe bat cochlea lacks efferent supply of outer hair cells (Bruns and Schmieszek, 1980). In the horseshoe bat, there are no postnatal changes in the tunnel of Corti and secretion of tectorial membrane is complete at the day of birth. Such baso-apical gradients in proceeding maturation can therefore not account for the physiological findings. As in other mammals, a thick TCL is attached to the BM of newborn bats. This is the only structure for which we could demonstrate pronounced postnatal changes. The time course in structural reorganization of the TCL correlates with stage 1 and 2 of physiological development. We speculate that the TCL influences the mechanical tuning characteristics of the specialized cochlear regions in horseshoes bats in early postnatal life. While this layer is present, no sharply tuned responses can be recorded, although BM- specializations are established. The additional mass of cells attached to the BM should influence resonance frequency, but more important might be the longitudinal orientation of tightly interwoven cell bodies and processes which could influence the coupling of neighboring BM-regions and possibly limit specialized mechanical oscillations. So far, we were unable to define structural correlates for the shift in BF of sharply tuned responses occuring in the third week. The fact that these responses were tuned to lower frequencies (maximum

16%) than in the adult might be explained by differences of BM-stiffness, which are not revealed in the morphological picture.

To summarize, evidence reported here supports the notion that in postnatal development of mammals the high frequency regions of the cochlea change frequency mapping pattern. The development of the non-specialized low frequency range of horseshoe bats remains to be studied.

Acknowledgements

We thank M.Kössl, B.Grothe and G.Neuweiler. Supported by SFB 204, DFG RU 390-1, & VW I-63742

References

Arjmand, E., Harris, D. and Dallos, P. (1988) Developmental changes in frequency mapping of the gerbil cochlea: Comparison of two cochlear locations. Hearing Res. 32, 93-96.

Bruns, V. and Schmieszek, E. (1980) Cochlear innervation in the Greater horseshoe bat: demonstration of an acoustic fovea. Hearing Res. 3:27-43

Feng, A.S. and Vater, M. (1985) Functional organization of the cochlear nucleus of rufous horseshoe bats (Rhinolophus rouxi): Frequencies and internal connections are arranged in slabs. J. comp. Neurol. 235, 529-555.

Harris, D.M. and Dallos, P. (1984) Ontogenetic changes in frequency mapping of a mammalian ear. Science 225, 741-743.

Lippe, W. and Rubel, E.W. (1983) Development of the place principle. Science 219, 514-516

Manley, G.A., Brix, J. and Kaiser, A. (1987) Developmental stability of the tonotopic organization of the chick's basilar papilla. Science 237, 655-656.

Romand, R. (1983) Development of the cochlea. In: Development of auditory and vestibular systems (Ed. Romand, R.) Academic Press, New York, pp. 47-88.

Rübsamen, R. (1987) Ontogenesis of the echolocation system in the rufous horseshoe bat, Rhinolophus rouxi (Audition and vocalization in early postnatal development). J. comp. Physiol. 161, 899-913.

Vater, M. (1987) Narrow-band frequency analysis in bats. In: Recent advances in the study of bats (Eds. Fenton, M.B., Racey, P., and Rayner, J.M.V.) Cambridge University Press, Cambridge, pp.200-226.

Vater, M. (1988) Lightmicroscopic observations on cochlear development in horseshoe bats. In: Animal sonar systems (Ed. Nachtigall, P.) Plenum Press, New York, London (in press).

Vater, M., Feng, A.S., and Betz, M. (1985) An HRP-study of the frequency place map of the horseshoe bat cochlea: Morphological correlates of the sharp tuning to a narrow frequency band. J. comp. Physiol. 157, 671-686.

Comments and Discussion

KIM

Your data indicate that the sensitivity of the horseshoe bat cochlear nucleus neurons is enhanced by about 50dB over a few weeks after birth. I would interpret this as a result of the postnatal maturation of a mechanically active outer-hair-cell mechanism rather than as a result of changes in passive mechanical properties of the cochlear partition.

Do you agree with this interpretation?

PUJOL

Your results on the development of the cochlea of the horseshoe bat do not disagree too much with what we know about cochlear development in other mammals.

1. The main morphological changes in the mammalian cochlea occur before and not after the onset of cochlear function (Pujol and Hilding, 1972). Then they should appear in your species around birth, as you could probably get cochlear responses in the very first postnatal days, using appropriate stimulation (around 100 dB SPL).

2. Moreover, the part of the cochlea you are referring to is to be compared with the hook region of other mammals where few morphological changes concerning OHC can be observed during development: they do not elongate much and they do not get many efferents.

3. The role of efferents in the development of the cochlea is not critical in other mammals either. Actually an early section of the vestibular nerve has no effect on the morphological development of the organ of Corti (Pujol and Carlier, 1982).

4. The basal to apical gradient of cochlear development is still valid for the first steps (onset of function, gross morphology). But it has been clearly demonstrated that the active mechanisms, as tested by distortion products, are the last event of physiological maturation: the bigger this active mechanism, the later the end of maturation. To summarize: the basal cochlea starts its maturation first and it is also the last to get completely mature (see Shuenson and Pujol, 1982; Lenoir and Puel, 1987).

VATER

We agree with comments that cochlear maturation of horseshoe bats essentially conforms to a general mammalian scheme. The participation of active processes in cochlear maturation of the horseshoe bat or in cochlear processing in the adult bat is an intriguing hypothesis but their nature remains to be determined. So far there are no ultrastructural data on outer hair cells in this species and it is unknown whether outer hair cell motility (slow or fast; e.g. Zenner et al.; Ashmore; this volume) occurs in the frequency range in question.

ON THE ORIGIN OF INTERSPECIFIC DIFFERENCES IN AUDITORY SUSCEPTIBILITY

L. Décory, A. Guilhaume*, A. Dancer and J.-M. Aran*

French-German Research Institute of Saint-Louis
68 301 Saint-Louis, FRANCE
**Laboratory of Experimental Audiology*
INSERM U229, Hôpital Pellegrin, Place Amélie Raba Léon
33 076 Bordeaux Cedex, FRANCE

Introduction

Noise-induced hearing losses have been widely studied over the past decades. But the different animal species and experimental conditions used rarely allowed interspecific correlations or extrapolation of the results to the human species.

The aim of this work is to study, on a quantitative point of view, the physiological and anatomical consequences of identical acoustical overstimulations in three well-known species of mammals: guinea-pig, chinchilla and cat and to relate the interspecific differences to the characteristics of the external, middle and inner-ear of each species. In all cases the same experimental conditions were used: continuous pure tone overstimulations were applied in closed sound system. Physiological auditory effects of such stimulations were evaluated by N1 audiograms threshold shifts and anatomical alterations were assessed by scanning electron microscopy.

Methods

N1 AUDIOGRAMS

Young animals of both sexes and free of middle-ear infection were used in this study. After premedication with sedative and anticholinergic agents, they were deeply anesthetised with ketamine (for guinea-pigs and chinchillas) or pentothal (for cats).

Pinnae were sectionned bilaterally and after a postero-lateral surgical approach, the right bulla was exposed. An electrode was acutely implanted on the round window. Bulla was kept open, but between two measurements a cotton plug was left on the opening to prevent cochlea from cooling. Normal body temperature was kept constant thanks to a rectal temperature probe and a heating-pad.

The animals were placed in a ear bar head-holder system which consisted on the left-hand side in a solid conical bar and, on the right-hand side, in a hollow cone made of Altuglass®. This hollow cone allowed the insertion of different sound sources and of a probe-tube connected to a 1/2" Brüel and Kjaer condenser microphone for the measurement of the acoustic level in front of the tympanum (about 1.5 mm).

A first audiogram was obtained for each animal by averaging N1 thresholds in response to tone-pips with a Gaussian enveloppe and a constant number of periods, over the frequency range 1-32 kHz.

Each animal was then exposed to a continuous 4 or 8 kHz pure tone for 20 minutes. The SPL of the pure tone was measured in front of the eardrum and controlled with a precision of 1/2 dB. It ranged from 82 to 132 dB SPL.

Twenty minutes after the end of the stimulation, another N1 audiogram was made and its difference with the first one gave the Threshold Shifts (TS). Given the short post-trauma period, these TS can be considered as partially temporary.

Immediatly after the end of this audiometry (30 minutes after the end of the overstimulation) the animals were decapitated and their bulla removed. The cochlea was then prepared for observation in scanning electron microscopy of the first two turns. Cochlear frequency maps were made according to previous studies: Wilson and Johnstone (1975), Johnstone (1977) and Cody and coll. (1980) for the guinea pig, Eldredge and coll (1981) for the chinchilla and Liberman (1982) for the cat. All normal-looking, altered as well as missing hair cells were counted within samples of 1/5 mm. For each exposure condition we used average groups of 5 to 10 animals.

Results

POST-TRAUMATIC THRESHOLD SHIFTS

Figure 1 shows average TS and standard deviations measured for each species 20 minutes after a 20 minutes 8 kHz pure tone overstimulation at 105 dB SPL.

One can observe the well known "half-octave shift" between the stimulation frequency (8 kHz) and the frequency for which the TS is maximum (11,3 kHz). The

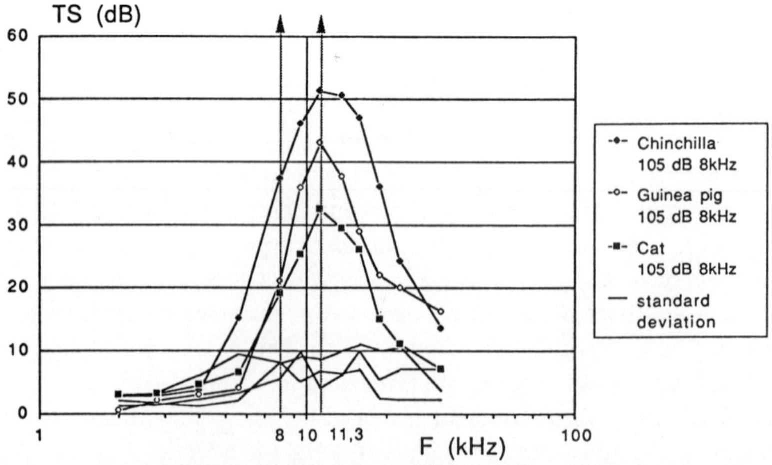

FIGURE 1 Average maximum TS measured after a 8 kHz 105 dB SPL overstimulation Lower curves are standard deviations.

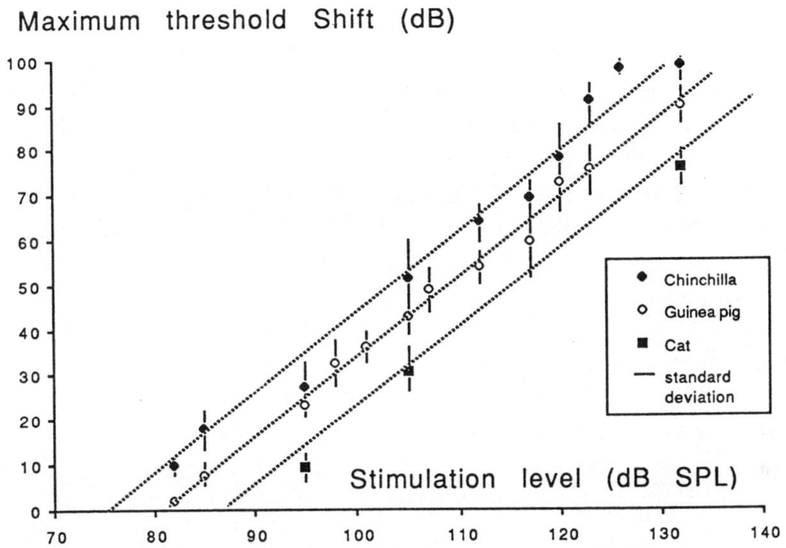

FIGURE 2 Mean maximum TS measured after 8 kHz stimulations. Dotted lines are idealise curves and bars are standard deviations.

chinchilla shows a 52 dB maximum TS and values for the guinea pig and the cat are 43 and 32 dB respectively. On a statistical point of view, these differences are significant (at the level of 95 %). Figure 2 shows for each species the average maximum TS plotted as a function of SPL of the 8 kHz stimulation at the eardrum.

For the overstimulating pure tone of 8 kHz the slopes of the idealised lines are very similar (1.8 dB of increase in maximum TS for each extra dB SPL at the eardrum). These results show an average decrease of 5 dB in susceptibility from the chinchilla to the guinea-pig, and another 5 dB decrease from the guinea-pig to the cat.

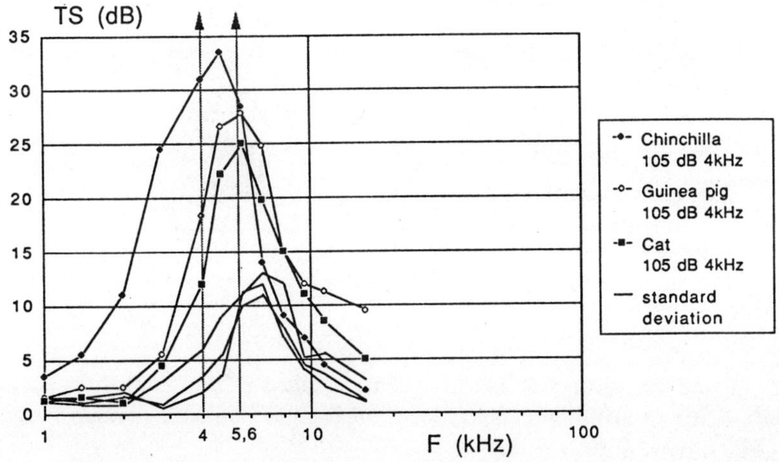

FIGURE 3 Average maximum TS measured after a 4 kHz 105 dB SPL overstimulation.

With a 4 kHz overstimulating pure tone, smaller TS and slighter interspecific differences than for the 8 kHz stimulation were found. Figure 3 shows average TS measured in each species 20 minutes after a 20 minutes 4 kHz pure tone overstimulation at a SPL of 105 dB SPL. The shapes of these curves are rather similar but in this case the shift between the stimulation frequency and the audiometric frequency showing the maximum TS is only 1/4 octave in the chinchilla. Again the chinchilla shows greater TS than the other two species, but these differences are not significant on a statistical point of view and in the present state of our experiment we can't conclude as precisely as for the 8 kHz stimulation.

HAIR CELL LESIONS

For overstimulating frequencies of 8 or 4 kHz all the lesions were located in the basal two turns of the cochlea. We present here average cochleograms for guinea pigs and chinchillas stimulated at 8 kHz.

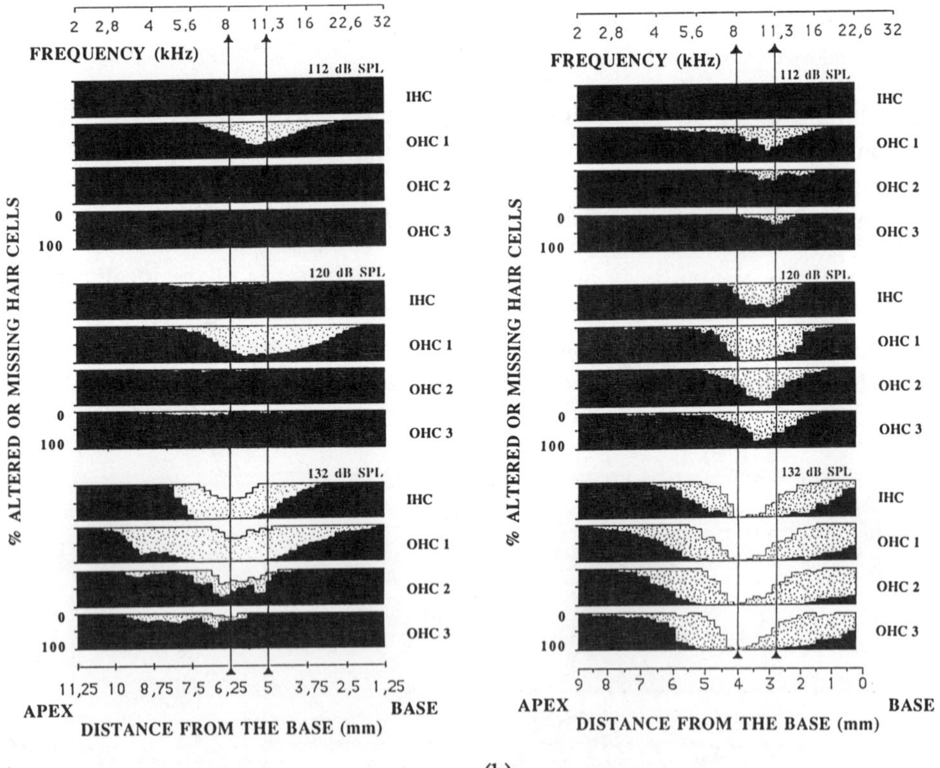

FIGURE 4a and 4b Average cochleograms obtained in the guinea pig (a) and in the chinchilla (b) after 8 kHz stimulations. Black areas show normal, dotted areas show altered and white areas show missing hair cells.

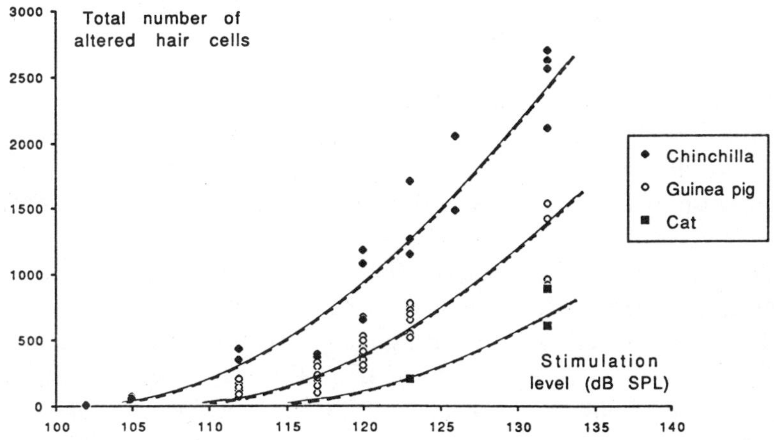

FIGURE 5 Individual total numbers of altered hair cells observed after 8 kHz stimulations Dotted lines are idealised cuves.

Figure 4a shows the results obtained in the guinea pig for three different SPLs: 112, 120 and 132 dB. The first row of outer hair cells (OHC 1) is the most sensitive to pure tone exposure, as previously described by several authors (Robertson and Johnstone, 1980). For intensities just above the threshold of lesion (here 112 dB SPL) a half-octave shift can be observed between the stimulation frequency and the Characteristic Frequency (CF) corresponding to the area of maximum stereocilia damage. For higher intensities, the amount and the severity of hair cell damage increase whereas the frequency shift decrease: for a stimulating level of 132 dB SPL, all hair cell rows show very severe disturbance, especially in the area situated 6.25 mm from the base (CF=8 kHz).

Figure 4b shows the results obtained in the chinchilla in exactly the same conditions. The pattern of lesions looks like the one observed in the guinea pig. The OHC 1 row is still the most sensitive but the sensitivity of the other three rows is higher than in the guinea pig. Again an half octave shift can be observed, just above stereocilia lesion threshold. This shift decreases as the stimulation level grows up.

On a quantitative point of view we compared the total number of lesionned hair cells in all three species. Figure 5 shows these results for each animal stimulated at 8 kHz, i.e. the total number of altered hair cells, plotted as a function of the SPL.

As observed from the threshold shifts, one can find a decrease of 5 dB in sensitivity from the chinchilla to the guinea pig, and another 5 dB decrease from the guinea pig to the cat. Across the species there is a good quantitative correlation between those lesions and the TS we measured 20 minutes after the end of the stimulation.

For animals stimulated at 4 kHz, individual and average cochleograms are not yet completed, but interspecific differences seem less important.

INTRACOCHLEAR ACOUSTIC PRESSURE MEASUREMENTS

Now how can we explain the interspecific susceptibility differences to a given acoustic exposure indicated by these first results. Being given the fact that in our experimental conditions, the influence of the external ear of each species could be neglected, a first hypothesis could be that the residual interspecific differences in sensitivity to noise exposure are due to the characteristics of the middle ear of each species.

The input to the cochlea (acoustic pressure at the base of scala vestibuli) depends on the transfer function of the middle ear (including the input impedance of the cochlea). This transfer function can be measured by recording the acoustic pressure at the base of scala vestibuli as a function of frequency for a given acoustic level in front of the eardrum. Following Nedzelnitski (1980) in the cat and Dancer and Franke (1980) in the guinea pig, we measured this transfer function from 100 Hz to 20 000 Hz in each species (average groups of 10 animals) in the same experimental conditions as for noise exposures.

The intracochlear sound pressure was measured with a piezo-resistive transducer (Kulite) fitted with a calibrated silicon fluid-filled probe (Dancer and Franke, 1980). The signal-to-noise ratio of the recorded signals was improved by narrow-band filtering allowing measurements for stimulus levels ranging from 50 to 100 dB SPL.

Figure 6 indicates average values and standard deviations of the amplitude of the middle ear transfer function for the guinea pig, the chinchilla and the cat. This amplitude is comprised between 10 and 40 dB for frequencies from 0,1 to 10 kHz, and between 25 and -10 dB above 10 kHz. In the guinea pig and the chinchilla, no noticeable difference in amplitude can be found between 1 and 10 kHz.

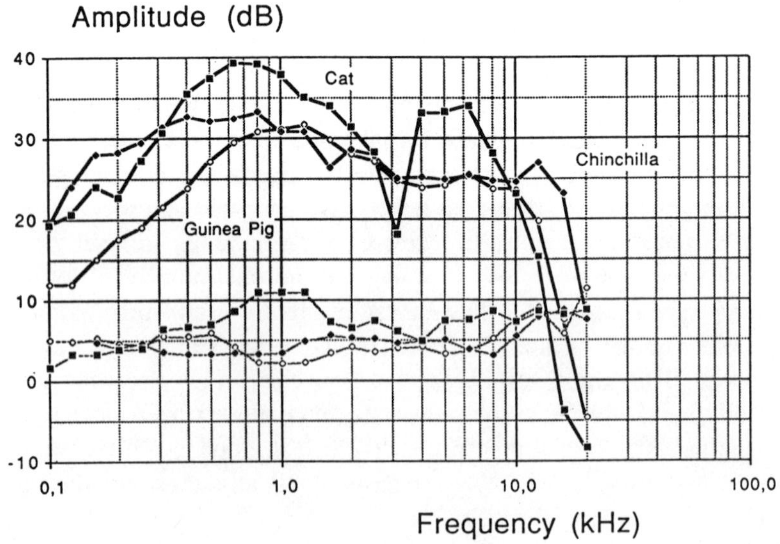

FIGURE 6 Mean amplitude of the middle ear transfer function. Lower curves are standard deviations.

The amplitude differences of the transfer functions in the three species at 4 and 8 kHz cannot explain the electrocochleographic measurements and the histological observations. According to these transfer functions, the cat receives more energy than chinchilla and guinea pig and should present more TS and more damage. Nevertheless, due to the fact that the pressure measurements are not performed at the very base of scala vestibuli but at a given distance from the oval window (5 mm in the guinea pig, 5.5 mm in the chinchilla and 8 mm in the cat), the values obtained at 8 kHz must be considered with caution.

Discussion

We have shown that even when placed in exactly the same experimental conditions, anesthetised, restrained and pinnaectomised animals still presented interspecific differences in susceptibility to pure tone exposure. These differences are particularly noticeable for an overstimulating frequency of 8 kHz. The origin of these differences or similarities is not clear.

The shape of the behavioral auditory threshold curves is mainly due to the combined effects of the external and middle ear of each species. On a quantitative point of view, Rosowski and coll. (1985) have shown that the acoustic power at the entrance to the cochlea at the threshold of hearing in man, guinea pig and cat, is the same and is constant whatever the frequency may be. One can wonder whether in the same way at the threshold of "auditory dysfunction", a given acoustic level at the entrance to the cochlea could induce the same threshold shift or the same hair cell lesion, whatever the frequency or the species may be.

If this was the case, the interspecific differences in susceptibility to noise would then be due to the respective influence of the transfer function of the outer and middle ear. Up to now our TS results, histological observations and intra-cochlear acoustic pressure measurements don't confirm this hypothesis.: for example the cat which has a lower behavioral threshold than the other two species and which presents the highest amplitude of the middle ear transfer function is less sensitive to noise exposure.

Due to the technical difficulties it is in fact uneasy to interpret correctly the intracochlear pressure measurements above 5 kHz for all these species. That's why the more complete results presented here for 8 kHz stimulations should be completed with further observations at 4 kHz and 2 kHz.

The origin of interspecific differences in susceptibility to noise exposure seem to be as diverse as one could have expected. The tempting assumption that the threshold of auditory dysfonctions could be constant whatever the frequency and the species considered, may not be as easy to achieve as we hoped: some important cochlear interspecific differences may exist. However even if further observations don't confirm our working hypothesis, it will be possible to define more precisely the influence of each element: outer and middle ear-inner ear on the interspecific differences in auditory susceptibility.

References

Cody, A.R. and Robertson, D. (1983) Variability of noise-induced damage in the guinea pig cochlea: Electrophysiological and morphological correlates after strictly controlled exposures Hearing Res.9, 55-70.

Cody, A.R., Robertson, D., Bredberg, G. and Johnstone,B.M.(1980) Electrophysiological and morphological changes in the guinea pig cochlea following mechanical trauma to the organ o: Corti. Acta Otolaryngol. 89,440-452.

Dallos, P.(1973) The auditory periphery. Acad press. New-York and London.

Dancer, A. and Franke,R. (1980) Intracochlear sound pressure measurements in guinea pigs. Hearing Res.2,191-205.

Eldredge, D.H. Miller, J.D. and Bohne, B.A. (1981) A frequency-position map for the chinchill: cochlea. J. Acoust. Soc. Am. 69, 1091-1095.

Johnstone, J.R.(1977) Properties of ganglion cells from the extreme base region of the guinea pig cochlea. Psychophysics and Physiology of Hearing (Ed. E.F.Evans and J.P.Wilson),p89, Academic Press, London.

Liberman, M.C. (1982) The cochlear frequency map for the cat: Labelling auditory-nerve fibers (known characteristic frequency. J. Acoust. Soc. Am. 75, 1441-1449.

Lynch, T.J., Netzelnitski, V. and Peake, W.T.(1982) Input impedance of the cochlea in cat., J.Acoust.Soc.Am.,72,108-130.

Nedzelnitsky, V. (1980) Sound pressure in the basal turn of the cat cochlea. J. Acoust. Soc. Am 68, 1676-1689.

Robertson, D. and Johnstone, B.M.(1980) Acoustic trauma in the guinea pig cochlea: early changes in ultrastructure and neural threshold. Hearing Res.3,167-179.

Rosowski, J.J., Carney, L.H., Lynch, T.J. and Peake, W.T.(1985) The effectiveness of external an(middle ears in coupling acoustic power into the cochlea. in: Lectures Notes in Biomathematics Peripheral Auditory Mechanisms, Springer Verlag, 3-12.

Wilson, J.P. and Johnstone, J.R.(1975) Basilar membrane and middle ear vibration in guinea pig measures by a capacitive probe. J.Acoust.Soc.Am.,57,705.

Comments and Discussion

WHITEHEAD

From your figure 4 it appears that, both in guinea pig and chinchilla, there is the characteristic half-octave shift present for hair cell damage, but not for hair cell loss, after exposure to intense pure-tones at 8 kHz. As the hair cell loss occurs after the more intense exposures, this suggests that at these very high levels the place of maximum vibration in the cochlea moves apically with increasing level, whereas the half-octave shift itself is thought to be due to a basal shift of excitation with stimulus level. Do you have any thoughts on why this should be so?

DÉCORY

This phenomenon may be related to the half-octave shift observed between the overstimulating frequency and the audiometric frequency showing maximum TS. H. Davis postulated in 1983 that it could be due to a shift towards higher frequencies that may exist between the location of the maximum amplitude of the so-called "travelling wave" of the basilar membrane, and the location of the additive motion due to the "Cochlear Amplifier", in an active cochlea. In an injured, passive cochlea, the motion of the basilar membrane could then be described by the "travelling wave" alone, and the maximum vibration would shift back towards a more apical region.

DANCER

Another explanation could be found if we considered the cochlea working as a series of resonators:

a) For a given resonator, when the damping increases, the frequency of the maximum amplitude shifts to lower frequencies (the increase of damping could be correlated to the high level of the acoustic over-stimulation). This could explain that the first lesions occur towards the base (referred to the CF place).

b) For even higher acoustic levels and because of the destruction of the hairs, linking the reticular lamina and the tectorial membrane, the damping could decrease severely: the maximum displacement, and the hair cell lesions and losses, would then shift back to the CF place. This hypothesis needs no active mechanism nor cochlear travelling wave.

RESPONSE PROPERTIES OF TURTLE AUDITORY AFFERENT NERVE FIBERS: EVIDENCE FOR A HIGH ORDER TUNING MECHANISM

Michael Sneary and Edwin R. Lewis

Department of Electrical Engineering
and Computer Sciences
145 Cory Hall
University of California
Berkeley, CA 94720 USA

Introduction

An early selective advantage of acoustic senses clearly was remote detection of predators (or other dangers) and prey. Therefore, one would expect evolution to have sculpted acoustic receptors for maximum sensitivity. The ultimate limitation on sensitivity is noise, and acoustic receptors must deal with both internal noise (arising from thermal energy within the ear) and external noise (arising from environmental sources, such as the wind). If the spectrum of a signal is different from that of noise, then the signal can be extracted by means of high-resolution spectral filtering; and if the spatial distribution of a signal source is different from that of the environmental noise, then the signal can be extracted by spatial filtering. Given its parallel processing capability and the presence of two ears, the vertebrate CNS is especially well adapted for spatial filtering . Available evidence indicates that this is achieved in large part by temporal correlation (Knudsen, '82). Therefore, for maximum sensitivity we expect acoustic sensors to have evolved with peripheral filters that combine high spectral resolution with high temporal resolution. The best way to achieve this combination of properties is to employ a filter with high-order dynamics that produce a relatively broad pass band with sustained, steep high-frequency rolloff and nearly linear phase-vs-frequency. Acting alone, a filter with second-order dynamics, such as those derivable from a simple resonance, cannot do this; indeed it cannot provide high temporal resolution and high spectral resolution at the same time (Lewis '87). Therefore, a second-order resonance, acting alone as the peripheral tuning element, appears to be inappropriate for acoustic sensors.

Interestingly, electrical resonances have been found in three nonhomologous acoustic receptors in lower vertebrates; the frog saccular macula (Lewis and Hudspeth, '83; Ashmore,'83), and amphibian papilla (Pitchford and Ashmore, '87) and the turtle basilar papilla (Fettiplace and Crawford, '78). Viewed as a neuroelectric process, each of these resonances appears to exhibit second-order dynamics. For two of the three receptors (those in the frog), there already is strong evidence that tuning is not accomplished by these resonances acting alone (Lewis, '84, '87; Hillery and Narins '84). Instead, the elements of several or many resonances apparently are linked (so that they exchange signal energy) to form filters with very high-order dynamics leading to broad pass bands with sustained, steep high-frequency rolloff and nearly linear phase-vs-frequency. Indeed, the linkages evidently are so strong that the resonances observed in isolated hair cells are totally obscured in the filter dynamics of the intact ear (Lewis '88). In this paper, we turn our attention to the third receptor, the turtle basilar papilla.

Hair cells in the auditory receptor of the red-eared turtle have been the subject of intensive electrophysiological studies by Crawford and Fettiplace('80,'81,'85) and their colleagues (Art and Fettiplace,'87; Art, Fettiplace and Fuchs, '85). In addition, the structure of the basilar papilla at the light microscopic, SEM and TEM levels is well understood (Wever, '78; Miller, '78; Sneary, '88a,b). As a result of this attention from a variety of perspectives, a meaningful picture of the overall properties of the receptor as an auditory signal analyzer is now beginning to take shape.

Crawford and Fettiplace ('81) have interpreted response data from individual hair cells to indicate that the peripheral filter is composed of two parts: a narrow band electrical resonance imposed upon a broad band residual filter. For the residual filter, they proposed that the high-frequency rolloff might be attributed to the action of the middle ear and the low-frequency rolloff might be attributed to the helicotrema. In this study we present evidence suggesting that the elements responsible for high frequency rolloff in this filter are situated in the receptor itself, rather than in the middle ear. Furthermore, we suggest that the data of Crawford and Fettiplace and colleagues imply that the electrical resonances in the turtle papilla are linked to other elements (perhaps those of neighboring resonances) in an energy-sharing manner. The net result appears once again to be a filter with high-order dynamics, yielding a broad pass band with sustained steep high-frequency rolloff and nearly linear phase-vs-frequency over much of its range. The difference between what has been observed in the other two receptors and what is seen here is that, in the turtle, the properties of the individual resonance may remain conspicuous in the overall high-order filter properties in the intact ear.

Methods and Results

Our experimental preparation is adapted from that of Crawford and Fettiplace ('78); however the red-eared turtles used by us have plastron lengths of at least 100 mm. The isolated half-head of the animal is placed in a small chamber with a moist, oxygenated atmosphere. Steady-state sinusoidal stimuli are delivered through a closed-field acoustical driver and monitored through a calibrated microphone and probe tube inserted close to the tympanum. Individual auditory fibers are penetrated with 60 to 100 megohm microelectrodes filled with 4M potassium acetate. The electrode is driven into the posterior branch of the eighth nerve near its point of exit from the otic capsule. During an

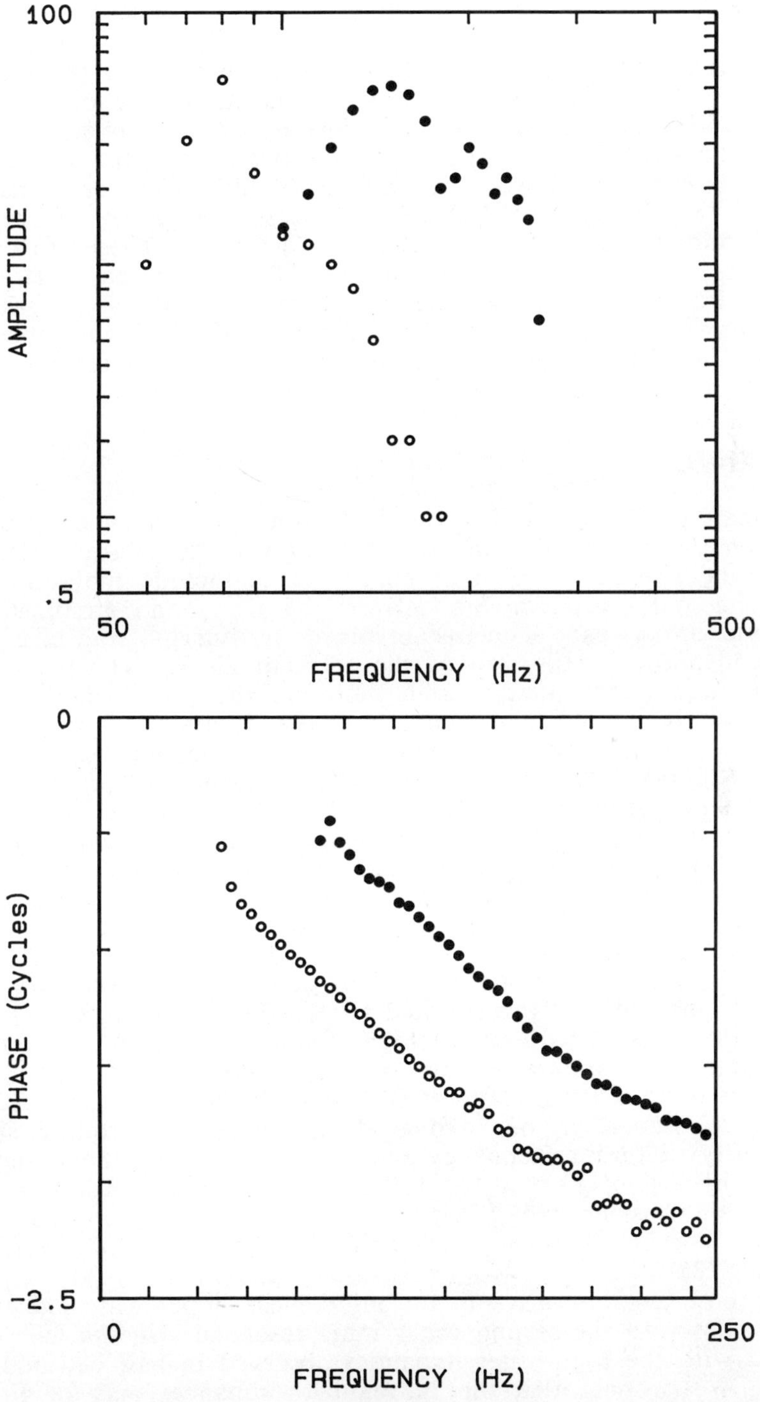
100
.5
AMPLITUDE
50
500
FREQUENCY (Hz)
0
-2.5
PHASE (Cycles)
0
250
FREQUENCY (Hz)

FIGURE 1

electrode pass, individual auditory units are located with a fast sweep of frequencies which encompass the known range of the turtle receptor (20-2000 Hz). In the present study a very slow sweep (4 octaves per minute) was used to collect spike data. The amplitude of the acoustic stimulus was constant to within approximately +/- 2dB over the response ranges of the fibers. From experiment to experiment, stimulus intensities ranged approximately between 50 and 70 dB SPL. The spike data were converted to conventional phase ("cycle") histograms, from which amplitude and phase tuning properties are deduced. These are displayed in fig. 1 for two fibers. Notice that each fiber's response shifts through more than 1.5 cycles (implying that the dynamical order is at least seven) and that the sustained, steep high-frequency rolloff of one fiber begins below the CF of the other. The slope of that rolloff is steeper than -6, again implying that the dynamical order is at least seven.

Discussion

The phase shifts observed in turtle afferent fibers must be imposed by elements in the chain of sound energy transfer which are peripheral to the recording site in the papillar nerve. These include the following: 1) the experimental setup for the delivery of the sound stimulus, 2) the middle and inner ear elements involved in energy transmission and transduction and, 3) a portion of the afferent fiber. The placement of the probe tube microphone, which monitors the phase of the stimulus close to the tympanic membrane, and the location of the recording electrode less than one millimeter from the receptor ensure a total (acoustic + spike) delay of less than one millisecond. Therefore, vitually all of the slope seen in the afferent fiber phase shift response can be presumed to result from the dynamic elements within the ear itself.

Acting independently, individually or in parallel, second-order resonances can produce a total phase shift of no more than one-half cycle. The more than one full cycle of additional phase shift that we observed in the axonal responses was also seen by Crawford and Fettiplace ('81) in the responses of hair-cell receptor potentials. They explained it in terms of the residual filter. In addition, Crawford and Fettiplace ('81) postulated that the high frequency rolloff observed in the receptor-potential response of individual hair cells (and observed here in the response of individual afferent fibers) could be a result of middle ear function. However, in our axonal data, we see the rolloff spanning conspicuously different frequency ranges for different fibers, suggesting different physical origins of the rolloff in each case. Additionally, we found sustained steep rolloff at frequencies well below 500 Hz, the middle-ear corner frequency according to the data of Moffat and Capranica ('78).

We propose an alternative to the middle-ear hypothesis. The question at hand is how can the second order ionic resonances in the hair cells be reconciled with the high order dynamics observed in hair cell and axonal tuning? We propose that the individual resonances may be linked in cascade, so that energy can be passed back and forth between them. This would produce a network with high-order dynamics, potentially capable of the observed phase shifts and high frequency rolloffs. This hypothesis rests upon the bidirectional coupling observed by Crawford and Fettiplace ('85) between the electrical and mechanical sides of the the papillar hair cells. As a consequence of the bidirectionality of this coupling, if several hair-cell electrical resonances are linked to a common mechanical structure, then they will share energy with one another as required in our hypothetical cascade network. Consistent with this notion is the evident difference in Q values between isolated hair cells and those cells in the intact receptor, the latter apparently being conspicuously lower (Crawford and Fettiplace, '80; Art and Fettiplace, '87). The lower Q values in the intact receptor indicate that some of the energy stored in the ionic resonance is being transferred out of the hair cell cycle by cycle. The hair cell bundles of the intact receptor are in contact with the tectorial plate (Sneary '88a), which could serve as the mechanical route for energy sharing.

One thus can imagine a situation analogous to the popular critical-layer resonance type of model of the mammalian cochlea (Lighthill,'81). The hair cell resonances might play the role of the local mechanical resonances of the basilar membrane, and the tectorial plate might play the role of cochlear fluid coupling those resonances.

As a takehome message, we offer the following conjecture: in different species of vertebrates, evolution seems to have converged on a common design for peripheral filtering in acoustic receptors (i.e., a filter with high-order dynamics, sustained steep high-frequency rolloff, and nearly linear phase-vs-frequency); but the realization of that design employs markedly different biophysical elements in the different species. The adaptive value of the design is its ability to provide good spectral resolution and good temporal resolution. These in turn serve to defeat noise and thus to enhance sensitivity.

References

Art, J.J. and Fettiplace, R. (1987) Variation of membrane properties in hair cells isolated from the turtle cochlea. J. Physiol. 385, 207-242.

Ashmore, J.T. (1983) Frequency tuning in a frog vestibular organ. Nature 304, 536-538.

Crawford, A.C. and Fettiplace, R. (1980) The frequency selectivity of auditory nerve fibres and hair cells in the turtle. J. Physiol. 306, 79-125.

Crawford, A.C. and Fettiplace, R. (1981) An electrical tuning mechanism in turtle cochlear hair cells. J. Physiol. 312, 377-412.

Crawford, A.C. and Fettiplace, R. (1985) The mechanical properties of ciliary bundles of turtle cochlear hair cells. J. Physiol. 364, 359-379.

Fettiplace, R. and Crawford, A.C. (1978) The coding of sound pressure and frequency in cochlear hair cells of the terrapin. Proc. R. Soc. Lond. B. 203, 29-218.

Hillery, C.M. and Narins, P. (1984) Neurophysiological evidence for a traveling wave in the amphibian inner ear. Science. 225, 1037-1039.

Knudsen, E.I. (1982) Auditory and visual maps of space in the optic tectum of the owl. J. Neurosci. 2, 1177-1194.

Lewis, E.R. (1987) Speculations about noise and the evolution of vertebrate hearing. Hear. Res. 25, 83-90.

Lewis, E.R. (1988) Tuning in the bullfrog ear. Biophys. J. 53, 441-447

Lewis, R.S. and Hudspeth, A.J. (1983) Frequency tuning and ionic conductances in hair cells of the bullfrog sacculus. In: Hearing-Physiological Bases and Psychophysics, pp. 17-24. Editors: R. Klinke and R. Hartmann. Springer-Verlag, Berlin.

Lighthill (1981) Energy flow in the cochlea. J. Fluid Mech. 106, 149-213.

Miller, M.R. (1978) Scanning electron microscope studies of the papilla basillaris of some turtles and snakes. Am. J. Anat. 151, 409-435.

Moffat, A.J.M. and R.R. Capranica (1978) Middle ear sensitivity in anurans and reptiles measured by light scattering spectroscopy. J. Comp. Physiol. 127, 97-107.

Narins, P.M. and Gleich, O. (1986) Phase response of low-frequency cochlear ganglion cells in the starling. In: Auditory Frequency Selectivity. (Eds. Brian C.J. Moore and Roy D. Patterson) Plenum Publishing Corp. pp. 209-216.

Pitchford, S. and Ashmore, J.F. (1987) An electrical resonance in hair cells of the amphibian papilla of the frog Rana temporaria. Hearing Res. 27, 75-84.

Sneary, M. (1988a) The auditory receptor of the red-eared turtle: I. general ultrastructural organization. J. Comp. Neurol. (In Press).

Sneary, M. (1988b) The auditory receptor of the red-eared turtle. II. ultrastructure of afferent and efferent synapses and innervation patterns. J. Comp. Neurol. (In Press).

Wever, E.G. (1978) The Reptile Ear. Princeton. Princeton University Press.

COCHLEAR FILTERING: A VIEW SEEN THROUGH THE TEMPORAL DISCHARGE PATTERNS OF SINGLE COCHLEAR NERVE FIBRES

E. F. Evans

Department of Communication and Neuroscience
University of Keele, Keele, Staffs., ST5 5BG, U.K.

Introduction

While the mechanisms underlying cochlear filtering are no doubt non-linear, a number of investigations have indicated that cochlear spectral analysis behaves surprisingly linearly. As seen by individual fibres of the cochlear nerve, with due allowances for transducer and synaptic (no memory type) non-linearities, the filtering of broad-band and multi-component stimuli is, to a first approximation at least, well modelled by linear filters. This has been shown in discharge rate terms for broad-band noise stimuli, in the predictability of noise thresholds from pure tone thresholds (yielding measures of effective bandwidths - Evans and Wilson, 1971), and, for comb-filtered noise stimuli in terms of the predictability of response 'contrast' (Wilson and Evans, 1971).

The major problem facing assessments of cochlear filtering as seen through the responses of cochlear fibres, concerns the non-linearities inherent in the processes of transduction and synaptic spike generation. These result in the compressive, saturating relationship between discharge rate and stimulus level, restricting severely the dynamic range over which rate-based measures can be utilized. However, providing the transducer-synaptic non-linearities are of the no-memory type, they can be circumvented or minimised either by utilising constant output measures (as in determining frequency threshold or tuning curves, FTCs), or by adopting the weighting of stimulus components shown in the temporal discharges of cochlear fibres. The former can be used over all frequencies, but only over a limited dynamic range (on average, about 40 dB), whereas the latter is restricted to frequencies below about 3 kHz in the cat (less in the guinea-pig), but over an apparently unlimited dynamic range.

The first method employed to study cochlear filtering, as seen through the temporal discharge patterns of cochlear fibres, was the Reverse Correlation (REVCOR) method of De Boer (1969). De Boer and Kuyper (1968) have shown that, providing the non-linearities associated with transduction and spike generation are of the no-memory type, the method, equivalent to cross-correlation between spike output of a single cochlear nerve fibre and the Gaussian noise signal stimulating the ear, yields the impulse response of the linear filter preceding the cochlear fibre. De Boer (1973) obtained close correspondence between the filtering revealed by this method and that represented by the pure tone derived (FTC) tuning curve. This has been shown to be the case over a surprisingly wide dynamic range, by Evans (1977, 1981) in the cat. Here, for some 40-60 dB above noise threshold, the REVCOR filtering is identical to that reflected in the FTCs and is relatively invariant of stimulus level. At higher stimulus levels, however, systematic changes occur in the filtering : for fibres having characteristic frequencies (optimal frequency, CF), below 1 kHz, the CF shifts upwards with level and the low frequency cut-off reduces somewhat in slope with little or no increase in bandwidth. For fibres with CFs above 1 kHz, the CF shifts downwards with level and the low frequency cut-off reduces in slope, the high frequency cut-off sometimes increasing in slope. At CFs of about 1 kHz, often very little change in CF, slope or bandwidth occurs. Increases in half-power bandwidth at other CFs are by a factor of 1.1-2.5 at the highest sound levels (100-110 dB SPL; Evans, 1977, 1981). In the guinea-pig (Harrison and Evans, 1982; Cooper and Evans, unpublished data), the dynamic range, over which little or no change in filtering characteristics occur with level, is more restricted, typically to around 30 dB. Thereafter, similar changes occur to those found in the cat.

Other methods that have been employed to assess cochlear filtering (as seen through the temporal discharge patterns of cochlear fibres) have used multi-component stimuli (e.g. harmonic complexes) with the extraction of the weighting of the frequency components reflected in the relative phase-locking of the discharges to each component. This is most straight-forwardly extracted by fast Fourier transform (FFT) of the period histogram (PH) of the spike discharges. Again, the weightings determined in this manner correspond remarkably well with the pure tone FTC, over a remarkably wide dynamic range in the cat. This has been shown for stimuli consisting of 10 harmonic components having the fundamental suppressed (Evans, 1981), for click trains (Evans, 1983a, 1984a, 1985, 1986), and for stimuli consisting of 2 frequency components, by Greenberg et al (1986).

The present paper summarizes the outcome of more detailed measurements using broad-band noise, and two types of multi-component stimulus over a wide range of stimulus levels in the cat.

Methods

The details of the stimulation and recording techniques, physiological controls, and of plotting the FTCs are given in Evans (1979). Briefly, micropipettes are used for recording the activity of single fibres in the cochlear nerve of pentobarbitone-anaesthetised cats. The cats were selected for freedom from middle ear disease and great care was taken to minimise noise exposure during the surgical preparation by avoiding drilling and bone snipping. The threshold of the gross cochlear action potential to tone pips from 0.4-40 kHz was automatically monitored (Evans 1984b) at intervals throughout the experiments and did not deteriorate. The bulla was intact but vented to atmospheric pressure.

Reverse correlograms, period and autocorrelation histograms were computed on-line and off-line by a Computer Automation Alpha 2/40 minicomputer system also used for the synthesis of the stimuli. A "SILO" DAC and hardware spike clock (Cambridge Electronic Design Limited 502 system) enabled synthesis of stimuli to be effected while logging spike data with a resolution of 1 us (Evans, 1983b). Each histogram was computed on 4096 spikes, with typically 256 bins of width 78 us. FTCs were obtained by an on-line up/down threshold tracking method described in Evans (1979) in response to 50 ms tone bursts having 5 ms rise/fall times.

For the reverse correlograms, the stimuli was continuous Gaussian white noise, low-pass-filtered at 4 kHz. This was digitized with a sample period of 78 us and stored in a circular buffer. Each time a spike event was discriminated, 20 ms of the buffer immediately preceding the spike was added to a double-precision summing register. The result of the successive summations represents the impulse response of the cochlear filter reversed in time. Reversing this, gave the impulse responses (IRs) shown in Fig. 1. This method has significant advantages over the original method of De Boer (e.g. 1969) and used by Evans (1977), utilizing an averaging computer, in that *all* spikes are used, and the result is not subject to the small but systematic biasses noted by Wilson and Evans (1975). Typically, 5000 or more spikes were used for each analysis. FFTs were made after rectangular windowing of the reverse correlograms.

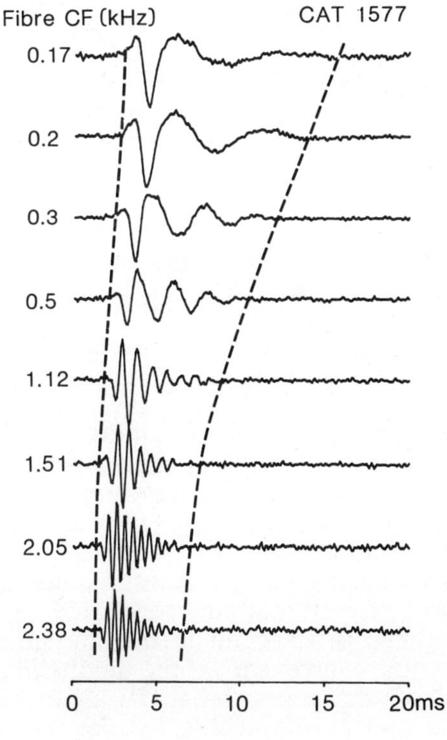

FIGURE 1 Impulse Responses, derived from Reverse Correlograms, of 8 cochlear nerve fibres in the cat, having the characteristic frequencies (CF) indicated.

For the filter derivations from phase-locking measures in response to harmonic complexes, two types of stimuli were used. The first was a continuous train of 100 us clicks at a repetition rate of 100 Hz . The second was a continuous complex tone consisting of the sum of 50 harmonics of 100 Hz fundamental mixed in equal amplitude, sine phase. The stimuli were synthesized by the Alpha 2/40 computer.

All stimuli were presented closed-field to the ear by a Bruel and Kjaer 4134 condenser driver system with compensation for distortion.

For comparisons with the pure tone frequency threshold curves, FFTs were constructed from the period histograms after utilizing a Hamming window across the full width of the histogram. The autocorrelograms were likewise windowed, but in most cases the *square root* of the FFT was taken for comparison with the FTCs, because the autocorrelogram gives squared spectral estimates (see Johnson, 1974). The results of comparisons between these measures and the FTCs are shown in Fig. 2.

Results and Discussion

COCHLEAR NERVE FIBRE DATA

Fig. 1 shows the time-reversed REVCORS, ie the impulse responses derived from 8 cochlear fibres with CFs ranging from 0.17 to 2.38 kHz. Each impulse response (IR) consists basically of two components: a delay (indicated to the left of the first dashed line), and a ringing response characteristic of multiple pole band-pass filters having Qs (Quality factors) in the region of 3 for the lowest CF fibres through 5 in the range 0.5-1 kHz, to 10 for the highest CF fibres. The delay ranges from 1.1 ms at 2.38 kHz to 2 ms at 0.5 kHz and 3 ms at 0.17 kHz. This delay presumably represents that of the travelling wave of the cochlear partition, followed by the second component due to the ringing of the cochlear filter at the place from which the cochlear fibre emanates. The latter component has a duration of between 5.1 ms at the highest CFs to 13 ms at the lowest CFs. This 'ringing time' corresponds well (Evans, 1985) with the values obtained from human psychophysical determinations of the temporal resolving power of the auditory system, e.g. from measurements of gap detection (FitzGibbons and Wightman, 1982). Duifhuis (1973) first suggested that the 'ringing time' of the cochlear filters must limit the temporal resolution of the auditory system.

While the IRs of fibres with CFs above about 0.5 kHz have ringing characteristics, following the delay, reminiscent of 1/3 octave filters, the situation is more complex for fibres with CFs below about 0.5 kHz. The IRs of the lowest CF fibres show an additional component. An earlier brief high frequency component is followed by a longer duration lower frequency component (see upper three IRs in Fig. 1). These two components are consistent with the finding in these fibres of FTCs (tuning curves) having two major frequency-selective components, as in the case of the left-most FTC of Fig. 2. It is almost invariably found that for fibres with these low CFs, there is a second frequency selective process between half an octave and an octave above the main CF. It seems likely that it is the ringing of the more broadly tuned higher frequency frequency selective process that is responsible for the fast early component of the IR, whereas the more sharply tuned low frequency CF component is responsible for the lower frequency, more protracted component. At high stimulus levels, the lower CF process dominates the IR, as it shifts upwards in frequency, and the higher frequency process becomes progressively attenuated (see thin line in upper left section of Fig. 2). While middle ear resonances can not be responsible for the two frequency selective processes, it is an interesting question whether separate, and different cochlear mechanisms could be.

Fig. 2. shows the results of the comparisons between the pure tone FTCs (thick continuous lines), the FFTs of the REVCORs (thin continuous lines) and the frequency weighting of the individual frequency components reflected in the phase locking in reponse to the 100 Hz click trains (crosses) and sine-mixed harmonics with 100Hz fundamental (open circles). The data are shown for three cochlear fibres having low (0.5 kHz), mid (1.12 kHz) and high (2.05 kHz) CFs at two stimulus levels. In the lower half of the figure, stimulus levels are within 10-20 dB of threshold, and in the upper half, above 50 dB above threshold. At the lower stimulus levels (lower half) there is excellent agreement between all of the derived measures and the pure tone FTCs. At higher levels, (upper half) the agreement is still good, but there are the systematic

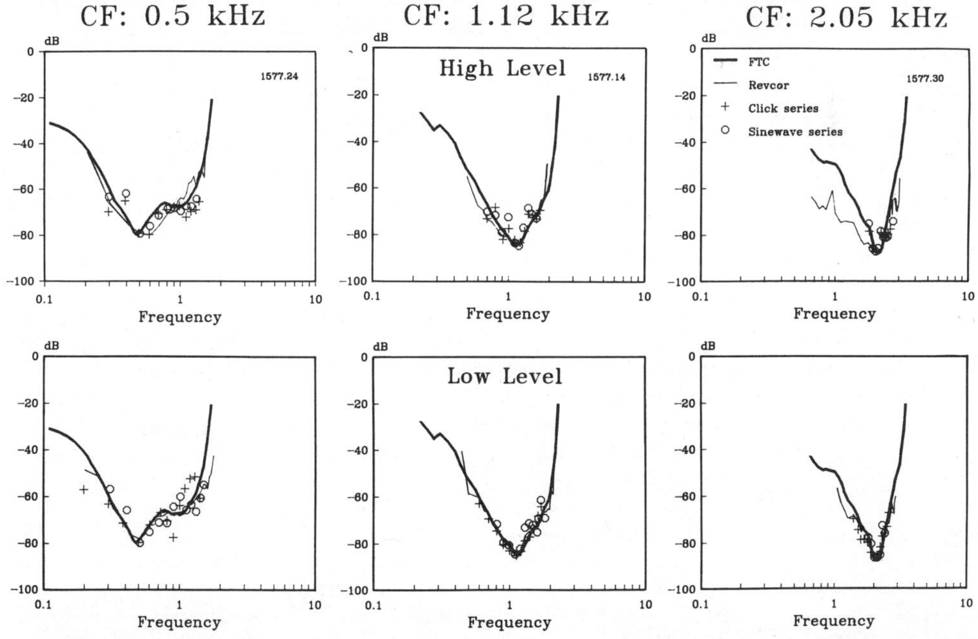

FIGURE 2 Comparison of three derivations of cochlear filtering seen by cat cochlear nerve fibres of low, middle and high CF, near threshold (lower half) and at stimulus levels 50 dB or more above threshold (upper half). Thick lines: pure tone Frequency Threshold Curves (FTC); thin lines: derived from Reverse Correlograms; crosses and circles : derived from weighting measures from temporal synchrony in response to click trains and sine phase mixed tone complexes, respectively.

deviations in tuning from the FTCs reported previously. For fibres with low CF (upper left hand corner of Fig. 2), the REVCOR filtering and that of the click and sine wave series show a systematic shift of CF upwards by about 20%, together with some reduction in the slope of the high frequency cut-off. The low frequency cut-off for the click and sine wave series, however, is slightly sharper than the FTC. The fibre with the intermediate CF (1.12 kHz) shows relatively little change in the filtering characteristics over a very wide range of levels (70 dB). If anything, there is some evidence in the click and sine wave series of an increased high frequency cut-off slope at the higher levels. In the case of the fibre with the highest CF, there is, in the REVCOR, clear evidence of a reduction in the low frequency cut-off at the higher stimulus levels and (not clearly seen in the figure) a systematic downward shift in CF of about 5%. Interestingly, the data from the click and sine wave series do not show, in this fibre, such pronounced changes in cut-off slopes. In other words, the frequency selectivity is well preserved with these stimuli.

One problem with the fitting of these data is that, in the illustrated case, they are derived from autocorrelograms. As has been indicated in the Methods section, autocorrelograms give squared spectral estimates of tuning and this has to be compensated for by taking the square root of the FFT. The matches described above are obtained with the square root of the FFT, in all of the cases described, apart from the two lower left hand (lower level) cases. Here, in the case of the click and sine wave series, the 'straight' FFTs of the autocorrelograms give the best fits. (In other words, the tuning seen through the temporal discharge patterns is less sharp than that of the FTC when using near-threshold stimulus levels, as shown already with period histogram analyses, Evans, 1981). In fact, for the fibres having the CFs much below 1 kHz, this holds for the first 30 dB or so above threshold. This anomalous behaviour may be possibly accounted for by spike generation being a threshold-crossing operation as opposed to the more generally accepted probabilistic spike generation which appears to be the case in the fibres of higher CF.

Models of cochlear filtering, therefore need to incorporate, at positions corresponding to CFs of about 0.5 kHz and below, processes not readily apparent at higher CFs. These processes include the double frequency selective components and the additional non-linearities implied by the near-threshold phenomena, alluded to above. In addition, fibres of these low CFs show anomalous 'remote' suppression with high-

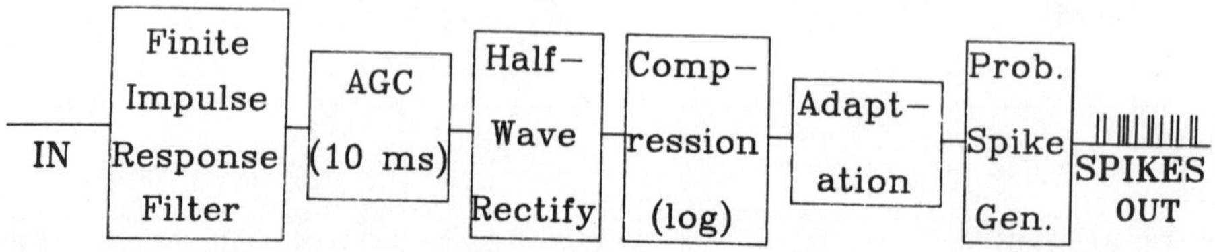

FIGURE 3 Model of cochlear filtering and cochlear nerve, accounting for many of the phenomena discussed here (From Evans, 1980).

pass noise maskers (Evans & Elberling, 1982) and an extensive frequency range of synchrony and rate suppression (Parker & Evans, 1987).

MODELLING

Apart from the systematic shifts in CFs and in cut-off slopes with level, all of the above findings can be predicted by a model (Evans, 1980) of the cochlea and cochlear nerve employing linear 'front-end' filtering followed by the non-linear elements depicted in Fig. 3. The linear filter employed is a finite impulse response filter, loaded with the impulse response of a given cochlear nerve fibre, derived by reverse correlation as in Fig. 1. This is followed by an automatic gain control (AGC) having a time constant of about 10 ms. This is then followed by stages of ideal half-wave rectification, log compression, adaptation and probabilistic spike generation designed to simulate the processes of hair cell transduction and synaptic impulse generation (Evans, 1980). With this model, the temporal discharge patterns of cochlear nerve fibres to a very wide variety of stimuli have been predicted without requiring non-linear 'front-end' filtering (Evans, 1978, 1983a, 1985, 1986, 1987, 1988).

While the model does incorporate the double frequency-selective processes found in fibres with the lowest CFs (through employing the appropriate REVCOR), it is not intended, of course, to simulate the additional non-linearities found in these fibres. However, the model (inadvertently) also gives better fits, near threshold, between the 'straight' FFT of the autocorrelogram and the FTC, like cochlear nerve fibres of lower CFs. This may be because, in a limited range of intensities near response threshold, the model inevitably has threshold- crossing behaviour rather than the intended probabilistic spike generation behaviour. Probabilistic spike generation was used in the model, because it has the important and necessary effect (together with the AGC) of retaining the charactistics of period and post-stimulus time intervals to sine wave and click stimuli over a very wide range of stimulus levels. This unexpected behaviour of the model near threshold possibly suggests that, while spike generation in cochlear nerve fibres is generally probabilistic (multiplicative), near response threshold, particularly for low CF fibres, there may be an additional threshold crossing (additive) component.

Acknowledgements

This work is supported by the Medical Research Council. I am indebted to Mr. N.P. Cooper for drawing attention to the nature of the spectral estimates arising from autocorrelograms.

References

de Boer, E. (1969). Reverse correlation II. Initiation of nerve impulses in the inner ear. Proc. Kon. Nederl. Akat. Wet. 72, 129-151.

de Boer, E. (1973). On the principle of specific coding. J. Dynamic Systems Measurement & Control. Sept, 265-273.

de Boer, E. & Kuyper, P. (1968). Triggered correlation. IEEE Trans. Biomed. Eng. 15, 169-179.

Duifhuis, H. (1973). Consequences of peripheral frequency selectivity for non-simultaneous masking. J. Acoust. Soc. Am. 53, 1471-1488.

Evans, E. F. (1977). Frequency selectivity at high signal levels of single units in cochlear nerve and nucleus. In: Psychophysics and Physiology of Hearing: E.F. Evans and J.P. Wilson eds., Academic Press. London, 185-192.

Evans, E. F. (1978). Place and time coding of frequency in the peripheral auditory system: some physiological pros and cons. Audiol. 17, 369-420.

Evans, E. F. (1979). Single unit studies of the mammalian auditory nerve. In: Auditory Investigations: The Scientific and Technological Basis. H.A. Beagley ed, Oxford University Press. Oxford, 324-367.

Evans, E. F. (1980). An electronic analogue of single unit recording from the cochlear nerve for teaching and research. J Physiol. 298, 6-7P.

Evans, E. F. (1981). The dynamic range problem: place and time coding at the level of cochlear nerve and nucleus. In: Neuronal Mechanisms of Hearing:J Syka and L Aitken ed, Plenum Press. NY, 69-85.

Evans, E. F. (1983a). Pitch and cochlear fibre temporal discharge patterns. In: Hearing - Physiological Bases and Psychophysics: R.Klinke and R.Hartmann eds., Springer Verlag. Berlin Heidelberg New York, 140- 145.

Evans, E. F. (1983b). Computer-controlled synthesis of acoustic stimuli and analysis of single unit responses. Brit J Audiol. 17, 120-120.

Evans, E. F. (1984a). Spectral analysis of complex sounds at the auditory periphery. Proc Institute of Acoustics Spring Meeting 1984, Institute of Acoustics. Edinburgh, 431-438.

Evans, E. F. (1984b). A method for automatically determining the frequency threshold of the gross cochlear action potential ("the AP audiogram"). Brit J Audiol. 18, 246-247.

Evans, E. F. (1985). Aspects of the neuronal coding of time in the mammalian peripheral auditory system relevant to temporal resolution. In: Time Resolution in Auditory Systems: 11th Danavox Symposium: A.Michelsen ed, Springer Verlag. Berlin Heidelberg New York, 74-95.

Evans, E. F. (1986). Cochlear nerve fibres:temporal discharge patterns, cochlear frequency selectivity and the dominant region for pitch. In:Auditory Frequency Selectivity:BCJ Moore and RD Patterson eds, Plenum Press. New York and London, 253-264.

Evans, E. F. (1987). Modelling cochlear nerve fibre responses to complex pitch-producing stimuli. Brit J Audiol. 21, 311-311.

Evans, E. F. (1988). Cochlear nerve discharge patterns in response to complex stimuli:Model predictions and neural data. Brit J Audiol. 0, 0- 0.

Evans, E. F. & Elberling, C. E. (1982). Location-specific components of the gross cochlear action potential: an assessment of the validity of the high-pass masking technique by cochlear nerve fibre recording in the cat. Audiol. 21, 204-227.

Evans, E. F. & Wilson, J. P. (1971). Frequency sharpening of the cochlea: the effective bandwidth of cochlear nerve fibres. Proc. 7th Internat. Cong. on Acoustics: Akademiai Kiado, Budapest. 3, 453-456.

Fitzgibbons, P. J. & Wightman, F. L. (1982). Gap detection in normal and hearing-impaired listeners. J. Acoust. Soc. Am. 72, 761-765.

Greenberg, S., Geisler, C. D. & Deng, L. (1986). Frequency selectivity of single cochlear nerve fibers based on the temporal response to two- tone signals. J. Acoust. Soc. Am. 79, 1010-1019.

Harrison, R. V. & Evans, E. F. (1982). Reverse correlation study of cochlear filtering in normal and pathological guinea pig ears. Hearing Research. 6, 303-314.

Johnson, D. H. (1974). The response of single auditory-nerve fibres in the cat to single tones: Synchrony and average discharge rate. Unpublished Ph.D.Thesis. M.I.T., 1-280.

Parker, D. J. & Evans, E. F. (1987). The frequency: Intensity distribution of excitation and suppression in terms of firing rate and synchrony of discharges in cat cochlear nerve fibres. Brit J Audiol. 21, 104-104.

Wilson, J. P. & Evans, E. F. (1971). Grating acuity of the ear: psychophysical and neurophysiological measures of frequency resolving power. Proc. 7th Internat. Cong. on Acoustics: Akademiai Kiado, Budapest. 3, 397-400.

Wilson, J. P. & Evans, E. F. (1975). Systematic error in some methods of reverse correlation. J. Acoust. Soc. Am. 57, 215-216.

Comments and Discussion

HORST

You suggest that for multicomponent stimuli the spectral content of the response is fairly independent of level. Several investigations (e.g. Young and Sachs; 1979; Sinex and Geisler, 1984; Horst, Javel and Farley, 1985, 1986a) have shown that this is not generally the case. Our data (Horst, Javel and Farley, 1985, 1986b) show for example that one can get very wild changes in the response spectra with level when the spectral content of the stimulus varies during the fundamental period.

Horst, J.W., Javel, E. and Farley, G.R. (1985) Extraction and enhancement of spectral structure by the cochlea. J. Acoust. Soc. Am., 78, 1898-1901.

Horst, J.W., Javel, E. and Farley, G.R. (1986a) Coding of spectral fine structure in the auditory nerve. I. Fourier analysis of period and interspike interval histograms. J. Acoust. Soc. Am., 79, 398-416.

Horst, J.W., Javel, E. and Farley, G.R. (1986b) Effects of phase- and amplitude spectrum in the nonlinear processing of complex stimuli in single fibers of the auditory nerve. In: Auditory Frequency Selectivity, B.C.J. Moore and R.D. Patterson (eds.), Plenum Press, New York and London, 229-239.

Sinex, D.G. and Geisler, C.D. (1984) Comparison of the responses of auditory nerve fibers to consonant-vowel syllables with predictions from linear models. J. Acoust. Soc. Am., 76, 116-121.

Young, E.D. and Sachs, M.B. (1979) Representation of steady-state vowels in the temporal aspects of the discharge patterns of populations of auditory nerve fibers. J. Acoust. Soc. Am., 66, 1381-1403.

EVANS

What I have shown is that for a wide variety of stimulus waveforms, *having a flat spectrum*, the spectral content of the response is surprisingly independent of level. It is also true of some stimuli having a non-flat spectrum (Evans, 1978, 1983a, 1984, 1985). I agree, that for certain stimuli having spectral discontinuities, important level-dependent effect disturb this preservation of tuning. However, at least some of these effects can be accounted for by a model (Evans, 1980) having a linear front-end filter, particularly your own stimuli and responses (Horst *et al*, 1985, 1986) as recently shown (Evans, 1987, 1988).

HORST

It seems to me that there is enough evidence that the front end of the transduction in the cochlea is not linear? Why then are you stressing the linearity of the front-end filter in your model?

EVANS

First, for simplicity and practicality. For building hardware models, linear front-end filters are both readily available, and, if they are finite impulse response filters (as in my hardware model) they can be fitted with different impulse responses in order to model more accurately the level-dependencies of Revcors over a very wide dynamic range. Most, if not all models of the peripheral auditory system (acting as input to speech recognition models for example) utilise linear front-end filters. I am concerned to explore how valid is their use for a wide variety of generalisable stimuli.

Secondly, because the use of a linear front end filter, followed by appropriate non-linear elements in the transduction process can model a surprisingly wide range of cochlear fibre data including those appearing to implicate non-linear filtering (see references in my paper).

COCHLEAR NONLINEARITIES IMPLIED BY THE DIFFERENCES BETWEEN TRANSIENT ONSETS AND OFFSETS TO A TONE BURST

Kenneth R. Henry and Edwin R. Lewis*

Department of Psychology
University of California
Davis, California, USA 95616
**Electronics Research Laboratory*
University of California
Berkeley, California, USA 94720

Introduction

A trapezoidal tone burst (Figure 1) is equivalent to a sum of four ramp-modulated sinusoids. The response of any linearly operating spectral filter (or tuning structure) to a single ramp-modulated sinusoid is made up of two families of components: (a) for each natural frequency of the filter itself, a transient excitation equivalent to that which would have been produced by an impulse occurring precisely at the time of the onset corner of the ramp, and (b) with the same frequency as the stimulus, a step modulated sinusoid and a ramp modulated sinusoid, each beginning precisely at the time of the corner of the stimulus ramp. The amplitude of the transient excitation of each of the filter's natural frequencies is directly proportional to the slope of the ramp and depends on the frequency of the stimulus relative to the natural frequency being excited (Lewis and Henry, '88). When the frequency of the stimulus sinusoid is close to or within the pass band of the filter, the transient excitations of the filter's natural frequencies combine with the responses at the stimulus frequency to produce a "delayed" version of the input waveform. In that case, the transient excitations are manifested merely as the "delay" itself.

If the filter is of high-order, and the frequency of the stimulus sinusoid is well outside the pass band of the filter, then the second family of response components may be attenuated sufficiently to allow the transient excitations to stand alone, providing a sharp temporal marker at the corner of the ramp. In that case, the trapezoid tone burst will yield four transient excitations, one for each corner. Although, strictly speaking, these excitations are time-domain phenomena, one might equate them, loosely, with spectral splatter (a frequency- domain concept). On the other hand, treating them in the time domain will provide insights not available from the frequency domain.

Deviations from the stereotypic "primary type" response to trapezoidal tone bursts have been reported recently (Geisler and Sinex, '82; Rhode and Smith, '85; Fay, '86). These deviations involve exaggerated responses to the stimulus onset and offset, often associated with decreased firing during the plateau portion of the stimulus. In this paper, we examine such responses from cochlear afferent axons of the gerbil, and interpret our results in terms of time-domain responses to ramp-modulated sinusoids. We find that some onset and offset responses are consistent with linear operation; others imply the presence of nonlinearities.

Methods

The VIIIth nerve was exposed close to the round window of healthy, young adult mongolian gerbils that had been anesthetized with ketamine. Single cochlear afferent axons within the first 0.25 mm of the surface of the nerve were impaled by 50 to 150 megohm glass micropipettes filled with 3.0M NaCl. Spike activity was recorded in response to trapezoid tone bursts, with different rise and decay (r/d) times and different plateau amplitudes. For each r/d time and each amplitude, at least 40 tone bursts were presented, with the onsets of the envelopes occurring at random phases of the stimulus sinusoid. Thus, in the course of these presentations, the corner of each of the four ramp-modulated sinusoids making up the trapezoid spanned the full range of phases; and for linear operation, the data accumulated over the presentations reflect responses to essentially identical sets of stimuli. All tone bursts were presented at a rate of 5 per s. For the data displayed in Figures 2, 3 and 4, the r/d time was 0.3 ms. For those of Figure 5 the r/d times were 2, 4 and 9 ms. In each of those figures, the timing of the tone burst is depicted by an outline of the stimulus envelop.

Results

The peristimulus time histograms (PSTHs) of Figure 2 show approximately equal responses to the onset and offset of the tone burst, and little or no response to the plateau. If we assume that the onset response was in fact the combined responses to corners 1 and 2 of the trapezoid (those corners being too close in time to elicit separate responses), and that the ofset response was the combined responses to corners 3 and 4, then the data of Figure 2 are consistent with the response of a linearly operating filter excited by a tone burst with a frequency well outside the filter's pass band. Thus, one might attribute these neural responses simply to spectral "splatter" in the stimulus.

The same interpretation cannot be applied to the PSTHs of Figures 3-5. The upper left-hand panel of Figures 3 shows a primary-type response pattern in an axon stimulated at its characteristic frequency (CF). As the stimulus intensity was increased, distinct onset and offset responses emerged. This will not happen in a linearly responding filter stimulated by a trapezoid tone burst with a frequency inside the filter's pass band (Lewis and Henry, '88). The nonlinearity that sets the onset response apart seems to be adaptation; but the source of the more diffuse offset response is not clear. One might attribute it to some sort of

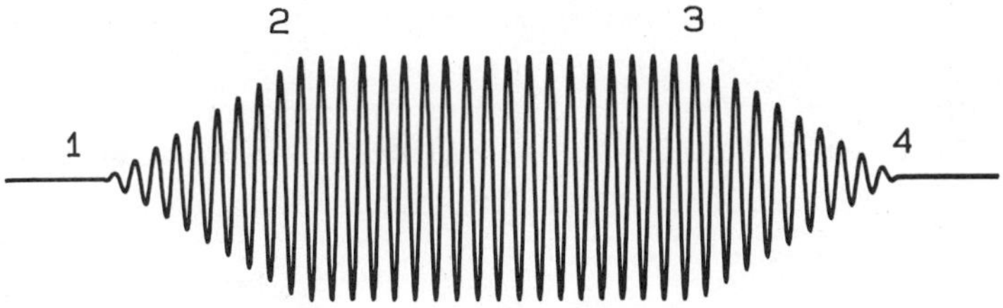

FIGURE 1 A trapezoidal tone burst comprises four ramp modulated sinusoids, one beginning at each of its four corners.

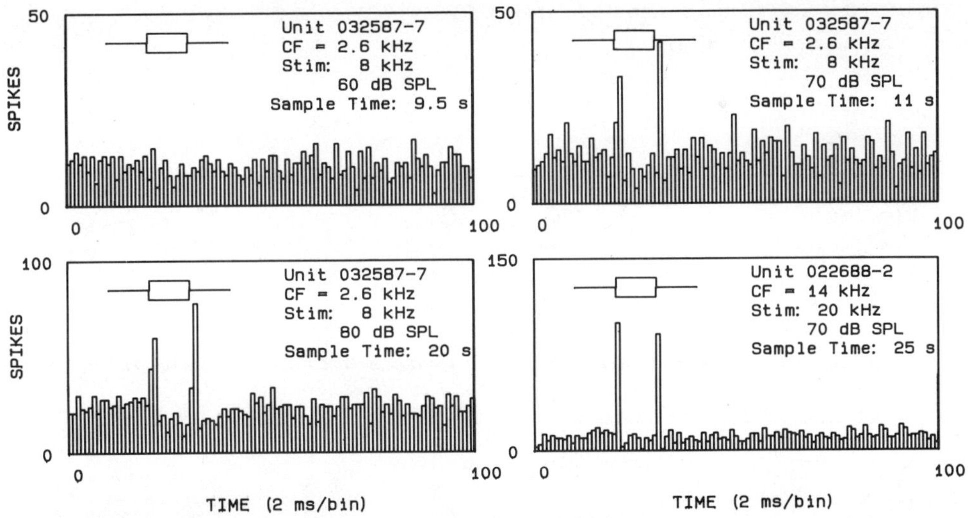

FIGURE 2 PSTHs for two units stimulated at frequencies above CF. Threshold at CF was approximately 25 dB SPL for unit 032587-7 and approximately 15 dB SPL for unit 022688-2.

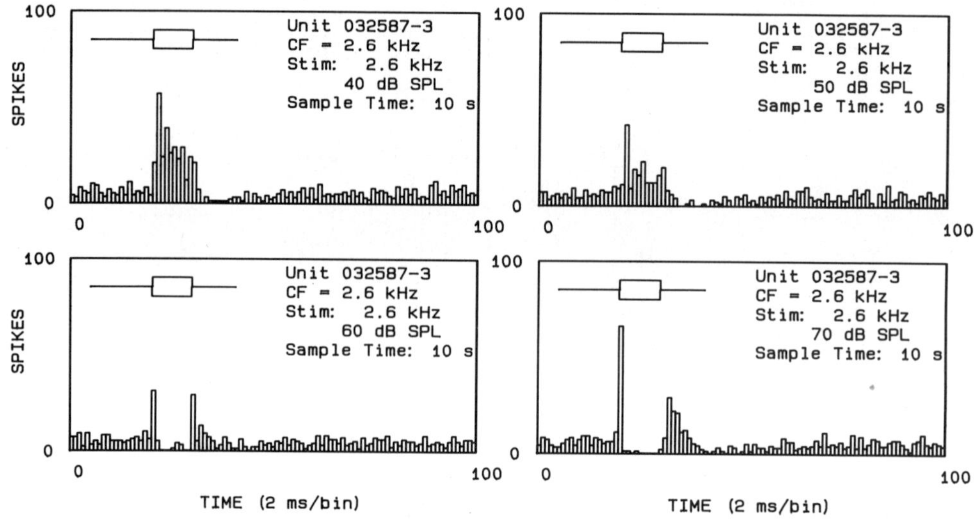

FIGURE 3 PSTHs for a unit stimulated at CF. Threshold at CF was approximately 20 dB SPL.

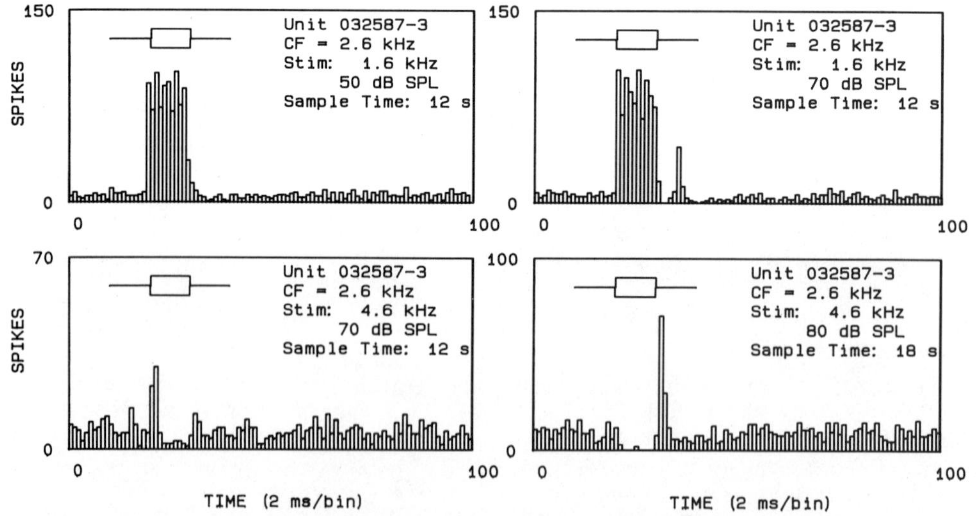

FIGURE 4 PSTHs for the unit of Figure 3, stimulated at frequencies below and above CF.

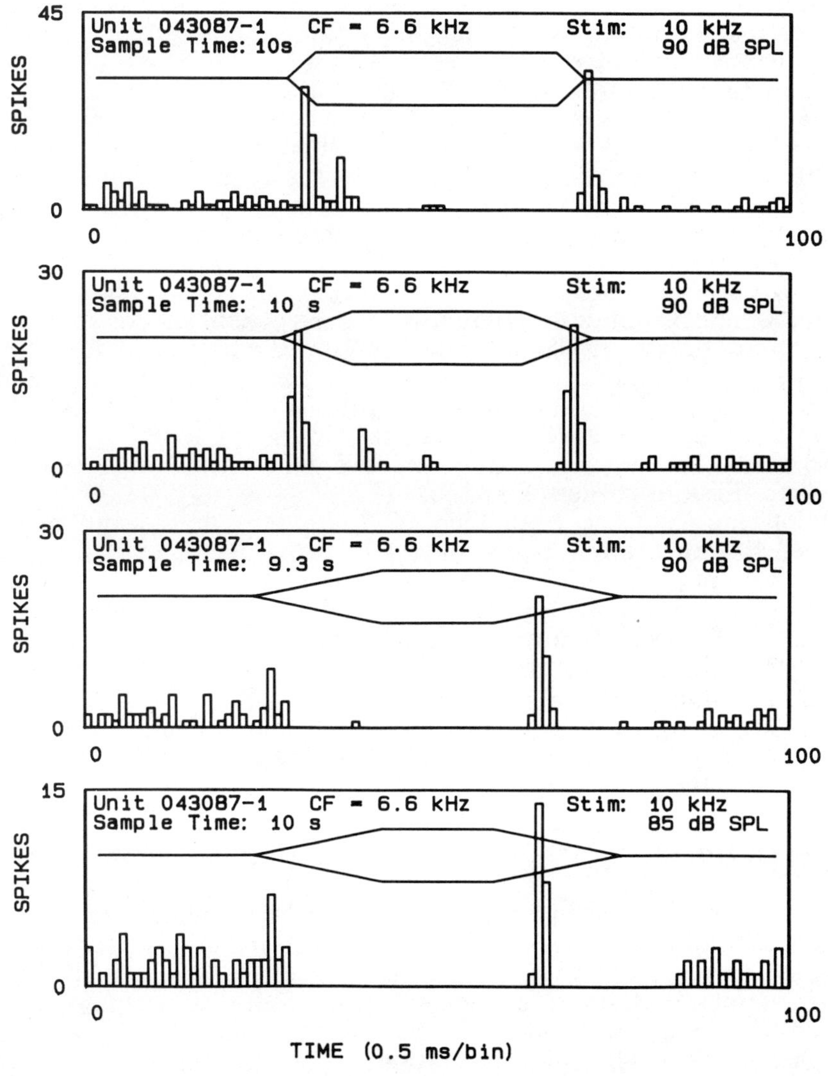

FIGURE 5 PSTHs produced by tone bursts with longer r/d times, to clarify relationships between trapezoid corners and transient responses. Threshold at CF was less than 10 dB SPL.

rebound from adaptation. However, in the top two panels of Figure 4 we see a similar, diffuse offset response develop without conspicuous evidence of adaptation. The very slow time courses of the offset response and the period of low spike acitivity following it in the upper right-hand panel of Figure 4 suggests the possibility of oscillations at the spike initiator of the afferent axon. However, the differences between that panel and the lower right-hand panel of Figure 3 (for the same axon) argue against this interpretation.

The lower panels of Figure 4 show an effect that we frequently encounter. As the stimulus intensity is increased, the onset reponse appears at lower levels and then is supplanted by the offset at higher levels. Because the onset and offset portions of the tone burst represent identical pairs of stimuli when applied to a linearly operating filter, this distinction between onset and offset responses could not occur in such a filter.

The r/d times employed for the experiments of Figure 5 were sufficiently long to allow separation of the responses to the four corners of the trapezoid, all of which would be equivalent stimuli to a linearly operating filter. In order to obtain offset reponses with these longer r/d times, we found it necessary to use higher stimulus intensities. In the upper two panels of Figure 5, we see responses to corners 1, 2 and 3 of the trapezoid. The latency of the response to corner 3 is conspicuously longer than those to corners 1 and 2.

The plateau response (reduction of spike rate to a level below the spontaneous rate) to a tone well above CF, which is apparent in Figure 5, has been common at high stimulus intensities among the gerbil auditory axons we have studied. For those who might suspect that this is a consequence of nonlinear interaction between the applied stimulus and the ambient acoustic noise in our test chamber, we report that the ambient noise for frequencies between 500 Hz and 20 kHz was less than 1.4×10^{-6} Pa/Hz$^{1/2}$. We also would point out the prolonged reduction in spike rate that follows the offset response and extends past the termination of the stimulus.

Conclusions

Our data imply that in some cases, when the frequency of the tone burst is well outside the pass band of the axon, transient onset and offset firing patterns of cochlear axons can be explained satisfactorily in terms of linear operation (via a phenomenon analogous to spectral splatter). However, in many instances, observed transient firing patterns are wholly inconsistent with linear operation. The qualitative nature of these nonlinear response patterns depends upon both the stimulus intensity and the stimulus frequency relative to CF. Nonlinear onset responses generally appear at stimulus intensities that are lower than those required to produce nonlinear offset responses. At higher intensities, nonlinear offset responses often remain robust when nonlinear onset responses have disappeared. Presently even the locations of the mechanisms underlying these phenomena are unknown. Whatever those mechanisms may be, they evidently increase the complexity of primary afferent auditory signals well beyond that of the traditional "primary response pattern."

References

Fay, R.R. (1986) Frequency selectivity, adaptation, and suppression in goldfish auditory nerve fibers. In: Frequency Selectivity in Hearing (Eds.: Moore, B.C.J. and Patterson, R.D.) Plenum Press, New York, pp. 137-145.

Geisler, C.D. and Sinex, D.G. (1982) Responses of primary auditory fibers to brief tone bursts. J. Acoust. Soc. Am. 72, 781-794.

Lewis, E.R. and Henry K.R. (1988) Time domain analysis of tone bursts and their responses. Submitted to Hearing Research.

Rhode, W.S. and Smith, P.H. (1985) Characteristics of tone-pip response patterns in relationship to spontaneous rate in cat auditory nerve fibers. Hearing Res. 21, 91-95.

Research supported in part by Grant 12359 from NINCDS, National Institutes of Health.

Comments and Discussion

PATUZZI

Your unusual finding that a pure tone burst presented above threshold reduces neural firing below "spontaneous" rate (even in a cell with a CF of almost 7 kHz) suggests that there may be an extraneous stimulus elevating firing rate in the absence of an intentional stimulus. If this were the case, many of the complicated effects you have observed may be explainable in terms of transient suppression and subsequent recovery. Were these results obtained in a sound proof room and, if so, are you confident that no low-level sounds, perhaps from the animal itself, were not confounding your results?

LEWIS

The level reported in the text was measured in the acoustic chamber at large; that reported verbally (for an added chamber within the original chamber) was estimated by extrapolation. Unfortunately, the sound pressure level in the chamber at large does not tell us how much acoustic input to the cochlea is derived from the animal's respiration, blood flow, gastric activity, and the like. With appropriate sensors and intervention, one should be able to eliminate or greatly reduce inputs from those sources. The issue, however, seems to be the discrepency between our observations and those of investigators who have not used such intervention.

"PEAK SPLITTING": INTENSITY EFFECTS IN COCHLEAR AFFERENT RESPONSES TO LOW FREQUENCY TONES

Mario A. Ruggero and Nola C. Rich

Department of Otolaryngology
University of Minnesota
Minneapolis, MN 55414, U.S.A.

Introduction

In 1972, Kiang and Moxon noted that a notch can sometimes be measured in the rate-intensity function of cochlear-afferent responses to tones over restricted ranges of high intensities. It has been subsequently shown that, for low-frequency tones, the notch is found in association with bimodality of period histograms ("peak splitting") and/or with a rapid shift in response phase (Gifford and Guinan, 1983; Kiang, 1984). In the present paper we present preliminary results from a systematic study of the intensity dependence of the magnitude and phase of responses of chinchilla cochlear afferents to low-frequency tones. Low-frequency stimuli are used to facilitate precise timing of the excitation of cochlear afferents relative to basilar membrane (BM) motion (Ruggero and Rich, 1987; Ruggero et al., 1986b). Our present findings, for responses to 200 - 600 Hz tones, agree with and extend our previous results for 100 Hz tones (Ruggero and Rich, 1988): within each stimulus cycle, there appear to exist two distinct preferred times for inner hair cell (IHC) excitation of cochlear afferents. Relative to BM motion, one corresponds to displacement or velocity toward scala tympani (ST) and the other is synchronous with maximal velocity toward scala vestibuli (SV). Which of these two response phases predominates depends on cochlear location (or, equivalently, characteristic frequency: CF) and on stimulus level, but does not depend significantly on stimulus frequency.

Methods

Electrophysiological recordings were made from single cochlear axons in chinchillas. Stimuli consisted of 5 repetitions of 100 - 600 Hz tones (100 ms on, 200 ms off) presented at even-dB stimulus intensities in random order. Responses were analyzed by means of period histograms and dot displays for individual responses (Fig. 1) and contour plots for averages of responses from many neurons (Figs. 2-4). In the dot displays, the abscissa indicates sound pressure level and the ordinate time modulo the stimulus period (i.e., phase), with the density of dots reflecting instantaneous discharge rate. The contour plots are similar, with various shadings coding for discharge rate ranges.

Results

Nonmonotonic behavior of rate-intensity functions is demonstrable for only a small fraction of chinchilla cochlear afferents (Fig. 1). Within the range of 85 to 105 dB SPL, response rate decreases over a narrow range of intensities, sometimes approaching spontaneous rates. When the stimulus is a low-frequency tone, as in Fig. 1, the drop in discharge rate is invariably accompanied by a change in the preferred response phase. In contrast with the low prevalence of rate notches, phase shifts occur in the vast majority of cochlear afferents at adequately high stimulus levels.

THE INTENSITY DEPENDENCE OF COCHLEAR NERVE EXCITATION PHASE RELATIVE TO BASILAR MEMBRANE MOTION IS NEARLY INVARIANT FOR FREQUENCIES 100 - 600 HZ IN APICAL COCHLEAR REGIONS

Figure 2 shows contour plots for the responses of neurons with CFs of 800-1600 Hz, corresponding to cochlear locations approximately 6.5 - 9 mm from the apex. Various delays intervening between the arrival of a pressure wave at the eardrum and the time of spike recording at the microelectrode tend to obscure the presumed orderly relationship between (IHC) depolarization and BM motion. The effects of these delays are greatest for lower CFs and for higher stimulus frequencies. In order

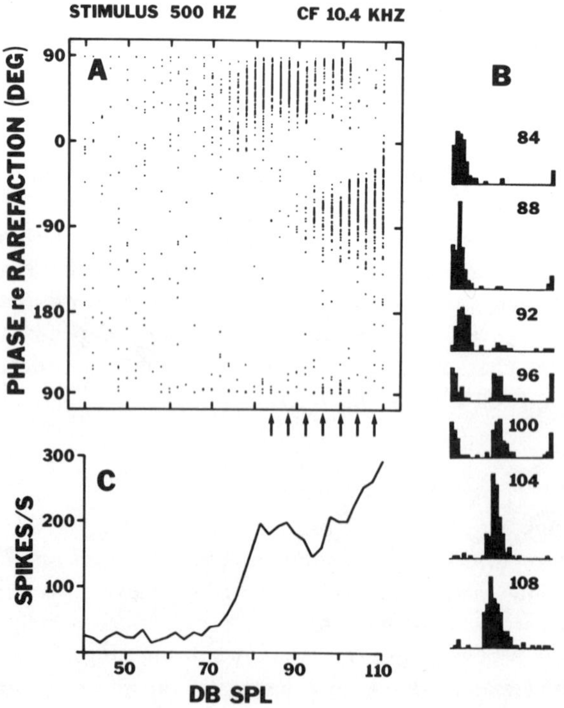

FIGURE 1. Intensity dependence of responses of a cochlear afferent to 500 Hz tones. A: Dot display showing the responses phase of each action potential relative to rarefaction (ordinate) vs. sound level (abscissa). B: Period histograms constructed for responses at selected stimulus intensities, indicated by arrows under panel A. C: Rate-intensity function for the data of panel A. Note the bimodality of response phases at 94-102 dB SPL (panels A and B) and the rate notch at the same stimulus levels (panel C).

to remove these effects, to uncover the underlying relationship between IHC depolarization and BM motion, the cochlear nerve responses have been corrected for middle-ear, synaptic and neural-travel-time delays and BM travel time before contour plot construction (Ruggero et al., 1986b; Ruggero and Rich, 1987). The ordinates, therefore, indicate the BM phase corresponding to neural excitation or,

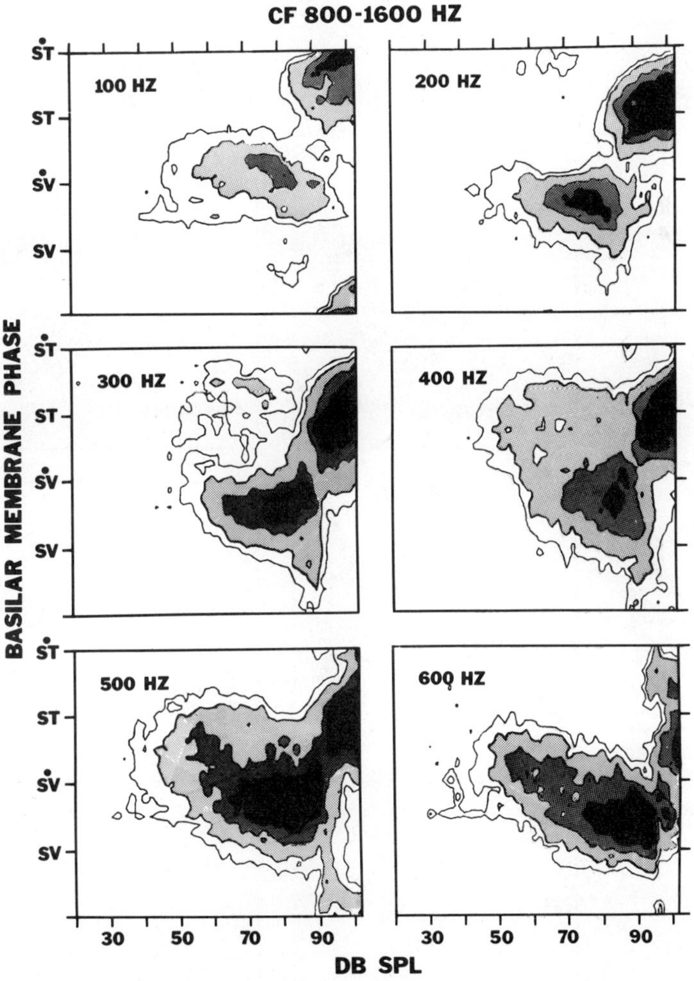

FIGURE 2. Contour plots for averaged responses of apical cochlear afferents (CFs 800 - 1600 Hz) to tones with frequencies 100 - 600 Hz. In each plot the abscissa indicates stimulus intensity and the ordinate shows the phase of BM motion: ST, maximal displacement toward scala tympani; ṠT, maximal velocity toward scala tympani; SV, maximal displacement toward scala vestibuli; ṠV, maximal velocity toward scala vestibuli. Contour lines are drawn for firing rates of 100, 150, 250 and 350 spikes/s. The black area represents rates higher than 350 spikes/s, the darker gray represents rates between 250 and 350 spikes/s, and so on. The plot for each frequency represents responses of many neurons from several chinchillas. 100 Hz: 57 neurons (from 10 chinchillas); 200 Hz: 51 (12); 300 Hz: 41 (11); 400 Hz: 44 (10); 500 Hz: 33 (8); 600 Hz: 18 (10).

more precisely, IHC depolarization. Thus, comparisons are possible between responses to tones with different frequencies and among neurons with widely varying CFs.

For the 100 Hz stimulus, clear phase locking begins at 50 dB SPL, with the peak of excitation synchronous with maximal velocity of the BM toward SV. This phase remains relatively constant to about 80 dB SPL. Between 80 and 98 dB SPL an abrupt response transition takes place and two peaks of excitation are apparent

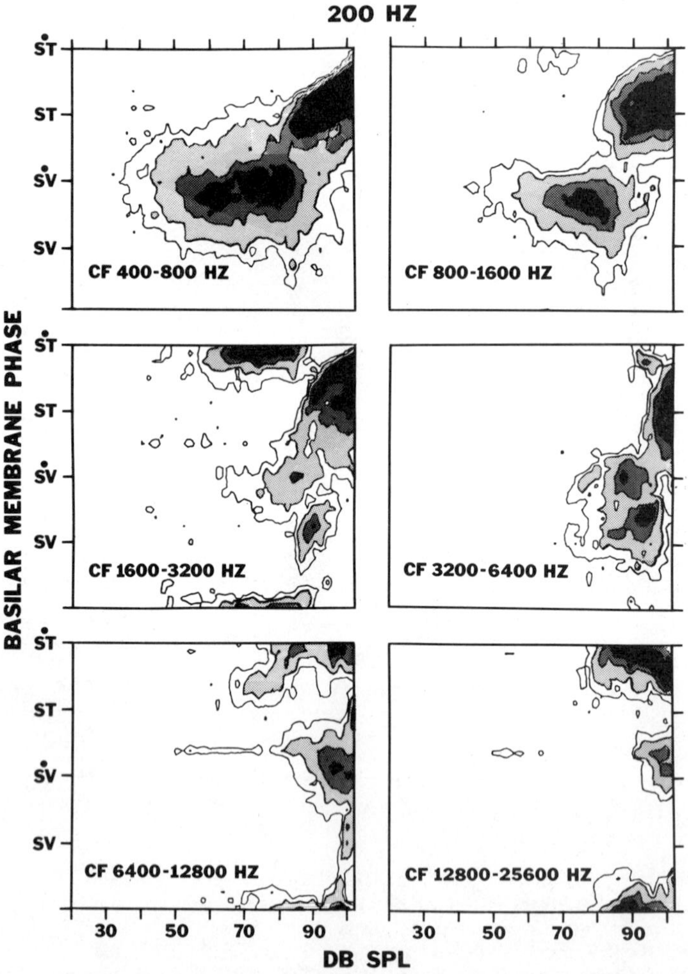

FIGURE 3. Contour plots for responses to 200 Hz tones of cochlear afferents innervating inner hair cells throughout the cochlea. Responses have been averaged over 1-octave CF ranges (indicated in each plot). CFs 400-800 Hz: 23 neurons (from 12 chinchillas); 800-1600 Hz: 51 (12); 1600-3200 Hz: 19 (9); 3200-6400 Hz: 13 (6); 6400-12800 Hz: 27 (10); 12800-25600 Hz: 17 (6). Other details as in Fig. 2.

through much of this range. Analysis of individual period histograms (not shown) indicates that the two peaks coexist in individual responses; i.e., "peak splitting" occurs, similar to that illustrated in Fig. 1. At stimulus levels above the transition, phase remains constant at some 60 degrees leading maximal BM displacement toward ST.

The contour plots for the 200-Hz through 600-Hz stimuli are similar in most respects to those for 100 Hz. In particular, the response phases at lower stimulus levels, the level at which the phase transition occurs and the phase for the high-level responses correspond closely to their counterparts for the 100-Hz contour plot. There is a seemingly systematic, but small, phase lag as stimulus frequency increases. Such phase lag may result from a small error in the delay corrections, which must translate into proportionally larger errors for higher frequencies.

COCHLEAR NERVE EXCITATION PHASES RELATIVE TO BASILAR MEMBRANE MOTION ARE STRONGLY DEPENDENT ON CHARACTERISTIC FREQUENCY

Figure 3 presents responses to 200 Hz tones for 6 1-octave bands spanning the CF range of 400 - 25600 Hz. In contrast with the relative invariance of response phase re BM motion as a function of stimulus frequency for a single 1-octave CF band (Fig. 2), substantial variation exists across CF bands. For the lowest CF bands (400-800 and 800-1600 Hz), the lower-level responses peak close to velocity of BM toward SV. Between 80 and 90 dB SPL two peaks are evident in the contour plots and, at the highest intensities, responses span a phase range between maximal ST displacement and velocity. This mode of high-level response is also evident in the panels for the 1600-3200 Hz and the 3200-6400 Hz bands for intensities above "peak splitting" (i.e., above 85 and 95 dB SPL, respectively). For intensities below "peak splitting", responses are detectable between maximal SV displacement and velocity. However, many neurons in the 1600-3200 Hz CF band also respond strongly at a phase just lagging maximal velocity toward ST. This is the BM phase at which the lowest level responses occur for the two high-CF ranges (6400-12800 and 12800-25600 Hz). At the highest intensities, for high-CF neurons, a second preferred response phase appears, which lags the near-threshold response by some 90-130 degrees. This second response phase of basal neurons corresponds to the low-level responses of apical neurons. In most respects, the transition of response modes as a function of CF depicted in Fig. 3 for 200 Hz is representative of frequencies 100 -600 Hz.

THE INTENSITY DEPENDENCE OF COCHLEAR NERVE EXCITATION PHASE RELATIVE TO BASILAR MEMBRANE MOTION IS NEARLY INVARIANT FOR FREQUENCIES 100 - 600 HZ IN BASAL COCHLEAR NEURONS

Figure 4 presents contour plots for responses to 100 - 600 Hz tones in the CF band 12800 - 25600 Hz, corresponding to neurons innervating the basal end of the cochlea. For all stimulus frequencies the near-threshold responses occur at 75-80 dB SPL and are synchronous with velocity of BM toward ST. At levels of 90-100 dB SPL responses shift to a BM phase intermediate between BM velocity toward SV and displacement toward ST.

Conclusions and discussion

Our findings on the intensity dependence of responses to low-frequency tones strengthen our contention that, in spite of the lack of direct information on the motion of the BM at other than basal locations, it is nevertheless possible to derive BM travel times (and, therefore, BM response phases for low-frequency stimuli) for most of the extent of the cochlea from a combination of measurements, for the same species, of BM motion at the base and latencies of cochlear-afferent responses to high-intensity

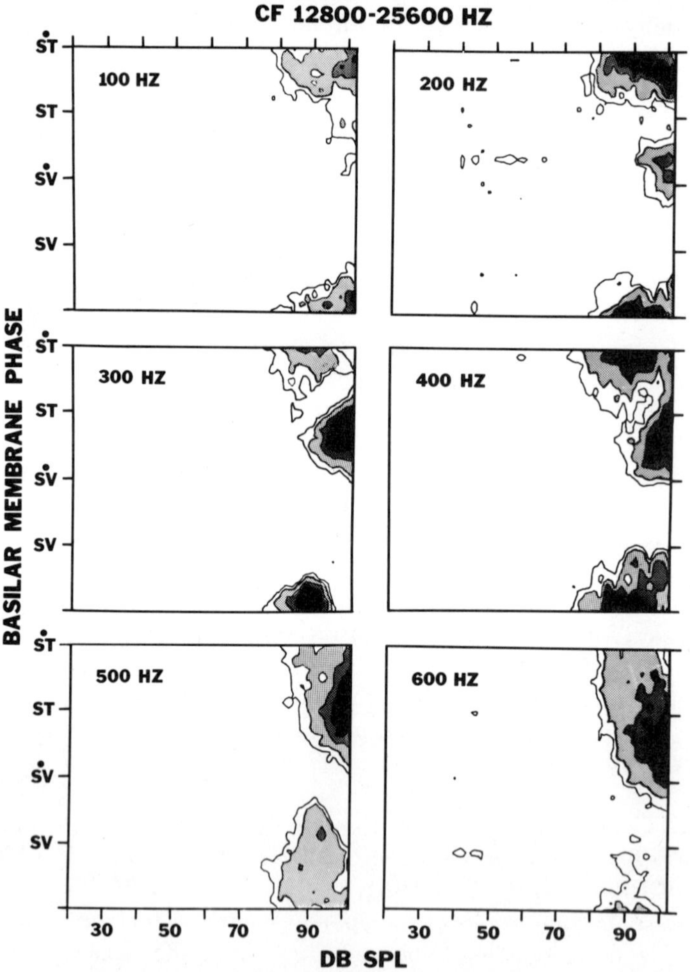

FIGURE 4. Contour plots for responses of basal cochlear afferents (CFs 12800 - 25600 Hz) to tones with frequencies 100 - 600 Hz. 100 Hz: 24 neurons (from 7 chinchillas); 200 Hz: 17 (6); 300 Hz: 14 (6); 400 Hz: 19 (7); 500 Hz: 23 (6); 600 Hz: 13 (6). Other details as in Figure 2.

clicks (Ruggero and Rich, 1987). We previously used such an approach to conclude that near-threshold responses of basal and apical neurons to low-frequency tones, relative to BM motion, occur some 130-180 degrees out-of-phase, with apical neurons responding nearly in phase with maximal velocity of BM toward SV (Ruggero and Rich, 1987). We now have shown that, for the vast majority of both basal and apical neurons, a sharp shift in response phase occurs at high intensities (80-90 dB for apical afferents, 90-100 dB for basal afferents). In the small proportion of cases where notches exist in the rate-intensity function, they occur at exactly the same intensities where the phase transition or "peak splitting" occurs. The phase transitions do not quite amount to phase reversals and occur in opposite directions for the two halves of the cochlea: in basal neurons the high-level responses *lag* threshold responses by some 110-130 degrees; in apical neurons, high-level responses *lead* low level responses by similar amounts.

The most parsimonious interpretation of our results is that there exist in the cochlea two distinct modes of IHC response, with phases of IHC depolarization (and cochlear-afferent excitation) corresponding in one case to BM displacement or velocity toward ST and in the other to BM velocity toward SV. [An alternative interpretation, for which there is some evidence from round window recordings (Ruggero et al., 1986a), is that there are *three* distinct response phases, at ST velocity, ST displacement and SV velocity.] Which response mode is dominant depends strongly on cochlear location and stimulus intensity, but only weakly or not at all on stimulus frequency, at least in the range 100-600 Hz. Counterparts for the phase shifts in cochlear afferent responses appear to have been recently identified in the intracellularly-recorded responses of IHCs, both basal and apical (Cody et al., 1986; Dallos et al., 1986). However, while the phase of the low-level response of apical cochlear afferents seems well accounted for by IHC recordings (Dallos, 1985), no appropriate IHC counterparts have yet been found for the response phase of basal afferents below "peak splitting" levels (Russell and Sellick, 1983; Nuttall et al., 1981).

The origin of "peak splitting" is unclear. Sellick et al. (1982) and ourselves (Ruggero and Rich, 1983; Ruggero et al., 1986a) have suggested that outer hair cells might electrically affect the response of IHCs, leading both to "peak splitting" and to the CF dependence of phases of cochlear afferent responses to very-low-frequency tones (< 100 Hz). In the light of newer evidence that shows that the CF-dependence is not confined to very low frequencies, but rather extends to stimulus frequencies at least as high as 500 Hz (Ruggero and Rich, 1987), and on the presumption that electrical interactions between hair cells must be very weak at such frequencies (Dallos, 1983), we now think it more likely that both "peak splitting" and the CF dependence of response phases have a mechanical origin (Ruggero and Rich, 1987). Indeed, there is a suggestion that a cochlear microphonic counterpart of "peak splitting", presumably of outer hair cell origin, can be recorded from the scala media of gerbils (Zwislocki, 1986). Since microphonics provide, in many respects, a faithful version of mechanical cochlear events at low frequencies (Ruggero et al., 1986b), this evidence might indicate that "peak splitting" exists at the level of BM macromechanics or, perhaps more likely, at the level of subtectorial-space micromechanics.

Acknowledgments

Ms Laura House helped with data processing and artwork. We were supported by NIH Grants NS-25012 and NS-12125, and NSF Grant BNS-8304587.

References

Cody, A.R., Mountain, D.C. and Russell, I.J. (1986) Acoustically evoked potentials in the basal turn of the guinea pig cochlea. In: IUPS Satellite Symposium on Hearing, Univ. of California, San Francisco, p. 24.

Dallos, P. (1983) Some electrical circuit properties of the organ of Corti. I. Analysis without reactive elements. Hear. Res. 12, 89-119.

Dallos, P. (1985) Response characteristics of mammalian cochlear hair cells. J. Neurosci. 5, 1591-1608.

Dallos, P., Cheatham, M.A. and Oesterle, E. (1986) Harmonic components in hair cell responses. In: Auditory Frequency Selectivity (Eds: Moore, B.C.J. and Patterson, R.D.) Plenum, London, pp. 73-80.

Gifford, M.L. and Guinan, Jr., J.J. (1983) Effects of crossed-olivocochlear-bundle stimulation on cat auditory nerve fiber responses to tones. J. Acoust. Soc. Am. 74, 115-123.

Kiang, N.Y.S. (1984) Peripheral neural processing of auditory information. In: Handbook of Physiology. The Nervous System. Sensory Processes. (Ed: Darian-Smith, I.) American Physiol. Soc., Bethesda, MD, pp. 639-674.

Kiang, N.Y.S. and Moxon, E.C. (1972) Physiological considerations in artificial stimulation of the inner ear. Ann. Otol. Rhinol. Laryngol. 81, 714-730.

Nuttall, A.L., Brown, M.C., Masta, R.I. and Lawrence, M. (1981) Inner hair cell responses to the velocity of basilar membrane motion in the guinea pig. Brain Res. 211, 171-174.

Ruggero, M.A. and Rich, N.C. (1983) Chinchilla auditory-nerve responses to low-frequency tones. J. Acoust. Soc. Am. 73, 2096-2108.

Ruggero, M.A. and Rich, N.C. (1987) Timing of spike initiation in cochlear afferents: dependence on site of innervation. J. Neurophysiol. 58, 379-403.

Ruggero, M.A. and Rich, N.C. (1988) Responses of cochlear afferents to low-frequency tones: intensity dependence. In: Auditory Pathway - Structure and Function (Eds: Syka, J. and Popelar, J.) Plenum, N.Y., in press.

Ruggero, M.A., Robles, L. and Rich, N.C. (1986a) Cochlear microphonics and the initiation of spikes in the auditory nerve: correlation of single-unit data with neural and receptor potentials recorded from the round window. J. Acoust. Soc. Am. 79, 1491-1498.

Ruggero, M.A., Robles, L. and Rich, N.C. (1986b) Basilar membrane mechanics at the base of the chinchilla cochlea. II. Responses to low-frequency tones and relationship to microphonics and spike initiation in the VIII Nerve. J. Acoust. Soc. Am. 80, 1375-1383.

Russell, I.J. and Sellick, P.M. (1983) Low-frequency characteristics of intracellularly recorded potentials in guinea-pig cochlear hair cells. J. Physiol. (Lond.) 338, 179-206.

Sellick, P.M., Patuzzi, R. and Johnstone, B.M. (1982) Modulation of responses of spiral ganglion cells in the guinea pig cochlea by low frequency sound. Hear. Res. 7, 199-221.

Zwislocki, J.J. (1986) Comments on "Basilar membrane motion and spike initiation in the cochlear nerve" (Ruggero, M.A., Robles, L., Rich, N.C. and Costalupes, J.A.). In: Auditory Frequency Selectivity (Eds: Moore, B.C.J. and Patterson, R.D.) Plenum, London, p. 197.

Comments and Discussion

PATUZZI

Q1. The low frequency neural response, at least in the basal turn, is complicated by fast adaptation which would bias the results towards a phase lead. Is it possible that the scala tympani velocity response you report is not a scala tympani response that is adapting during firing to appear more as a velocity response?

Q2. The "peak splitting" described by Mountain and Cody is more likely to be a correlate of the very complicated, very high intensity histograms we reported previously (Sellick et al., 1982). They are unlikely to be related to the ST and SV velocity response we reported at lower intensities and should be considered, I believe, as a separate phenomenon.

It should also be noted that the transition of the intra-cellular inner hair cell response from a maximum depolarization during scala vestibuli, to one during scala vestibuli displacement (Patuzzi and Yates, 1987; Russell and Sellick, 1983) at higher frequencies, will complicate the neural response in the basal turn above about 400-1000 Hz.

In addition, the changes we have observed in the period histograms after acute acoustic trauma (Patuzzi, Sellick and Johnstone, 1983) suggest that two excitatory mechanisms may operate simultaneously. We require a better understanding of these traumatic changes if we are to understand the origin of the phase changes in the normal cochlea.

RUGGERO

A1. No! The phase lead of approximately 45-60 degrees relative to maximal displacement toward scala tympani was measured at near-threshold levels, when adaptation should be minimal.

A2. No comment.

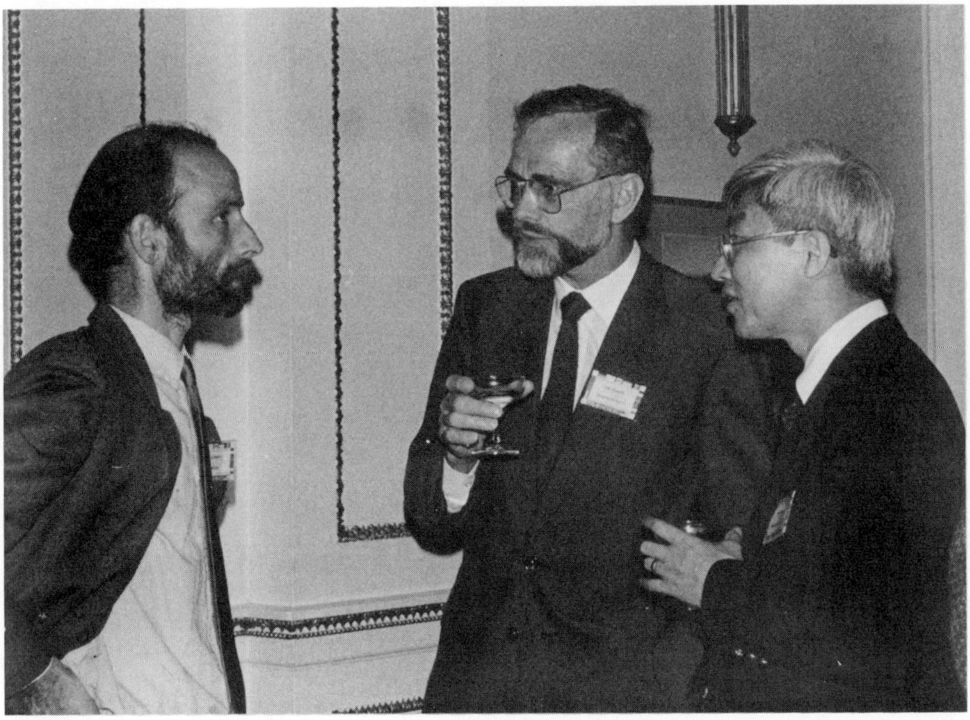

J.F. Ashmore, C.R. Steele and D.O. Kim

4. DISCUSSION SESSION I

DISCUSSION SESSION I

Chairman - Peter Dallos

This tape transcript has not been checked by all contributors. Whilst all speakers knew that the workshop was being recorded, the decision to publish the discussion sessions came after the meeting. In view of this, and the spontaneous nature of the discussion, the dialogues reported below may not represent the actual or considered or final view of the named participants on any matter. The editors thank the participants for supporting (or at least tolerating) the publication of this debate, and apologise for any inaccuracies in transcription.

DALLOS Ladies and gentlemen, you have kindly supplied a substantial number of questions for discussion tonight. Here is the list -

Many questions concern outer hair cell properties, motility and feedback.

1 What is the real voltage sensitivity of the motile response?

2 What is the real frequency limit of effective feedback from the outer hair cells?

3 Is it possible to have a bat at 80kHz, whose frequency selectivity is aided by wiggling hair cells?

4 What is the frequency limit of the spontaneous acoustic emissions?

5 OHCs show voltage related expansion and contraction cycles ... how are those movements coupled to the basilar membrane/tectorial membrane complex? What is the mechanism of coupling?

6 Is there a consenus on slow motility - is it an actin-myosin reaction and if so where is the myosin?

7 Why do OHC have W-shaped stereocilia configurations, and IHC straight configurations? Then there is the topic - mammals versus other creatures. There are a whole host of questions under that heading.

8 Adaptation has be shown very elegantly in various non-mammalian hair cells. Does it exist in mammalian haircells and how can this be demonstrated?

9 Some people would like to see a census on ion channels in various types of hair cell. Certain types that have been patch clamped, voltage clamped etc., and "put through the wringer" - we have a good idea of the variety of ion channels that exist in them but that's mostly submammalian species. Can we get some kind of an overview? What are the commonalities of existing ion channels and what are the differences?

10 What messages from lower creature results can be carried over to the mammals or do we have to rediscover everything over again when we study a new species?

11 What is the real speed of transducer channels? In bats we have microphonic responses at 100kHz. What is the evidence that ion channels do open and close at those rates? And if they don't, what are those microphonics doing and where do they come from, and if they do, what is their kinetics and how do they do it?

12 What determines the asymmetry of the transducer function? e.g., in most *in vivo* experiments, it's asymmetrical, showing hard saturation, and in many *in vitro* experiments it is more symmetrical. What is the mechanism of this difference? What determines the hard saturation for example?

13 The multiplicity of mechanisms! Only a decade ago we thought that all ears work the same way. But now we think differently. That Australian skink we heard about with two differents kinds of papillae, and the alligator lizard is another well known example but there are others where, within a particular auditory organ, there are apparently separate mechanisms. Why? What is nature accomplishing by this, and can you carry this to the mammalian organ? Does the apex function differently from the base?

14 Finally we should talk about the vulnerability of the cochlea. Why when you open it and do something nasty to it, such as put a radioactive source on the basilar membrane, does it start to deteriorate?

The Role of the Motile Response

So, we begin with question 1. What is the real voltage sensitivity of the motile response? Ashmore and others have given us some figures. An electromechanical conversion ratio of 20nm/mV. With a capacitive high frequency roll-off of potential, at 15kHz that's 0.2nm and at 80kHz that's 0.03nm. Is that big enough to do anything? Are the numbers right? Can we assume that what we see *in vitro* can be translated to the *in vivo* conditions? Are the numbers we have misleading?

ALLEN I remembered from Joe Santos, 30nm/mV max, 15 on average. You have then to include the loading by the cochlea...then the frequency response.

DALLOS The loading? You can't include that because you don't know the numbers. I just picked 500Hz as the corner frequency of the outer hair cell for the frequency response of the membrane filter.

ASHMORE One of my slides showed the figure 20nm/mV and this was the mean for apical cells. For basal cells the figure is slightly smaller. The next slide suggests that for the apical cells, the frequency break point at about 150Hz. Basal cells which appear to have a larger input conductance may have a breakpoint of 500Hz.

PARTICIPANT Is this the time constant of the movement or the membrane?

ASHMORE The membrane!

DALLOS The maximum receptor potential is 30mV, so you can take the cut-off of 500Hz and 20nm/mV, go up to 15kHz and you get 0.2nm movement.

RUSSELL But that's for the most apical turn haircell!

DALLOS So, I'm being optimistic!

PARTICIPANT But what is the time constant of the movement itself? 1ms, 2ms? That's 80 Hz so the limiting factor is the time constant of the movement

ASHMORE Well I don't think we should be talking about length changes, rather forces.

ALLEN Look if you can't produce a displacement with *no load* that's greater than 0.2nm, who cares what the force is!

PARTICIPANT The displacement might not be the right thing to look at. You've got to see how much energy this cell can feed back into the system at a certain frequency, and if you assume that mechanism instantaneously follows the voltage, then you see that the energy the mechanism can feed back into the system is independent of frequency. Because if you assume a viscous load, the energy depends on the velocity, not the displacement. On the this model the velocity is independent of frequency.

DALLOS Everybody understood that?

MOUNTAIN The load is always going to be greater than the load of the cell itself. As Jont Allen says, if it can produce no more than 2/10nm movement it's not going to create any more when it's got a load on it.

ALLEN Well what we're missing here is the nanometer displacement of the basilar membrane at threshold. You've just estimated the largest displacement under the largest stimulation conditions - now let's get the lowest bound of the basilar membrane at threshold at the same frequency. I've been hearing 1/2 nm.

DALLOS No, I translated my figures down to threshold.

PARTICIPANT The basilar membrane is a passively resonant structure alright, so that means you don't have to generate all this displacement you need by the haircell, you only have to compensate the losses. You have a lot of cycles to build up the displacement.

MOUNTAIN But the BM is probably critically damped!

ZWISLOCKI It seems to me that it's energy not displacement we should look at. What we want is the energy lost through viscosity.

KIM So let's get the force and the displacement - both of them, and that will allow us to get the energy.

DALLOS We know displacement, I'm not sure how you're going to get the force.

ALLEN The viscous drag? - that's not easy to estimate.

ASHMORE Well you can make a crude estimate of the force these cells can produce, and I thought this was about 200pN for 100mV command step. That's the maximum force of elongation in isolation for a step input.

KIM Let's say at 100Hz - what would be the displacement? A micron?

ASHMORE Yes, that's based on the maximum rate of elongation of the cell.

ALLEN You've got to be pushing against something to measure this displacement. The impedance is going to be a factor. You don't want to take the open circuit displacement - but the loaded displacement.

KIM So the viscosity of the medium has to come in.

ASHMORE And that's what it's based on. It seems to me that we can make crude estimates of force in the cell.

DALLOS Well, do we know what sort of energy requirement we have?

DEBOER Could we guess how many haircells would be on just one millimeter of the basilar membrane, estimate what we know of the stiffness of the basilar membrane, to have an idea of the impedance against which this cell is working. Taking this force per cell, find out if the energy that can be given to the basilar membrane is worth all the trouble.

ZWISLOCKI That's the *imaginary* part. You have to include the viscosity.

DALLOS I don't think we're going to do this calculation tonight!

DEBOER Yes, but this is what we have to do, and then we can answer the question. We have enough information! From modellers, we know the range of impedances of the basilar membrane. So everybody can go home, for this question at least, and come back in a couple of years, and we can see if there is a consensus!

DALLOS Please send me your results!

ALLEN Well let's say all this works out - this cell, under *open circuit* conditions, puts out 0.2nm and the basilar membrane wants to move more than that at threshold! So you're going to be stretching the cell beyond what it wants to drive! OK?

KEMP But doesn't this energy go in before the peak though, so we are talking about a place where the displacement is a lot less than that?

DEBOER Yes, and that's why we can estimate what the impedance of the basilar membrane would be, roughly.

DALLOS Joe, you look dissatisfied!

ZWISLOCKI Well what is the purpose of all this feedback if not to counteract energy losses - that are converted to heat, and so impedance won't tell you anything except if you calculate what the resistance is! You have to know the resistance of the partition, and the velocity, and then you can calculate the energy loss in the basilar membrane motion, then you can compare that to the energy given by the hair cell, and for that you will need to know the impedance of the hair cell! The haircell must be considered as a source with an impedance, and energy will be lost in that too! You have to know all these things, and I don't think we know them.

DALLOS I agree with you!

JONES We can't use the result of this experiment (hair cell contraction) because its going to produce maximum energy when its working into a similar impedance - that is the resistive part - and we don't know if that is the case. In fact it would be a coincidence! So it might be able to generate considerably more power.

KOLSTON Shouldn't we look at the position of the OHC in the organ of Corti and see if this movement could actually produce the changes in responses that are observed.

NEELY In vitro is it generally agreed that this hair cell is working against its own a viscous load?

SEVERAL PARTICIPANTS Certainly!

NEELY If the displacement falls off at 6dB/oct what happens to the velocity with frequency? - It stays constant! And how much energy is this outer hair cell putting into the fluid *in vitro*? - it's the constant viscous damping times the velocity - that's constant?

DEBOER No Steve, this is all for constant displacement, not velocity. If you're talking about energy or power, you have to relate velocity with pressure and not displacement - so you get 12dB/oct. The force delivered by the hair cell, for high frequencies, is 1/frequency times the displacement. Displacement is 1/frequency times the velocity so the force is 1/frequency *squared* times the velocity. That makes it pretty bad for high frequencies!

ALLEN If I have to drive a radio which needs 110v with an oscillator that gives only 1v, but plenty of power - well I have to have a transformer. So I have to amplify the displacement. You've got to find a way of amplifying the displacement - a transformer which will have the mechanical advantage of allowing you to step it up to the kind of displacements you can use - otherwise you can't use that power.

JONES A transformer *or* a resonant circuit!

ALLEN/TUBIS Transformer, resonators, it doesn't matter!

DEBOER We have the levers in the system! What we are concerned about is that at these high frequencies, the cell can deliver enough force to compensate for lost energy.

MOUNTAIN This discussion is missing a really key point. Jonathan has stated that above 60Hz or whatever, the cell is operating against its own viscosity, and not the external viscosity and so that viscosity appears in parallel with any spring or mass that you may want to calculate. It's adding to the damping of the system. If it can't compensate for its own damping how's it going to overcome the additional damping in the system?

DEBOER That means we have to measure the internal mechanical impedance of the cell!

KIM We need the Thevenin equivalent expression of the cell, i.e., the internal force generator and internal impedance. This could be measured by putting too different values of outside load.

MOUNTAIN Above 60Hz we don't have to worry about its stiffness or mass, only its viscosity - and the mechanical impedance which appears across that cell in its environment.

ASHMORE I've done experiments to determine those numbers.

KIM You mean the source impedance is already known?

ASHMORE It hasn't been calculated yet!

KIM So then when we have that result, we can plug in the *in vivo* organ of Corti parameters and we can see what they do!

DALLOS Have you all had enough of this question? I think we are in agreement that certain measurements have been made, but they have to be made use of and we may very well have some answers. On the other hand - from what I have heard it's still pretty grim! (for cancelling high frequency damping).

The Mechanical Coupling of Hair Cells

DALLOS Now to another question. Supposing we have OHCs with enough energy, how's it coupled back in? Is there any kind of a mechanical lever that can be made use of? Any insights?

ALLEN Look at this sketch of the pillar cells, supporting cells, and hair cells. There is a triangle. Basilar membrane motion is applied to the stereocilia and tectorial membrane through this transformer but it's not a large displacement. I calculated 50um to 60um. This means it's applying a force to the tectorial membrane but not a large displacement. Now you need some resonance to build it up. You've got three rows of OHCs, three linear arrays that are acting so ....

DIUFHUIS Why do you need the larger displacement of the tectorial membrane?

ZWISLOCKI How did you decide on the point of rotation?

ALLEN Arbitrarily!

PUJOL The only problem is, that this triangle doesn't exist, it exists only at the apex. At the base and at second turn you have a different configuration - outer hair cells and Deiters' cells are linearly arranged.

PARTICIPANT What is wrong with the original idea that the cell shortens and just pulls the basilar membrane closer to the tectorial membrane? And that will also generate a movement of the basilar membrane.

ALLEN It all depends on the relative impedances of the reticular lamina and the basilar membrane, as to what's going to move. So you squeeze that - how does that generate any shear?

GEILSER No, not necessarily any shear, but a movement of the basilar membrane, because the tectorial membrane is not in line with....

ALLEN But there is the pillar cell, directly in parallel with it.....

COTANCHE Has anyone measured the compressabilities of the Deiters' cells from the top down?

DALLOS Are you kidding?

COTANCHE Well if it's not a solid object, the haircell could pull up and down and it's not going to have any affect on the basilar membrane!

HUDSPETH What's missing morphologically is a compelling demonstration of any attachment whatsoever between the base of the OHC and the Deiters' cells - particularly as that area is absolutely studded with efferent synapses, which are not noted for mechanical strength. The mere fact that the OHCs can be isolated by just tweaking it does not speak well for a firm bond with the Deiters' cells!

PUJOL I think there is a kind of attachment, and this is not just a normal apposition of membranes, it's not a tight junction, it's something else. A lot of microtubles in Deiters' cells make a firm attachment with the basilar membrane.

KOLSTON That's a good cushion for the OHCs, but what happens when it pulls up?

FURNESS There are also microtubules around the inside of the hair cell around that membrane area - margin upwards.

DALLOS But there is nothing in the gap, is there?

PUJOL There *is* a kind of a dense material.

DENK There is a another point. If you look at the morphology, then you see that the Deiters' cell is connected to the next outer hair cell so that what really happens is, that if the outer hair cell shortens, then you get a change in the spatial derivative of the basilar membrane displacement. It doesn't couple to basilar membrane displacement, more to it's derivative along the travelling wave.

KOLSTON It's so complicated all this geometry that I think you only really benefit if you can do in situ experiments of hair cell motility.

JONES Well there's a related problem that bothers me - Let's assume that the tectorial membrane is more flexible than the basilar membrane. If so, well how do you generate spontaneous otoacoustic emissions? When these things are being generated it looks like the tectorial membrane is vibrating but as a dipole in the worst possible orientation - pushing fluid out on the top, sucking it in on the bottom! Well how do you get anything out of the cochlea?

ALLEN I think you've got the wrong geometry in mind. We are looking for shear between the tectorial membrane and the reticular lamina, not vertical motions. You can't get vertical motions because the fluid that's trapped in that space won't allow it.

JONES I think we are in agreement then - how are we going to get spontaneous emission?

ALLEN Not that way!

JONES Well I don't think you're going to get them any way! What I'm saying is - you're not going to move the basilar membrane. You're not going to move the tectorial membrane much - but if anything's going to move, it's the tectorial membrane, because of the difference in stiffness, and that's not going to generate acoustic emissions.

WIT I think at this point it's good to remember that frogs also have spontaneous emissions, and they have quite different structures inside their ears!

MANLEY Not only frogs but caiman, and birds as well!

KOLSTON It would be really easy if the active process - or whatever you liked to call it - manifested itself by the stereocilia bending, rather than through the length changes, because it's then directly coupled both to the shear motion - i.e., the neural tuning - and to the basilar membrane motion of the cochlea and organ of Corti.

ASHMORE But that's not what happens!

KOLSTON Well, what about the tilting of the cuticular plate?

GEISLER Going back to the mammalian cochlea for a minute, in '86 I published a model that obeyed all of Newton's 14 equations!!! At least I think it's an accurate model - I've never been challenged on it - and you can get, if you assume the reticular lamina can pivot about the tip where it attaches to the top of the pillar cells, you can get the proper phase of the force which opposes viscous friction. Now that's a beautiful theory that was slain by an ugly fact! When Jonathan Ashmore published his work the phase *lead* I was looking for, to make it work, turned out to be a phase *lag*! And unless you entertain such things as "a 270 degree phase lag amounts to a phase lead" then that configuration won't work! I would like to suggest that the tipping of the cuticular plate that Zenner has seen is, both a more efficient way of doing things, and one that might work very well and in the right direction. Because, if you look at that structure, having to push the whole reticular lamina up and down requires a certain amount a force, whereas tipping the cuticular plate inside the hair cell, it seems to me, will require a great deal less force, and will do the proper thing. It will change the angle of the stereocilia relative to the cuticular plate and if you've got them attached to the tectorial membrane, and you rock the cuticular plate, well that's a very efficient way of changing the angle.

DALLOS Is my recollection correct that that's not an observation that is universally supported?

GEILSER It doesn't have to be very big! We're talking about minute angles.

JONES But it seems too slow. How fast is it?

REUTER We see it by a stroboscopic method at 500Hz, and there is no reason to think we would not see it at 2000Hz.

DEBOER Is that [tilting] linear - is it for small displacements, a linear function of the (cell apex) displacement?

REUTER This I cannot say, but it is visible at 500Hz, and it is not an artifact! It could be demonstrated after or during slow motility, after changing the potassium and after treatment with ATP, and with calcium. In my talk I showed an example up to a 500Hz measurement.

DEBOER But that was from an extreme elongation of the cell.

REUTER No, not always so.

DALLOS So, there *is* a potential for pivoting!

KOLSTON It seems strange that Zenner's group see this, but Ashmore says he's never seen it. What's the difference?

ALLEN - and another thing bothers me - if all your forces are up at the cuticular plate and you're swinging this great big hair cell body down there in order to move a few little stereocilia at the top - well it's going to have a lot of viscous drag on the pivot itself.

ZWISLOCKI Well I have to call your attention to the fact that Zenner's experiments were done *not* in the presence of the tectorial membrane so whatever the tectorial membrane does, it's a fact that the tips of the stereocilia were not embeded in the tectorial membrane.

DALLOS Time to move on! Slow motility! Is it a dead horse? Is it an actin-myosin reaction for sure? Where is the myosin? Anybody any insights? Anybody want to discuss it? ...... Nobody cares about slow motility!

Contractile Proteins

RUGGERO There was a poster yesterday which told us where abouts myosin was ... where are the authors?

FURNESS The myosin localisation that was shown on that poster - we used a myosin antibody raised against human blood platelet myosin and we found staining in very similar regions to where the actin is located. We subsequently did a second myosin localisation, using a different myosin antibody and obtained a very different result. In the first case we found it in the stereocilia, which agrees with Macartney et al. 1980, in the second case we did not find any staining in the stereocilia, and this agrees with the Drenkhahn result, and directly contradicts the other result. So we can't really say where the myosin is.

HACKNEY But we can suggest that the variability of the results in the literature might be as a result of either, the antibodies acting on different portions of the myosin molecule, or not being as specific as they have been intended to be. In the absence of detailed biochemistry on those antibodies, it's very difficult to say how specific that was.

FURNESS So we may be saying either different sorts of myosin are at different positions in the cell, or that we are not actually sure which is the myosin that we are staining up.

HACKNEY And actually that criticism applies to all the antibody, cytoskeletal protein work that's been done. For example Flock and Slepecky have suggested tropomyosin is in the stereociliary rootlets, and we would like to see other people repeat that for the same specificity reasons. It's a very difficult experiment to be certain of.

HOLLEY It's a strange cell that doesn't contain actin and possibly a strange cell that doesn't contain myosin! Finding simply the *presence* of actin and myosin gets you nowhere! The only thing that will get you somewhere is if there is an acto-myosin interaction, shown to work with an ATP and possibly calcium dependance, and that those filaments are in a position to do work. The gut brush border people with their (motile/non-motile) microvilli know this to their cost! A lot of work went into that. They said "we have actin and myosin, therefore we have movement, and a non-reversible response". That was a disaster! You really *have* to have more than just actin and myosin.

HACKNEY I agree entirely with that. You don't know whether these proteins are just structural or whether they are involved in any motility. The antibodies we use are from human platelets, which are not well known for their ability to move!

PARTICIPANT Yes they *do* move!

PICKLES Can I put a point in? That same reaction (to antibodies) is in the heads of the pillar cells - and we don't expect they are motile!

FURNESS I think one of the points though, is that since actin-myosin is such an important system in some forms of contraction, one can't just brush it aside.

HOLLEY Yes, but you must test the critical thing - involved with movement!

FURNESS Sure! I agree.

SAUNDERS From a structural basis in the stereocilia, there is no way you can have myosin inside the actin bundle. The only other option is that it's somehow associated with the sides of the actin bundle, and I think in the case of microvilli, it's been somewhere indicated, that the 1-10KD sidelinker proteins are a variety of myosin, and I think if there is myosin indicated (in stereocilia) then it might be this 1-10KD side linker, which would be a different kind of myosin, and not involved in contraction, but with the actin crystal in the membrane itself.

Micromechanics

NEELY Can I just address the question about the W shape of OHC stereocilia. I have here a model made from a piece of paper. [Holds up folded paper]. The W shape, made by folding makes it quite stiff [along the direction of the folds] - excellent for moving the tectorial membrane. In contrast the unfolded "inner hair cell" stereocilial bundles is quite complaint, quite floppy, which would be quite good if you wanted to couple all the displacement to the channels.

DANCER The movement of the outer haircell - how is it possible that one hair cell is moving much more than it's neighbour? For example if you consider the high frequency cut-off of the tuning curve on the basilar membrane, at a high number of dB per octave it means that displacement of one haircell to another is very different. e.g., 30% or 50% less displacement from one to another. How is this possible?

RUSSELL The tectorial membrane is built up of striations, which are lined up with the plane of maximum excitation of the OHCs. The striations are made up of collagen fibrils. Between them, in fact wrapped round each fibril is a band of non-collagenous protein. This is a very viscous substance and so the tectorial membrane is likely to exert radial forces in the excitatory plane of the OHCs and not much in the lateral direction.

ZWISLOCKI I'm sorry, but it doesn't work that way! We measured stiffnesses directly: the stiffness of the tectorial membrane, longitudinally and radially. It's pretty much the same! I don't understand why - logically you're right but....

Models and Irregularities

MOUNTAIN An observation - I think several modellers will agree with me that if you want a model which can produce the sharp tuning which we think is normal in the cochlea, then you have to go to 2000-3000 sections as a minimum to reduce reflections. It's intersting because this starts corresponding to the number of "ranks" of outer hair cells that one sees in a real cochlea. This correspondance makes me think that these roll-offs are quite reasonable.

RUGGERO Yes, but you have too many [sections?]

KOLSTON No, that's only if your model reduces the damping.

MOUNTAIN No, this is for an active model. Does anyone disagree with me?

ASHMORE Is there a consensus on this amongst modellers that that statement is true?

SEVERAL MODELLERS No, I disagree!

ALLEN I think this is just a conjecture.

KOLSTON If the active process is reducing the resistive part, which most people seem to assume, but in fact it may not be true, then yes, David Mountian is correct. Because then you're talking about a model which has very low resistance in each section and you have to have very many sections to stop reflections.

GEISLER I've been playing with 1400 section models, and I don't get reflections with very very high Qs, and we are modelling a full cochlea.

ALLEN I think you are confusing a numerical issue, with a physical energy problem....

TUBIS No, it has to do with the discontinuities in impedance. Reflections due to mathematical artifacts can be of very low level, and they can be distinguished from physical effects.

ZWICKER Maybe I can say a little bit about modelling now! I've been quiet so far! Now you have to be very careful if you raise the Q to very high values in models - when you come very close to oscillation - Q to infinity so speak! Now if you consider discretisation - what you have to avoid is any significant step in impedance from one section to the next. The higher the Q, then the smaller the subdivisions required to avoid reflection. These lead to otoacoustic emission delays which are greater for more sections. Twenty milliseconds is too short to see the DEOAEs for a 500-section model. About 100ms may be necessary. On the other hand, in turtles or chicken, where there only 200 to 400 haircells and no travelling wave, I don't see how you can dissect this. I don't have any idea how you can dissect it in a way that is meaningful for the mammalian cochlea. In nonmammalians, the whole of the basilar membrane is moving, in phase, and what we are looking for is some kind of resonance system which can either be electrical, inside the cell or mechanical, or a combination of both, where the tectorial membrane may be of influence. But I don't see what you can do to make any reasonable sectionalisation for modelling.

DEBOER But in that case also the discretisation along the length is dictated by the number of elements, i.e., hair cells, that are available.

ZWICKER I agree. I would very much like to see whether the membrane or the tissue in which the hair cells are resting - in a frog or another animal that is producing spontaneous emissions - is the whole thing moving? What exactly is going on there? This would be very useful for our thinking. To me there seems a big difference between what's going on in a frog, and a human in which you have a cochlea where travelling waves occur.

DENK There seem to be two things. We are talking first about a discretisation, i.e., if you want to solve this differential equation then you have to put a sort of grid on it and you have to put a certain number of points on it, OK? Then there is a different question - you have the equations actually representing a continuous system and then you *add on* an active feedback, as discrete elements - actually in the physical system discrete elements - these are different issues.

VIERGEVER Does anybody have a decent estimate of the wavelength in the travelling wave in recent tuning curve? Spatially, because the number of points [in a model] should be such that you have approximately 10 points/wavelength, to avoid reflections - 20 if you want to get rid of them all.

REUTER For the pigeon we can say that the smaller and taller cells don't elogate like the guinea pig. We have measured and we see no response in an electric field.

DALLOS So bird "outer hair cells" don't move!

ALLEN Do they have emissions?

MANLEY We've published a paper demonstrating simultaneous emissions in birds. I don't know of any other experiments in birds.

WIT Well we've looked for it in pigeon and we haven't found it.

DALLOS I think the "quantisation" issue has been exhausted for the moment. What about the frequency limit of spontaneous emissions! Do we have any input on that? What shall we say! Do I hear 60kHz?

WHITEHEAD The *lowest* frequency spontaneous emission I've seen is 500Hz. Has anyone seen one lower? This was in a frog, and I could see evoked emission lower, so it wasn't the noise floor.

Hair Cell Adaptation

DALLOS Well that covers the frequency range [for otoacoustic emissions]!. Now Jim Hudspeth and others have shown a fascinating self adjustment or adaptation in the responses of the saccular hair cells and in turtles. Is there any evidence of it in mammalian hair cells and how would you measure it?

HUDSPETH There are two things we could look at. One is the so-called automatic gain control in the cochlea, which might be adaptation, and the other is the issue of adaptation, that is, time dependent diminution of VIIIth nerve fiber responses. Could either or both of these come from [mechanical] adaptation - particularly since Russell has now seen it in mammalian hair cells?

RUSSELL I've seen that if you give a sustained push to the stereocilia of outer hair cells, they are initially 50% stiffer than at about 30ms later. The voltage response of outer hair cells to a step displacement of the stereocilia is initially large, which then decays, in around 30ms. I've not looked at the resetting of the responses with incremental displacements.

DALLOS Have you ever seen it in *in vivo* experiments?

RUSSELL No, but the way to do that is to put a trapezoid sound pressure wave in and record CM, or OHC response.

DALLOS But if the definition of adaptation is a diminution of the response in a sustained stimulus, then it does not seem to happen [in CM] *in vivo*.

RUSSELL If it's a phasic stimulus then it's difficult to say if it's the same as a step. If you put a sustained *displacement* on OHC stereocilia and saw the same effect, then that could be adaptation.

DENK The cells that Ian Russell works with are not quite mature yet, so they may show an adaptation which a mature cell doesn't show. In putting the system together you might expect certain adaptations, which might vanish at later stages.

DALLOS I think it is more important in those preparations that there is no tectorial membrane and you are driving the cilia directly. But if you want to ask the question is there anything in the vivo recording of receptor potentials that's analogous to adaptation in the neural response - the answer is no! Neither the DC nor AC receptor potentials show any semblance of adaptation.

Organ of Corti Irregularities, Otoacoustic Emissions and Delay

ALLEN Going back to an earlier issue, it seems to me that there's growing evidence that spontaneous emissions are associated with discontinuities in the system, at least in the animals with travelling waves. A correlate of that is that there are multiple emissions around one frequency region with periodic spacing that is dependent on the round trip travel time of the system. Do people generally agree with that model first proposed by David Kemp? For me that model is not violated by

Bialek and Wit's experiment [where they were] making a probability distribution of the emission. All that result says is that it's a nonlinear emission and reflection at the site of the proposed discontinuity.

ZWICKER My paper will consider this. There's a big difference between what we call travel time along the basilar membrane - in humans maybe 1.5ms for 1500Hz - twice this for the round trip - and the delay of otoacoustic emissions which is 10-11ms. There's a factor of 3 to 4!. So from that point of view I disagree with Allen.

WHITEHEAD Where did you get your 1.5ms? Is that for a high level stimulus?

ZWICKER Yes! That's what we are talking about.

ALLEN The travelling wave delay drops with higher levels!

WHITEHEAD - and emissions are a low level phenomenon!

DEBOER - and you have the build up of the resonance at that frequency - which is several cycles of 1500Hz. The delay would be several multiples of 0.6ms anyway. 1.5ms is too small certainly. The low level action potential has about half the delay of the evoked emission approximately. So that tallies.

DALLOS So, issue number 1 is the delay time; how long does it take to make the trip? Issue 2 - do the spontaneous emissions really correspond to presumed micropathologies [discontinuities]?

ALLEN - and issue 3 is - how else do you account for multiple emission that seem correlated to each other?

RUGGERO I'd like to answer Bert de Boer's point. We have to distinguish between different kinds of delays. Today there was discussion of a paper that caused confusion because the paper was talking about *group* delays of several milliseconds when I think the question which had motived the discussion referred to what is called in some circles *signal front* delay. This is only one third or one fourth as long. In other words [we need to remember] the delay between the beginning of the response to an impulse and the weighted average which follows several milliseconds after. Now I think that in discussing the delayed evoked emissions the correct thing to be talking about is group delay - but I'm not sure. So now - the low level AP response - I think the CAP are close to worthless! You should look at the delays you get from the single unit responses - for the shortest possible delays.

DEBOER Not the *shortest* delay, but the delay to the peak of the response; and not for intense clicks but for weak clicks...

RUGGERO - but my point is this. Nelson Kiang has a paper in which he has shown very well the relation between the single unit response and the AP. As far as I can remember, what it comes down to is that the AP [near threshold] corresponds relatively well to *group* delay. All you are getting is the center of the response - but that tells you nothing about how fast things can travel along the basilar membrane.

DEBOER Sorry, but the [threshold] *click* AP is not the right thing to talk about because that is a question about which [frequency] fibres are excited. It just happens to be at a certain intensity that at a certain frequency the system is first excited. That's a very complicated thing. I think we should talk about the APs produced by weak *tone* burst stimuli that have been designed in such a way as to give the right trading of frequency and time. *Then* I say that the delay will be about 5ms for 1500Hz.

RUGGERO - but that's the *group* delay!

JONES Yes! There's confusion over group delay and phase delay. Anything that carries information is a group delay - even including the wave front!

DEBOER - but the centre of gravity is the group delay - and that is about 5ms, which is about half the emission delay - as we expect. So I would like to know what Zwicker has to say about this.

ZWICKER I agree that if you lower the level, then you come closer to where we have sharper tuning. Now if you assume you are close to [generating] a spontaneous emission - not quite oscillating - then Q maybe around 100 or so. What kind of a group delay do you expect? It's long, very long, greater than observed otoacoustic latencies! Now all kinds of otoacoustic emission, I think, have the same origin. The difference is that we can look in the time domain (DEOAE) or frequency domain (SOAE). As the feedback changes, the Q value can rise to infinity leading to oscillation (SOAE). I have been surprised that if you measure with electrodes you get 5ms delay time! This must occur somehow by accident! If you go down by 10dB you may get 10ms, and if you go down lower, maybe 20ms.

DEBOER Yes, and that can be nicely modelled, and there is no doubt that it will be in that kind of region. Now your arguement about the high Q would be valid were it not for the fact that the actual [emission] reflection might well take place just where the discontinuity is, or just where the system becomes nonlinear. The local build-up time may not correspond to that high Q - that may explain [the problem you described].

ALLEN The problem I have with what you are proposing here is that Zwicker is thinking of a high Q oscillator - so you should have a delay that is very very long. What I'm talking about [in the model for closely spaced spontaneous emission frequencies] is a delay line with a reflection close to one so the high Q is a result of passing a signal repeatedly between the ear canal and the reflection. That gives you multiple high Q oscillations, but the delay in this case is [still] going to be 5ms [each way].

JONES It's a combination of the two.

ALLEN [Yes]. One way you can separate the two is by controlling the impedance of the transducer that you put in the ear, because that's one of the things that determines the reflection coefficient. [If you made the impedance exactly match the line] and put your pulse in then you won't get all these high Q things and you'll be able to measure the reflection coefficient properly.

DALLOS One final comment on this issue...?

ZWISLOCKI I would like to ask - what creates this discontinuity and how much is it, in terms of the impedance?

ALLEN - only an experiment can determine it!

ZWISLOCKI If there is auditory pathology, what is the first thing that happens in the ear? Outer hair cells are shot! Now how much does this change the impedance of the basilar membrane? I would say very little!

DALLOS That's a very good question.

RUGGERO In the animal that Pat Zurek and Duck On Kim had, there was a tiny, very short [OHC] wipe out and clearly that wipe out was somehow related to the generation of the spontaneous emission in one chinchilla.

DALLOS But isn't it also true that there are many animals where there is no such correlation?

RUGGERO I think that it was a bit too much for chance in the fact that they had measured the animal before, among many that did not have the emissions. They had two with emissions.

ZWISLOCKI Well if there is a wipe out, then the mass of the organ of Corti will be decreased, and that will be a substantial difference [in impedance]. My understanding is that emissions happen very nicely with small damage. Well then there is practically no difference in the impedance then!

ZWICKER Well I agree completely with your feelings - for high levels. When we go to low levels what I think then is that we should not only look at the basilar membrane but also its load, producing the travelling wave. At low levels, we have along with all that, a complete series of negative resistive parts, or feedback loops which produce a different kind of a travelling wave. And if you have a reduction of feedback, this gives you a discontinuity!

ZWISLOCKI We modelled all that, from a simple concept. We said that the feedback system is close to instability, that's how you get the most energy transfer - and if you get a little damage, you start to oscillate. To give you a little hint, in a model we have positive feedback and we don't change at all the energetics of the feedback - what we do is to change the stiffness of the stereocilia in the model - and it oscillates!

Speed of Transducer Channels

DALLOS Time to move on folks! How about *speed of transducer channels*? Back to cell biology! The question is this - what kind of a mechanism is it, that a channel is capable of being excited at 200kHz? Anyone have any ideas?

HUDSPETH Well it's easily done! Reaction times, such as that for channels rattling back-and-forth between two configurations, are set by a rate that's given by Eyring rate theory. The rate at which these can rattle back and forth depends on how big one supposes the gate, which cause the opening and closing of channels, to be. But from molecular spectroscopy it's know that relaxations in large proteins can occur on a nanosecond scale, and I mean substantial changes. By this I mean that movements of amino acid side chains *can* take place in nanoseconds; movements of an arm of a protein or something like that, can take microseconds. [As to the size of the channel], in principle all one needs to block is a pore that, for a haircell's transduction channel, need be no larger than 0.7nm. That's an order of magnitude, based on the largest permeant molecule. That puts it in the realm of say amino acid side chains.

EDITORS [This view met with some opposition - it was agreed that no known channel works at such high speeds. In response the point was made that we were not yet able to measure operationally speeds of 100kHz, for technical reasons, e.g., owing to membrane capacitance. The need to distinguish cause and effect was emphasised - the opening of the channel was the cause under discussion, and measurements tended to be about what happens to the membrane afterwards, when you observe it. Others felt that if known channels could open in a couple of microseconds, then operation at 100kHz was feasible. The question was raised - can a channel open *and* close at a 100kHz rate, as some felt that the closing time was the slow part of the cycle. If the system had to respond at 100kHz then maybe not every channel responded in each cycle....]

HUDSPETH I don't see any difficulty. If the transition to the open state can occur in one or two microseconds, then it seems to me that you can close the channel in one or a few microseconds. Most channels may not want to do that; a voltage-activated channel such as a sodium channel wants to be open long enough to allow an event [the action potential] as long as a millisecond to occur. It would be very inefficient if it should close again in, say, three microseconds. But in fundamental molecular terms there's no difficulty in making a channel that can open and close in a few microseconds. I agree that there is no precedent for it!

Transducer Function Asymmetry

DALLOS What determines the asymmetry of transducer functions? Most that you see have hard saturation on the hyperpolarised side. What is the mechanism? Is it trivial?

NEELY Jim Saunders probably gave us the answer. All channels are not treated equally - different stereocilia undergo different displacements. If the tallest stereocilia are activated by the mechanical stimulus, then you've got different stereocilia undergoing different displacements, or different tip links or whatever. You've got different populations of channels appearing in sections of the stimulus....

EDITORS [A participant who had explored this approach reported that it did not work].

PARTICIPANT Well the problem is that for the *in vitro* preparations, you tend not to see this [asymmetrical] pattern. You tend to get a more symmetrical pattern than you get in the more normal situations. It probably could be that in the *in vitro* situations you are exciting the channels all together - they really are simple two state channels and that in our intact organs we're getting a little different mode of excitation, and were getting a bit of a distribution of forces exerted on the different channels.

EDITORS [In contradiction to this it was reported by another participant that there that some assymetry *was* present in isolated cells].

SAUNDERS Well it depends what you mean by asymmetry. The stiffness gradients of the stereocilia for the displacements in the excitatory and the inhibitory direction appear to be the same. So we can rule out one element - the mechanical input to the hair bundle. Even though the hair bundle exhibits this very interesting asymmetry, its mechanical properties are such that they respond symmetrically to excititory and inhibitory displacements.

RUSSELL We're not sure about that.

SAUNDERS Well you've got data that suggests that -

RUSSELL - not the onset, no. At the onset in the excititory direction they are stiffer.

SAUNDERS - and that's for static displacement?

RUSSELL That's at the onset of dynamic displacement. If you talk about static displacement then I'd agree with you.

SAUNDERS ...at 20Hz or 50Hz or what?

RUSSELL Just a step displacement so far, with a cut-off of about 1400Hz.

SAUNDERS Well certainly high frequency displacements suggest it's symmetrical.

DEBOER Could anybody guess what we would measure if only one tip link would have survived? Would it be asymmetrical or not?

HUDSPETH It would be very small!! On average you'd expect the identical, asymmetrical behaviour. There is one way that could arise that would give a single, exponential relaxation: if the tip link went slack on pushing in a negative direction. Imagine protracting the [input-output] curve down into a symmetrical, Boltzman-like relation, but then falling off it because the linkage goes slack, because an elastic link my be able to bear extension, but not compression.

PATUZZI It seems to me that the assumption of symmetry is based on the fact that the potential energy bias that you propose is directly proportional to displacement. That's a huge assumption! You're dealing with a protein moving next to these gates and changing the potential energy and it's just a huge assumption that displacement of the protein near to those channels will linearly modulate the potential energy!

ZWICKER A comment - If you model the cubic difference tone which is present in the human cochlear, and you use the assumption that what is occurring internally, as determined by the cancellation method, is produced there, then you to have a relatively symmetrical saturation curve, saturating at around 20-30dB on both sides! So I'm very much puzzled that I don't find in the literature, that kind of input-output curve!

FAHEY The asymmetrical curve will produce a difference tone! It has odd and even parts.

ZWICKER Yes, but not in the amounts we want!

FAHEY You expect to see more even products...

ZWICKER The curve presented here has the wrong shape for what we observe psychoacoustically.

ALLEN You are seeing the distortion from the *outer* hair cells, which are symmetrical I think -

DALLOS This is not so in the frequency range where Zwicker makes his observations - around 1000Hz in human beings. You don't see cubic difference tones above 4000Hz do you?

BROWN Yes, up to 7000Hz!

DALLOS Little bitty ones, yes?

ALLEN No! They may be little bitty in the human but in the cat they are much bigger. They are [all] from the outer hair cells as far as I am concerned.

PATUZZI You have to make sure that you're not confusing asymmetry of the [haircell input-output] curve with the operating point on the curve. Also, we've measured in our lab, distortion tones in guinea pig up to 20kHz.

SAUNDERS There's an interesting corollary here - that curve is an asymmetrical curve and one thing we have to realise - with the exception of the squid, the cuttle fishes and the octopuses, all hair cell bundles are staircased - always! Now the staircase varies morphometrically across the organ of Corti in many species, and the question I would like to ask is - do we have any inkling as to what the role of this staircase organisation is? We could start simply and say - well it's there to hang the tip links on so they pass to the body of the adjacent hair, but I think there are other reasons.

KOLSTON In a paper by T. Wright in Hearing Research, he did an analysis of the change in stiffness of the whole bundle along the cochlea of the whole bundle, rather than just the longest one. I think the buttress part is more or less the same length - the longest stereocilia change in length. He found the variation in stiffness of the whole bundle (you assume that the buttress is rigid) is about the same as the stiffness gradient along the basilar membrane.

SAUNDERS I take some issue with those data. The heights of the second, third fourth and fifth rows in vertebrates change across the length of the organ....

KOLSTON - but as much as the length of the long ones?

SAUNDERS No, the changes are complex. It's not a simple ratio. Wright was looking at human data. Those conclusions may not be universal.

DALLOS Now, we are coming to the end; are there any burning issues we forgot, or you'd like to add?

Comparative Aspects

MANLEY One of the questions we've left out is - how much comparative data can be applied to mammals. I'd like to pass on some data that is interesting. We've shown that all active [afferent] auditory fibres in birds innervate only tall hair cells. In other words its like in mammals - that the active fibres only go to the hair cells on the neural side of the papilla. In birds of course you have very many more hair cells in one cross section and you have in one location, maybe a dozen tall hair cells which are innervated by fibres which obviously pass information to the brain. If you look across from the neural [side] to the middle of the papilla the threshold goes up steadily. In other words the hair cells on the most neural side which are furthest from the basilar membrane are the *most* sensitive and those fibres innervating cells which are near the basilar membrane but still not on it, have a threshold of above 90dB! In other words, we have something which makes us think again about the mechanisms of stimulating hair cells. None of these hair cells are on the basilar membrane.

PATUZZI You must be careful in interpreating that because you don't know at this stage whether it was the synapses that were shut off.

MANLEY No, I don't want to imply that the mechanics were necessarily different at all these different cell [positions] but it gives you something to think about. There is obviously something going on which is also going on in mammals. I think the bird as a model system is more attractive in that sense.

Tectorial Membrane

DEBOER I think we forgot one thing about the link between OHC motility and cochlear modelling - that is resonance of the tectorial membrane. Could it resonate? Are people who are assuming that it takes part in cochlear mechanics using the right coefficients, and so on. What does everybody think about that?

DALLOS Well, Joe Zwislocki has had to go, and he's the one to ask! Does anyone wish to address the question?

KOLSTON Am I right in assumming that if the neural tuning is the same as the mechanical tuning, then there is no *resonant* tectorial membrane? Because it implies that the shear motion in the subtectorial space is the same as the deformation of the basilar membrane.

DALLOS - not if you had feedback!

WIT Another question about the tectorial membrane - could it change its stiffness when the temperature changes, or when you inject current into it?

RUSSELL Well, Judith Hasko and Guy Richardson in my lab have been investigating the structure of the tectorial membrane. The collagen composition is fairly well known but there is an unknown matrix which wraps around the collagen fibres. A very strange structure. We nickname it "taglietellin" because that's what it looks like - like a tape. The tape is formed by alternating light and dark fibrils which run parallel to one another within the plane of the sheet. The spacing between the fibrils and the existance of the tape itself is calcium dependent. So if calcium is removed, the tape disrupts, and if calcium is replaced, the tape is recomposed. The matrix is heavily charged and other evidence, for example from Karen Steel, Nottingham, shows that the tectorial membrane can sustain Donnan equilibrium. So, the matrix is not a simple gel, it could also be temperature sensitive. No measurments have been made.

MANLEY In that direction, Kronester-Frei shows that if you put the tectorial membrane in endolymph with EGTA it swells dramatically, and it you put the calcium back again it returns to its original size. In contrast, sodium has an irreversible shrinkage effect - at least in mammals. That's something we should also remember. Thalmann has shown that in bird the structure of the tectorial membrane is probably substantially different at the molecular level.

RUSSELL The matrix of the avian tectorial membrane is different.

Role of the EP

SAUNDERS Another interesting thing that struck me is that - if you're dealing with dissociated hair cells, or hair cells in culture medium, with bird cochleae, or intact mammalian cochleae or vestibular organs - the endocochlear potential surrounding the apical pole is tremendously different [in all these cases] and we've not addressed at this conference, what the implications of that might be. The birds exhibit frequency selectivity and sensitivity comparable to that of mammals, with an EP that is substantially smaller.

DALLOS Well the driving force of course is the sum of the EP and the cell polarisation.

RUSSELL If Brian Johnstone were here I think he would say that the [addition of an] EP simply gives you a 6dB increase in sensitivity. Another suggestion, made in fact by von Bekesy, was that the role of the endolymph was to preserve the structure of the tectorial membrane. Keith Bosher for example, has shown that the calcium concentration of the endolymph is very highly controlled - it's only 30 micromolar - but it must be secreted against a gradient to be 30 micromolar. So maybe the whole of the endolymph is not primarily to provide the driving force but to preserve the tectorial membrane.

PATUZZI [On the point about 6dB]. It may just be 6dB to us auditory physiologists but for say a resistor - it's a doubling - and in a mammal cochlea, if you wipe-out the EP [you reduce the driving force by 50%] in an animal that has an active process, then you'd expect a 40dB change in sensitivity! The fact that there *is* no EP in the bird might mean that the "active process" is not active at all!

DALLOS I think that's a pretty good place to stop! Thank you all!

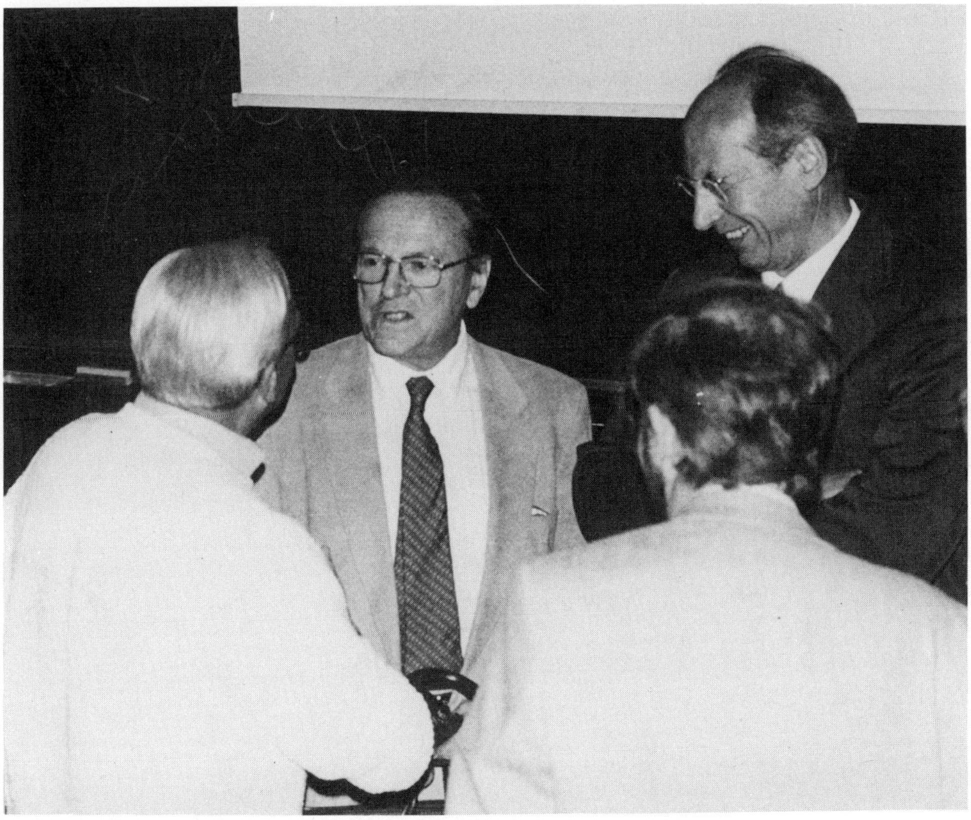

J.J. Zwislocki, T. Gold, D.T. Kemp and E. Zwicker

5. OTOACOUSTIC EMISSIONS

HISTORICAL BACKGROUND TO THE PROPOSAL, 40 YEARS AGO, OF AN ACTIVE MODEL FOR COCHLEAR FREQUENCY ANALYSIS

T. Gold

Center for Radiophysics and Space Science
Cornell University, Ithaca, N.Y. 14853

Editorial Note

Professor Thomas Gold, FRS, is best known for his work in astronomy and cosmology - particularly the theory of continuous creation of matter, the nature of pulsars as rapidly-rotating high-density neutron stars, and his controvertial non-biological hypothesis for the origin of oil, currently receiving supporting evidence from a 6 km deep borehole in Sweden. He did, however, start his research career in hearing and published papers [1,2, see also 3] which although prophetic, were not accepted by the auditory establishment at the time.

With an important emphasis of this meeting clearly on motile cellular mechanisms and the role of active mechanical processes, it seemed appropriate to the organisers of this Workshop to invite Prof Gold to relate to us the atmosphere in hearing research 40 years ago. We reproduce his talk substantially verbatim with notes, references and additions in square brackets.

Gold

Thank you Dr. Kemp [for your introduction]. You don't know what a pleasure it is for me to see what a change has overcome the fraternity that works on hearing. I got into this field in 1946, immediately after the war. During the war my good friend R.J. Pumphrey was a quite senior person - even though he was a biologist! - working on radar - and in fact he became very knowlegeable on all the sophistications of radar. I had made my way in the Admiralty Signals Establishment also, and was in charge of a laboratory called "New Devices" - that is - radar devices, and I'd just built a successful radar Doppler set so I was into, at that time, very forward thinking electronics.

When I returned to Cambridge after the war, Pumphrey was working in the Zoology lab in Cambridge and I had a job in the Cavendish, building the world's largest magnetron. While I was building this magnetron I was seduced to become, so to speak, the "tame physicist" in the Zoology lab. I was handed around from one person to another, through Pumphrey, to explain to one person after another all kinds of trickeries of physics which they thought that I understood! In the course of this, Pumphrey confronted me with a number of puzzling things about the mechanism of hearing, and the next thing was that I got a grant from the Medical Research Council to actually work with Pumphrey, and I worked for two years with him. Pumphrey taught me how to anaesthetise guinea pigs and to shove little electrodes into their eighth nerve and record their responses. We became quite proficient -` Pumphrey was a very good experimenter - at repeating experiments that were done at the time on cats, etc. Then I started to think - in my capacity as a tame physicist - I started to think "well what could such a mechanism - the hardware of the ear - what could it do?" . And I concluded very quickly that the degree of resonance that could be achieved in a passive system was of course limited. The sharpest limitation that was easy to calculate was just from the viscosity of water. But of course I realised that there would be other limitations that might be equally or more important but the viscosity of water alone was quite sufficient to persuade me that one could not obtain anywhere near the sharpness of frequency discrimination that we subjectively had - nor the sharpness of frequency discrimination that comes from the masking curves. We did quite a bit of work on masking. We saw how sharply masking cuts off on the high frequency side, and that sharpness fitted quite well with the subjective frequency discrimination one had. We thought that that really meant that the cochlea must possess a mechanical response system which was as sharp as these observations indicated, and that was just not compatible with the viscous damping.

Well, I puzzled very much about that for some time, and then one day when I was sitting in a colloquium in the Cavendish - listening to an extremely dull physics colloquium - nothing to do with this subject - and my mind strayed, and I said to myself - "Boy! If the thing only had a positive feedback in it, all these problems would disappear wouldn't they?' And then, well, I thought that biology is awfully clever usually. If some mechanism can use energy from the body to overcome the damping in the system - to make it more sensitive, and to make the frequency discrimination better - then surely, it would have invented that.

Since I knew about regenerative receivers and all that kind of technology in radio, I was quite aware of the fact already in 1947 that one would not wish to put a "detector" at the front end of a receiver. It was pretty clear to me that you had to have some kind of amplification using body energy rather than to have a nonlinear detector as the first element. So I said to myself "surely nature can't be as stupid as that to go and put a nerve fibre - that is a detector - right at the front end of the sensitivity of the system". So I quickly convinced myself within the time of that dull colloquium that I was right. I went storming into Pumphrey and told him and he immediately said "Yes, of course you're right, why didn't we think of this earlier". Then I wrote this up as a dissertation for a Trinity Fellowship, which I received, because William Rushton, a great physiologist of the day, and a very clever man, saw there was a merit to this story. He propelled me through the fellowship election and that set me up in a big way, and I could then work with Pumphrey for some time.

I did work for some time on this subject but, the dilemma was that for a young man to work in a field were there was no audience - was *very* difficult. The kind of audience I had? For example, I remember giving a lecture in London - *very well attended* - to the otologists in London, Harley Street, in one of the big buildings there. All the ancient otologists and neurologists in London were assembled there. And as I looked over my audience I noticed that there were two kinds of people there; those that had a twitch, and those that had an ear trumpet! Well I suppose I'm as ancient now as most of those people were then but they looked to me very ancient at the time! It was absolutely hopeless to put these sophistications across to them. And I got very discouraged, and instead invented theories of cosmology and one thing and another and drifted out of the hearing field.

Well it really took thirty years from that time before I saw there was any kind of an understanding of the complexities of this subject. I was greatly helped in recent years by Charles McCutchen who works at the Public Health, Bethesda, Maryland, and he kept me informed over the years of new discoveries. Initially he wrote to me "Prof Frisch told me years ago that you had a theory of hearing that said roughly - frequency discrimination is good, yet the physical mechanism has high damping, therefore there must be positive feedback somewhere in the mechanism". So he knew that, and understood, and kept me informed and one of the items of information that he sent me was the Rhode paper [4] which I was jubilant about of course!

We had written in the 1948 paper on the physical basis of the action of the cochlea and we clearly spelled out that when you observed it on a live cochlea the frequency response curve you would see would be a curve that rises steeply and cuts off very steeply. I had discussed at length in 1948 with von Békésy at Harvard, that the observations that he made on the dead cochlea [5] were unrepresentitive. But he wouldn't have that! He thought that there must have been some cunning neural mechanism that somehow steepens up the subjective response. He knew it was already sharp in the VIIIth nerve. But he thought that maybe there was something in the nerve net in the cochlea that intervened and made some cunning trickery that sharpened up the response curve going to the nerve. And I told him at the time "Look what enormous amplitude discrimination you would need to possess in order that the flat curves you produce could be identified not only with one note present - but in the presence of many notes which overlapped on your curves enormously!" - but he didn't have any evidence for it - and then to work out where the little wiggles were on that curve, that was phenomenal! But he said "well maybe the amplitude discrimination is not carried into the central nervous system but its available out there locally".

Well, I couldn't believe that! Then Pumphrey and I actually did an experiment on what we called the phase memory of the ear. What we did was to create pairs of pulses of a few cycles of oscillation, separated by several milliseconds of nothing, with the phase of the pulse continuous across the empty interval or with the phase reversed. How well could we tell the difference as a function of the length of the empty interval? How long could that interval be so that you could tell the difference whether the phase was this way up or the other way up. That, you now all understand clearly, but at the time only we understood that, I think, and no-one else. That was of course the same thing as saying that I'm making an overall frequency curve which is an interleaved set of wiggles [1, Fig. 9]. If you Fourier analyse this situation it is the most confusing that you could make for an intrinsically wide-band receiver, for singling out the individual frequencies. So we looked at that and we convinced ourselves that, yes you have to be dealing with an effective Q of the order of 100-200 rather than a Q of about 5 which was the absolute maximum that I could get from any kind of a passive system in the presence of the viscosity of water.

But Békésy also, I must say, seemed quite unaware of the necessity to apply the correct physical scaling laws between the large models that he built and the observations on the cochlea that he had. I explained to him that Q is really the same as a Reynold's number and Reynold's number is proportional to L, the linear dimensions. In his model he had his model dimensions 55 times larger, or something, and that made a big difference with the same viscosity. So I returned from my meeting with Békésy even more convinced that I was correct because, before I met him, I may have had the viewpoint that well, maybe these great men they have something up their sleeve that we don't know about that I don't understand. But when I really came face to face with him I became more convinced that really we had to pursue this.

Well then, over the years the various predictions that we had made at the time came to pass one by one. The predictions that we made in the 1948 paper, if I may be so blatant as to remind you of them we said that:

1) there should be active fibres in the position of some of the hair cells.

2) the mechanical observation of the live cochlea should give a narrow band response, quite unlike the wide response that Békésy observed, and especially the sharp cut off on the one side.

3) it would be very unlikely for a positive feedback system to be *always* stable and we therefore expected that there must be pathological cases where the stability mechanism didn't work right and therefore there should be objective tinnitus. We had tried to induce objective tinnitus in one way or another. Actually we did the wrong thing, you see we took aspirin, which I learned today stops emissions! But whatever we did we couldn't measure it. We wrote that we if we had more sensitive instrumentation than we had at our disposal we might be able to measure it.

4) And then we also said that, of course, such a system with positive feedback must have a nonlinearity in it and if it has a nonlinearity in it then it will explain in the right sense the apparent change in frequency [pitch] with loudness.

These were the four points that came out of that paper - three of them being predictions. And they came, one after the other, to pass. It was Rhode [4] who demonstrated in the first place the mechanical tuning situation in the live cochlea. There was that family that was reported, the baby having a 14 kHz noise coming out of its ears and the father also had noises coming out of his ears, and one could easily measure them [7]. That paper was sent to me by McCutchen. Then came the story [8] that the outer hair cells were motile units that were active. We had said in

1948 that we know that there is the microphonic potential - we measured it on our rabbits very well. We judged that the amount of energy in the cochlear microphonic potential was more than the incoming sound. It was not easy to be firm about that, but we were pretty sure that was so. Therefore, we only needed a transducer going from electricity back into mechanics to complete the cycle and we thought that that was probably one set of the hair cells. Well, I think that's probably the right story!

I'd like to show you what we then understood about the full mechanics. I wrote a paper together with Ben Noble in 1948-9, to say that instead of individual (resonant) elements we should look at it as a transmission line and of course, being at that time an electrical engineer, I thought in terms of electrical equivalents and it is generally easier to think in terms of an electrical analogue. We called voltage- pressure difference, current- volume current, capacitance- volumetric compliance, and inductance- volumetric inertia. I showed Pumphrey, when he asked me "why is the input at the high frequency end" and I said "well it has to be at the high frequnecy end because such a transmission line looks like this. It is a transmission line only up to the point of resonance and then it becomes an inductance network beyond the point of resonance which is an attenuator at frequencies above the frequency of resonance, so the signal doesn't run over in that direction, so that it's a unidirectional system. So the input has to be at the high frequnecy end. The largest current will flow at the place of resonance". We worked out various things about the characteristic impedance, which is the square root of the distributed inductance over the distributed capacity. The velocity, as a function of frequency at a point, showed a peak for certain parameters and we compared this to the physical quantities. The Q of a physical system would scale the same as Reynold's number as I said, and we checked that the impedance values were approximately correct, to see if this kind of a model could give you the right answer for the match to the air outside and so on. The impedance of air is 41.5 in cgs units, the eardum size was known, the compliance was approximately known, and it matched the air very well. The best match for transferring the sound inside would be 10 cgs units, and the velocity that the cochlear would have going through the stapes, with the matching taken into account. It would all tell you what the velocity of propagation would be of this transverse wave running over the basilar membrane. That came to 12.5 mm/ms which was later observed by Rhode, so we were very close. My friend at the time - Ben Noble - who was a mathematician, took this model at my request and calculated on a differential analyser (that's all that we had!) the different response curves that you would get for the various unknowns, Q for example, and what sort of sideways coupling between the fibres. We calculated the displacement of the line at one point for various frequencies and for different coupling sideways.

Now if you have very little coupling then you have almost independent curves like you would have when you shout into your piano - where there is very little coupling beteen the strings. If you increase the amount of coupling between one fibre and the next then you will come to a curve where the peak is less high but the cut off is much sharper on the high frequency side.

Unfortunately Ben Noble then got a job somewhere else and left before the paper was quite finished and it was never published! I'm sure that by now much more sophisticated similar computations have been made, and I'm sure the results will agree with what is nowadays observed. And that's really all that I wanted to tell you.

Perhaps I should tell you of some of the contacts of recent times. I was particularly delighted to have, not long ago, a very generous letter from Halliwell Davis, the old man of hearing, who is now 92. He had had correspondence with Pumphrey and me in 1948 and he at that time was not very benevolent to our viewpoint! So it was particularly nice to receive a letter from him saying that he is now writing up some historical material and he points out that the active cochlea is now clearly a proven fact!. He said "I'm sure your 1948 paper is now a collector's item!". That was very nice of him.

So where do we go from here? Of course, I've been following the recent progress. McCutchen told me of the possibility of producing a stimulated emission [9]. I must admit that I was too negative on that - that one could evoke an emission. He had thought that you should get an emission out for a time as long as the effective Q of the fibres implied. I wrote back and I said - "well that's wrong. You would only get it out for the inaccuracies of the frequency response of the cochlea. If the neighbouring fibres were neatly overlapping as they ought to be, to make a smooth curve, then you would get practically nothing out. The individual fibres would all oscillate for some time, as predicted by the Q, but they will all cancel their outputs. Neighbouring fibre outputs would cancel. The overall response would be given by the overall input response - and that's wide - and if it's wide then there's no long time constant involved". That was difficult to swallow but that's how it has to be. That fact that we now produce the evoked sound, the evoked sound coming out, it is the inaccuracies of the system that account for the time constants of that sound - and not the intrinsic time constants. I'm sure that you are mostly aware of that [10]. But that was a very difficult thing to put across to people. But what I said was that if you take a piano and clap your hand you hear all the ringing of all the strings, but if you go and put 20 times the number of strings into a piano and clap your hands in it - you won't hear its response! That's a little tricky!

Well thanks very much for listening to me, and its very nice of you to have invited me.

References and notes

1. Gold, T. and Pumphrey, R.J. (1948) Hearing I. The cochlea as a frequency analyzer. Proc. Roy. Soc. B, 135, 462-491.
2. Gold, T. (1948) Hearing II. The physical basis of the action the action of the cochlea. Proc. Roy. Soc. B, 135, 492-498.
3. Gold T. (1988) The theory of hearing. In Highlights in Science, Ed H. Messel, Pergmon Press, Sydney, pp. 149-157.
4. Rhode, W.S. (1971) Observations on the basilar membrane in the squirrel monkeys using the Mössbauer technique. J. Acoust. Soc. Am., 49, 1218-1231.
5. Békésy, G. von (1949) On the resonance curve and decay period at various points on the cochlear partition. J. Acoust. Soc. Am. 21, 245-254.

6. See ref. 1, Fig. 9.
7. Glanville J.D, Coles R.R.A. Sullivan B.M. (1971). A family with high-tonal objective tinnitus. J. Laryngol. Otol. 85, 1-10. See also - Wilson, J.P. and Sutton, G.J. (1983) "A family with high-tonal objective tinnitus" - an update. In: Hearing - Physiological Bases and Psychophysics (Eds: Klinke, R. and Hartmann, R.) Springer, Berlin, pp. 97-103.
8. Brownell, W.E. (1983) Observations on a motile response in isolated outer hair cells. In: Mechanisms of Hearing (Eds: Webster, W.R. and Aitkin, L.M.) Monash Univ. Press, Clayton, pp. 5-10. See also - Brownell, W.E., Barder C.D., Bertrand D., DeRibaupierre Y., (1985) Evoked mechanical responses of isoloated cochlear outer hair cells. Science 227, 194-196.
9. Kemp, D.T. (1978) Stimulated acoustic emissions from the human auditory system. J. Acoust. Soc. Am., 64, 1386-1391. See also - Kemp D.T. (1987) Hearing in Focus? In Royal Institution Proceedings Vol 59. Ed. D. Phillips, I. Williams, S.T. Nash, pp. 185-213.
10. These ideas were later independently developed in - Wilson, J.P. (1980) Model for cochlear echoes and tinnitus based on an observed electrical correlate. Hear. Res., 2, 527-532. Wilson, J.P. (1980) Model for cochlear function and acoustic re-emission. In: Psychophysical, Physiological and Behavioural Studies in Hearing. (Eds: G. van den Brink and F.A. Bilsen) Delft University Press, pp.72-73. Sutton, G.J. and Wilson, J.P. (1983) Modelling cochlear echoes: the influence of irregularities in frequency mapping on summed cochlear activity. In: Mechanics of Hearing (Eds: E. de Boer and M.A. Viergever) Delft Univ. Press, pp. 83-93.

CM AND OAE CHANGES FOLLOWING TRANSIENT EFFERENT EXCITATION

D.T. Kemp and M. Souter

Functional Analysis Laboratory
Audiology Department
UCMSM Institute of Laryngology and Otology
330 Gray's Inn Road, London WC1X 8EE

Introduction

Electrical stimulation of the efferent system produces changes in both electrical and mechanical cochlear responses. The AP is depressed, CM is enhanced and otoacoustic emissions (OAEs) are modified (Fex, 1962, Mountain, 1980, Siegal & Kim, 1982, Wiederhold, 1969, Wiederhold & Kiang, 1970, Robertson & Gummer, 1985). Most published data shows post stimulation changes that last for about 200ms following 100-200ms of 400 shocks/second COCB excitation (see Wiederhold & Kiang, 1970).

The temporal fine structure of efferent action on the cochlea has only recently been investigated. Kemp and Souter (1988a,b) examined post efferent cochlear response changes with a 1ms temporal resolution and with transient electrical excitation at lower intensities than used by previous workers; more compatible with physiological activity levels (Robertson & Gummer, 1985). They discovered a rapid onset of effect within 12ms of the efferent excitation, followed by a rapid fall towards 30ms with a tendency to form a notch. The subsequent slower decay with a 200ms time constant was as reported by previous workers.

Detailed observations of the way that CM and OAEs are dynamically modulated by mild transient efferent stimulation are of value in allowing us to explore the functioning dynamics of the cochlear-neural control system, and its possible role in maintaining cochlear mechanical responsivity. In this paper we seek to further delineate the changes in the cochlear microphonic and otoacoustic emission caused by transient efferent stimulation. In particular we examine the induced amplitude and phase changes as a function of time and two tone interactions.

Methods

Guinea pigs were used for this study. All measurements were made under neurolept anaesthesia and Flaxedil was used to eliminate electrically evoked muscle spasms. Electrical stimulation was delivered to the COCB as described in Kemp and Souter (1988a). It consisted of 10v, 100us pulses applied to the COCB via a bipolar electrode. Each pulse was separated from the next by 2.5ms, and a typical transient burst consisted of 5 pulses, lasting 10ms in total. A time between 100 and 200ms was left between burst applications. Acoustic stimulation was delivered by a speculum, at 2000Hz 80dB SPL plus in two tone experiments a second tone at 2200Hz, 80dB. A round window electrode and an ear canal microphone provided the signals for analysis. Two complementary signal analysis methods were employed to derive amplitude and phase information as a function of time for the CM and OAE responses.

Analysis method one was designed to give medium time resolution (down to 15ms) maintained over periods of minutes. Several minutes of raw response data were recorded on digital tape (122us per pair of data points, acoustic and CM). Recording was in 100 or 200ms blocks triggered 15ms after cessation of the shock burst (to avoid electrical artifacts). A free running oscillator provided the acoustic stimulus. Recorded data was then replayed in sections into a software based, spectrum analyser. With this we could track the amplitude and phase of the stimulus tone, or (in two tone work) every primary and distortion product, as a function of time, by analysing serial time sections. We used sub and supra burst interval time sections. The analyser was capable of multicomponent phase and amplitude distortion component analysis, with vector averaging. The phase reference for each sample was taken from primaries on the acoustic recording channel. (3).

Analysis method two was designed to give high amplitude and temporal resolutions over small time window (0.01dB and 1ms) within a limited post excitation time window (100-200ms). It has been described Kemp and Souter 1988a. It consisted of synchronous differential averaging of the wide band response to a single continuous tone (phase locked to the trigger pulse). Response samples (100-200ms long) were taken after each efferent shock burst. A long averaging time (256 sums) was needed to extract the OAE effect from the ear canal sound field. The differential technique served to eliminate the large part of the CM/Ear canal acoustic signal which was not affected by the efferent stimulation and cancelled most of the electrical artefact allowing data within 3 ms of shock burst termination to be obtained. Modulations of less than 0.01dB to be seen but with this method, high resolution is at the expense of failing to register any slow changes, lasting longer than the sample duration(ie 100-200ms).

Results

A) THE ENVELOPE OF EFFERENT EVOKED COCHLEAR PERTURBATIONS

Sustained efferent stimulation by 5 shock bursts repeated at 100-200ms intervals caused a mean elevation in the CM of between 1 and 3dB. Figure 1a shows the CM elevation envelope during an episode of efferent stimulation obtained by method one with 100ms resolution. It reveals a rounded onset covering 10-20 shock burst presentations. The initial rise following the first shock bursts was only 2/3 of the final value of 1.2dB, achieved after about 2 seconds. This does not however imply a 2 second onset time for the primary efferent effect. Using smaller time sections for analysis, (15ms/point) (see fig 1b) we can see that between

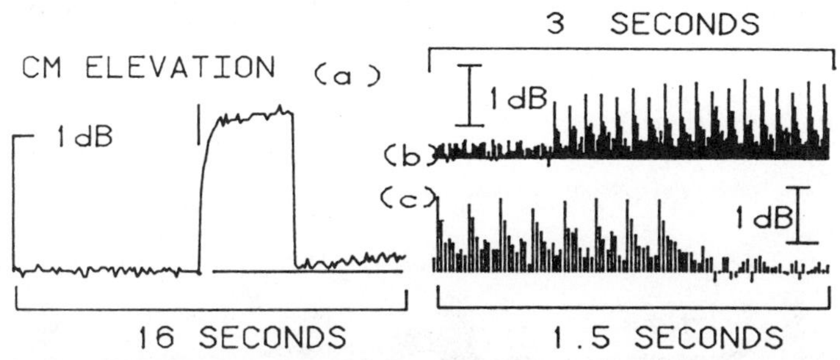

FIGURE 1. Efferent induced CM elevation as a function of time, obtained by method 1. (a) Mean elevation between shock bursts (8 shocks/second). Close up (from another animal) of the onset (b) and termination (c) of stimulation, with ordinates giving the CM elevation every 15ms.

each shock burst the effect is strongest in the first 15ms section displayed then decays rapidly. The time constant is of order 45ms. The rise in elevation can be traced in fig 1b.

To explain the slow mean elevation rise (fig 1a) we could propose that the residual elevation per shock burst decayed with a time constant of around 2 seconds and that the effect of each new burst was additive with respect to the residual. This longer time constant should also be seen as an off decay. Fig 1c shows the elevations at burst termination. The residual effect decays with time constant of only 200ms to the pre base line plus about 0.1dB. This post stimulation level then increases at about 0.04dB/second for tens of seconds. (see fig 1a). This overshoot could indicate that some longer term adaptation of the system had occurred, but it does not explain the onset rise. Our data is consistent with the hypothesis that it is the increment/burst which rises over 2 seconds with repeated bursts, not simply the residual base line.

Using the highest temporal resolution available with method one (15ms as in fig 1 band c) and averaging post shock perturbation decays over the whole of the plateau period to in increase precision we were able to define the amplitude and phase deviation of CM as a function of post efferent time. (fig 3a and b). Figure 3c and d is the vectorially derived deviation ie the pre and post shock CM vector difference. The decay of the disturbance between bursts is seen to be not a simple exponential decay but possibly a two stage decay. The initial decay has a slope suggesting 30ms time constant the rest, 75ms.

No efferent evoked changes in the ear canal sound level could be detected by method one, down to the practical measuring limit of 0.01dB. This was expected as the primary otoacoustic emission level in the meatal coupling used was 40dB below the acoustic stimulus. A 1dB change in emission would thus cause only a 0.01dB change in ear canal sound.

Having established the overall envelope of the changes occurring we used method two to examine inter-burst changes in more detail, and to obtain the sensitivity to see OAE changes. Figure 2 shows the differential waveform envelopes obtained. Fig 2a shows the differential

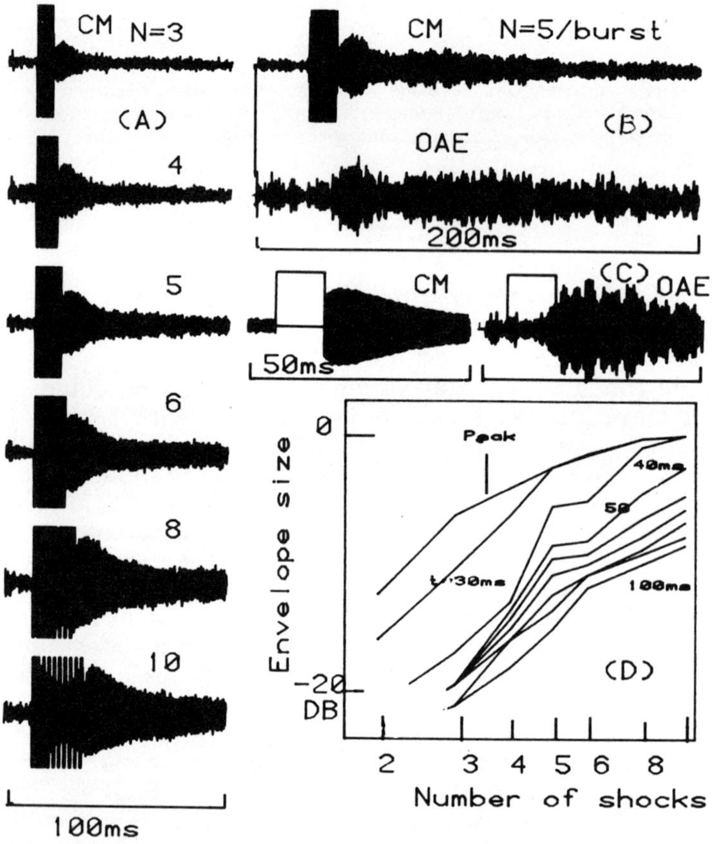

FIGURE 2. (a) Left column of CM differential waveform envelopes for 6 shock burst lengths (3-10). The artefact marks the stimulation. (b) For another animal CM and OAE 5 shock envelopes show initial burst (as in (a) N=3) and a long tail (as in (a) N=10) with a notch between. (c) Another CM OAE pair show the rise time of the effect. (d) From (a) a log-log plot of envelope size with burst size for various points in the envelope.

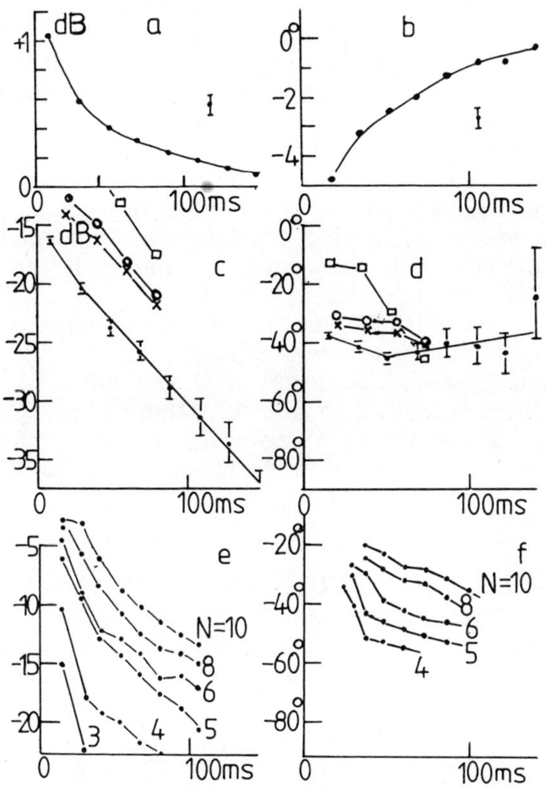

FIGURE 3. Shows intensity (left) and phase (right) as a function of post efferent burst time. (a and b) Perturbed re unperturbed CM from data in 1b. (c and d) solid line. Same data after vector subtraction of unperturbed CM. Circle and cross, data from another animal with (squares) 2f1-f2 data re pre shock DP. (e and f) From experiment in 2a, CM perturbation vector as a function of shocks/burst.

CM (ie the change in CM) for different shock burst lengths. The detailed form of the envelopes differs from animal to animal but CM and OAE envelopes are usually very similar as illustrated by 2b and 2c.

There is some evidence of a two part growth feature of the disturbance at each post shock time as a function of shock number. Figure 2d shows the perturbation (envelope) size as a function shock number/burst for each 10ms period measured from the start of the burst. From 1-5 shocks/burst the growth is fastest, growing roughly as N squared for all time periods. Beyond 5 shocks/burst growth nearly proportional to N. The boundary between the two is marked by a "corner" on all but the most latent points. Clearly data is not available when the burts spreads into the response. The observable peak is plotted and shows near saturation after 5 shocks. The "corner" coincides with the condition that the duration of the shock burst (5 shocks) is 10ms, is of the order of the rise time of the effect, visible in fig 2b and c OAE and confirmed elsewhere by single shock data. This time might be the integration time of the responding system (OHCs) and it is clearly not linear. It appears to be a function of the power (N squared) delivered. As the burst lengthens it runs beyond this time and into the fast decay period. From here effects add linearly.

The growth of effect with N has been further analysed in figure 3e to test the hypothesis that there are two inherent inter-burst time constants. It shows the envelope size as a function of time from first shock onset for various shock numbers. From 2 to 8 shocks there is a rapid initial decay, time constant about 25ms, up to 35-55ms from onset. After 50ms from onset the decay is slower, with a time constant of 100ms. By 10 shocks/burst only this slow decay component is visible beyond the shock artefact.

B) PHASE CHANGES AND VECTOR ANALYSIS

Fig 3b shows the efferent induced phase change in the whole CM as a function of time between bursts, from method one. There is an initial phase change of about -5 degrees (lag), associated with a 1.2dB intensity increase ie the CM is marginally delayed. Both amplitude and phase disturbances appear to decay exponentially with a time constant of about 45ms. By employing vector subtraction of the pre excitation CM the efferent induced disturbance can be extracted as a new response component initially -15dB below normal CM, and then decaying. Its phase remains relatively constant at about -40 degrees re CM (see fig 2d). Thus although the resultant CM rotates back to normal as the perturbation decays this is largely due to the decay in the magnitude of a fixed phase component. We have found similar underlieing phase angles, -30 to -50 degrees relative to the total CM, in each of 5 animals studies with 5 shock bursts. The phase angle does show an small increase with time, and a decrease with increasing shocks/burst. This is shown in fig 3f, using data from method two for various burst durations. The angle with the CM is thus smallest when the strongest effect is taking place.

For otoacoustic data the vector derived efferent component phase was found to be -90degrees re the normal (suppressible) otoacoustic emission component of the ear canal sound field, and this too increases (more negative) with decreasing efferent effect (see fig 3d).

C) EFFERENT EVOKED EFFECT ON TWO TONE INTERACTIONS

Using two tone acoustic stimuli we observed the effect of efferent stimulation using method one. Introducing a second acoustic stimulus tone (f2) ,equal to the first (fl) but of frequency 2200Hz, itself suppressed the CM by 1.8dB. ie comparable to the increase due to the efferent stimulation. Significantly the phase change in CM caused by accoustic suppression was only +1.4 degrees, compared to -5 degrees with efferent stimulation. Unsuppression (ie removal of f2) caused intensity and phase changes in the same sense of efferent stimulation. However expressed as a vector addition, unsuppression added a component -12.6dB re L1,and at -7.5 degrees, whilst efferent excitation added a component -15.3 below, at -32.3 degrees. The efferent effect is thus not simply the opposite of suppression, the former has more effect on phase. This may be related to the fact that CM enhancement by efferent stimulation elevates CAP threshold, whilst unsuppression obviously lowers it.

Both primary tone CM response components suffered equal amounts of change with efferent stimulation. The magnitude of the efferent effect was only marginaly greater (0.1dB) with one tone present than with two. The distortion products generated were also enhanced by efferent stimulation in both the CM and OAE responses. The $2f_1-f_2$ and $2f_2-f_1$ components showed a greater intensity enhancement than the primaries (typically 50-80% more). The phase change was -4 to -5 degrees, not significantly larger. Vector subtraction (fig 3c and d) showed the introduced distortion components to be about 10dB below the distortion normally present, which was in turn 20dB below the primaries. The phase of the added component was -20 degrees re the phase of the distortion normally present. The inter-shock burst decay of the distortion products appear similar to that of the primary disturbance. Resolution was less good with DPs because of the lower signal, and it was not possible to examine these in as much detail as the primaries.

Discussion and Summary

Vector analysis of efferent evoked changes in the CM, OAE and cubic distortion products has shown that the efferent effect could be described as an addition of a small response component at a relatively stable and "universal" phase angle of -45 degrees to the full CM, and -90 degrees to the OAE. Substantial phase angles were *not* found in suppression experiments causing similar intensity changes.

We have called the vector efferent increment an addition because the CM clearly increases. However our results equally support the hypthothesis that a small component approximately *out of phase* (-135 degrees) with the majority of the CM at 80dB has been *suppressed* by the efferent activity. This could be the correct interpretation since low level AP is depressed by efferent stimulation.

We have described several new features of the rise and fall of efferent evoked changes in the cochlea's CM and OAE responses. They span a wide time scale range. We have previously discussed the rapid (10ms) rise and initial fall (30ms) of efferent effect, and the bimodal envelope features which apply after each shock burst. We have here reported an initial sensitisation to individual bursts occuring over a 2 second time scale, and a post stimulation overshoot over a time scale of tens of seconds. We have also discussed the shock integration time. All these features may relate to specific physiological features of the action of individual neural pulses on the OHC mechanism. From the data presented it would be possible to build a model displaying the same dynamics as seen in the efferent-cochlear system, and this may be useful in suggesting further experiments.

Acknowledgements

This research was supported by the Hearing and Speech Trust and the Medical research Council. The authors would also like to thank Prof Ian Russell.

References

Fex J. (1962) Auditory activity in centrifugal and centripetal cochlear fibres in cat. A study of a feedback system. Acto Physiol. Scand. 55, 1-68 (suppl.)

Kemp D.T. and Brown A M. (1986) Wide Band Anaylsis of otoacoustic intermodulation. In: Peripheral Auditory Mechanisms, Springer Verlag. pp 306-313

Kemp D.T. and Souter M. (1988a) A new rapid component in the cochlear response to brief electrical efferent stimulation - CM and otoacoustic observations. Hearing Research 34, 49-62.

Kemp D. T. and Souter M. (1988b) The dynamics of cochlear perturbations following brief acoustic and efferent stimulation - otoacoustic and CM data. In: Basic Issues in Hearing. Eds: Duifuis, Horst & Wit, Academic Press, pp 116-123

Mountain D.C (1980) Changes in endolymphatic potential and COCB stimulation alter cochlear mechanics. Science 210, 71-72.

Robertson, D. and Gummer M, (1985) Physiological and morphological characteristics at efferent neurones in the guinea pig cochlea. Hearing Res. 20, 63-77.

Siegal J.H. and Kim D.O. (1982) Efferent neural control of cochlear mechanics? Olivocochlear bundle stimulation affects cochlear biomechanical nonlinearity. Hearing Res. 6, 171-182.

Wiederhold, M.L. (1969) Variations in the effect of electrical stimulation of the COCB on cat single nerve fiber responses to tone bursts. J. Acoust. Soc. Am. 48, 966-977.

Wiederhold, M.L. and Kiang, N.Y.S (1970) Effects of electrical stimulation at the COCB on single auditory nerve fibres in the cat. J.Acoust. Soc. Am. 48, 950-965.

Comments and Discussion

WIT

You observe changes in otoacoustic emissions evoked with 80 dB SPL tones. Is not the term OAE misleading in this case? Would it not be better to speak of impedance changes?

KEMP

Yes, I agree. We did not distinguish between delay emissions and "simple" evoked changes in mechanical input impedance.

EFFECT OF VISUAL SELECTIVE ATTENTION ON OTOACOUSTIC EMISSIONS

J.-L. Puel, G. Rebillard, P. Bonfils and R. Pujol

INSERM - U. 254, Laboratoire de Neurobiologie de l'Audition, Hôpital St. Charles, 34059 Montpellier Cedex , France

Introduction

Otoacoustic emissions have been demonstrated to have a cochlear origin (Kemp, 1978; Wilson, 1980; Kemp, 1986). They may reflect the existence of an active mechanism (Davis, 1983), which is responsible for the exquisite sensitivity and frequency discrimination of the cochlea. This active mechanism is probably based upon the motile properties of outer hair cells (OHCs) (Brownell et al., 1985; Zenner, 1986). The neurons of the medial efferent system (Warr and Guinan, 1979) form huge synapses, probably cholinergic (Eybalin and Pujol, 1987), with the OHC base, in such a way that a modulation of some of the OHC motile properties could well be postulated. Indeed, an electrical stimulation of the crossed part of the medial efferent bundle has been found to modify cochlear mechanics (Mountain, 1980; Siegel and Kim, 1982). In addition, a section of the same bundle alters the masking phenomènon (Carlier and Pujol, 1982; Bonfils et al., 1986; Bonfils and Puel, 1987).

Could the central nervous system, by using the medial efferents to OHCs, change the cochlear mechanics? To check this hypothesis, we have recorded OAEs, both evoked (EOAEs), and spontaneous (SOAEs), in human subjects before, during, and after a visual selective attention task. Previous data, both in human and animal, have indicated that such a task has an effect on the afferent auditory pathway (Hernandez-Peon et al., 1956; Oatman, 1971; Picton and Hillyard, 1974; Oatman, 1976; Glenn and Oatman, 1977; Lukas, 1980), and possibly on the cochlea (Hernandez-Peon et al., 1956; Lukas, 1980).

Preliminary results have already been presented as a short note (Puel et al., 1988).

Methods

Twenty volunteers (8 males, 12 females), between 18 and 39 years of age, participated in the study. All had normal vision and were not on any medication. These subjects had normal otoscopy and normal hearing. Auditory thresholds were better than, or equal to, 10 dB HL at frequencies ranging from 0.25 kHz to 8 kHz. The subjects were experimentally naive and were not informed about the particular hypothesis under investigation. They were simply asked to pay attention to the task. The experimental protocol chosen was the "look" condition as proposed by Lukas (1980). Visual stimuli consisting of two letters (O and Q) were randomly presented on a TV screen for a duration of 120 ms and at the rate of 2/s. Subjects were required to mentally count the target letter (Q) and report at the end of the trial how many times it had occurred. At the same time, the subjects had to push a button when the target letter (Q) appeared; the test lasted 5 minutes. Prior to the experiments the subjects were searched for possible SOAEs.

Acoustic emission recordings were made using a small acoustic probe containing a microphone (Knowles, BT 1751) and a miniature speaker (Knowles, BK 2615). The probe was fitted into the external ear canal and needed no external support. For EOAE recordings, as well as for synchronized SOAEs, the stimuli consisted in clicks (100 us duration) delivered at a rate of 21/s. The level of stimulation was set 15 dB above the perceptual threshold of the subject. The acoustic events in the closed ear canal were recorded in a 30 ms window starting 5 ms after stimulus onset to eliminate the artifact of stimulation. After amplification and band-pass filtering (high-pass: 250 Hz, 16 dB per octave; low-pass: 8 kHz, 16 dB per octave), the signal was averaged (512 repetitions). Spectral analysis was performed by using a Brüel & Kjaer (2033) spectrum analyser. The effect of visual attention on EOAEs and eventual synchronized SOAEs was analyzed by measuring the variation of the amplitude of the main spectral peaks. Three series of 5 minute-recordings were made: before, during and after the task. In each series, at least 6 recordings were obtained. The average amplitude obtained before the attentional task was taken as a reference (0 dB). The amplitude obtained during and after the task was then expressed relative to this reference. From each subject the mean values for each series were then combined to evaluate the general effect of an attentional tasks on EOAEs. When SOAEs were recorded separately, the experimental protocol was the same except for the fact that no acoustic stimulation was presented and that the low-pass filtering was extended to 32 kHz. Statistical analysis of data was done by the Student t test.

Results

Selective attention and EOAEs

In 17 out of the 20 subjects tested (85%), the amplitude of the dominant frequency of the EOAE spectrum significantly decreased during the attentional task. This decrease was highly significant ($p < 0.0001$). The mean ± SEM of the EOAEs amplitude recorded in all the 20 subjects is

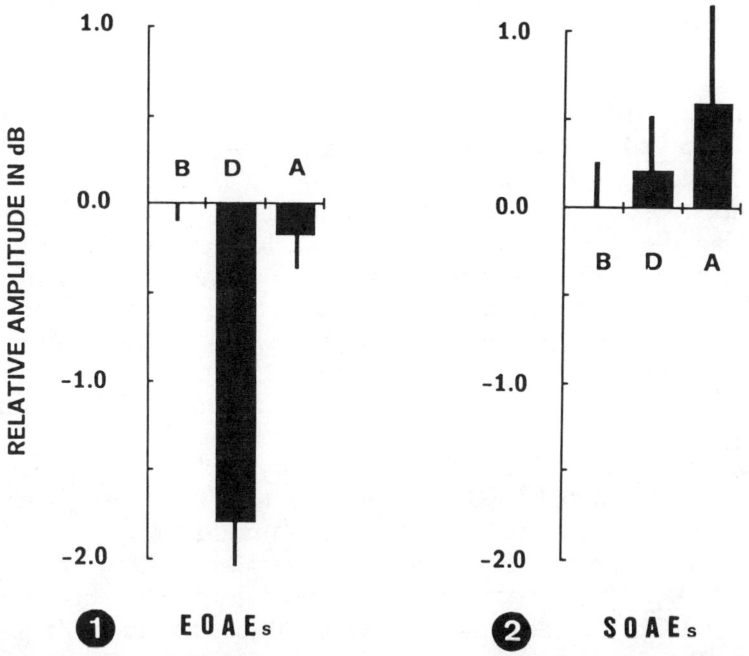

FIGURE 1 Relative amplitude of the EOAEs recorded in 20 subjects before (B), during (D), and after (A) the visual attentional task. The mean amplitude of the dominant frequency recorded before the task as been taken as the reference (0 dB). During the task (D) a significant decrease is observed ($p < 0.0001$). After the task (A) the amplitude recovers its initial value. Bars represent the SEM.

FIGURE 2 Relative amplitude of the SOAEs recorded in 6 subjects before (B), during (D), and after (A) the visual attentional task. No significant difference is observed.

shown in Fig. 1, in each tested condition (i.e., before, during, and after the task). The time course of the EOAEs changes was similar in the 17 subjects presenting a positive response to the test: the amplitude of the EOAEs quickly decreased during the first minute of the attentional task, and did not vary during all the visual stimuli presentation. Recovery of the initial amplitude was rapidly observed after the end of the task.

Selective attention and SOAEs

Six of the subjects, presenting a positive response to the previous test, also presented SOAEs. In three of these subjects, the amplitudes of the synchronized SOAEs were studied at the same time as EOAEs. In the others, the SOAEs were recorded directly (i.e., in the absence of any acoustic stimulation) by using the same attention procedure. The results obtained with both experimental techniques were similar and no significant variations were observed on any of the SOAEs frequency components (Fig. 2).

Discussion

A first question arises when trying to interpret the decrease observed in EOAEs during the visual selective attentional tast. Is the inner ear really involved? To answer this question, two different arguments can be taken. First, control recordings were done to assess variations of middle ear transmission: neither tympanometry nor acoustic reflex thresholds varied during the task. Moreover, it is unlikely that the middle ear muscle reflex plays a role with the level of stimulation used in this study (i.e., 15 dB SL). Second, in the 6 subjects where both EOAEs and SOAEs were recorded, only EOAEs varied during the task. A middle ear impedance variation, if involved, would have affected both OAEs, although not necessarily to the same extent. Especially significant in this respect are the results on the 3 subjects with synchronized SOAEs, as both recordings were done simultaneously. The fact that these synchronized SOAEs did not vary during a variation of EOAEs indicates that the effect is unlikely to be due to changes in transmission through the middle ear.

Since the report of Hernandez-Peon et al. (1956) suggesting that an attentional task may decrease cochlear potentials, the effects of attention on afferent auditory information has been subject to much discussion. All the subsequent human research essentially has used auditory evoked potentials as the measured parameter. However, different and contradictory results have been obtained. Picton and Hillyard (1974) observed a decrease of long-latency cortical evoked response to a variety of tasks and failed to demonstrate an effect on auditory brainstem responses (ABRs) during a "read" condition task. On the other hand, Lukas (1980) found that while subjects were focusing on a visual task the first and the fifth peaks of scalp-recorded ABRs were reduced in amplitude and increased in latency.

Our results provide the first evidence from human subjects that concentrated visual attention can modify EOAEs. Compared with ABRs and other measured parameters, EOAEs are a more sensitive measurement (i.e., EOAEs can be recorded below audiometric thresholds) (Kemp, 1978; Kemp, 1986), and the level of stimulation used in this study to obtain a significant result was very low: 15 dB SL versus 80 dB SL in experiments using ABRs (Lukas, 1980).

It is likely that these changes in the EOAEs were mediated by the OHCs of the cochlea. The EOAEs are considered to be the result of an active cochlear mechanism which is expressed through the OHCs (Kemp, 1978; Wilson, 1980; Davis, 1983; Kemp, 1986), and reflect their motile properties (Brownell et al, 1985; Zenner, 1986). Our results may indicate that the central nervous system uses the medial efferent pathway leading to OHCs (Warr and Guinan, 1979) to change the mechanical properties of the cochlea during a selective attention task. This action, resulting in decreased EOAEs, could well be mediated via some slow motile process of OHCs (see: Zenner, 1986), or via an overall electrical change of the OHCs, driven by the efferent synapses.

Finally, the fact that changes can be observed in the EOAEs without changes in the SOAEs in the same ear suggests that different mechanisms may be involved in the production of the two emissions. This difference may also indicate that SOAEs originate from OHCs which lack efferent synapses, and therefore are not subject to the influence of the CNS.

Acknowledgements

Thanks are due to R. Patuzzi for his helpful comments, to J.-P. Piron and P. Sibleyras for technical assistance, and to A. Bara for editorial work.

References

Bonfils, P., Remond, M.-C. and Pujol, R. (1986) Efferent tracts and cochlear frequency selectivity. Hearing Res. 24, 277-283.

Bonfils, P. and Puel, J.-L. (1987) Functional properties of the crossed part of the medial olivo-cochlear bundle. Hearing Res. 28, 125-130.

Brownell, W.E., Bader, C.R., Bertrand, D. and de Ribaupierre, Y. (1985) Evoked mechanical responses of isolated cochlear outer hair cells. Science 227, 194-196.

Carlier, E. and Pujol R. (1982) Sectioning the efferent bundle decreases cochlear frequenncy selectivity. Neurosci. Lett. 28, 101-106.

Davis, H. (1983) An active process in cochlear mechanics. Hearing Res. 9, 79-90.

Eybalin, M. and Pujol, R. (1987) Choline acetyltransferase (ChAT) immunoelectron microscopy distinguishes at least three types of efferent synapses in the organ of Corti. Exp. Brain Res. 65, 261-270.

Glenn, J.F. and Oatman, L.C. (1977) Effects of visual attention on the latency of auditory evoked potentials. Exp. Neurol. 57, 34-40.

Hernandez-Peon, R., Scherrer, H .and Jouvet, M. (1956) Modification of electrical activity in cochlear nucleus during "attention" in unanesthetized cats. Science 123, 331-332.

Kemp, D.T. (1978) Stimulated acoustic emissions from the human auditory system. J. Acoust. Soc. Am. 64, 1386-1391.

Kemp, D.T. (1986) Otoacoustic emissions, travelling waves and cochlear mechanisms. Hearing Res. 22, 95-104.

Lukas, J.H. (1980) Human auditory attention: The olivo-cochlear bundle may function as a peripheral filter. Psychophysiology 17, 444-452.

Mountain, D.C. (1980) Changes of endolymphatic potential and crossed olivocochlear bundle stimulation alter cochlear mechanics. Science 210, 71-72.

Oatman, L.C. (1971) Role of visual attention on auditory evoked potentials in unanesthetized cats. Exp. Neurol. 10, 341-356.

Oatman, L.C. (1976) Effects of visual attention on the intensity of auditory evoked potentials. Exp. Neurol. 51, 41-53.

Picton, T.W. and Hillyard, S.A. (1974) Human auditory evoked potentials. II. Effects of attention. E.E.G.. Clin. Neurophysiol. 36, 191-199.

Puel, J.-L., Bonfils, P. and Pujol, R. (1988) Selective attention modifies the active micromechanical properties of the cochlea. Brain Res. 447, 380-383.

Siegel, J.H. and Kim, D.O. (1982) Efferent neural control of cochlear mechanics? Olivocochlear bundle stimulation affects cochlear biomechanical nonlinearity. Hearing Res. 6, 171-182.

Warr, W.B. and Guinan Jr., J.J. (1979) Efferent innervation of the organ of Corti: two separate systems. Brain Research 173, 152-155.

Wilson, J.P. (1980) Evidence for a cochlear origin for acoustic re-emissions threshold fine-structure and tonal tinnitus. Hearing Res. 2, 233-252.

Zenner, H.P. (1986) Motile responses in outer hair cells. Hearing Res. 22, 83-90.

Comments and Discussion

WHITEHEAD

I routinely measure the amplitude and frequency of spontaneous otoacoustic emissions (SOAEs) in the ear canal both before and after experiments upon otoacoustic emissions. Analysis of these data has shown that the majority of SOAEs are larger after experiments than before; typically by less than 2 dB, but occasionally by over 15 dB! Consistent with this I am often able to measure SOAEs after experiments that were not detectable before-hand. Often associated with these changes are shifts in SOAE frequency, which can be in either direction but are typically downwards, and always less than 1% of the emission frequency. For any one SOAE, these amplitude and frequency shifts are repeatable between experiments.

Experiments on SOAEs demonstrating this effect particularly robustly have demonstrated:

(1) that it does not depend on stimulation of the ear by acoustic stimuli; it is of equal magnitude upon recording in silence.

(2) that the amplitude (and frequency) changes are approximately exponential in form with the majority of the shifts occurring in the first 10-20 minutes after insertion of the microphone probe into the ear canal.

(3) that this effect is not due to some "warm-up" effect altering the microphone characteristics.

(4) that these changes are very much reduced if the microphone probe is removed from the ear for the period between the "before" and "after" recordings.

(5) that the changes are equally strong when the microphone is left in the ipsilateral ear between the "before" and "after" recordings, and when it is removed and placed in the contralateral ear between these recordings.

These results indicate that the amplitude and frequency shifts are not due to a "whole-body" change (e.g. a temperature change) associated with being in the sound proof room, or due to a direct physical effect of the microphone on the ear (e.g. a temperature change or alteration of ear canal static pressure) occurring over the first few minutes of recording.

Similar amplitude and frequency shifts are measurable in the cancellation of a swept frequency sinusoidal acoustic stimulus in the ear canal by the stimulus frequency emission evoked by this stimulus.

A possible explanation of these data is that the changes represent an efferent influence on the emission generator associated with increased auditory selective attention.

HORNER

Q1. Does the amplitude of evoked otoacoustic emissions change after the subject has fallen asleep - measurements in the same subject before and after onset of sleep?

Q2. Does contralateral masking noise (or pop music) have an effect on the evoked emissions? (Contralateral masker at a low enough level not to evoke the middle ear reflex.)

Q3. Does the argument of the effect of discontinuities of hair cells upon the spectrum of spontaneous emissions - not get back to the older suggestion (Wit *et al.* 1983) that the fine structure of the audiogram is related to the spectrum of the emissions? Have neonates more dips in the fine structure of the audiogram?

PUJOL

Q1. We have not looked systematically, but during some recordings subjects go to sleep, and no variation can be observed, other than respiratory artifacts.

Q2. We have no data of our own on this point.

Q3. The only thing I could add about supernumerary OHCs is that they seem to lack efferent innervation.

WHITEHEAD

I have measured six spontaneous otoacoustic emissions (SOAEs) from two ears (of different subjects) over a period in which the subjects passed from wakefulness, through over an hours sleep, including REM sleep, and back to wakefulness again. The measured variations in SOAE amplitude and frequency were entirely consistent with the variations seen over an equivalent period of wakefulness; there appeared to be no changes in SOAE properties correlated with level of conciousness.

Also, measurement of SOAEs before, during and after psychoacoustical threshold fine-structure determinations (which require considerable concentration on the part of the subject) (also) revealed no corresponding changes in their amplitude or frequency. This may be taken as evidence that increased auditory selective attention does not influence SOAEs, and is consistent with your finding that visual selective attention did not appear to have any effect on SOAEs.

However, as I noted previously, increases in amplitude, sometimes accompanied by changes of frequency, do occur for most, but not all, SOAEs over the first few minutes of recording. These changes are typically smaller than 2 dB, although they can be much larger. I have suggested that these result from an increase in auditory selective attention associated with the act of recording from the ear canal. If this is so, further attempts to increase auditory selective attention may well have no effect. The threshold fine-structure measurements noted above were carried out after these initial drifts in SOAEs had asymptoted. The experiments in which SOAEs were measured during sleep involved SOAEs in which these drifts were too small to be reliably detected. In ears with SOAEs showing large drifts, I have found that removing the microphone after the drifts have asymptoted, and re-inserting the microphone to record only briefly at several minute intervals, allows a gradual recovery of the SOAEs to their initial frequency and amplitude. A similar phenomenon was described by Zurek (1981) for the frequency decrease of an SOAE. It would be of interest to determine whether SOAEs demonstrating large drifts in frequency and amplitude during the first few minutes of recording show a return to their initial state when the subject falls asleep, and is presumably no longer attending to the microphone.

Zurek, P.M., Spontaneous narrow-band acoustic signals emitted by human ears, J. Acoust. Soc. Am. 69, pp. 514-523, 1981.

TRACKING AND INTERPRETIVE MODELS OF THE ACTIVE-NONLINEAR COCHLEAR RESPONSE DURING REVERSIBLE CHANGES INDUCED BY ASPIRIN CONSUMPTION

A. Tubis, G.R. Long*, S. Sivaramakrishnan*, and K.L. Jones†

Department of Physics, Purdue University
West Lafayette, IN, USA
**Department of Audiology and Speech Sciences*
Purdue University, West Lafayette, IN, USA
†Division of Otolaryngology
University of Connecticut, Health Center
Farmington, CT, USA

Introduction

Aspirin consumption in humans has been found to reversibly reduce delayed-evoked and synchronous-evoked otoacoustic emisions, and to reversibly reduce and subsequently abolish spontaneous emissions (Johnsen and Elberling, 1982; McFadden and Plattsmier, 1984; Long, Tubis and Jones, 1986; Probst et al., 1986; Pasanen et al., 1987; Long and Tubis, 1988a; Long et al., 1988).

Long et al. (1986) and Long and Tubis (1988a,b) also showed that aspirin consumption produced correlated changes in the psychoacoustic threshold microstructure associated with the emissions. In particular, the initial change in threshold microstructure in most instances was a trend to increased sensitivity with the greatest change near threshold maxima. Further reduction in the levels of the evoked emissions was accompanied by the eventual elevation of all thresholds (reduced sensitivity) to levels slightly above threshold maxima in pre-aspirin measures.

Studies of the statistical properties of spontaneous emissions before and during aspirin-induced level reduction (Long et al., 1988) show that the emissions are manifestations of noisy self-sustained or limit-cycle oscillations of an active-nonlinear cochlea (Bialek and Wit, 1984; Wit, 1986) and are not associated with the selective amplification of narrow bands of noise. These limit-cycle oscillations may be entrained or frequency locked by external tones, with the minimum external-tone level required for locking, at different frequencies, constituting a tuning curve (Zwicker and Schloth, 1984). Aspirin consumption results in a broadening of this tuning curve (Long et al., 1988).

These reversible effects of aspirin consumption on the properties of otoacoustic emissions and their associated psychoacoustic threshold microstructure provide an important channel of information concerning nonlinear-active cochlear function. At present we have little knowledge concerning the biochemical effects of aspirin in the cochlea, and only tentative understanding of active cochlear response (cf., Geisler, 1986; Neely and Kim, 1986; Ashmore, 1987). We therefore focus on those aspects of the subjective and objective data which may be simply interpreted on the basis of some gross features of the effective cochlear macromechanical response.

Van der Pol Model for a Spontaneous Emission

For simplicity, we will confine the present discussion to models based on the Van der Pol cochlear-partition damping function:

$$R = -r_1(x) + r_2(x)y^2; \qquad (1)$$

x = distance from the basal end of the cochlea;

y = basilar membrane (BM) displacement;

where $r_2(x)$ is positive and $r_1(x)$ may be positive along various sections of the cochlear partition. The latter situation corresponds to net negative damping for some range of BM displacement.

Such models embody many of the essential features of more elaborate nonlinear-active micromechanical ones, and have in various simplified forms, been used to simulate: 1) the statistical properties of spontaneous emissions (Bialek and Wit, 1984; Wit, 1986); 2) their interaction with external tones (Long et al. 1988; Diependaal et al., 1987; van Dijk and Wit, 1988); and 3) their self interactions (Jones et al., 1986).

A simple unforced Van der Pol oscillator satisfies the dynamical equation,

$$\frac{d^2y}{dt^2} + w_o^2\, y + (-r_1 + r_2y^2)\frac{dy}{dt} = 0, \qquad (2)$$

which has the approximate limit-cycle solution (c.f. Hanggi and Riseborough, 1983):

$$y(t) = 2\sqrt{\frac{r_1}{r_2}}\sin(w_o t + \phi), \qquad (3)$$

$$\phi = \text{const.}$$

If this oscillator is embedded in a cochlear model, e.g. if there is a small region of the cochlear partition where $r_1 > 0$, with place frequency $f_o = w_o/2\pi$, a spontaneous emission will result with an ear-canal pressure variation of the form given by Eq. (3) (c.f., Koshigoe and Tubis, 1983).

In Fig. 1a, the spatial variation of the basilar membrane vibration amplitude is plotted for the case of a 967 Hz spontaneous emission, which is calculated using a one-dimensional cochlear model with a localized region where $r_1 > 0$. For comparison, Fig. 1b shows the basilar membrane vibration amplitude which results when the active region is eliminated from the cochlea, and the cochlea is driven externally at 967 Hz.

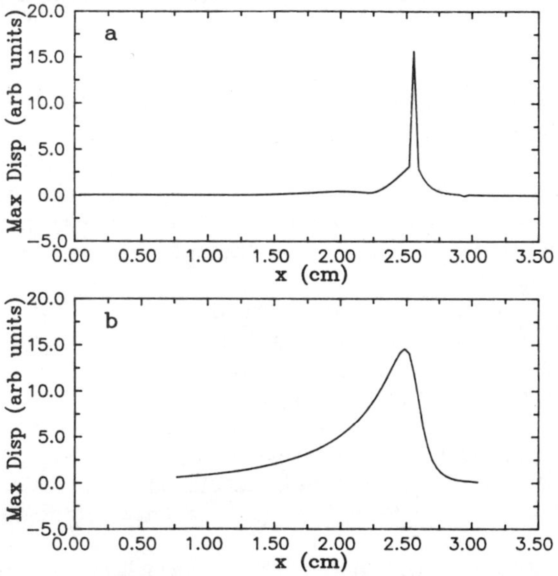

FIGURE 1 a) Cochlear model simulation of peak BM displacement associated with a 967 Hz, 10 dB simulated spontaneous emission. The BM areal mass, stiffness and damping functions are given (in c.g.s. units) by: $M = 0.15$; $K = 10^9 e^{-2x}$; $R = 200$ ($0<x<2.555$, $x>2.590$), $-100 + 10^{16}y^2$ ($2.555<x<2.590$). The BM width is 0.1 cm, and the lengths of the cochlea and capped ear canal are 3.5 and 1.5 cm, respectively. The middle-ear model is the one used by Matthews (1980). b) Simulation of the peak BM displacement associated with external driving at 967 Hz, for a linear passive periphery model, which is the same as the one used in obtaining Fig. 1a except that $R = 200$ for all x.

Variation of Threshold Microstructure during Aspirin Consumption

The initial trend, during aspirin consumption, to reduced thresholds (increased sensitivity) around threshold maxima in the neighborhood of a spontaneous emission, has been speculated (Long et al., 1986; Long and Tubis, 1988a) to be due to the reduction of masking (or other interference) by the emission. The observed eventual elevation of all thresholds to levels above threshold maxima in pre-aspirin measures may possibly be associated with the overall net increase in cochlear damping (due to the aspirin-induced weakening of the processes such as hair-cell motility, which may underlie the active cochlear response).

The situation is more complicated near threshold minima which occur at the spontaneous emission frequencies. Threshold detection of a tone very close in frequency to an emission is associated with a tonal percept, i.e. the emission is frequency-locked to the tone (Long and Tubis, 1988b). By assuming that: 1) threshold detection occurs when basilar-membrane vibration amplitude is greater than that for a spontaneous emission; and 2) the cochlear partition damping, under aspirin consumption, evolves from an initial active-nonlinear form of Eq. (2), with $r_1 > 0$, to an eventual linear-passive form ($r_1 < 0$, $r_2 = 0$), Long and Tubis (1988a) have shown that it is plausible that the threshold very close to the emission could initially decrease and eventually increase as seen experimentally.

External-tone Synchronization of Spontaneous Emissions

As the swept frequency of a low-level external tone approaches that of an emission, the ear canal signal in a narrow band containing the emission frequency approximates simple beating which disappears when the external tone is sufficiently close to the emission so as to entrain it (Long et al. 1988; Zwicker and Schloth, 1984). A closer examination of the ear-canal signal during a sufficiently slow sweep reveals a transition region of asymmetric beating just prior to entrainment (Long et al., 1988). Typical results are shown in Fig. (2).

This behavior is a general feature of externally-driven limit-cycle oscillators (c.f., Stratonovich, 1963; Machlup and Sluckin, 1980). The output (peak vibration displacement) of a computer simulation of the response of a Van der Pol oscillator to a frequency-swept, external sinusoidal driving force, corresponding to Fsin(w(t)t) on the right hand side of Eq. (2), is shown in Fig. (3) for various values of F. The results were obtained using the first-approximation of the averaging method of Krylov and Bogoliubov (c.f., Hanggi and Riseborough, 1983). Similar results have been calculated for the peak ear-canal pressure in a model of the auditory periphery used in obtaining the results of Fig. (1).

The finding of Long et al. (1988) that the frequency-locking tuning curve is broadened as a result of aspirin consumption, may be correlated with the behavior of the driven Van der Pol oscillator. The frequency-locking tuning curve, for $F^2 > \dfrac{32\, w^2 r_1^{\,3}}{27\, r_2}$,

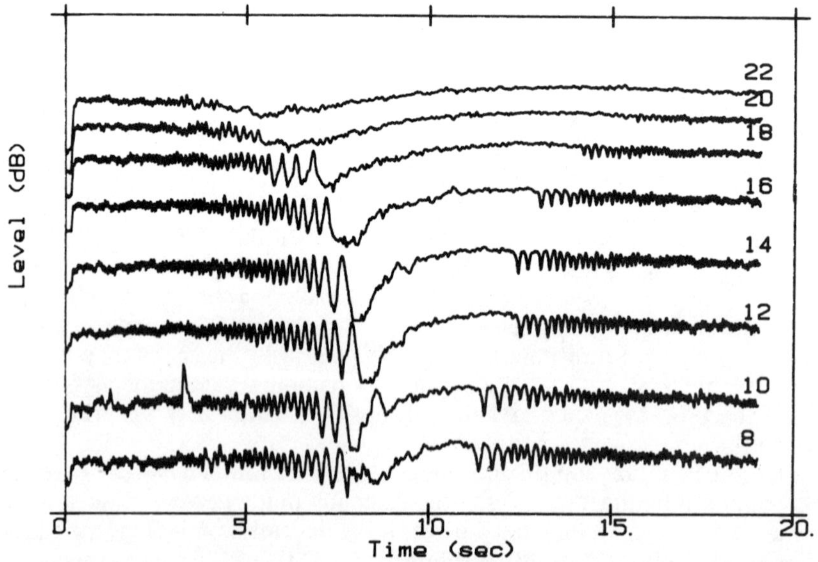

FIGURE 2 RMS level of the filtered (31.6 Hz bandwidth) ear-canal signal in the right ear of JN when tones (levels in dB SPL indicated above the traces) were swept from 1610 Hz to 1640 Hz past a 1625 Hz, 11.5 dB SPL emission. Traces are shifted vertically to avoid overlap.

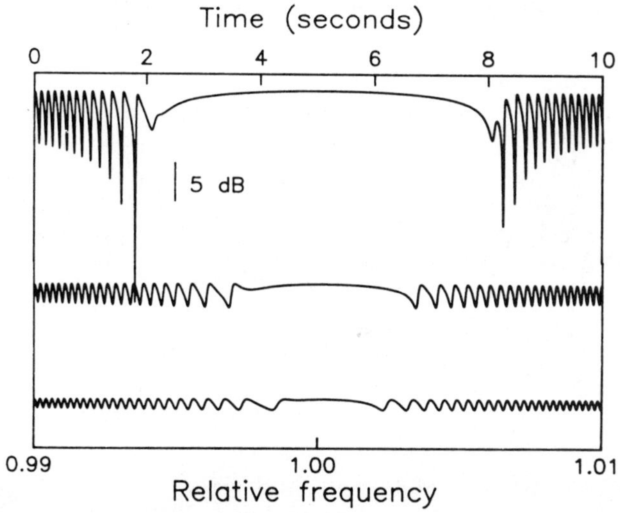

FIGURE 3 Simulation of the peak displacement response of a Van der Pol oscillator to driving forces of amplitude F = 0.8, 0.4, 0.2, swept from 0.99 to 1.01 of the limit-cycle frequency, $w_o/2\pi$. The Van der Pol parameters used were $w_o = 2\pi$, $r_1 = 0.1$, $r_2 = 0.1$. Traces are shifted vertically to avoid overlap.

is given by (cf., Hanggi and Riseborough, 1983):

$$|w - w_o|^2 = \frac{F^2}{2w^2A^2} - \frac{r_2{}^2A^4}{256}, \qquad (4)$$

where $A = 2\sqrt{\frac{r_1}{r_2}}$, the limit-cycle amplitude when F = 0. Thus if "aspirin-induced" changes in r_1 and r_2 are such that A and r_2 are decreased, corresponding to decreases in the level of the emission and the nonlinear response, then the frequency locking, for a fixed F, occurs at a larger value of $|w - w_o|$ relative to that before aspirin-induced changes in r_1 and r_2. Similar results are obtained using a cochlear model.

External-tone Suppression of Spontaneous Emissions

A detailed study of external-tone suppression of spontaneous emissions during aspirin consumption is in progress. Typical results implied by our simple Van der Pol model of cochlear partition damping are illustrated in Fig. 4, which shows 3-dB suppression tuning curves for an emission before and after assumed aspirin-induced changes (reduction in r_1) in the active-cochlear response. For comparison, 3-dB suppression tuning curves for a spontaneous emission with a frequency at approximately 1630 Hz and level varying between 11 and 12 dB SPL before aspirin consumption are shown in Fig. 5. During aspirin consumption, an initial

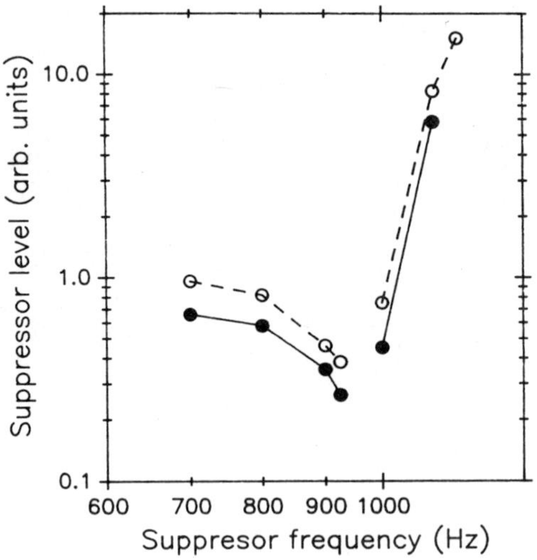

FIGURE 4 Cochlear model simulation of the 3-dB suppression tuning curves for a 967 Hz spontaneous emission, calculated with: 1) the same cochlear parameters used in obtaining Fig. 1a (dashed line), and 2) the same cochlear parameters used in obtaining Fig. 1a (solid line) except for $R = -65 + 10^{16}\ y^2$ (2.555<x<2.590), which gives a 5 dB reduction of the emission level.

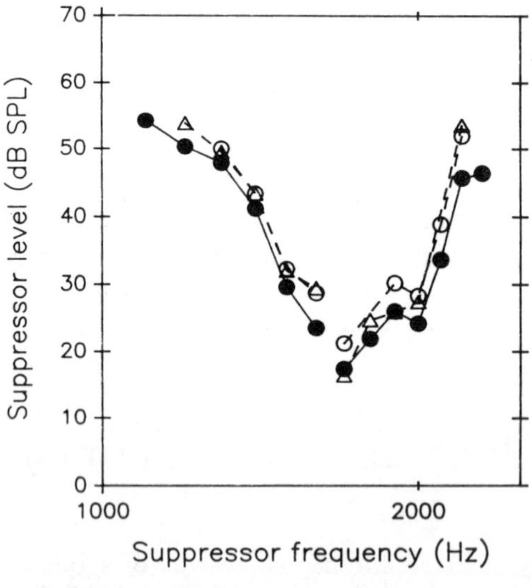

FIGURE 5 3-dB suppression tuning curves for a 1628 Hz spontaneous emission of subject JN with pre-aspirin level of 11-12 dB SPL. The open-circle data was taken before aspirin consumption during a one-hour session. The open-square was similarly taken two weeks later just prior to the beginning of aspirin consumption. The solid-circle data was similarly taken after the start of aspirin consumption when the emission level was reduced to values fluctuating between 8-10 dB SPL. The flattened tips of the tuning curves between 1800 and 2000 Hz may be due to evoked emissions.

depression of the emission level to 8 dB SPL followed by an increase to 10 dB SPL, during the measurement session, was correlated with a downward trend of the tuning curve which was similar to the trend of the model simulations.

Discussion

The studies described or referenced in this paper suggest: 1) some aspects of spontaneous otoacoustic emissions may be modelled as limit-cycle oscillations of the cochlear partition; 2) these oscillations may be roughly described in terms of the nonlinear-active cochlear-partition damping function of Eq. (1); and 3) the effects of aspirin on spontaneous emissions may be modelled in terms of smooth changes in the parameters of the damping function.

Acknowledgements

This work was supported by NINCDS Grant NS22095 and Purdue University. The authors wish to thank William J. Murphy for help in the preparation of the manuscript, Elizabeth Marrs and Lidia Lee for help in analyzing data and making the figures, and Professor Aditya P. Mathur for helpful discussions on vectorizing cochlear model calculations and arranging for cpu time on the Alliant FX/8 vector multiprocessor of the Purdue University Computer Science Department.

References

Ashmore, J.F. (1987) A fast motile response in guinea-pig outer hair cells: The cellular basis of the cochlear amplifier. J. Physiol. 388, 323-347.

Bialek, W.S. and Wit, H.P. (1984) Quantum limits to oscillator stability: theory and experiments on acoustic emissions from the human ear. Phys. Lett. 104A, 1973-1978.

Diependaal, R.J., Duifhuis, H., Hoogstraten, H.W. and Viergever, M.A. (1987) Numerical methods for solving one-dimensional cochlear models in the time domain. J. Acoust. Soc. Am. 82, 1655-1666.

Geisler, C.D. (1986) A model of the effect of outer hair cell motility on cochlear vibrations. Hear. Res. 24, 125-131.

Hanggi, P. and Riseborough, P. (1983) Dynamics of nonlinear dissipative oscillators. Am. J. Physics 51, 347-351.

Johnsen, N.J. and Elberling, C. (1982) Evoked acoustic emissions from the human ear. I. Equipment and response parameters. Scand. Audiol. 11, 3-12.

Jones, K.L., Tubis, A., Long, G.R., Burns, E.M. and Strickland, E.A. (1986) Interactions among multiple spontaneous otoacoustic emissions. In: Peripheral Auditory Mechanisms (Eds: Allen, J.B., Hall, J.L., Hubbard, A.E., Neely, S.T. and Tubis, A.) Springer Verlag, Berlin, pp. 266-273.

Koshigoe, S. and Tubis, A. (1983) A nonlinear feedback model for outer-hair-cell stereocilia and its implication for the response of the auditory periphery. In: Mechanics of Hearing (Eds: de Boer, E. and Viergever, M.A.) Delft University Press, Delft, pp. 127-134.

Long, G.R. and Tubis, A. (1988a) Modification of spontaneous and evoked otoacoustic emissions and associated psychoacoustic microstructure by aspirin consumption. J. Acoust. Soc. Am., submitted.

Long, G.R. and Tubis, A. (1988b) Investigations into the nature of the association between threshold microstructure and otoacoustic emissions. Hear. Res., submitted.

Long, G.R., Tubis, A. and Jones, K.L. (1986) Changes in spontaneous and evoked otoacoustic emissions and the corresponding psychoacoustic threshold microstructure induced by aspirin consumption. In: Peripheral Auditory Mechanisms (Eds: Allen, J.B., Hall, J.L., Hubbard, A.E., Neely, S.T. and Tubis, A.) Springer Verlag, Berlin, pp. 213-218.

Long, G.R., Tubis, A., Jones, K.L. and Sivaramakrishnan, S. (1988) Modification of the external-tone synchronization and statistical properties of spontaneous otoacoustic emissions by aspirin consumption In: Basic Issues in Hearing (Eds: Duifhuis, H., Horst, J.W., and Wit, H.P.) University Press Groningen, The Netherlands, in press.

Machlup, S. and Sluckin, T.J. (1980) Driven oscillations of a limit-cycle oscillator. J. Theor. Biol. 84, 119-134.

Matthews, J.W. (1980) Mathematical modeling of nonlinear phenomena observed in the peripheral auditory system. Ph.D. thesis, Washington University, St. Louis, MO.

McFadden, D. and Plattsmier, H.S. (1984) Aspirin abolishes spontaneous otoacoustic emissions. J. Acoust. Soc. Am. 76, 443-448.

Neely, S.T. and Kim, D.O. (1986) A model for active elements in cochlear biomechanics. J. Acoust. Soc. Am. 79, 1472-1480.

Pasanen, G., Weir, C.G. and McFadden, D. (1987) Reciprocal relation between the growth of an emitted cubic distortion product and the suppression of a spontaneous otoacoustic emission. J. Acoust. Soc. Am. 81 Suppl. 1, S8.

Probst, R., Coats, A.C., Martin, G.K. and Lonsbury-Martin, B.L. (1986) Spontaneous click- and toneburst-evoked otoacoustic emissions from normal ears. Hear. Res. 21, 261-275.

Stratonovich, R.L. (1963) Topics in Theory of Random Noise, Volume II, Gordon and Breach, New York, pp. 222-276.

van Dijk, P. and Wit, H.P. (1987) Phase-lock of spontaneous otoacoustic emissions to a cubic-difference tone. In: Basic Issues in Hearing (Eds: Duifhuis, H., Horst, J.W. and Wit, H.P.) University Press, Groningen, The Netherlands, in press.

Wit, H.P. (1986) Statistical properties of a strong spontaneous otoacoustic emission. In: Peripheral Auditory Mechanisms (Eds: Allen, J.B., Hall, J.L., Hubbard, A.E., Neely, S.T. and Tubis, A.) Springer Verlag, Berlin, pp. 221-228.

Zwicker, E. and Schloth, E. (1984) Interaction of different otoacoustic emissions. J. Acoust. Soc. Am. 75, 1148-1154.

Comments and Discussion

PATUZZI

From the data we have presented at this meeting (Patuzzi et al) it is quite probable that the nonlinearity you have described in the van der Pol formulation of the oscillator responsible for spontaneous emissions is the saturating mechano-electric transduction channels at the apex of the outer hair cells.

WHITEHEAD

What frequency changes in spontaneous otoacoustic emissions do you find during and after aspirin consumption?

TUBIS

With few exceptions, the aspirin-induced amplitude reduction of spontaneous emission levels was accompanied by a decrease in the emission frequencies up to about 10 Hz. These frequency shifts correlated with shifts in the minima of the threshold microstructure. After recovery, the emission frequencies generally approached their pre-aspirin values.

ANALYSIS AND INFLUENCE OF LIDOCAINE ON EVOKED OTOACOUSTIC EMISSIONS FROM TINNITUS SUFFERERS

B. Kollmeier and S. Uppenkamp

Drittes Physikalisches Institut, Universität Göttingen
Bürgerstr. 42-44, D-3400 Göttingen, FRG

Introduction

The discovery of otoacoustic emissions (Kemp, 1978) raised hope that some kind of tinnitus (that is, subjective sensations of sound without acoustical or electrical stimulation) could be attributed to mechanical hyperactivity in the inner ear. For this reason, the relation between tinnitus and spontaneous otoacoustic emissions (SOAEs) has been investigated by several authors (c.f. Wilson and Sutton, 1981, Hazell, 1984, Penner and Burns, 1987). Their findings of no affirmative relation between both phenomena could have been affected by two circumstances: First, a relation between otoacoustic emissions and tinnitus might only occur if both effects originate from roughly the same location within the auditory pathway. Therefore, only cases of "peripheral" (sensorineural) tinnitus should be considered if a reliable distinction between central and peripheral tinnitus can be made at all. Second, tinnitus is often associated with hearing impairment whereas otoacoustic emissions (OAEs) are rarely found in hearing-impaired subjects (Kemp, 1978). This fact might be due to attenuation in the middle ear (primarily for conductive hearing losses), the altered mechanical (back-)propagation in the basal turns of the cochlea and alterations in the "active" cochlea feedback mechanisms. In order to obtain information on these neuro-mechanical mechanisms even in hearing-impaired tinnitus sufferers in a reproducible way, we decided to record evoked otoacoustic emissions (EOAEs). In addition, we attempted to classify the probable origin of the tinnitus clinically and by the effect of lidocaine, a drug that prolongs the refractory period and hence reduces the activity of certain neurons: A subjective change in the perceived tinnitus after an infusion of lidocaine (2mg/kg body weight) indicates a peripheral (sensorineural) origin (Shulman and Seitz, 1981). In addition, a lidocaine effect on the EOAE would provide further evidence that OAEs in humans are generated by an active feedback mechanism which is controlled by neural activity. Last, a correlation between the lidocaine effect on EOAEs and tinnitus would help to clarify the origin of tinnitus.

Recording Method

Recording of EOAEs was part of the diagnostics for tinnitus sufferers in the ENT clinic Göttingen. Each patient underwent a clinical and audiological examination, tinnitus matching experiments, tinnitus masking experiments (Feldmann, 1971) and evoked response audiometry (ERA). Essentially the same apparatus was used for the recording of EOAEs and ERA (Computer PDP 11/34, Madsen audiometer ER074, B&K measurement amplifier). The stimulus was a click of .5 ms duration (one period of a sinewave at 2 kHz) at a repetition rate of 8 Hz. It was amplified, emitted by a hearing-aid speaker and fed into an elastic rubber tube (length 26 cm, diameter 2 mm) leading to a metal probe tube (length 3.5 cm, diameter 1 mm). A metal jacket of 3 mm diameter enclosed this tube as well as the recording metal probe tube of the same kind. Its end was inserted into the external meatus which was occluded by a rubber seal. The acoustic level of the click was approximately 20, 40 or 60 dB SL. The evoked emissions were recorded at the outer end of the recording tube by a Knowles EA-1843 miniature microphone. They were amplified, lowpass-filtered (3 kHz), converted to digital by a 12-bit-A/D-converter at a sampling rate of 10 kHz and digitally averaged over 2000 sweeps.

One severe problem for the recording of EOAEs was the large hearing loss of some patients (more than 40 dB). In most of these cases, the stimulus level had to be raised to 60 dB SL to be audible to the patients. The "passive" response of the apparatus, which decays exponentially after the offset of the click, increasingly obscures the "active" response of the cochlea which is observable approximately 10 ms later. This effect as well as the maximum output power of the speaker limited the stimulus level to a maximum of 60 dB SL. Two examples of the curves obtained with this stimulus level (subject JZ) are given in Fig. 1. Fig. 1a shows the curve before and Fig. 1b after infusion of lidocaine. In order not to overload the recording system, the first 10 ms (or 15 ms, respectively) of the recorded signal was set to zero by an electronic gate switch.

Analysis Method

In order to quantify the amplitude of observed EOAEs, an average power spectrum is computed. Successive 12.8 ms sections of the average signal in the range between 10 and 60 ms are weighted by a Hamming-window (128 points), fouriertransformed and the power of each frequency channel is averaged over successive

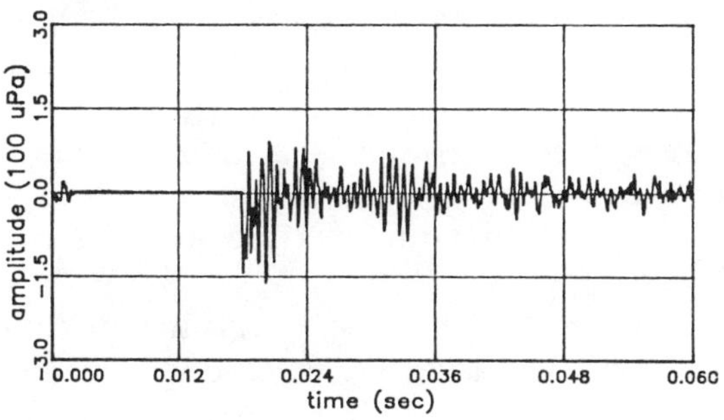

FIGURE 1a Evoked oto-acoustic emission (EOAE) recorded from subject JZ's right ear at a stimulus level of 60 dB SL before the infusion of lidocaine. The stimulus starts at 1.8 ms after the beginning of the recording interval. During the first 15ms following the stimulus onset, the recorded signal is set to zero by an electronic gate switch.

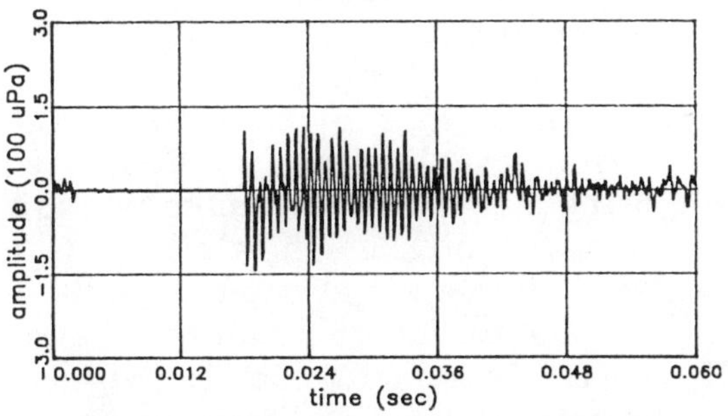

FIGURE 1b Same as Fig. 1a, but after the infusion of lidocaine (2mg/kg body weight).

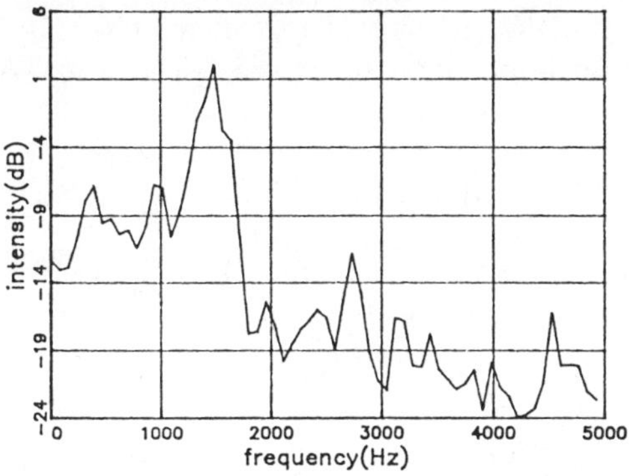

FIGURE 2a Average power spectrum of the section between 10ms and 60ms of the curve from Fig. 1a (i.e., before the infusion of lido-caine). 0 dB denotes 0 dB SPL.

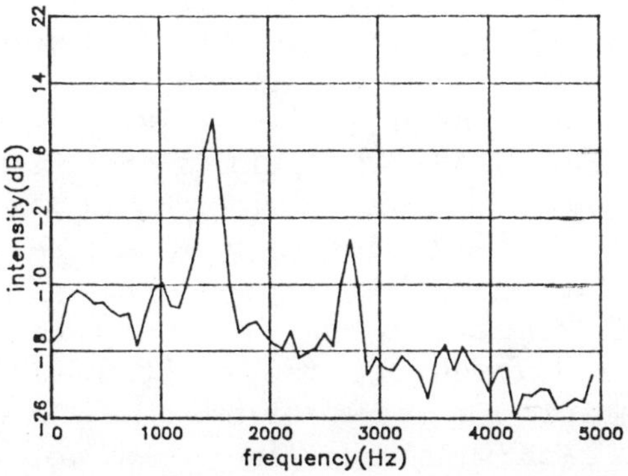

FIGURE 2b Same as Fig. 2a, but after the infusion of lidocaine (power spectrum of Fig. 1b).

samples. The results for the signals from Fig. 1 are shown in Fig. 2 (a: before, b: after lidocaine). In order to obtain information about the frequency contents and the temporal structure of the EOAE simultaneously, short-time spectrograms are computed: A 12.8-ms- section of the signal is weighted by a Hamming window, fouriertransformed and displayed as a function of time every 2 ms (Fig. 3a:before, b: after lidocaine).

Since the frequencies in EOAEs might not be constant during the short time of their occurences, the inverse relation between temporal resolution and spectral resolution in short-time fourier analysis is disadvantageous for the structural evaluation of EOAEs. However, a better compromise between temporal and simultaneous spectral resolution is obtained by the Wigner Ville distribution (c.f. Claasen and Mecklenbräuker, 1980). For signals of finite duration, the frequency distribution at a certain instant of time t is computed from a signal segment z(t) by weighting z(t) with a Hamming window $h(\tau)$ and fouriertransforming the product $h(\tau)z(t+\tau)h(-\tau)z(t-\tau)$ as a function of the delay τ. The result is displayed at time t and the window is shifted to the next instant of time where again the distribution function is evaluated. The result is named "Pseudo-Wigner-Ville-Distribution" (PWVD). In order to evaluate this distribution for time-discrete signals up to half the sampling frequency, the signal must first be oversampled at twice the sampling rate by a sin(x)/x-interpolation. In addition, the interpretation is faciliated if the PWVD is smoothed over successive instants of time by a smoothing window g(k). Therefore, the resulting formula is:

$$PWVD(t,f) = 2 \sum_{k=-M}^{M} g(k) \sum_{\tau=-N}^{N} |h(\tau/2)|^2 z(t+kT+\tau/2)\, z^*(t+kT-\tau/2)\, e^{-2i\pi f\tau}$$

The length of each signal segment was N=128 points, smoothing included seven successive frames (i.e., M=3) and the distance between successive instants of time was T= 2 ms. The results for the curves from Fig. 1 are given in Fig. 4 (a: before, b: after lidocaine). In this figure, the maximum of the PWVD is normalized to one. The temporal developement of the main spectral component (c.f. Fig. 2) is clearly visible. In addition, large contributions of the PWVD occur at the frequency 0 Hz whenever the main component is prominent. These contributions arise from the pronounced periodicity at these instants of time since the Wigner-Ville-Distribution of a periodic signal is known to have a contribution at 0 Hz.

When interpreting the PWVD one has to bear in mind that its integral over the whole time and frequency range reflects the total energy of the signal. However, in some regions the PWVD may be less than zero so that each function value must not be directly interpreted as an energy. In addition, it is not possible to plot the PWVD on a logarithmic scale comparable to the plot of the short-time fourier spectra in Fig. 3. Therefore, the linear

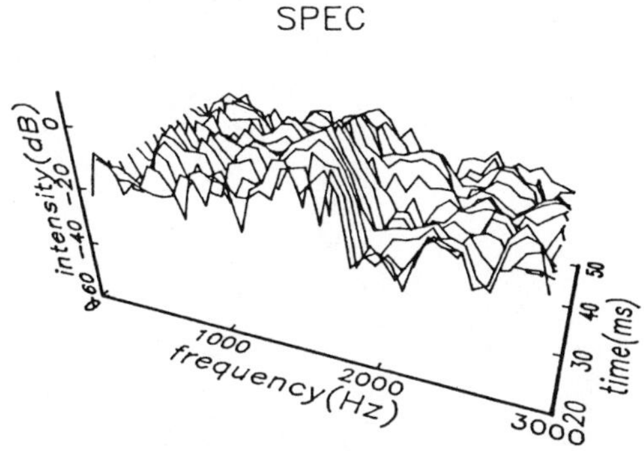

FIGURE 3a Short-time spectrogram of the curve from Fig. 1a. The time axis denotes the time after the stimulus offset. The intensity has been normalized to the maximum of the spectrogram.

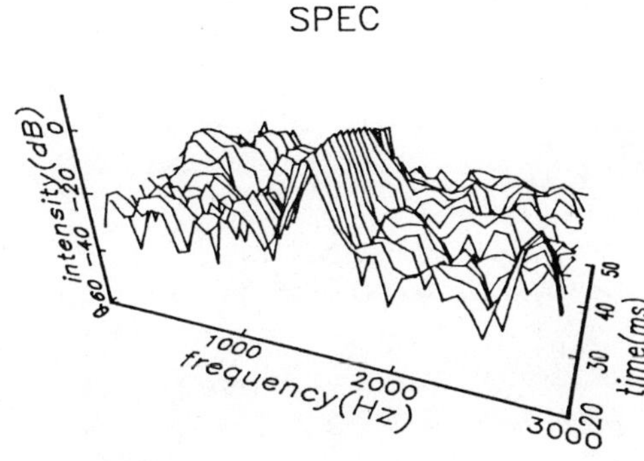

FIGURE 3b Same as Fig. 3a, but after the infusion of lidocaine (spectrogram of the curve from Fig. 1b).

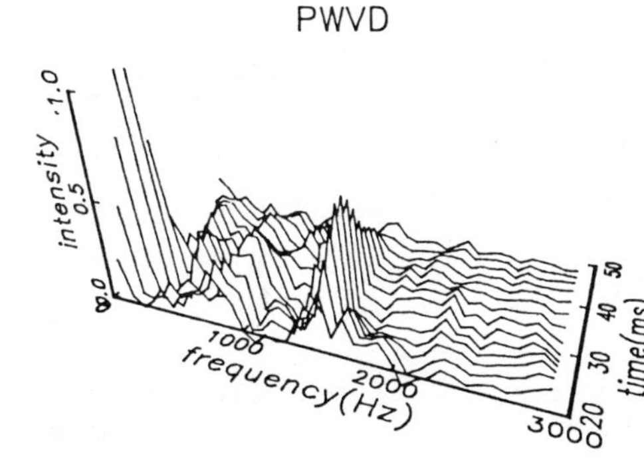

FIGURE 4a Pseudo-Wigner-Ville-Distribution (PWVD) of the curve from Fig. 1a (before lidocaine). The time axis denotes the time after the stimulus offset. The amplitude has been normalized to the maximum amplitude.

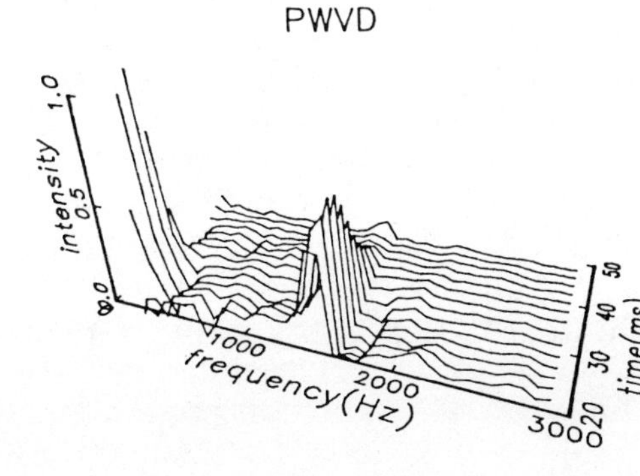

FIGURE 4b Same as Fig. 4a, but after the infusion of lidocaine (PWVD of the curve from Fig. 1b).

plots of the PWVD as given in Fig. 4 were used to specify the occurance and the structural details of the EOAEs qualitatively whereas the logarithmic plots of the average power spectra (Fig. 2) were used for the quantitative evaluation of the influence of lidocaine on the EOAEs.

TABLE I Clinical and experimental findings for all tinnitus patients. "Ø" indicates that no tinnitus and "–" that no EOAE was observed. The lidocaine effect on the EOAE is reported if it exceeds 2 dB.

subject	side	subjective kind of tinnitus	hearing loss at 2 kHz	EOAE	lidocaine effect on tinnitus	lidocaine effect on EOAE
HW	r	whisper	25 dB (hf loss)	yes	yes	0
	l	Ø	30 dB (hf loss)	yes	Ø	0
GN	r	Ø	normal	yes	Ø	0
	l	tonal at 4kHz	normal	yes	yes	0
IS	r	tonal at 6kHz	50 dB (hf loss)	yes	yes	0
	l	Ø	50 dB (hf loss)	yes	Ø	- (7.0dB)
EW	r	Ø	20 dB (hf loss)	yes	Ø	0
	l	noise, whisper	60dB (flat)	yes	yes	0
JZ	r	tonal at 8 kHz	40dB (flat)	yes	yes	+(7.5 dB)
	l	noise at 1.5kHz	40dB (flat)	yes	yes	0
RS	r	noise, whistle	40dB (dip)	yes	yes	+(9.5 dB)
	l	noise, whistle	40dB (dip)	no	yes	-
RY	r	Ø	30 dB (flat)	yes	Ø	+(4.5 dB)
	l	noise	> 90 dB	no	yes	-
US	r	Ø	normal	yes	Ø	0
	l	noise	10 dB at 4kHz	no	yes	-
MH	r	ringing	30 dB (hf loss)	yes	no	- (4.0dB)
	l	ringing	35 dB (hf loss)	yes	no	- (7.0dB)
LP	r	noise at 250 Hz	10 dB (hf loss)	yes	no	0
	l	tonal at 2 kHz	10 dB (hf loss)	yes	no	0
HG	r	tonal at 4 kHz	{normal up to 3 kHz}	yes	no	- (4.4 dB)
	l	tonal at 6 kHz		yes	no	- (3.5 dB)
HH	r	Ø	20 dB at 4 kHz	yes	Ø	+ (4.0 dB)
	l	noise, whistle	60 dB (flat)	yes	yes	+ (4.5 dB)
DH	r	Ø	normal	yes	Ø	0
	l	tonal at 750 Hz noise at 6 kHz	20 dB (hf loss)	yes	yes	+ (4.0dB)

Results

Fifteen subjects with normal hearing (aged 22 to 28) and 20 tinnitus sufferers (aged 24 to 80) were included in this study. For ten normal-hearing subjects, clear EOAEs were recorded, that is, at a stimulation level of 20 dB the level of the EOAEs exceeded 0 dB SPL. For another four normal-hearing subjects, the emissions were less than 0 dB SPL and no emission at all was found for only one normal-hearing subject. As already reported in the literature (cf. Kemp, 1978, Zwicker, 1985), the occurance of EOAEs is the normal case for normal ears.

For the least stimulus level (20 dB SL), EOAEs could only be detected for very few patients with tinnitus. Due to this lower limitation of the stimulus level and its upper limitation at 60 dB SL, saturation of the EOAE amplitude with increasing stimulus level could not be demonstrated for all patients. For five tinnitus sufferers, no emission at all could be detected even for the largest stimulus level. One important reason is the sensorineural hearing loss that accompanies tinnitus in many cases. A lidocaine test was performed for eleven of the remaining patients and two of the tinnitus sufferers without EOAEs (RY, US). Table I shows the individual results for both ears of each of the thirteen patients. A short description of the subjective tinnitus and its dominating frequencies from the matching experiment is given as well as the hearing loss at 2 kHz and a coarse classification of the individual audiogram. The subsequent columns report the occurence of an EOAE and a subjective change of the tinnitus after the infusion of lidocaine. The last column finally gives the quantitative change of the main spectral component of the EOAE under the influence of lidocaine if this effect exceeds 2 dB.

One example of an EOAE amplification after the infusion of lidocaine has been given in Figs. 1 to 4 (subject JZ, stimulus level 60 dB SL). In Fig. 2, the dominant component of the average spectrum of the EOAE around 1.5 kHz increased from 2.5 dB SPL before lidocaine to 10 dB SPL after lidocaine without alterations in the frequency of the main components. The temporal changes of the spectrum are visualized in Figs. 3 and 4 where the amplitudes have been normalized by their respective maximum. The influence of lidocaine on the EOAE is most clearly shown by the PWVD where the main spectral component becomes more distinguishable from the background after the infusion of lidocaine (Fig. 4b). The clinical data on this patient's tinnitus (different tinnitus in both ears, maskability of the tinnitus, subjective change in tinnitus quality after lidocaine) all indicate that the tinnitus is of peripheral, i.e. sensorineural origin.

TABLE II Influence of lidocaine on tinnitus and on EOAEs. The number of only those patient's ears from Tab. I is reported in the respective classification, where an EOAE could be recorded.

Lidocaine effect on:	EOAE		
Tinnitus	Amplification	No effect	Attenuation
subj. change	4	5	0
no change	0	2	4
ear w/o tinnitus	2	5	1

In order to investigate the relation between the effect of lidocaine on the EOAE and the origin of the tinnitus (i.e., the effect of lidocaine on the tinnitus), the data from Tab. I is recollected in a different way in Tab. II: Each patient's ear has been classified according to the effect of lidocaine on the tinnitus and the effect of lidocaine on the EOAE: In presence of lidocaine, the EOAEs remain essentially unchanged in ears without tinnitus whereas both groups of ears with tinnitus deviate significantly in opposite directions from this balanced distribution of the effect on EOAEs.

Conclusion

Evoked otoacoustic emissions could be measured in fourteen of fifteen normal hearing subjects and in the majority of tinnitus patients even with hearing impairment. The occurence of changes in EOAEs after an infusion of lidocaine provides further evidence that EOAEs are controlled by neural activity. In addition, the different lidocaine effect on EOAEs for ears with and without tinnitus indicates that tinnitus involves some of the neurons that constitute the neuromechanical feedback generator of OAEs. The opposite direction of the average lidocaine effect on EOAEs for ears with and without a change in tinnitus (i.e., peripheral vs. central tinnitus) suggests an inhibitory vs. excitatory influence on the efferent control of OAEs which might also be found in theoretical or animal models of tinnitus or OAEs. However, since an unambigous relation between EOAEs and tinnitus is not apparent in our data, the clinical measurement of EOAEs does not seem to be a sufficient criterion for the classification and topodiagnostic of tinnitus.

References

Claasen, T.A.C.M., Mecklenbräuker, U.F.G. (1980) The Wigner Distribution - a tool for time-frequency analysis. Philips J. Res. 35, 217-250.

Feldmann, H. (1971) Homolateral and Contralateral Masking of Tinnitus by Noise-Bands and by Pure Tones. Audiology 10, 138-144.

Hazell, J.W.P. (1984) Spontaneous cochlear acoustic emissions and tinnitus: Clinical experience in the tinnitus patient. J. Laryngol. Suppl. 9, 106-110.

Kemp, D.T. (1978) Stimulated acoustic emissions from within the human auditory system. J. Acoust. Soc. Am. 64, 1386-1391.

Penner, M.J., Burns, E.M. (1987) The dissociation of SOAE's and tinnitus. J. Speech Hear. Res. 30, 396-402.

Shulman, A., Seitz, M.R. (1981) Central Tinnitus-Diagnosis and Treatment. The Laryngoscope 91, 2025-2036.

Wilson, J.P., Sutton, G.J. (1981) Acoustic correlates of tonal tinnitus. In: Tinnitus (Eds: Evered, D. and Larenson, G.) Pitman, London, pp. 82-100.

Zwicker, E. (1985) Das Ohr als aktives schallverarbeitendes und schallaussendendes System. In: Fortschritte d. Akustik, DAGA'85, DPG-Verlag, Bad Honnef, FRG, pp. 29-44.

Comments and Discussion

PUJOL

6 out of your 26 cases shown in table I presented a hearing loss of 40dB or more: it seems then surprising that you recorded EOAEs. According to our (and others) experience, no EOAE can be recorded when the hearing loss exceeds 30dB.

EDITORS

We also feel that the author cannot have distinguished between the linear, passive ear canal and middle ear ringing and that of a nonlinear delayed OAE, for this result to have been obtained.

AN ELECTRICAL CORRELATE OF SPONTANEOUS OTOACOUSTIC EMISSIONS IN A FROG, A PRELIMINARY REPORT

H.P. Wit, P. van Dijk and J.M. Segenhout

Institute of Audiology
University Hospital
Postbox 30.001
9700 RB Groningen
The Netherlands

Introduction

Amphibians are the lowest class of vertebrates equipped with a specialized hearing organ for airborne sound. In comparison with the highly specialized inner ear of humans the amphibian inner ear is rather primitive. (Lewis et al., 1985). Therefore it is of interest that both human ears and amphibian ears produce spontaneous otoacoustic emissions (Palmer and Wilson, 1981; Wilson et al., 1986); and furthermore that there are no essential differences between emissions from human ears and from amphibian ears (Van Dijk and Wit, 1987). In both cases the acoustic emission signals are the product of a self-sustained oscillatory process (Long et al., 1988; Van Dijk and Wit, 1988), most likely in the inner ear.

Because of its relative simplicity in comparison with the human ear, study of (the generation of emissions by) the frog's inner ear might bring us closer to an understanding of the process by which otoacoustic emissions are generated.

This process must be active in the sense that energy is supplied to it to compensate for losses in its resistive elements. In the recent past it has been proposed by many authors that such an active mechanism may play an important role in the inner ear's transduction process. (For a review see: Mountain, 1986). One of the elements of the mechanism could be "nonlinear feedback, from physiological events back to cochlear mechanisms" as discussed by De Boer (1980) at the first conference fully devoted to active mechanic processes in the cochlea. Evidence for a relation between (evoked) otoacoustic emissions and a physiological event was first given by Wilson (1980), who measured cochlear microphonic responses from the round window of the cat, together with tone-burst evoked acoustical responses from the earcanal. Excellent agreement between envelope and phase delays appeared to indicate that both responses arose from the same site. Therefore Wilson (1980) considered the possibility that the measured microphonic response was an electrical correlate of the cochlear echo.

We report here the simultaneous measurement of spontaneous otoacoustic emissions from the tympanic membrane and "spontaneous microphonics" from the perilymphatic space of a frog's ear. Both signals are strongly related.

Material and Methods

Spontaneous otoacoustic emissions were recorded from six green frogs (Rana esculenta), using a sensitive condenser microphone (Van Dijk and Wit, 1987). One frog, which showed relatively strong emissions (fig. 1) was selected for further measurements. Under anaesthesia, after immersion in a o.1 % MS 222 solution, a small hole was made in the cranial side of the otic capsule, approximately halfway between the tympanic membrane and the midline of the skull. A teflon coated (except for the tip) o.13 mm diameter platinum wire was placed into this hole and fixed to the skull with dental cement. In this way the frog was supplied with a permanent electrode which contacts perilymph at the tip and protrutes from the skin at the other side.

Preceding a recording session the frog, which lives in a terrarium together with other frogs, was again lightly anaesthetized in MS 222. During a session acoustical signals were recorded from the middle ear cavity through a silastic tube gently fitted into the Eustachian tube through the mouth. (This connection to the ear has two advantages: acoustical signals are recorded from only one ear, and the tympanic membrane is free for manipulations as described in the Results section). Electrical signals were differentially recorded between the permanent otic capsule electrode and a needle electrode under the skin. The frog was placed in an electrically shielded PVC box during the measurements, inside a soundproof booth.

Electrical signals were amplified with an Ithaco 1201 low-noise preamplifier. Both acoustical and electrical signal were (simultaneously) recorded on videotape after pulse code modulation with a Sony digital audioprocessor and analyzed off-line with a Unigon 4512 real-time spectrum analyzer. This analyzer was also used to monitor the signals during recording.

Results

Figure 2 gives frequency spectra for the spontaneous otoacoustic emission signal (measured with the microphone) and the spontaneous microphonic signal (simultaneously measured through the implanted electrode) from the same (right) ear of the frog. Apart from differences in amplitude these spectra are equal, making it very likely that acoustic and electric signal are related. Extra evidence for such a relation is given by the fact that increase of body temperature (which is known to increase otoacoustic emission frequency in the frog; Wilson et al., 1986) produces identical shifts in the frequency spectra of the acoustic and the electric signal.

After 1 minute of acoustic overstimulation, with a 90 dB SPL pure tone of 1.6 kHz produced by a loudspeaker, the spontaneous microphonic

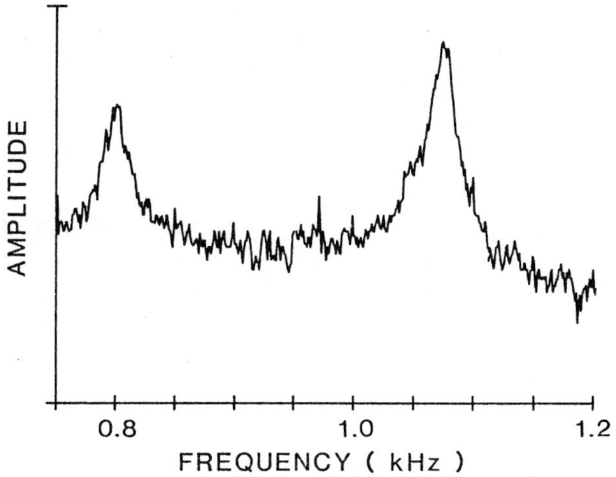

FIGURE 1. Frequency spectrum of spontaneous otoacoustic emission signal (averaged in frequency domain; log. vertical scale). Two emission peaks are visible: at 0.80 and at 1.08 kHz. The larger peak has an amplitude of 5 dB SPL and rises approximately 15 dB above the noise level of the measuring microphone.

signal has disappeared. Recovery of the signal occurs within approximately 1 minute (fig. 3). During this recovery process the external tone of 1.6 kHz. was still present at a level of 70 dB, producing the "ordinary" microphonic peak in the frequency spectra of figure 3. This ordinary microphonic signal is not affected by the acoustic overstimulation.

Contacting the tympanic membrane with the tip of a lucite rod (carefully placed with a micromanipulator), reduces the amplitude of the acoustic emission signal in the middle ear cavity (fig. 4). This reduction, however, has no large influence on the spontaneous microphonic signal.

Discussion

As far as we know, this is the first report on an electrical correlate of spontaneous otoacoustic emissions.

If the acoustic emission signal in the middle ear cavity were generated by some process outside of the frog's inner ear, reduction of the acoustic signal by damping the tympanic membrane vibration would also reduce the electric emission signal. (The electric signal would then simply be an "ordinary" microphonic signal produced by the tympanic membrane vibration). Figure 4 shows that this is not the case. This fact, and the close relation between acoustic and electric emission signal, as shown in fig 2, make it more likely that both signals have a common source, (or common sources) somewhere inside the inner ear. This source does not seem to be identical with the process that generates the "ordinary"

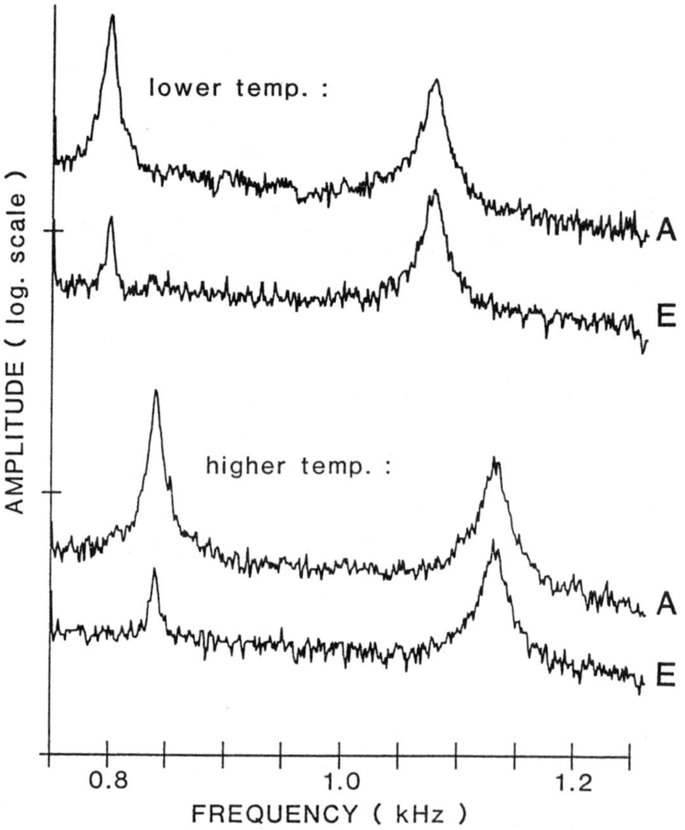

FIGURE 2. Frequency spectra of spontaneous oto-acoustic emission signal (A) and of spontaneous microphonic signal (E), before and after 2° centigrades increase of body temperature. The amplitude of the electric emission signal (E) around 1.1 kHz is 0.3 microvolt (RMS).

microphonic, because acoustic over-stimulation affects spontaneous microphonic and sound evoked microphonic signals in different ways (fig. 3). The spontaneous microphonic signal is more vulnerable.

Comparison of upper and lower traces in figure 4 shows that obstruction of tympanic membrane vibration causes a 3 percent increase for the frequency of the related spontaneous microphonic signal. (The sequence of measurements was such that a body temperature change is less likely for an explanation.) A similar frequency increase can be observed for spontaneous otoacoustic emissions in man, following a change in ear canal pressure (Schloth and Zwicker, 1983).

Acoustic overstimulation in man makes spontaneous otoacoustic emissions disappear for several minutes. And when the emission signal becomes measureable again it is at first slightly reduced in frequency (Norton et al., 1988). The frequency reduction at half a minute

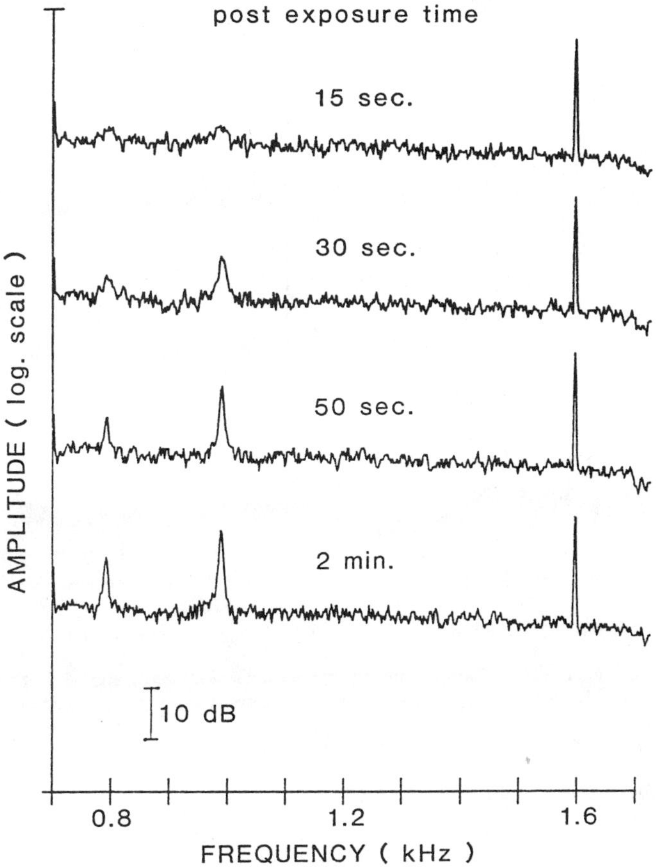

FIGURE 3. Recovery of spontaneous microphonics (Two peaks at the left) after acoustic overstimulation. The sharp peak at the right is a microphonics signal generated by the external tone. (The presence of this tone has shifted the spontaneous microphonics peaks somewhat along the frequency axis).

post-exposure time was approximately 1 percent in their study. No similar recovery from a frequency shift is observable in the frog after overstimulation. (fig. 3).

This makes generation of otoacoustic emissions by vibrating cilia of hair cells less likely, because hair stiffness is substantially reduced by overstimulation (Saunders and Flock, 1986), and we expect that this would lead to an easily observable decrease of oscillation frequency.

On the other hand, evidence for a possible involvement of haircells in the generation of acoustic signals in the ear canal (of gerbils) was given by Hubbard and Mountain (1983), who electrically stimulated scala media.

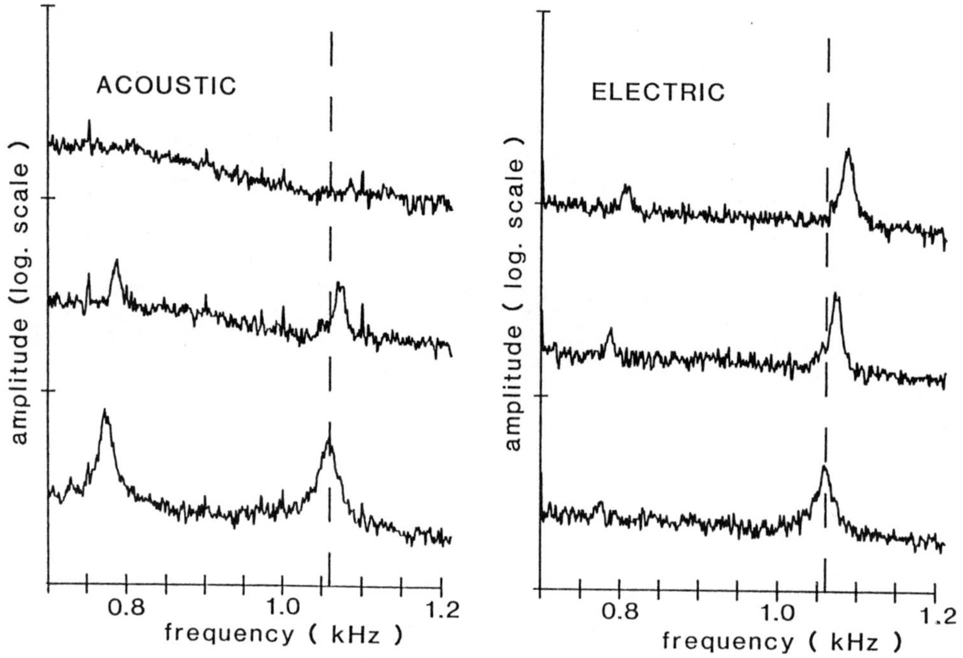

FIGURE 4. Frequency spectra of spontaneous otoacoustic emission signal (left panel) and of spontaneous microphonic signal (right panel) at different stages of obstruction of tympanic membrane vibration.
Upper traces: lucite rod firmly placed against tympanic membrane.
Middle traces: rod contacts membrane loosely.
Lower traces: no obstruction at all.

However, this evidence is rather indirect.

So, more experimental work needs to be done to shed more light on active processes in the inner ear. That further study of the frog's ear (because of its simplicity) may help us in this respect, was shown by the preliminary results reported in this paper.

References

De Boer, E. (1980). Nonlinear interactions and the "Kemp echo". Hearing Res. 2, pp. 519 - 526.

Hubbard, A.E. and Mountain, D.C. (1983). Alternating current delivered into scala media alters sound pressure at the eardrum. Science 222, pp. 510 - 512.

Lewis, E.R., Leverenz, E.L. and Bialek, W.S. (1985). The vertebrate Inner Ear, CRC, Boca Raton, Florida.

Long, G.R., Tubis, A., Jones, K.L. and Sivaramakrishnan, S. (1988). Modification of the external-tone synchronization and statistical properties of spontaneous otoacoustic emissions by aspirin consumption, Proceedings 8th International Symposium on Hearing, Paterswolde.

Mountain, D.C. (1986). Electromechanical Properties of Hair Cells. In: Neurobiology of Hearing. The Cochlea (Eds: Altschuler, R.A., Bobbin, R.P. and Hoffman, D.W.) Raven Press, New York, pp. 77 - 90.

Norton, S.J., Mott, J.B. and Neely, S.T. (1988). Changes in spontaneous otoacoustic emissions produced by acoustic stimulation. Proceedings 8th International Symposium on Hearing, Paterswolde.

Palmer, A.R. and Wilson, J.P. (1981). Spontaneous and Evoked Acoustic Emissions in the Frog Rana Esculenta, J. Physiol. 324, p. 66P.

Saunders, J.C. and Flock, A. (1986). Recovery of threshold shift in hair-cell stereocilia following exposure to intense stimulation. Hearing Res. 23, pp. 233-243.

Schloth, E. and Zwicker, E. (1983). Mechanical and acoustical influences on spontaneous oto-acoustic emissions. Hearing Res. 11, pp. 285-293.

Van Dijk, P. and Wit H.P. (1987) Temperature dependence of frog spontaneous otoacoustic emissions, J. Acoust. Soc. Am. 82 pp. 2147 - 2150.

Van Dijk, P. and Wit H.P. (1988). Phase-lock of spontaneous otoacoustic emissions to a cubic difference tone, Proceedings 8th International Symposium on Hearing, Paterswolde.

Wilson, J.P. (1980). Model for cochlear echoes and tinnitus based on an observed electrical correlate. Hearing Res. 2., pp. 527-532.

Wilson, J.P., Whitehead, M.L. and Baker, R.J. (1986). The effects of Temperature on Otoacoustic Emissions Tuning Properties. In: Auditory Frequency Selectivity (Eds: Moore, B.C.J. and Patterson, R.D.) Plenum, London, pp. 39 - 46.

Comments and Discussion

LEWIS

Based on the tonotopy in rana catesbeiana, the frequencies of emissions in your frog seem to correspond to the CFs of axons from the caudal extension of the amphibian papilla. That structure arose in the modern frogs (e.g. bufonids, hylids, micoohylids, dendrobatids, leptodactylids, ranids and rhacophorids) and is absent in the ancient frogs (e.g. leiopelmatids, pipids, discoglossids and pelobatids). It differs fom the rest of the papilla in the orientation of its hair cells (transverse rather than longitudinal) and perhaps in its lack of two tone suppression (Feng et al., 1975).

Feng, A.S., Narins, P.M. and Capranica, R.R. (1975) Three populations of primary auditory fibers in the bullfrog (R. catesbeiana): their peripheral origins and frequency sensitivities. J. Comp. Physiol., 100: 221-229.

WHITEHEAD

You have observed, in the cochlear microphonic (CM) of the frog, a difference tone apparently generated by an external tone and a spontaneous otoacoustic emission (SOAE) acting as primaries. The range of frequencies of the difference tone, external tone and SOAE fall within the region in which Baker et al (this volume) failed to detect otoacoustic difference tones upon stimulation by two external tones. Also, neurophysiological studies (e.g. Capranica and Moffat, 1980) have shown that primary afferents with best frequencies in this region show no difference tone excitation. It is surprising that this nonlinearity should be detectable in the CM response, but not in the otoacoustic or neural responses.

Capranica and Moffatt (1980) Nonlinear Properties of the Studies of Hearing in Vertebrates. Eds. Popper, A.N. Fay, R.R. Springer-Verlag, N.Y. pp. 139-165.

OTOACOUSTIC EVIDENCE FOR NONLINEAR BEHAVIOUR IN FROGS' HEARING: SUPPRESSION BUT NO DISTORTION PRODUCTS

R.J. Baker, J.P. Wilson and M.L. Whitehead

Department of Communication and Neuroscience
University of Keele, Staffs ST5 5BG, UK

Introduction

There is evidence that the mechanism responsible for the sharp auditory tuning in vertebrates may differ between classes. In mammals it has been shown, contrary to earlier indications, that the sharp tuning can be found at the level of the mechanical motion of the basilar membrane (Khanna and Leonard, 1982; Sellick *et al.*, 1982; Robles *et al.*, 1985). Such properties appear to be the result of the combination of passive basilar membrane mechanics and an active positive feedback mechanism which serves to sharpen the tuning of the basilar membrane motion. The presence of such sharp basilar membrane tuning negates the need for an additional filter within the mechanical to neural transduction mechanism.

In the alligator lizard, Weiss *et al.* (1978) demonstrated that the basilar membrane was untuned, but nevertheless, intracellular recordings from hair cells showed sharp tuning properties. In turtle hair cells, Crawford and Fettiplace (1981a) were able to demonstrate that tuning properties were determined electrically.

In the frog, *Rana temporaria*, Pitchford and Ashmore (1987) demonstrated the presence of an electrical resonance in an *in vitro* preparation of the amphibian papilla hair cells. The frequency distribution of these electrical resonators in the frog was shown to be in agreement up to 300 Hz with the tonotopic organization of the papilla innervation (Lewis *et al.*, 1982). It was also noted by Pitchford and Ashmore that the Q-factor of this electrical resonator corresponds closely to that recorded for afferent fibre tuning in the frog (Capranica, 1976). Such an electrical resonance does not appear to be present in mammalian hair cells.

The effect of variation of temperature on the auditory system provides further evidence for a difference in tuning mechanisms in mammals and lower vertebrates. The relative temperature independence of mammalian auditory tuning (Gummer and Klinke, 1983; Wilson, 1985) and the large temperature effects shown in lower vertebrates (Moffat and Capranica, 1976; Smolders and Klinke, 1984; Whitehead *et al.*, 1986) suggest that the latter rely on electrochemical rather than mechanical elements to determine tuning. The existence of otoacoustic emissions in frogs, however, is evidence that there is also a mechanical involvement. It is likely that otoacoustic emissions are closely linked to the auditory tuning mechanisms.

Nonlinear properties have been known to exist in hearing mechanisms for some time. Two ways in which they are manifested are in the change of response to one signal brought about by the presence of another signal, and in the existence in the output of distortion or intermodulation frequencies in addition to the two simultaneous input signals. The distortion products most frequently found, even at quite low levels of stimulation, are $2f_1-f_2$ and f_2-f_1, although many other components may also be present (Kemp and Brown, 1986).

Suppression curves have been shown for stimulated or spontaneous OAEs in a number of species: man (Kemp, 1979, Wit and Ritsma, 1979, Wilson, 1980, Zurek, 1981, Rabinowitz and Widin, 1984), guinea pig (Evans *et al.*, 1981), chinchilla (Zurek and Clark, 1981), dog (Ruggero *et al.*, 1984) and caiman (Strack *et al.*, 1981, see Wilson, 1984). Zurek (1981) showed using an external tone to suppress the SOAEs in his ears, that the tuning curves thus obtained were very similar to psychophysical tuning curves obtained in a masking experiment with the probe tone near the SOAE frequency and amplitude. Such a close match between these two curves suggests a close link between the mechanisms of OAE production and those of psychophysical, and thus neural, tuning in man.

In frogs the neural manifestations of such nonlinearities are limited to the low frequency population of fibres innervating the amphibian papilla (i.e. BEFs of 200-600 Hz). Such fibres can be excited by two simultaneous tones (which are ineffective in isolation) when the BEF is equal to the quadratic tone (f_2-f_1) but not $2f_1-f_2$. The suppressive effects of a second tone on neural activity are also restricted to this population of fibres and occur only if the suppressor tone is higher in frequency than the BEF of the fibre being measured (Capranica and Moffat, 1980).

The aim of this present sudy is to investigate the nonlinear properties of the frog otoacoustic emission generating mechanism by means of suppression of an SOAE by an external tone and by the acoustic response to a pair of tones. If the OAE generating mechanisms are as closely coupled to the tuning processes in frogs as they appear to be in mammals, we would expect the results to correspond to anuran neural tuning properties.

Methods

A total of 12 frogs (10 R. temporaria, 1 R. pipiens and 1 R. esculenta) were anaesthetised, with between 300 and 500 mg/Kg of MS222 injected i.p., for restraint purposes only. The animal was placed in an acoustically sealed measuring chamber within an anechoic, electrically screened room. A miniature thermocouple was placed in the frog's mouth, to monitor body temperature, and its body covered with moist gauze. Body temperature was held constant (±0.4 °C) in any experiment (range 17-21 °C). Heart rate was monitored from wire electrodes wrapped around the limbs.

The OAEs were measured using a low noise, B&K 4179 microphone coupled to the ear with 6 mm i.d. p.v.c. tube (acoustic path length 30 mm) and sealed with silicone grease. The stimulus generation system consisted of two SONY MDR-E242 earpieces, coupled to the p.v.c. tube via a metal holder with minimal enclosed volume. These were driven via attenuators or directly by low-distortion Levell TG150D oscillators for the distortion product measurements and by a B&K 1024 BFO for the suppression measurements, each monitored using digital counters. The microphone output fed, via a B&K 2660 microphone pre-amplifier at +20 dB gain with an internal two-pole 100 Hz HP-filter, into a variable phase and gain network which allowed cancellation of the stimulus components followed by a further switchable gain of 0 to +50 dB. The SOAE or distortion components were then measured by a quadrature pair of Brookdeal 401 lock-in amplifiers, the reference for which was taken from a Brookdeal 9471 VCO controlled by a multiturn pot. SOAE frequencies were measured by a frequency counter on the VCO when adjusted for a stationary spot on the XY storage display fed by the lock-ins. A SONY PCM 791ES and SL-HF100UB digital recorder was used to record SOAEs and the response to two stimulus tones for later analysis.

Results

DISTORTION PRODUCTS

In this part of the study 12 ears were investigated: 9 from *R. temporaria*, 2 from *R. pipiens* and one from *R. esculanta*. Two of the ears (one in *R. temporaria* and one in *R. esculenta*) had SOAEs present (949 Hz, -12 dB SPL and 886 Hz, -21 dB SPL respectively). The primary tone frequencies were arranged such that they both fell within the known sensitivity range of the amphibian papilla (200-1000 Hz) and that either or both of the quadratic (f_2-f_1) or the cubic ($2f_1$-f_2) difference tones fell within the frequency range (200-550 Hz) in which neural nonlinearities were found in American toads (Capranica and Moffat, 1980). The f_2/f_1 ratios used ranged from 1.1 to 1.8 although the majority were below 1.5. The stimuli used were always of equal amplitude and varied from 40 to 80 dB SPL.

In none of the experiments outlined above were the levels of distortion products (f_2-f_1, $2f_1$-f_2, $2f_1$, $2f_2$, $2f_2$-f_1) greater than the level of the system distortion measured with the microphone assembly sealed at the same position as the tympanic membrane. For 80 dB SPL stimuli the $2f_1$-f_2 and f_2-f_1 components were 70 dB below the stimuli, and for 60 dB SPL or below they fell below the noise floor (-20 dB SPL), and in some cases they were clearly more than 85 dB below the primaries.

SUPPRESSION OF SOAEs

Seven ears from fiye *R. temporaria* were used for these experiments, the SOAEs present ranging between 580 Hz and 930 Hz in frequency and -15 dB SPL and 5 dB SPL in level. Lower amplitude emissions were not used as measurements of such emissions were less precise and required much more time.

Experiment 1. For a set suppressor tone frequency the level was adjusted to obtain 5 dB suppression of the SOAE, the lock-in amplifiers being kept tuned to the SOAE frequency, and the SOAE frequency and suppressor level required for 5 dB suppression were noted. This was then repeated for different frequencies and the suppressor levels and SOAE frequency shifts (relative to the unsuppressed frequency) were plotted against suppressor frequency. Two of the five sets of results thus obtained for different ears are shown in fig. 1. These iso-suppression curves are asymmetrical with a mean low-frequency slope of -22 ± 3 (S.E.) dB/oct and a high frequency slope of 98 ± 13 dB/oct. The corresponding means from three human SOAEs given by Rabinowitz and Widin (1984) are -91 dB/oct and 234 dB/oct. Although the high and low-frequency slope values are smaller than for humans, the contours show a similar asymmetry. The frog contours appear not to be displaced towards a frequency slightly above the SOAE as in humans.

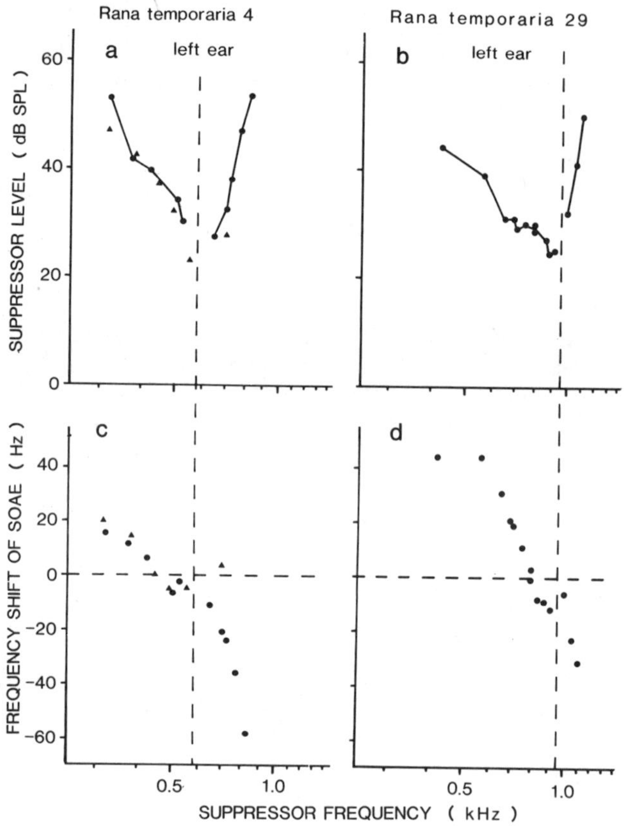

FIGURE 1. Iso-suppression contours (a and b) for two SOAEs for 5 dB of suppression shown as a function of suppressor frequency. (c and d) show the shift in SOAE frequency as a function of suppressor frequency for a constant 5 dB degree of suppression. The vertical dashed lines indicate the unsuppressed SOAE frequency. The dots and triangles represent data collected on different days. R. temporaria 4 SOAE: 580 Hz, 1 dB SPL, R. temporaria 29 SOAE: 930 Hz, -13 dB SPL.

The frequency shifting data (fig. 1) shows that suppressors above the SOAE frequency shift the SOAE down by as much as 10% and those below shift the SOAE frequency up by as much as 5% (for 5 dB suppression). These figures are much greater than the shifts found in humans (<1%) and which occur predominantly for higher frequency suppressors (Wilson and Sutton, 1981). The slopes of these frequency shift versus suppressor frequency functions, -0.11 ± 0.01 Hz/Hz for lower frequency suppressors and -0.21 ± 0.05 Hz/Hz, show a non-significant difference. The mean suppressor frequency for which the SOAE frequency shift is zero, is 99 Hz ± 16 Hz below the SOAE frequency. Apart from this narrow band between SOAE frequency and the zero shift point, and neglecting the narrow region where frequency-locking occurs, the suppressor always 'repels' the SOAE frequency.

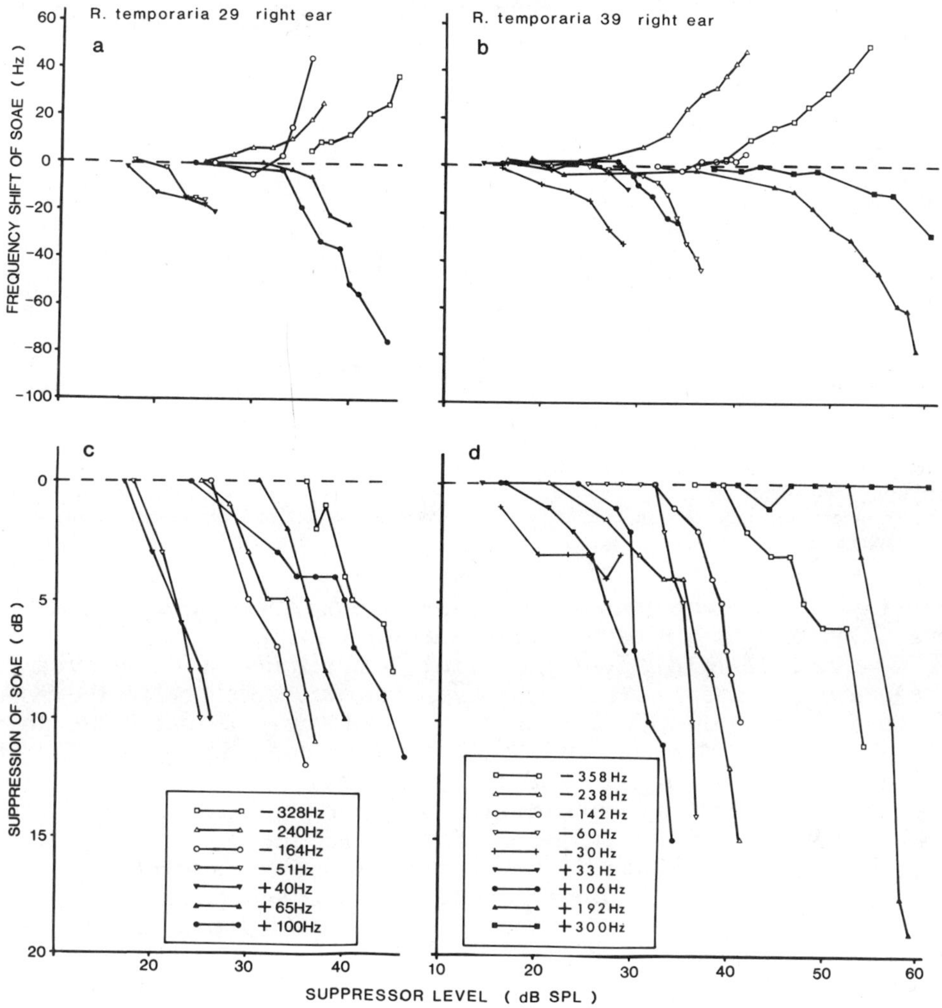

FIGURE 2. (a and b) show the shift in SOAE frequency as a function of suppressor level, with suppressor frequency as parameter. Suppressor frequency is indicated in the insets in (c and d). Note that most suppressors below the SOAE shift it upwards and vice-versa. (c and d) show the degree of suppression as a function of suppressor level with suppressor frequency as parameter. Note that there appears to be no consistent change in the shape of the suppression function with suppressor frequency. R. temporaria 29 SOAE: 840 Hz, -11dB SPL, R. temporaria 39 SOAE: 770 Hz, -2 dB SPL.

Experiment 2. The growth of suppression and the change in SOAE frequency were measured for fixed suppressor frequency as the suppressor level was varied. This is shown in figure 2 for a range of suppressor frequencies. The rate of growth of suppression was measured from the slopes of the lower graphs in fig. 2 for 3 dB or greater suppression. The mean slopes were -1.2 ± 0.2 dB/dB for *R. temporaria 29* and -1.7 ± 0.5 dB/dB for *R. temporaria 39*. There is no clear tendency for suppressors below the SOAE frequency to show a more

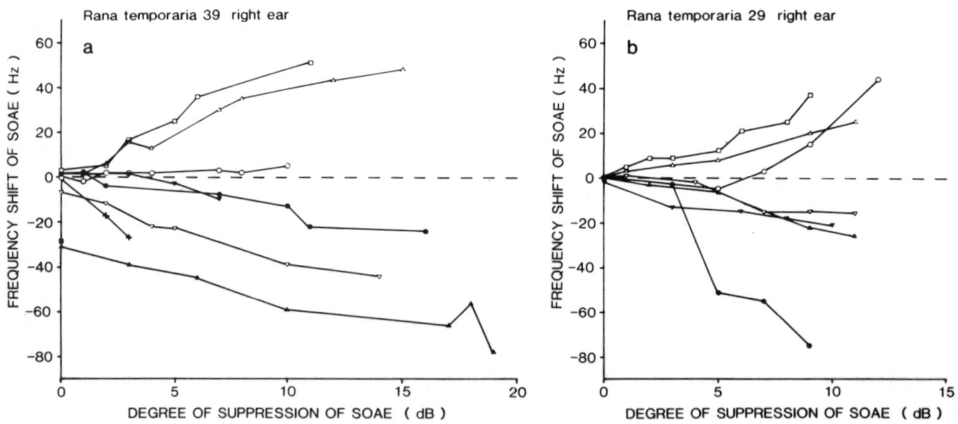

FIGURE 3. This shows frequency shifts from figure 2 (a and b) plotted as a function of degree of suppression from figure 2 (c and d, respectively). Note that in two cases frequency shift occurs before any suppression, whilst in other cases a few dB of suppression occurs before frequency shift.

rapid growth of suppression than those above as Zurek (1981) showed for man (approx. 5 dB/dB below and 0.75 dB/dB above).

The rate of SOAE frequency shift demonstrated a tendency to be frequency dependent. As noted above, suppressors well below the SOAE frequency cause the SOAE frequency to shift upwards and those above the SOAE frequency cause the SOAE to move down in frequency. The rate of change of frequency with suppressor level decreases between these two extremes, changing from positive to negative at a frequency of about 140 Hz below the SOAE frequency. Except near the cross-over point, the gradient of the frequency shift with suppressor level is greater than that shown by Wilson and Sutton (1981) for a 3 kHz suppressor and 2.6 kHz SOAE in a human, ranging from -9.5 Hz/dB to 7.9 Hz/dB depending on suppressor frequency.

Figure 3 shows the frequency shift of the SOAEs (given in fig. 2) as a function of the degree of suppression. It can be seen that in only 2 out of 16 suppressor frequencies (+192 Hz and -60 Hz) in *R. temporaria* does a frequency shift occur before the level of the SOAE is suppressed, which corresponds with the limited results presented by Rabinowitz and Widin (1984) in humans.

Discussion

The findings of Capranica and Moffat (1980) that neural distortion products and two-tone suppression are resistant to hypercapnia in anurans, suggest that the nonlinearities occur at the mechanical level for lower frequencies. The strong temperature dependence of OAEs implies an electrochemical tuning mechanism and their strength implies an efficient two-way coupling between this mechanism and mechanical processes. The failure to find distortion products in the present experiments may be due to their non-generation by higher frequency primaries where stimulus frequency emissions are measurable, and to poor mechanical coupling at low frequencies. This view is also supported by the failure of the present and previous studies (Whitehead *et al*, 1986) to find otoacoustic emissions below 500 Hz in frogs.

The presence of SOAE suppression does suggest nonlinearity at a peripheral location and its features suggest properties in common with mammalian tuning (further supported by the similarity of the compressive nonlinearity seen in EOAEs in frogs and humans, Whitehead and Baker, unpublished). One effect of a suppressor tone may be to introduce a d.c. bias to the hair cells whose polarity somehow depends on frequency position, i.e., on whether it is above or below the SOAE frequency (or more precisely, the frequency of zero shift just below the SOAE). For an electrochemical tuning mechanism this bias would change the tuning frequency (Crawford and Fettiplace, 1981b). This might explain the much greater frequency shifts in frogs compared to mammals, but might in turn suggest that the small frequency shifts found in mammals could be due to a small residual electrical component. Unfortunately, however, the effect of a suppressor tone above the CF of a hair cell appears to be depolarisation (Crawford and Fettiplace, 1981b) implying an *upward* shift in CF. The slight *downward* shift of tuning frequency of otoacoustic emissions as a function of level in humans (Wilson *et al*, 1988) and the corresponding upward pitch shift also appear to be in the wrong direction to support this view.

For human OAE iso-suppression curves (Wilson and Sutton, 1981; Wit, *et al*, 1981; Zurek, 1981; Schloth and Zwicker, 1983, and Rabinowitz and Widin, 1984) the mean low- and high-frequency slopes were estimated at -75,-70,-90,-85,-91 dB/oct. (mean -82 dB/oct.) and 97, 216, 123, 130, 234 dB/oct. (mean 158 dB/oct.) respectively. These slopes are steeper and less symmetrical than those from chinchilla (-42 and 57 dB/oct., Zurek and Clark, 1981), guinea pig (-65 and 47 dB/oct., Evans *et al*, 1981), and caiman (-25 and 40 dB/oct., Wilson, 1984). The slopes for neural tuning in frog, -30 and 35 dB/oct. (Narins and Hillery, 1983), are comparable to our data for the low frequency slopes but considerably less for the high frequency slopes.

The shape and asymmetry of the suppression pattern suggests a high-order filter in line with the neural findings of Narins and Hillery (1983) even if the elements in this filter are not mechanical as implied by the hair cell array being fixed to limbic tissue and not on a mobile basilar membrane. A tectorial membrane travelling wave may, however, exist to provide some mechanical filtering (Hillery and Narins, 1984).

References

Capranica, R.R. (1976) Morphology and Physiology of the Auditory system. In: Frog Neurobiology (Eds: Llinas, R. and Precht, W.) Springer-Verlag, Berlin, pp.551-575.

Capranica, R.R. and Moffat, A.J.M. (1980) Nonlinear Properties of the Peripheral Auditory System of Anurans. In: Comparative Studies of Hearing in Vertebrates (Eds. Popper, A.N. and Fay, R.R.) Springer-Verlag, N.Y. pp.139-165.

Crawford, A.C. and Fettiplace, R. (1981a) An electrical tuning mechanism in turtle cochlear haircells. J. Physiol., 312, 377-412.

Crawford, A.C. and Fettiplace, R. (1981b) Non-linearities in the responses of turtle hair cells. J. Physiol., 315, 317-338.

Evans, E.F., Wilson, J.P. and Borerwe, T.A. (1981) Animal models of tinnitus. In: Tinnitus. Ciba Found. Symp. 85. (Eds: Evered, D. and Lawrenson, G.) Pitman, London, pp.108-129.

Gummer, A.W. and Klinke, R. (1983) Influence of temperature on tuning of primary-like units in the guinea pig cochlear nucleus. Hear. Res.,12, 367-380.

Hillery, C.M. and Narins, P.M. (1984) Neurophysiological evidence for a travelling wave in the amphibian inner ear. Science 225, 1037-1039.

Kemp, D.T. (1979) Evidence of mechanical nonlinearity and frequency selective wave amplification in the cochlea. Arch. Otorhinolaryngol. 224, 37-45.

Kemp, D.T. and Brown, A.M. (1986) Wideband analysis of otoacoustic intermodulation. In: Peripheral Auditory Mechanisms (Eds. Allen, J.B., Hall, J.L.,Hubbard, A., Neely, S.T. and Tubis, A.) Springer-Verlag, N.Y., pp.306-313.

Khanna, S.M. and Leonard, D.G.B. (1982) Basilar membrane tuning in the cat cochlea. Science 215, 305-306.

Lewis, E.R., Leverenz, E.L. and Koyama, H. (1982) The tonotopic organization of the bullfrog amphibian papilla: An auditory organ lacking a basilar membrane. J. Comp. Physiol. 145, 437-455.

Moffat, A.J.M. and Capranica, R.R. (1976) Effects of temperature on the response properties of auditory nerve fibers in the American toad (Bufo americanus). J. Acoust. Soc. Am. 60, S80.

Narins, P.M. and Hillery, C.M. (1983) Frequency coding in the inner ear of anuran amphibians. In: Hearing - Physiological Bases and Psychophysics (Eds: Klinke, R. and Hartmann, R.) Springer-Verlag, Berlin, pp.70-76.

Pitchford, S. and Ashmore, J.F. (1987) An electrical resonance in hair cells of the amphibian papilla of the frog Rana temporaria. Hear. Res. 27, 75-83.

Rabinowitz, W.M. and Widin, G.P. (1984) Interaction of spontaneous otoacoustic emissions and external sounds. J. Acoust. Soc. Am. 76, 1713-1720.

Robles, L., Ruggero, M.A., and Rich, N.C. (1985) Mössbauer measurements of the mechanical response to single-tone and two-tone stimuli at the base of the chinchilla cochlea. In: Peripheral Auditory Mechanisms (Eds. Allen, J.B., Hall, J.L., Hubbard, A., Neely, S.T. and Tubis, A.) Springer-Verlag, N.Y., pp.121-128.

Ruggero, M.A., Kramek, B. and Rich, N.C. (1984) Spontaneous otoacoustic emissions in a dog. Hear. Res. 13, 293-296.

Sellick, P.M., Patuzzi, R. and Johnstone, B.M. (1982) Measurement of basilar membrane motion in guinea pig cochlea using the Mössbauer technique. J. Acoust. Soc. Am. 72, 131-141.

Smolders, J. and Klinke, R. (1984) Effects of temperature on the properties of primary auditory fibres of the spectacled caiman, Caiman crocodilus. J. Comp. Physiol. 155, 19-30.

Strack, G., Klinke, R. and Wilson, J.P. (1981) Evoked cochlear mechanical responses in Caiman crocodilus. Pflugers Arch. Suppl. 391, R43.

Weiss, T.F., Peake, W.T., Ling, A. and Holton, T. (1978) Which structures determine frequency selectivity and tonotopic organisation of vertebrate cochlear nerve fibres In: Evoked Electrical Activity in the Auditory Nervous System (Eds: Naunton, R. and Fernandez, C.) Academic Press, N.Y., pp.9-112.

Whitehead, M.L., Wilson, J.P. and Baker, R.J. (1986) The effects of temperature on otoacoustic emission tuning properties. In: Auditory Frequency Selectivity (Eds: Moore, B.C.J. and Patterson, R.D.) Plenum, London, pp. 39-46.

Wilson, J.P. (1980) Evidence for a cochlear origin for acoustic re-emission, threshold fine structure and tonal tinnitus. Hear. Res. 2, 233-252.

Wilson, J.P. and Sutton, G.J. (1981) Acoustic correlates of tonal tinnitus. In: Tinnitus. Ciba Found. Symp. 85. (Eds. Evered, D. and Lawrenson, G.) Pitman, London, pp.82-101.

Wilson, J.P. (1984) Otoacoustic emissions and hearing mechanisms. Rev. Laryngol. 105, (2) Suppl., 179-191.

Wilson, J.P. (1985) The influence of temperature on frequency-tuning mechanisms. In: Peripheral Auditory Mechanisms (Eds: Allen, J.B., Hall, J.L., Hubbard, A., Neely, S.T. and Tubis, A.) Springer-Verlag, N.Y., pp.229-236.

Wilson, J.P., Baker, R.J. and Whitehead, M.L. (1988) Level dependence of frequency tuning in human ears. In: Proceedings 8th. International Symposium on Hearing - Basic Issues in Hearing, Groningen, Academic Press, In press.

Zurek, P.M. (1981) Spontaneous narrowband acoustic signals emitted by human ears. J. Acoust. Soc. Am. 69, 514-523.

Zurek, P.M. and Clark, W.W. (1981) Narrow-band acoustic signals emitted by chinchilla ears after noise exposure. J. Acoust. Soc. Am. 70, 446-450.

Comments and Discussion

WIT

Increasing frequency shift of an SOAE for increasing level of a suppressor tone, as shown in Figs. 2a and 2b in the paper by Baker et al., can also be observed for the electrical correlate of a spontaneous otoacoustic emission in a frog (Wit et al., this volume). This is shown in Fig. 1.

Peak number 2 in the frequency spectra in this figure is a microphonics response to an external tone (1.79 kHz), produced by a loudspeaker. The level of this tone in dB SPL is given at the right side of the figure.

Peak number 1 is the electrical correlate of an SOAE. The figure shows what actually happens: For higher levels of the external tone an electrical distortion product (peak number 3) is created ($f_3 = f_2 - f_1$). This distortion product approaches the SOAE if the level of the external tone is increased. And finally distortion product and SOAE coincide: the emission generator is forced to oscillate at exactly half the frequency of the external tone. (Apart from $f_2 - f_1$, $f_2 + f_1$ and $2f_2$ are also present in the frequency spectrum, if the frequency range is extended from 2 to 5 kHz).

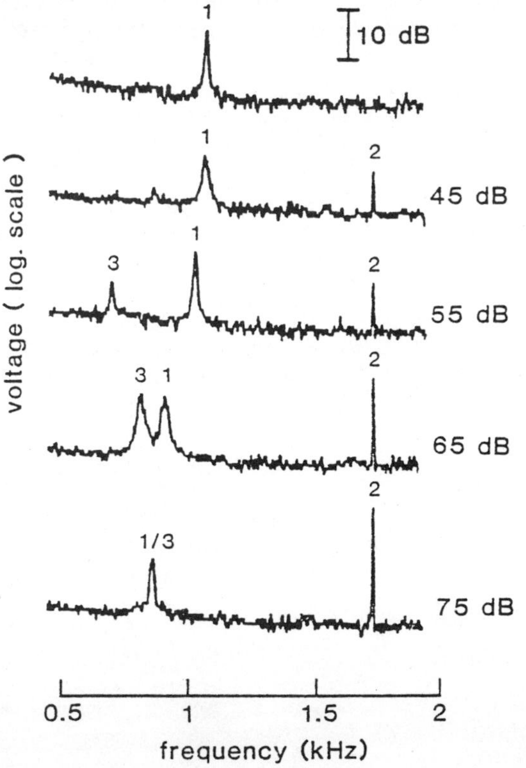

FIGURE 1. Upper trace: Electrical correlate of SOAE (1). Lower traces: External tone at 1.79 kHz (2) causes frequency shift of SOAE and generates electrical distortion product (3).

LEWIS

In our experimental animal, *Rana catesbeiana*, the order of the amphibian-papillar filter dynamics implied by phase data can be as high as twenty (Lewis, 1984; Lewis & Lombard, 1988). However, after carefully considering the possibility of a traveling-wave supported solely by the tectorial membrane of the frog amphibian papilla (Lewis and Leverenz, 1983), we rejected it on the grounds that it could not be consistent at once with both the observed tonotopy of the papilla and the observed morphology of the tectorium. Furthermore, the frequency dependence of the phase observed in cycle histograms showed systematic deviations from the linearity one would expect from a traveling wave in a continuous medium (Lewis, 1984, 1987). As an alternative hypothesis, we proposed that electrically resonant hair cells, bidirectionally coupled to each other through the micromechanical elements of the papilla (largely the tectorium) might provide the high-order dynamics of the filter. In effect, we proposed that the hair cells and the tectorium combine to yield a lumped-element traveling-wave structure. This could account for the strong temperature dependence of tuning seen in the axons of the amphibian papilla (Zakon & Wilczynski, 1988). It is interesting to note that acoustic sensors have arisen five or more times in the vertebrate ear (fish and amphibian saccule; clupeid utricle; elasmobranch macula neglecta; fish and amphibian lagena; amphibian papilla; basilar papilla/cochlea). In every instance in which the corresponding spectral filter has been examined carefully, it has proved to have high-order dynamics (in contrast to the low-order dynamics usually attributed to vestibular endorgans). Furthermore, the frequency dependence of the phase is usually nearly linear. This suggests that these sensors converged on a filter design that provided good temporal resolution as well as good spectral resolution.

Lewis, E.R. (1984) On the frog amphibian papilla. Scan. Electr. Microsc. 1984: 1899-1913.

Lewis, E.R. (1987) Speculations about noise and the evolution of vertebrate hearing. Hearing Res. 25, 83-90.

Lewis, E.R. and Lombard, R.E. (1988) The amphibian inner ear. In: The Evolution of the Amphibian Auditory System (Ed. B. Fritsch) Wiley, N.Y., pp. 93-123.

Zakon, H.H. and Wilczynski, W. (1988) The physiology of the anuran eighth nerve. In: The Evolution of the Amphibian Auditory System (Ed. B. Fritsch) Wiley, N.Y., pp. 125-155.

OTOACOUSTIC EMISSIONS AND COCHLEAR TRAVELLING WAVES

Eberhard Zwicker

Institute of Electroacoustics
Technical University München
Arcisstr.21, D-8000 München 2, F.R.Germany

Introduction

An interesting characteristic of human hearing is the frequency distance of extreme values of all three kinds of emissions, spontaneous (SOAE), simultaneous evoked (SEOAE), and delayed evoked (DEOAE) otoacoustic emissions. This preferred frequency distance was described as being frequency dependent. Transformed into the critical band rate, however, it shows a quite constant value. The first data collection (Zwicker and Schloth, 1984) pointed towards a characteristic value of about a half of a critical band width. Larger data collection (Dallmayr, 1985, 1987) for SOAE and SEOAE uncovered this characteristic value as being close to 0.4 Bark. This value seems to be very stable and quite independent of subjects. The reason for this value must be hidden somehow in the cochlear mechanics. It is the goal of this paper to search for such a relation.

Since direct physiological measurements on human inner ears are not possible, analog models like that of cochlear nonlinear preprocessing with feedback (Zwicker, 1985a) seem to be useful for comparisons and indirect conclusions. The subdivision of this model into sections was slightly refined and its frequency range somewhat enlarged. In order to simulate the original strategy even closer, the proposed lateral coupling (Zwicker, 1979) was also introduced.

The characteristic value of 0.4 Bark

The frequency distance of neighbouring spontaneous otoacoustic emissions (SOAE) transformed into corresponding critical band rate distance and outlined as probability (Dallmayr, 1985), is given in Fig. 1a. A distinct peak at 0.4 Bark indicates that this distance appears very often and independent of frequency. At frequencies around 3 kHz this distance is near 250 Hz, while it is only about 40 Hz near 500 Hz.

Simultaneous evoked otoacoustic emissions (SEOAE) are measured as ripple in the frequency response of the sound pressure in the closed ear canal for constant electrical input level of the probe's transducer. The frequency distance of neighbouring maxima or minima was again

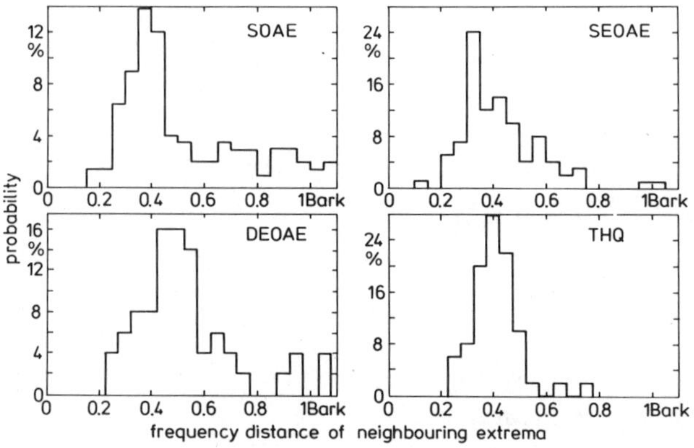

FIGURE 1: Frequency distance of SOAE and of neighbouring extrema of SEOAE, of the spectral content of DEOAE, and of threshold in quiet (THQ). Partly adopted from Dallmayr, 1985, 1987.

transformed into critical band rate distance (Dallmayr,1987). The result is shown in Fig. 1b and indicates again a strong concentration of the probability around 0.4 Bark.

Delayed evoked otoacoustic emissions (DEOAE) are commonly expressed as time functions. However, DEOAE's can be analyzed in frequency (see Zwicker and Schloth, 1985, Fig. 6). The spectra of DEOAEs obtained this way often show many distinct maxima. The frequency distance of these maxima was measured for three subjects without SOAEs but DEOAEs of considerable size. The corresponding critical band rate distance outlined in Fig. 1c shows a peak at about 0.45 Bark.

The close relation between otoacoustic emissions and the microstructure of threshold in quiet was already discussed in a former paper (Zwicker and Schloth,1985). Therefore, data of this microstructure available in our laboratory and in the literature (especially from Long, et al. 1986) have been used to search for a characteristic frequency distance. Most accurately describable are the minima in the frequency dependence of threshold in quiet. The frequency difference of neighbouring minima were transformed into critical band rate distance and statistically evaluated. The results of 8 subjects (Fig. 1d) show again a distinct peak close to the value of 0.4 Bark.

All four distributions shown in Fig. 1 indicate a clear emphasis of the probability near 0.4 Bark. This value seems to be unique for human cochlea processes which take place at low levels close to threshold and which need active feedback to be generated.

Level- and phase-place patterns in the model

The peripheral preprocessing model with nonlinear saturating feedback is described in detail elsewhere (Zwicker,1985a). The number of sections

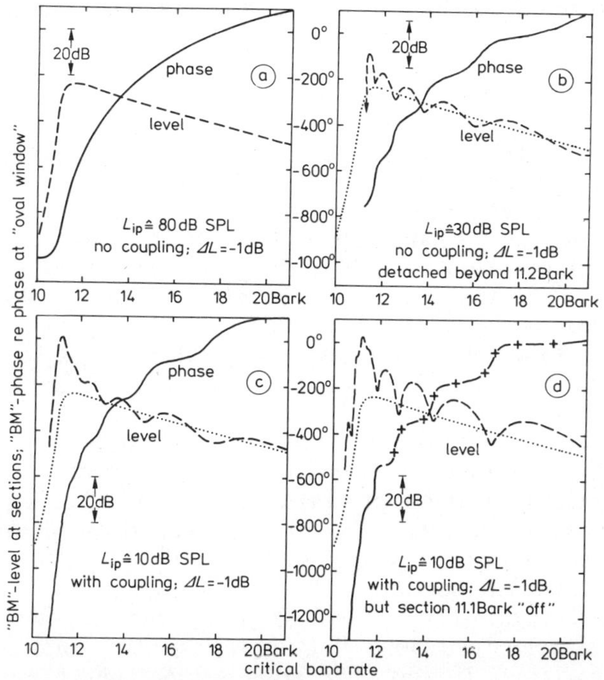

FIGURE 2: Level- and phase-place pattern, i.e. data as a function of the section number expressed in critical band rate. Frequency is 1505 Hz, corresponding to a characteristic critical band rate of 11.2 Bark. The parameter conditions are indicated. Subdivision in the model is 10 sections per Bark, i.e. per 1.3 mm.

has been enlarged from 90 to 150 with a section width corresponding to 0.1 Bark. The structure of the sections remained the same. The outer hair cells, stimulated by the vibration of the basilar membrane, are assumed to act as a saturating amplifier which feeds back to the vibration of the basilar membrane which is picked up and transformed into neural activity by the inner hair cells. This feedback can be effective only at low levels since the amplifier's gain is strongly reduced at high levels due to its saturation characteristic. Therefore, the system acts at high levels like the corresponding passive system, i.e. without feedback.

Fig. 2 shows the level and phase corresponding to the velocity of the basilar membrane as a function of the distance along the basilar membrane, expressed in critical band rate. One Bark corresponds to about 1.3 mm distance along the basilar membrane, i.e. the section width of 0.1 Bark integrates about 50 outer hair cells in three rows. Large Bark-values point towards the oval window. A 1505-Hz tone with a level corresponding to 80 dB SPL was used as stimulus. Its characteristic place is 11.2 Bark. The level-place pattern (broken in Fig. 2a) shows the expected increment towards helicotrema, i.e. smaller critical band rates, until a maximum is reached, beyond which the level strongly diminishes. The phase-place pattern shows decreasing phase with decreasing critical band rate, first slowly then rapidly, before it reaches a plateau. Both patterns correspond to those found in the passive system. The slope of the phase-pattern reaches a value of about 400 degrees per Bark at the steepest point which corresponds to the characteristic place.

Patterns for low levels with feedback on are shown in a former paper (Zwicker,1985a). For all data described here, the gain of the amplifiers is set at about 1 dB (DL = -1 dB) below that amplification which would just lead to self-oscillation. This creates a 20 dB larger level at 11.2 Bark in the level-place pattern in relation to that of Fig. 2a. Close inspection of the curves indicates a small ripple in the level pattern and of the phase pattern, with long place periods at large critical band rates and smaller place periods near the characteristic place. This ripple is due to the subdivision into sections which produces unwanted OAEs of small size. The steepest slope of the phase-place distribution increases a little compared to that of Fig. 2a to about 500 degrees per Bark.

A lateral coupling was installed in the model by two additional resistors in each section which connect the output of the amplifier to the two neighbouring points of basilarmembrane vibration. Such a lateral coupling can simulate the fact that electrical AC-fields produced in the outer hair cells show a lateral spread. The feedback factor which couples to the next neighbours was installed to be one third of the coupling towards the identical section. The consequence of this procedure is shown in Fig. 2c again for low levels. The effect is generally the same as found with simple feedback, but there are two interesting additional effects besides larger ripples: The enhancement at 11.2 Bark is not only larger (27 dB) but also broader reaching a frequency selectivity closer to what is measured in tuning curves. Additionally, the slope of the phase-place curve shows no plateau while its steepness is enlarged to about 800 degrees per Bark.

There are many possibilities to produce artificial discontinuities. Manley (1983) proposed them as the source of OAE. The most drastic discontinuity is that of totally cutting off the model at a certain place which would correspond to an elimination of the basilar membrane beyond that place. The result of such a cut beyond section 11.2 Bark in the model with simple feedback (no coupling) is shown in Fig. 2b for an input level of 30 dB. The level- and phase-place pattern clearly show a standing wave superimposed on the travelling wave. It produces a ripple along both patterns so that phase steps with a height of 180 degrees coincide with minima in the level pattern. Actually, the strong discontinuity leads to self-oscillation corresponding to a 15-dB spontaneous "otoacoustic" emission (SOAE). The SOAE disappears, however, for input levels as used in producing the data of Fig. 2c.

Less drastic discontinuities can be installed in the model by reducing the gain of the feedback amplifiers. The feed back of section 11.1 Bark, i.e. that following the characteristic place of 11.2 Bark for 1505 Hz, was chosen to be switched off. The consequence of this reduction is shown in Fig. 2d. The enhancement at 11.2 Bark increased to 30 dB; the ripple in the level-place curve is strongly enlarged; the ripple in the phase-place curve indicating a standing wave is not only enlarged, but the phase is reversed, i.e. the travelling wave is seen as a wave which travels towards the oval window (indicated by the "plus"-symbols). This means that more energy is produced within the model than is introduced to the model at the oval window.

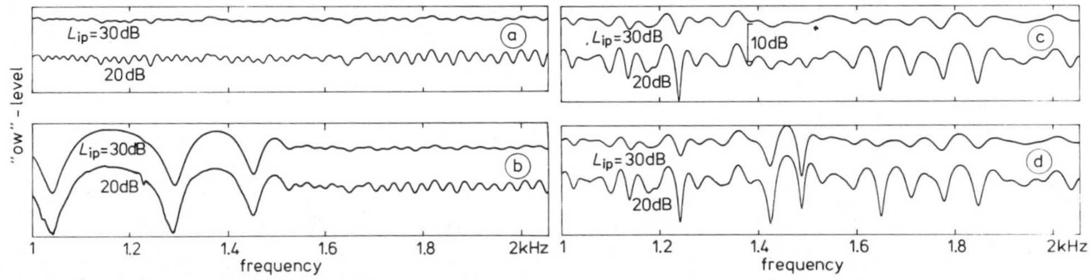

FIGURE 3: "SEOAEs" in the model, i.e. level of a tone at the "oval window" as a function of its frequency for given levels and four conditions. No coupling, no special discontinuity in (a); no coupling, model cut beyond 11.2 Bark in (b); with lateral coupling, no special discontinuity in (c); with coupling, feedback off in section 11.2 in (d).

"Otoacoustic" emissions in the model

Simultaneous evoked "otoacoustic" emissions (SEOAE) are measured in the model as the frequency dependence of the level picked up at the "oval window",i.e. the input of the model when fed through a matching resistive impedance. The traces shown in Fig. 3 belong to situations of low input levels and additionally to "no lateral coupling" in (a), with the model cut beyond 11.2 Bark in (b), "with lateral coupling" in (c), and" with lateral coupling and single discontinuity at 11.1 Bark (feedback off)" in (d). The ripple shown in (a) corresponds to the subdivision into sections which produces a frequency separation of neighbouring minima of about 30Hz near 1800 Hz correspondingto 0.1 Bark, which is the subdivision. Cutting off the model beyond 11.2 Bark produces very prominent ripple for frequencies below 1500 Hz due to the characteristic frequency of the last section before disconnection. The frequency distance between neighbouring maxima or minima increases with decreasing frequency from 125 to 160, 215, and 250 Hz. This is in contrast to the decrement of frequency distances with decreasing frequency observed for OAEs of subjects. The effect in the model is due to the drastic discontinuity which reflects the incoming travelling wave so that a wave travelling backwards to the oval window is superimposed. This super position produces maxima and minima at the oval window for frequencies which produce the proper phase-place pattern (corresponding to that shown for 1505Hz in Fig. 2a). The drastic discontinuity produces the wellknown effect of reflections along a mismatched line which, however, differs strongly from what is produced in SEOAEs and DEOAEs.

Installing lateral coupling in the model without special discontinuity (c) not only enlarges the ripple in comparison to (a) but also widens the distance between minima to 67 Hz at 1800 Hz. This ripple is still created through the 0.1- Bark subdivision and through the not exactly homogeneous distribution of the elements and of the coupling in the model. The homogenity seems to be better around 1500 Hz and consequently the ripple is smaller there. Therefore, section 11.1 Bark (corresponding to a characteristic frequency of 1475Hz) was chosen as the place for a distinct single discontinuity (feedback switched off). The

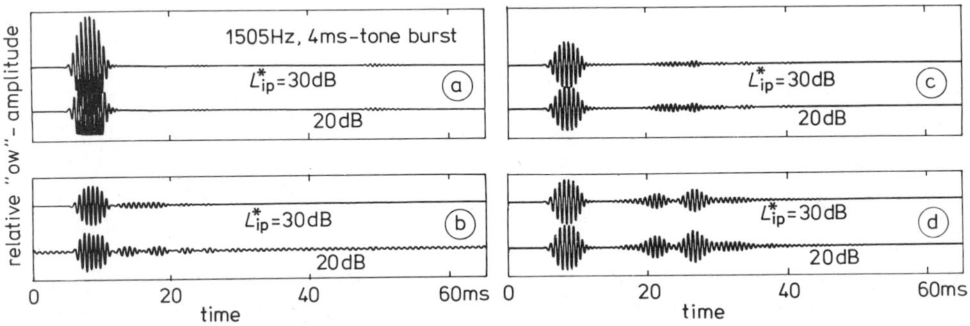

FIGURE 4: "DEOAEs" in the model, i.e. time functions of "oval window" - voltage with normalized amplitude as a response to a 1505-Hz tone burst of 4-ms duration and 2-ms Gaussian rise and fall time. Parameters as in Fig.3.

consequences are a maximum in between two distinct minima. The maximum appears at 1460 Hz and the frequency separation between the two minimais 65 Hz corresponding to a critical band rate distance of 0.28 Bark. This is the critical band rate distance needed to change the phase by 180 degrees in the phase-place pattern (Fig. 2d).

Delayed evoked "otoacoustic" emissions picked up in the model also at the "oval window" and for the same parameter conditions of Fig. 2 and Fig. 3 are shown in Fig. 4. Tone bursts with a duration of 4 ms, Gaussian rise/fall times of 2ms, and a tone frequency of 1505 Hz are used in order to concentrate the spectrum closely around the extrema produced by the discontinuities. DEOAEs produced in condition (a) are very small and show long delay time of about 40 ms corresponding to the ripple distance in Fig. 3a of 1/40 ms = 25 Hz. Disconnecting the part of the model beyond 11.2 Bark leads to atypical "DEOAEs". The time functions illustrated in Fig. 4c show no pause following the evoking burst indicating the difference from real DEOAEs. The time function superimposes with the occuring SOAE for the lower inputlevel. At large input levels, the response to a short DC-impulse shows a delay time of 3.6 ms as should be expected by assuming a single reflection at 11.2 Bark (travelling time 1.8 ms). For the condition "with coupling", Fig. 4c indicates larger DEOAE so that the gain of the registration could be reduced by a factor of two in comparison to panel (a). The delay time is about 18ms. The single discontinuity enlarges the DEOAE even further (Fig. 4d). Its time function shows two maxima, with delay times of about 14 ms and 19 ms. These values are correlated to the reciprocal values of frequency distances between the neighbouring minima or maxima (65 Hz and 55 Hz). All these data together confirm the formerly (Zwicker, 1985b) stated relation between DEOAE's delay time and SEOAE's frequency distance by simple reciprocity.

The frequency distances of neighbouring extrema in subjects are about 40 per cent larger than in the model. The delay time of DEOAE's are - in consequence of that - smaller for subjects than for the analog model. In order to produce model data which are more similar to those of subjects, the phase-place curves as indicated in Fig. 2 (solid) have to be changed a little. Such parameter variation, however, can be done much more easily in computer models of which we have two kinds available. One acts in the frequency domain (Lumer, 1987, Zwicker and Lumer, 1987), the other in the time domain (Peisl, 1988). Data from computer models are also interesting in view of a larger number of sections per Bark, so that the artifacts produced by the discretization become negligible.

Conclusion

The value of 0.4 Bark, characteristic for normal human hearing at small levels for which nonlinear active feedback in the cochlea has to be assumed, seems to be closely related to the phase-place patterns. Data produced in the model indicate that an almost homogeneous system with feed back is needed to produce the basis for the creation of OAEs. The reason for the characteristic value of 0.4 Bark is hidden in the system by the "450 degrees per Bark slope" of the phase-place pattern. Small discontinuities together with lateral coupling and with feedback conditions near oscillation create distinct SEOAEs and DEOAEs.

The travelling wave of the vibration of the basilar membrane seems to produce almost independent of frequency a pattern which is characterized by the fact that velocities 0.5 mm towards both sides of the place of maximum are out of phase relative to the velocity at the maximum. Therefore, it is possible to gain from OAEs indirect information about the hydromechanics of the human cochlea, at least in the frequency range between 500 Hz and 4 kHz.

Acknowledgements

This work was performed within the Sonder forschungsbereich 204 "Gehör", München, supported by the Deutsche Forschungsgemeinschaft.

References

Dallmayr, C. (1985) Spontane otoakustische Emissionen, Statistik und Reaktion auf akustische Störtöne. Acustica 59, 67-75.

Dallmayr, C. (1987) Stationary and dynamic properties of simultaneous evoked otoacoustic emissions (SEOAE). Acustica 63, 243-255.

Long, G.R., Tubis, A., and Jones, K. (1986) Changes in spontaneous and evoked otoacoustic emissions and the corresponding psychoacoustic threshold microstructure induced by aspirin consumption. In: Peripheral Auditory Mechanisms (Eds: J.B. Allen et al.) Springer Verlag, Berlin, pp. 213-220.

Lumer, G. (1987) Computer model of cochlear preprocessing (steady state condition) I. Basics and results for one sinusoidal input signal. Acustica 62, 282-290.

Manley, G.A. (1983) Frequency spacing of acoustic emissions: a possible explanation. In: Mechanisms of Hearing. W.R. Webster and L.M. Aitkin (Eds.), Monash-University Press, Melbourne, pp. 36-39.

Peisl,W. (1988) Simulation von zeitverzögerten evozierten oto-akustischen Emissionen mit Hilfe eines digitalen Innenohrmodells. In:Fortschritte der Akustik, DAGA'88, Verl.: DPG-GmbH, Bad Honnef. (in press)

Zwicker, E. (1979) A model describing nonlinearities in hearing by active processes with saturation at 40dB. Biol. Cybernetics 35, 243-250.

Zwicker, E. (1986a) A hardware cochlear nonlinear preprocessing model with active feedback. J.Acoust.Soc.Am. 80, 154-162.

Zwicker, E.(1986b) "Otoacoustic" emissions in a nonlinear cochlear hardware model with feedback. J.Acoust.Soc.A. 80, 163-176.

Zwicker, E. and Lumer, G. (1985) Evaluating traveling wave characteristics in man by an active nonlinear cochlear preprocessing model. In: Peripheral Auditory Mechanisms, (Eds: J.B.Allen et al.) Springer, Berlin, pp. 250-257.

Zwicker, E. and Schloth, E. (1984) Interrelation of different oto-acoustic emissions. J.Acoust.Soc.Am. 75, 1148-1154.

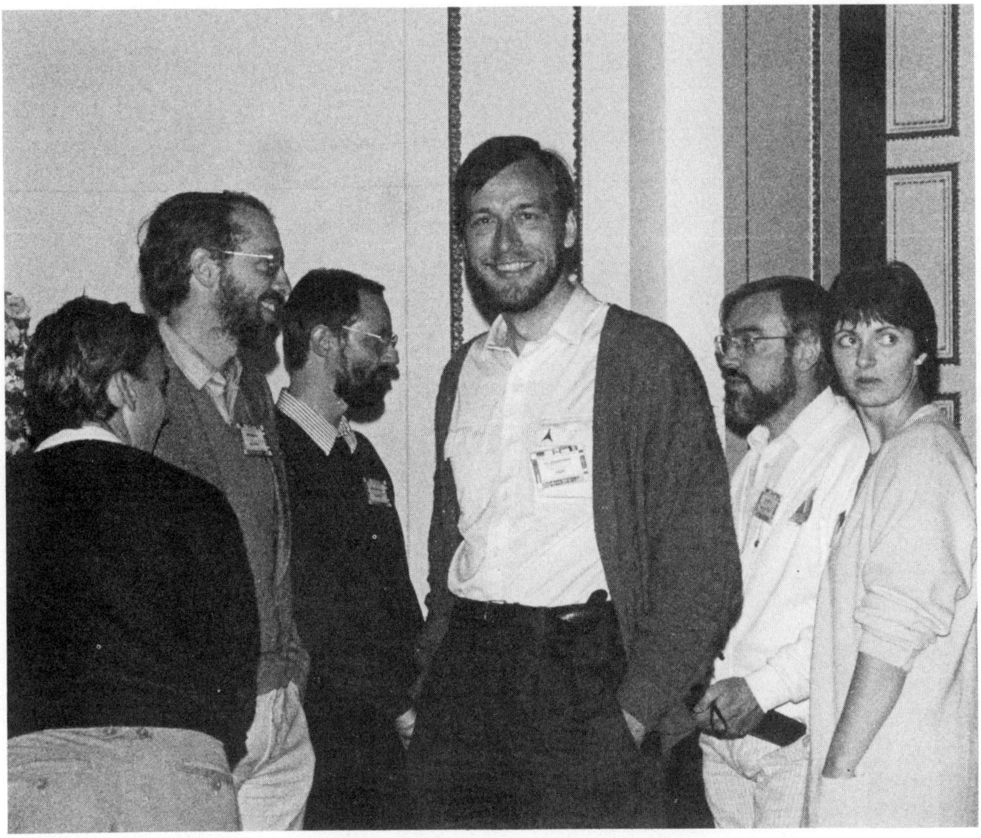

R.B. Patuzzi, A.W. Gummer, J.W.T. Smolders, R.J. Diependaal, G.A. Manley and C. Köppl

6. MACROMECHANICAL MEASUREMENTS

NONLINEAR INTERACTIONS IN THE MECHANICAL RESPONSE OF THE COCHLEA TO TWO-TONE STIMULI

Luis Robles, Mario A. Ruggero* and Nola C. Rich*

Departamento de Fisiología y Biofísica, Facultad de Medicina
Universidad de Chile, Casilla 70055, Santiago, Chile
**Department of Otolaryngology, University of Minnesota*
Minneapolis, MN 55414, U.S.A.

Introduction

The reduction of the auditory response to one tone due to the simultaneous presence of a second tone is known as two-tone suppression. This nonlinear cochlear response was first described by Galambos and Davis (1944) in electrophysiological recordings from the cat auditory nerve. Since then two-tone suppression has been extensively studied in cochlear afferents of mammals (Nomoto et al., 1964; Kiang et al., 1965; Hind et al., 1967; Sachs and Kiang, 1968) and also of amphibia (Frischkopf and Goldstein, 1963; Feng et al., 1975), birds (Sachs et al., 1974) and reptiles (Holton and Weiss, 1978). Two-tone suppression seems to be demonstrable in all well-studied cochlear fibers, for suppressors at frequencies on both sides of the tuning curve (Sachs and Kiang, 1968; Sachs, 1969; Abbas and Sachs, 1976), and has also been observed in guinea pig inner hair cells (Sellick and Russell, 1979).

The finding of a nonlinearity in the motion of the squirrel monkey basilar membrane (BM) (Rhode, 1971; Rhode and Robles, 1974) raised the possibility that two-tone interactions could in part be generated at the BM mechanics. Subsequent mechanical measurements (Rhode, 1977) showed the existence in the BM response of two-tone suppression by suppressors above characteristic frequency (CF, the most sensitive frequency for that position on the BM). However, these results were obtained at fairly high intensities (85-95 dB SPL for tones at CF; 70-120 dB SPL for suppressors) and cannot be directly compared to suppression measured in cochlear fibers at much lower intensities.

Recently, investigations using BM preparations in animals with minimal surgical damage (Sellick et al., 1982; Khanna and Leonard, 1982; Robles et al., 1986) have succeeded in demonstrating mechanical responses as sharply tuned as those from auditory nerve fibers innervating the same cochlear region. Two of these studies (Sellick et al., 1982; Robles et al., 1986) have confirmed the existence of nonlinearities, for frequencies around CF, even at low stimulus intensities (10 to 20 dB SPL). In addition, Patuzzi et al. (1984) have shown that phase-specific suppression effects of low-frequency tones upon cochlear-ganglion-cell and inner-hair-cell responses to near-CF tones substantially reflect similar phenomena observed in BM motion. In this paper we present mechanical measurements of two-tone suppression at the basal end of the chinchilla cochlea, obtained using the Mossbauer technique. Our results, for suppressor tones at above-CF frequencies, show suppression magnitudes and phase lags comparable to those of discharge-rate suppression reported for auditory nerve fibers at similar frequencies and intensities of stimulation.

Methods

All experiments were performed in chinchillas anesthetized with sodium pentobarbital (65 mg/kg intraperitoneally). A small hole was drilled in the basal turn of the otic capsule allowing direct visualization of the BM. A radioactive source (80 um square or 50 by 100 um, cut from a 6-um-thick rhodium foil doped with Co-57) was gently placed on the BM at a location about 3.5 mm from the base. A Fe-57-enriched palladium foil absorber mounted in front of the detector, a proportional counter, provided an isomer shift of 0.07 mm/s for the source-absorber combination. The 14.4-KeV Mossbauer radiation was selected by means of a single-channel analyzer and the times of occurrence of gamma rays were binned into 32-bin period histograms locked to the probe tone. Velocity and phase of the BM motion were estimated using a least-squares program. Stimulus tones were generated independently by uniform sampling and digital to analog conversion from a 16-bit, 8-K word read-only-memory containing a sine table. The two tones were delivered through Beyer DT-48 earphones mounted on the back of a plastic speculum, which was sealed to the bony ear canal by means of ear-impression compound. The sound pressure at the ear canal was measured using a miniature microphone. More details on methods can be found in Robles et al. (1986).

Results

The effect of a suppressor tone on the magnitude and phase of the response to the probe tone was measured at several combinations of frequencies and intensities of the two tones. Probe tones were set at frequencies at or near CF and at intensities that produced a clear response when presented alone (30 to 80 dB SPL). Suppressor tones were set at frequencies higher than CF (with a suppressor/probe frequency ratio of 1.18 to 1.4) and at intensities that did not produce a measurable response when presented alone (20 to 90 dB SPL). Two-tone suppression was demonstrated in five of the six animals studied.

Figure 1 shows BM-response suppression measured as the reduction in BM velocity of vibration in response to the probe tone due to the simultaneous presentation of the suppressor tone. Suppression was measured as a function of suppressor intensity for 8.5 and 9 kHz probe tones at 41 to 51 dB SPL. The suppressors used were 11 and 12 kHz tones at intensities ranging from 30 to 78 dB SPL. For all suppressors the curves obtained display an increase of suppression with suppressor intensity. They also show greater magnitudes of suppression for the suppressor (11 kHz) closer in frequency to the probe and for probe tones at lower intensities.

Due to the limited dynamic range of the Mossbauer technique, it is difficult to measure large magnitudes of suppression using the stimulation paradigm of Fig. 1 (i.e., fixed-level probes and varying suppressor intensities). Therefore, in some experiments we studied the effect of suppressor tones on the response to probe tones by observing the horizontal shift of the intensity function for the probe tone caused by the simultaneous presentation of a suppressor tone (Javel et al., 1978). Figure 2 displays intensity functions for the probe tone alone (solid symbols), and in the presence of a suppressor tone (open symbols). Time (referred to placement of the Mossbauer source) at which the intensity curves were obtained is indicated in the figure. In all three cases the suppressor tone produced a clear shift of the probe-tone intensity function to higher intensities (i.e., reduced sensitivity). The largest suppression obtained in this experiment, for the 12 kHz, 90 dB SPL suppressor, amounts to 21 dB at low probe levels and about 7 dB at higher ones. Due to this dependency of suppression magnitude on probe level, the effect of the suppressor on

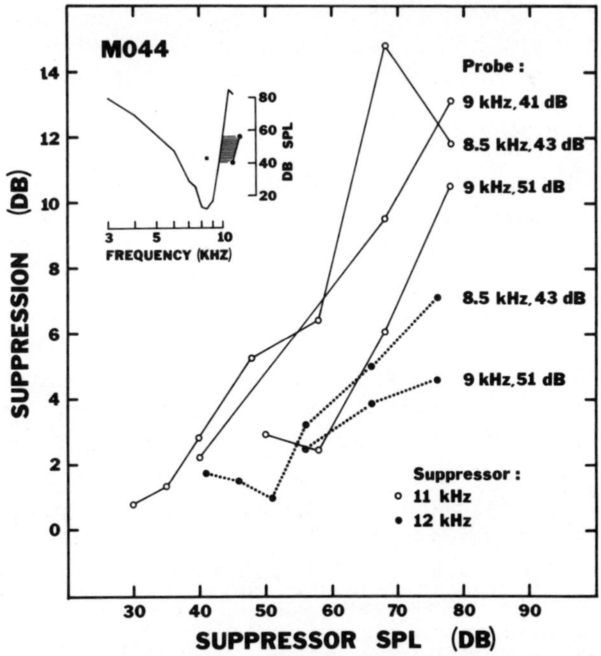

FIGURE 1. Suppression of the BM mechanical response to a probe tone (in dB relative to response to probe alone) as a function of intensity of a simultaneous suppressor tone. The inset shows an isovelocity (0.1 mm/s) tuning curve obtained earlier in the experiment, with CF at 8.5 kHz and minimum at 16 dB SPL. In the inset the solid square indicates the frequency (8.5 kHz) and intensity (43 dB SPL) of one of the probes used, and the solid circles show the corresponding 3-dB iso-suppression contour.

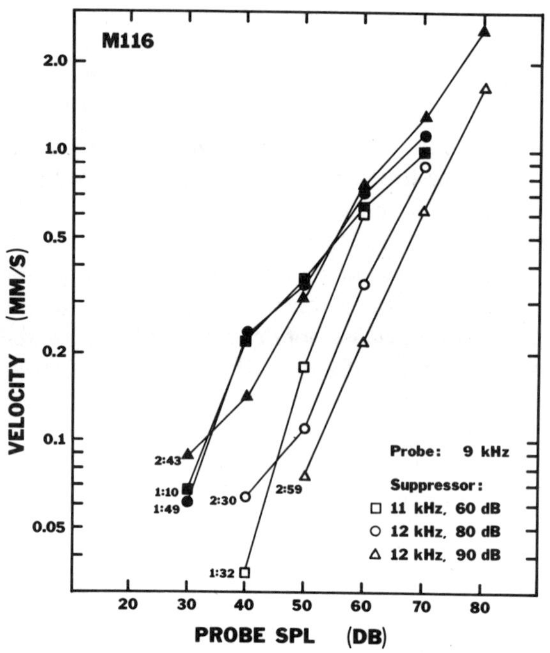

FIGURE 2. Effect of suppressor tones on BM intensity functions for probe tones. Solid symbols indicate BM intensity functions for the probe tone (9 kHz) alone and open symbols for the probe when presented simultaneously with a suppressor tone. Time (referred to placement of the source) at which the intensity curves were obtained is indicated for each intensity function. The suppressor tones produce a shift of the probe intensity functions to higher intensities and also an increase in slope.

the probe intensity functions is not only a reduction of sensitivity, but also an increase in slope, making them more linear.

In four of the five animals in which we were able to demonstrate suppression of the amplitude of the mechanical response to the probe tone, there were also phase effects produced by the suppressor tones. These effects on the phase of the probe response are shown in Fig. 3, for the same experiment depicted in Fig. 2. Panel A displays phase of the BM velocity responses (scala vestibuli velocity re rarefaction) to the probe tone alone (solid symbols) and when presented together with a suppressor (open symbols). The differences between the phase curves for the probe tones with suppressors and the corresponding curves for the probe tones alone have been plotted in Panel B. In all cases the suppressor produced a lag in the probe tone response, which increased with suppressor intensity.

Figure 4 shows the correlation between phase lag and suppression magnitude for the three experiments in which we studied the effect of suppressors on probe intensity functions. The scatter diagram displays (open symbols) phase lags from Fig. 3B, versus suppression magnitude (horizontal shifts of the probe-tone responses) caused by the corresponding suppressor tones in Fig. 2. The slope of regression for the data from this experiment (M116) is 2.1 deg/dB (correlation coefficient, $r = 0.73$). The solid symbols include similar data obtained in two other experiments. The solid squares (M114) follow a regression line (not shown in the figure) with a slope of 1.2 deg/dB

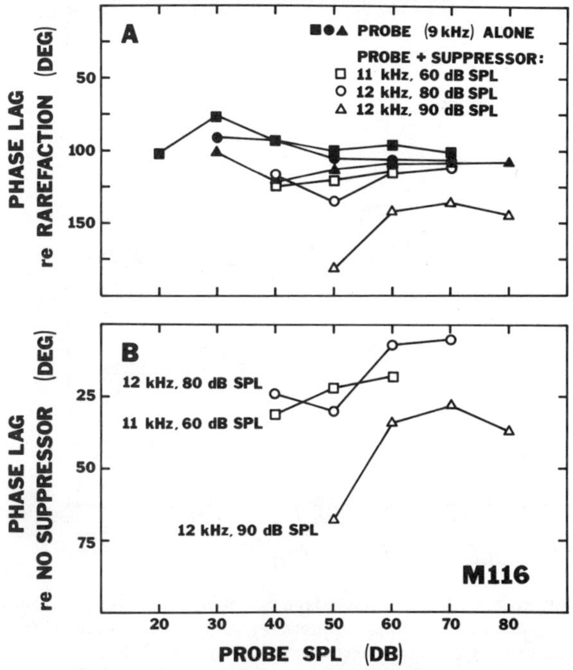

FIGURE 3. Effect of suppressor tones on the phase of BM mechanical responses to a probe tone. Panel A: Solid symbols indicate the phases when the probe tone is presented alone, open symbols when probe and suppressor tones are presented simultaneously. Panel B: Phase lags produced by suppressor tones, computed as the differences between the corresponding curves in panel A.

(r=0.61). The closed circles (M056) however show much smaller phase lags for the same suppression magnitudes, reducing the slope of the regression line computed for the pooled data for the three experiments to 1.2 deg/dB (r=0.52).

Discussion

We have demonstrated the existence of two-tone suppression in the basal region of the chinchilla BM at intensities as low as 20 dB SPL for probe tones and 30 dB SPL for suppressors. Our results extend those of Rhode (1977), which were obtained at much higher intensities in less sensitive preparations of the squirrel monkey BM. Mechanical two-tone suppression in the chinchilla BM, for above-CF suppressors, is similar to discharge-rate suppression in cochlear afferents of chinchilla (Costalupes et al., 1987) and of other species (Sachs and Kiang, 1968; Abbas and Sachs, 1976; Javel et al., 1978; Schmiedt, 1982; Deng and Geisler, 1985; Delgutte, 1986) in several respects:

1. Suppression is demonstrable at comparable probe tone intensities and at suppressor levels that by themselves do not evoke measurable responses;
2. Suppression magnitude increases with the level of the suppressor;
3. The rate of increase of suppression magnitude with suppressor intensity is less than 1 dB/dB;
4. Suppression diminishes as the frequency difference between suppressor and CF probe tone increases;

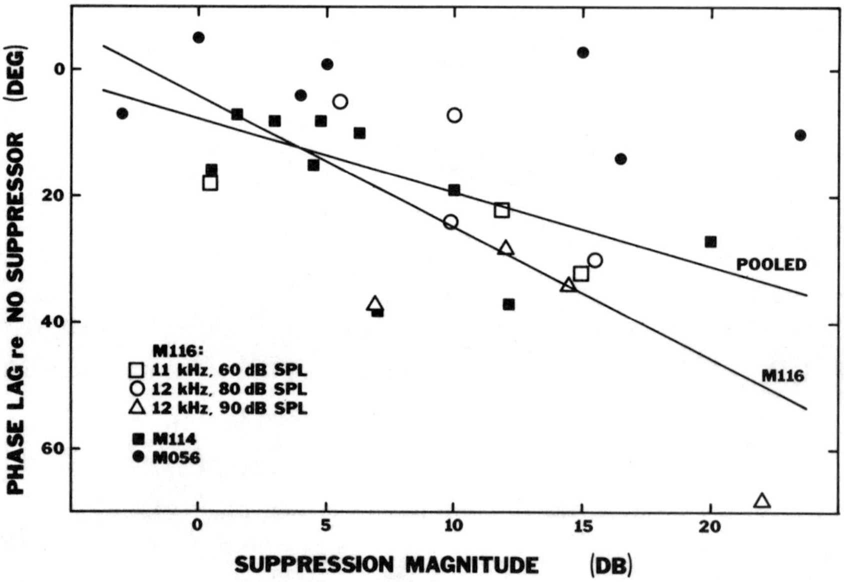

FIGURE 4. Correlation between suppression magnitudes and phase lags produced by suppressor tones. Open symbols: phase lag from Fig. 3B versus the corresponding suppression magnitudes computed from the horizontal shifts produced by the suppressors on the probe-tone responses in Fig. 2. Solid symbols: similar data obtained in two other experiments. Regression lines are shown for experiment M116 (open symbols) and for pooled data from the three experiments .

5. Magnitude-reduction suppression effects are correlated with phase lags in the probe responses.

However, two-tone suppression in the BM appears to differ from that in cochlear afferents in that its magnitude depends on probe level, whereas suppression in cochlear afferents is largely independent of probe SPL. Basilar membrane suppression obtained at low probe levels is comparable in magnitude (about 11 to 28 dB)with that seen in cochlear afferents in the same species (Costalupes et al., 1987) and in cat (Javel et al., 1978) at similar frequencies and intensities of stimulation. At higher probe levels BM suppression decreases, in clear contrast with suppression in cochlear nerve fibers.

Patuzzi et al. (1984) have shown that, for below-CF suppressors, the phase-specific two-tone suppression they measured in the guinea pig BM could largely account for parallel suppression phenomena in cochlear ganglion cells and inner hair cells. The present work suggests that, for suppressors above CF, the nonlinear motion of the BM contributes substantially to two-tone rate suppression in cochlear afferents.

Acknowledgments

This work was supported by FONDECYT Grant 1427, Chile and NIH Grants NS-25012 and NS-12125, and NSF Grant BNS-8304587, U.S.A.

References

Abbas, P.J. and Sachs, M.B. (1976) Two-tone suppression in auditory-nerve fibers: Extension of a stimulus-response relationship. J. Acoust. Soc. Am. 59, 112-122.

Costalupes, J.A., Rich, N.C. and Ruggero, M.A. (1987) Effects of excitatory and non-excitatory suppresor tones on two-tone rate suppression in auditory nerve fibers. Hear. Res. 26,155-164.

Delgutte, B. (1986) Two-tone rate suppression in auditory nerve fibers: Variations with suppressor level and frequency. Assoc. Res. Otolaryngol., Abstr. 9th Midwinter Meet., p. 65.

Deng, L. and Geisler, C.D. (1985) Changes in the phase of excitor-tone responses in cat auditory-nerve fibers by suppressor tones and fatigue. J. Acoust. Soc. Am. 78, 1633-1643.

Feng, A.S., Narins, P.M. and Capranica, R.R. (1975) Three populations of primary auditory fibers in the bullfrog (Rana catesbeiana): their peripheral origins and frequency sensitivities. J. Comp. Physiol. 100, 221-229.

Frischkopf, L.S. and Goldstein, M.H. (1963) Responses to acoustic stimuli from single units in the eighth nerve of the bullfrog. J. Acoust. Soc. Am. 35, 1219-1228.

Galambos, R. and Davis H. (1944) Inhibition of activity in single auditory nerve fibers by acoustic stimulation. J. Neurophysiol. 7, 287-303.

Hind, J.E., Anderson, D.J., Brugge, J.R. and Rose J.E. (1967) Coding of information pertaining to paired low frequency tones in single auditory nerve fibers of the squirrel monkey. J. Neurophysiol. 30, 794-816.

Holton, T. and Weiss, T.F. (1978) Two-tone suppression in lizard cochlear nerve fibers, relation to receptor morphology. Brain Res. 159, 219-222.

Javel, E., Geisler, C.D. and Ravindran, A. (1978) Two-tone suppression in auditory nerve of the cat: rate-intensity and temporal analysis. J. Acoust Soc. Am. 63, 1093-1104.

Khanna, S.M. and Leonard, D.G.B. (1982). Basilar membrane tuning in the cat cochlea. Science 215, 305-306.

Kiang, N.Y.S., Watanabe, T., Thomas, E.C. and Clark, L. (1965) Discharge patterns of single fibers in the cat's auditory nerve. MIT Press, Cambridge, MA.

Nomoto, M., Suga, N. and Katsuki, Y. (1964) Discharege pattern and inhibition of primary auditory nerve fibers in the monkey. J. Neurophysiol. 27, 768-787.

Patuzzi, R., Sellick, P.M. and Johnstone, B.M. (1984) The modulation of the sensitivity of the mammalian cochlea by low-frequency tones. III. Basilar membrane motion. Hear. Res. 13, 19-27.

Rhode, W.S. (1971) Observations of the vibration of the basilar membrane in squirrel monkeys using the Mossbauer technique. J. Acoust. Soc. Am. 49, 1218-1231.

Rhode, W.S. (1977) Some observations on two-tone interaction measured with the Mossbauer effect. In: Psychophysics and Physiology of Hearing (Eds: Evans, E.F. and Wilson, J.P.) Academic Press, London, pp. 27-41.

Rhode, W.S. and Robles, L. (1974) Evidence from Mossbauer experiments for nonlinear vibration in the cochlea. J. Acoust. Soc. Am. 55, 588-596.

Robles, L., Ruggero, M.A. and Rich, N.C. (1986) Basilar membrane mechanics at the base of the chinchilla cochlea. I.Input-output functions, tuning curves and response phases. J. Acoust. Soc. Am. 80, 1364-1374.

Sachs, M.B. (1969) Stimulus-response relation for auditory-nerve fibers: two-tone suppression. J. Acoust. Soc. Am. 45, 1025-1036.

Sachs, M.B. and Kiang, N.Y.S. (1968) Two-tone inhibition in auditory-nerve fibers. J. Acoust. Soc. Am. 43, 1120-1128.

Sachs, M.B., Young, E.D. and Lewis, R.H. (1974) Discharge patterns of single fibers in the pigeon auditory nerve. Brain Res. 70, 431-447.

Schmiedt, R.A. (1982) Boundaries of two-tone rate suppression of cochlear-nerve activity. Hear. Res. 7, 335-351.

Sellick, P.M., Patuzzi, R. and Johnstone, B.M. (1982) Measurement of basilar membrane motion in the guinea pig using the Mossbauer technique. J. Acoust. Soc. Am. 72, 131-141.

Sellick, P.M. and Russell, I.J. (1979) Two-tone suppression in cochlear hair cells. Hear. Res. 1, 227-236.

DETERMINANTS OF HIGH-FREQUENCY SENSITIVITY IN THE BIRD

A.W. Gummer, J.W.Th. Smolders* and R. Klinke*

Research School of Biological Sciences
Australian National University, Canberra, Australia
**Zentrum der Physiologie, J.W. Goethe Universität, FRG*

Introduction

In two previous publications (Gummer et al., 1986, 1987) we reported the presence of anti-resonances in the middle-ear transmission function of the pigeon. The anti-resonances were often associated with phase lags of up to 2 cycles at 11 kHz, which were so excessive that basilar membrane (BM) motion recorded in the basal region of the basilar papilla (BP) appeared to lead columella footplate (CFP) motion over an extended frequency range. In this paper we report on the results of experiments which lead us to the conclusion that since travelling waves cannot be launched on the pigeon BM above 6 kHz, the anti-resonances are the result of reflection of incident energy at the basal end of the BM back to the CFP so that the nett volume velocity of the CFP into scala vestibuli vanishes. This proposal may provide an important physical principle for defining the limit of high-frequency sensitivity.

Methods

Recordings of the motion of the CFP were made in the Nembutal anaesthetized pigeon (36 mg kg^{-1}) using the Mössbauer technique. The methods are extensively described in Gummer et al. (1987). In the present series of experiments measurements of CFP velocity were made with the cochlea in various states: (i) intact; (ii) fenestrated; (iii) fenestrated, BP extirpated and fluid filled; and (iv) as for (iii) but fluid drained. It suffices to emphasize that: (i) animals were paralyzed; (ii) the sound pressure level at the tympanic membrane (TM) was also measured after each structural manipulation of the cochlea; and (iii) the isomer shift of the Mössbauer source-absorber combination was non-zero, giving phase ambiguity of integral cycles only.

Results and Discussion

Columella footplate response - modified cochlea

The amplitude and phase of the velocity of the CFP at 100 dB SPL is shown in Fig. 1 for seven animals. The most striking feature of these responses is the presence of amplitude and phase irregularities at frequencies above 4 kHz, evident as amplitude notches, excessively large phase rotations (up to 2 cycles at 11 kHz) or negative group delays. At first sight these high-frequency effects may be considered anomalous and unimportant because the highest frequency represented on the BM is 6 kHz (Gummer et al., 1987). However, differences in phase responses from different animals already become evident at 2.828 kHz; responses are readily separated into two groups according to the phase difference between low and high frequencies (0.1 and 11 kHz); namely, 1 and 2 cycles. If a phase response from the 2-cycle group is used as a phase reference for BM motion recorded in the basal region of the BP then BM motion may appear to lead CFP motion at most frequencies (Gummer et al., 1987).

Both phase groups contain amplitude irregularities. The effects are found for both the intact cochlea and also for those cochleae in which BM recordings had been made prior to CFP recordings. No evidence of such irregularities was found in the BM motion when referred to sound pressure at the TM. The frequency resolution in Fig. 1 is so fine that there can be no likelihood of phase error arising from phase ambiguity.

The recorded CFP response was dependent on the orientation of the measurement axis in a way which could not be accounted for by the cosine-effect for frequencies above 2.828 kHz, but rather was indicative of interference between the presumed piston-like vibration mode of the CFP and other modes dominant at high frequencies.

Columella footplate response - intact cochlea

In order to elucidate the origin of the high-frequency irregularities the CFP response was recorded after having extirpated the BP, and with the cochlea either full of fluid or drained. The fluid came from within the cochlea and had the texture of perilymph; the fluid level remained constant at the level of the hole in scala tympani through which the BP had been extirpated. Since the recorded CFP response depended on the measurement axis, if possible we avoided moving the Mössbauer absorber after the initial recording for the intact cochlea. If it was necessary to shift the absorber between manipulations on the cochlea, it was returned to its original position. However, with some forethought and the use of a 350-mm objective lens it was often possible to leave the absorber undisturbed.

Representative data are displayed in Fig. 2. In general, the important results are that in the absence of the BP: (i) the amplitude notch vanished; (ii) the phase slope no longer exhibited significant positive values (i.e. no significant negative group delays); (iii) the phase difference between low and high frequency was always less than 1 cycle and up to 6 kHz it was no

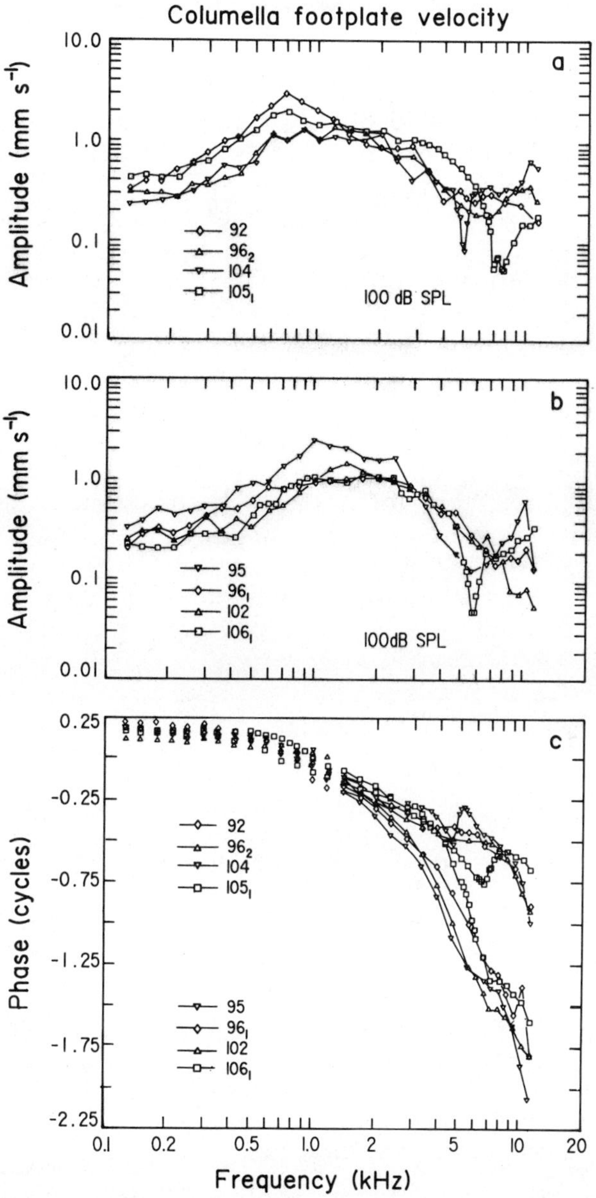

FIGURE 1. (a), (b) Amplitude and (c) phase of CFP velocity at 100 dB SPL as a function of frequency for 7 pigeons. The cochlea was intact for pigeon (PGN) 96, 102, 104, 105 and 106. BM motion was measured prior to measurement of CFP motion in PGN 92 and 95; abneural limbus motion had also been measured in PGN 95. For PGN 96 the Mössbauer absorber was shifted by 33° from its initial position (96_1), where the Mössbauer fraction was greatest, to a position where the measurement axis was more aligned with the surface normal of the CFP (96_2). Amplitude responses are grouped according to the high-frequency phase values.

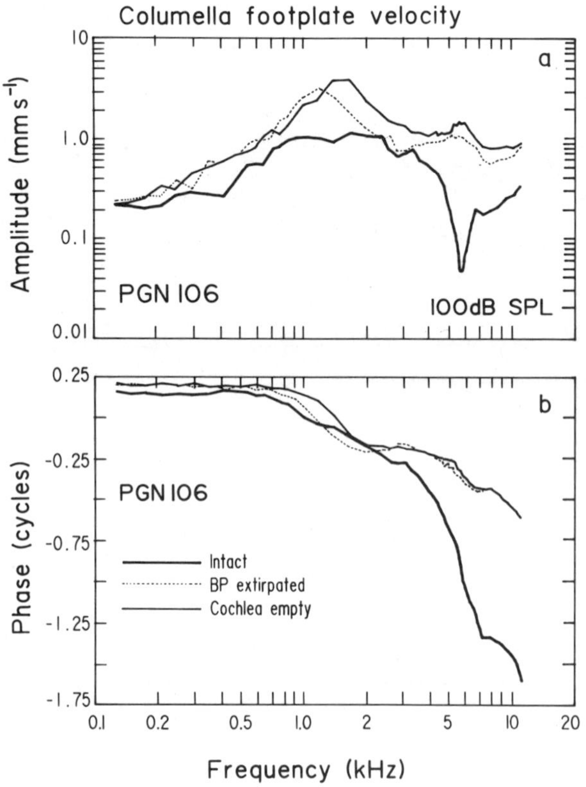

FIGURE 2 (a) Amplitude and (b) phase of CFP velocity at 100 dB SPL as a function of frequency for PGN 106 for: (i) intact cochlea; (ii) BP extirpated and cochlea filled with fluid (perilymph?); and (iii) BP extirpated and cochlea drained.

more than 0.5 cycles. The main difference between the drained and fluid filled conditions were the reduced resonant frequency and Q_{3dB} of the latter (0.34 oct and 16%, respectively, for PGN 106). The greatest inter-animal differences were to be found in the range of resonant frequencies (0.77-1.44 kHz) and Q_{3dB} (1.6-3.9).

Thus provided the condition of other structures were not altered by BP extirpation these results demonstrate that the high-frequency irregularities were dependent on the presence of the BP.

Input and output impedances of the cochlea

In order to understand the role of the BP in the production of the high-frequency irregularities the data contained in the preceding figure are presented in the form of impedance ratios. The procedure adopts a network model of the auditory periphery, which is a modified form of the ones which have been used by investigators for other species (Møller, 1961; Rosowski et al., 1985; Zwislocki, 1962). The available space does not permit a comprehensive presentation of the procedure. Briefly, the middle-ear transmission function, T, may be written as

$$T = \frac{U_c}{P_t} = \frac{z_{12}}{z_{11}} \frac{1}{Z_o + Z_c}$$

where U_c is the volume velocity of the CFP; P_t is the sound pressure at the TM; z_{12} and z_{11} are two of the open circuit impedance parameters characterizing the middle ear; Z_o and Z_c are the output and input impedances of the cochlea, respectively. The middle ear, which for present purposes may be considered to include the annular ligament and round window membrane, is presumed to be unchanged by the cochlear manipulations. By contrast, extirpation of the BP causes $Z_c = Z_v$, where Z_v is the combined impedance of scalae tympani and vestibuli; extirpation of the BP and draining of the cochlea gives $Z_c \sim 0$. Since U_c is proportional to the (mechanical) velocity of the CFP, T is proportional to our measured CFP response. Consequently, if T' is applied to the extirpated BP condition and T" to the extirpated BP and drained cochlea condition, the ratios Z_c/Z_o and Z_v/Z_o may be evaluated through the expressions

$$\frac{Z_c}{Z_o} = \frac{T''}{T} - 1$$

and

$$\frac{Z_v}{Z_o} = \frac{T''}{T'} - 1$$

where T and Z_c are henceforth applied exclusively to the intact cochlea condition.

The results of such an evaluation for PGN 106 are shown in Fig. 3 where the real and imaginary parts of Z_c/Z_o are displayed and in Fig. 4 where the magnitude and phase of Z_c/Z_o are compared with that of Z_v/Z_o. The most important finding is that the real part of Z_c/Z_o becomes negative with maximum absolute value at 5.657 kHz. Since Z_o is not the source of the anti-resonance, the negative real part for 3.364-6.727 kHz means that the BP is a source of energy in this frequency range. The frequency at which the imaginary part of Z_c/Z_o becomes zero, namely 5.5 kHz, is the true resonant frequency of the phenomenon.

Wilson and Johnstone (1975) reported a series of one to three sharp notches between 3 and 8 kHz in the amplitude response of the long process of the incus in the guinea pig, together with unusually steep high-frequency slopes above 20kHz. They mentioned that similar notches had been reported for other species where they had been attributed to the influence of Helmholtz resonators. The explanation was dismissed by their study

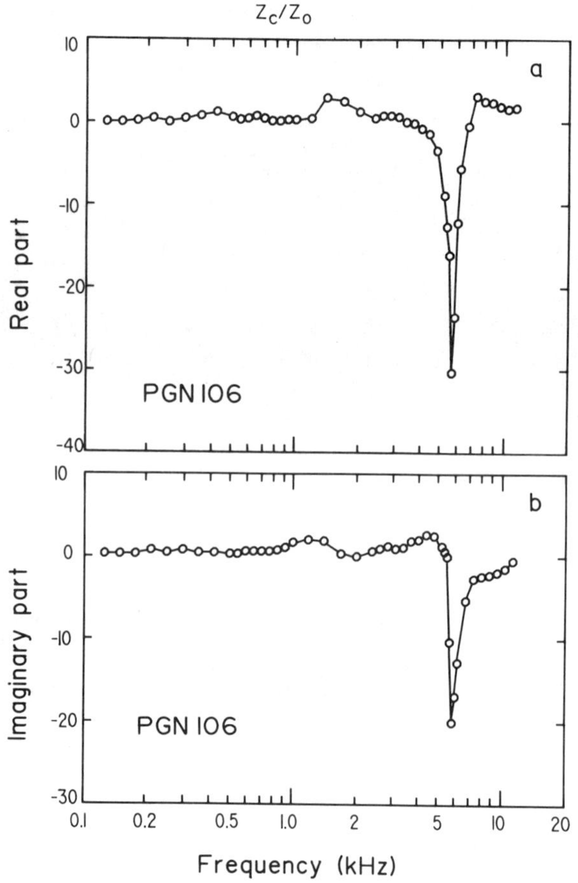

FIGURE 3. (a) Real and (b) imaginary parts of the ratio of the input and output impedances of the cochlea, Z_C/Z_O, for PGN 106.

because the notches were absent from the measured BM response; various vibration modes of the incus were proposed. However, provided that the middle ear was not damaged by our surgical procedures and modifications to the cochlea, an explanation for the observed effects in the present study must be sought primarily from within the cochlea. It is appropriate to mention that the model calculations of Geisler and Hubbard (1972) predicted a sharp resonance in the input impedance of the human cochlea near 10 kHz, which was due to the fact that the length of the human cochlea is equal to a quarter length of the average fluid pressure wave at that frequency. This condition is not applicable to the pigeon because the BM length of 4 mm (Takasaka and Smith, 1971) yields a quarter-wave frequency of 91 kHz! (Incidentally the quarter-wave frequency for the guinea-pig BM is 20 kHz).

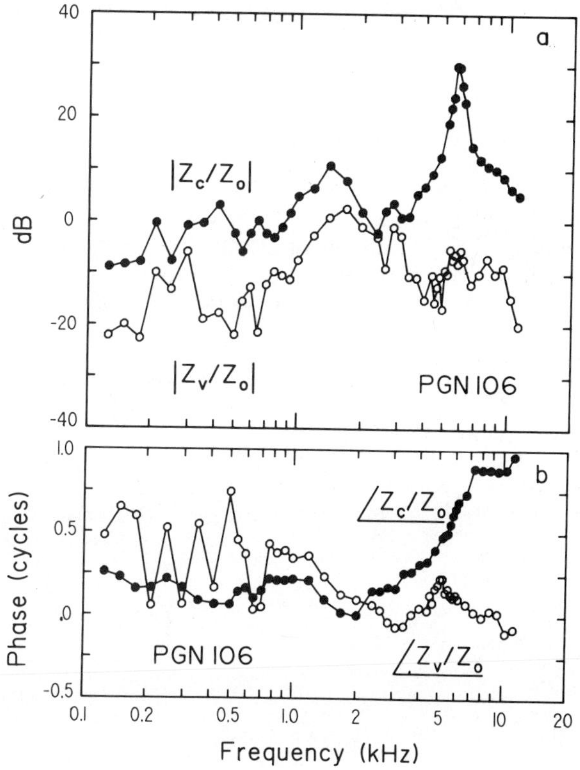

FIGURE 4 (a) Magnitude and (b) phase of Z_C/Z_O and Z_V/Z_O for PGN 106.

Our interpretation of the anti-resonance phenomenon in the pigeon relies on the fact that the resonant frequency is approximately equal to the maximum frequency represented on the BM, namely 6 kHz (Gummer et al., 1987). We propose that since a travelling wave cannot be launched on the BM for frequencies above 6 kHz, most of the incident energy near that frequency is reflected at the BM back to CFP, so that the nett volume velocity of the CFP into scala vestibuli is approximately zero. Presumably the largest reflection occurs at the boundary between the extreme basal end of the BM and the limbus where the impedance mismatch is greatest. Since a reflected wave will be out of (temporal) phase with the incident wave, both the amplitude and the phase of the recorded CFP velocity are dependent on the measurement axis.

Acknowledgements

The experiments were conducted at Zentrum der Physiologie, Frankfurt, and were supported by the Deutsche Forschungsgemeinschaft (SFB 45)

References

Geisler, C.D. and Hubbard, A.E. (1972) New boundary conditions and results for the Peterson-Bogert model of the cochlea. J. Acoust. Soc. Am. 52, 1629-1634.

Gummer, A.W., Smolders, J.W.Th. and Klinke, R. (1986) The mechanics of the basilar membrane and middle ear in the pigeon. In: Peripheral Auditory Mechanisms (Eds: Allen, J.B., Hall, J.L., Hubbard, A., Neely, S.T. and Tubis, A.) Springer-Verlag, Berlin, Heidelberg, New York, Tokyo, pp. 81-88.

Gummer, A.W., Smolders, J.W.T. and Klinke, R. (1987) Basilar membrane motion in the pigeon measured with the Mössbauer technique. Hearing Research, 29, 63-92.

Møller, A.R. (1961) Network model of the middle ear. J. Acoust. Soc. Am. 33, 168-176.

Rosowski, J.J., Peake, W.T., Lynch, T.J., III, Leong, R. and Weiss T.F. (1985) A model for signal transmission in an ear having hair cells with free-standing stereocilia. II. Macromechanical stage. Hearing Research, 20, 139-155.

Takasaka, T. and Smith, C.A. (1971) The structure and innervation of the pigeon's basilar papilla. J. Ultrastruct. Res 35, 20-65.

Wilson, J.P. and Johnstone, J.R. (1975) Basilar membrane and middle-ear vibration in guinea pig measured by capacitive probe. J. Acoust. Soc. Am. 57, 705-723.

Zwislocki, J. (1962) Analysis of the middle-ear function. Part I: Input impedance. J. Acoust. Soc. Am. 34, 1514-1523.

Comments and Discussion

MANLEY

The finding that inner ear characteristics are reflected in the transfer function of the pigeon middle ear is very interesting. It strengthens the impression gained from earlier work on lizards (Manley, 1972a,b) and mammals (Manley and Johnstone, 1974; Manley et al, 1972), each of which show dramatic slope changes in their transfer function at their respective upper frequency limits. In the guinea pig, we examined the high-frequency responses in some detail. Guinea pigs showed a sudden increase in slope of the transfer function for displacement amplitude of the malleus above approximately 30kHz; the slope increases from 6dB/octave to more than 30dB/octave. These data thus resemble those of Wilson and Johnstone (1975) . At these high frequencies in the guinea pig, there was both a 40dB difference in the displacement amplitudes and a large phase change between the malleus and the incus; the displacement amplitude recovered again at even higher frequencies. Although studied in less detail, the displacement amplitude of the malleus bat *Eptesicus pumilis* also fell off very rapidly above 70kHz. In the gekko *Gehyra*, there was a loss of transmission between the extracolumella and columella at frequencies above about 4kHz due to a flexing of the inferior process of the extracolumella. The flexing was not present after removal of the connection to the inner ear, suggesting that the transmission loss at high frequencies is due to a rising impedance of the columella/inner ear system (Manley, 1972b). It should be noted, however, that it is extremely unlikely that a travelling wave is present in *Gehyra*. Taken together with the findings of Gummer et al., the data indicate the general importance of the influence of the inner ear on the middle-ear transfer characteristics in three groups of vertebrates.

Manley, G.A. (1972a) The middle ear of the tokay gecko. J. Comp. Physiol. 81, 239-250.
Manley, G.A. (1972b) Frequency response of the middle ear of geckos. J. Comp. Physiol. 81, 251-258.
Manley, G.A., Johnstone, B.M. (1974) Middle-ear function in the guinea pig. J. Acoust. Soc. Amer. 56, 571-576.
Manley, G.A., Irvine, D.R.F., and Johnstone, B.M. (1972) Frequency response of bat tympanic membrane. Nature 237, 112-113.
Wilson, J.P. and Johnstone, J.R. (1975) Basilar-membrane and middle-ear vibration in guinea pig measured by capacitative probe. J. Acoust. Soc. Amer. 57, 705-723.

MECHANICAL RESPONSE OF THE OUTER HAIR CELL REGION OF THE ISOLATED GUINEA PIG COCHLEA IN VITRO

Shyam M. Khanna,[1] Mats Ulfendahl,[2] and Åke Flock[2]

[1]*Department of Otolaryngology, College of Physicians and Surgeons, Columbia University, New York, 630 West 168th Street, New York, N.Y. 10032, USA*
[2]*Department of Physiology II, Karolinska Institute, Stockholm, Sweden*

Introduction

The mechanical response of the guinea pig cochlea was measured utilizing a combination of an optical sectioning microscope (Koester, 1980) and a heterodyne interferometer (Willemin, Dandliker & Khanna, 1988). The optical sectioning microscope allowed visualization of the cochlear structure through the intact Reissner's membrane. Individual Hensen's cells could always be visualized. In favorable preparations individual rows of outer hair cells, pillar cells, inner hair cells and many other cochlear structures could also be seen.

The heterodyne interferometer allowed the measurement of vibration by means of a laser beam incident on the object through the objective lens of the microscope. The spot size of the beam is 5 µ. The optical sectioning depth of the interferometer is $\pm$ 10 µ. (The carrier to noise ratio is reduced by 10 dB when the object is moved $\pm$ 10 µ above or below the plane of focus.) The laser beam is visible in the microscope image. It is positioned on the cochlea by means of a two-axis goniometer system that provides tilting of the object around two mutually perpendicular axes. The object can also be positioned in the x, y and z planes with respect to the axis of the microscope by means of an x, y and z micromanipulator system. This x, y, z positioning system is mounted on the inner goniometer and tilts with it.

MOUNTING AND DISSECTION OF THE COCHLEA

Pigmented guinea pigs were anesthetized and decapitated. The temporal bone was removed and cemented to a metal tube so that the lateral side with the remaining auditory canal was facing the opening of the tube. The free end of the metal tube was connected to the sound source and the probe microphone system with rubber tubing. The metal tube was attached to a metal rod that could be rotated and tilted to change the orientation of the bone needed to view the apical part of the cochlea or the malleus. The bulla was then gently opened to expose the cochlea and the tympanic membrane. During these steps the temporal bone was moistened with tissue culture medium to prevent it from drying. After the temporal bone was transferred to the experimental chamber filled with tissue culture medium, the bony cochlea was opened by careful removal of the bone covering the apical turn(s), thus usually leaving the scala media intact.

MEASUREMENT TECHNIQUE

The temporal bone is attached to the x,y,z positioning and goniometer rotation system by means of a rod. It is positioned inside a clear plastic chamber filled with tissue culture medium so that the exposed apical turn of the cochlea faces the dipping cone of the water immersion objective lens of the microscope. The objective lens (20 X) fits into the side of the chamber with a fluid tight gasket and has a working distance of 4 mm.

The position of the bone is adjusted until the desired portion of the cochlear turn is visible. A sketch is made of identified cochlear structures. The measuring laser beam is turned on and positioned on the cellular region of interest. The diameter of the laser beam is small, therefore the beam can be placed on a single cell. Fine adjustments in the beam position and focusing are used to maximize the carrier to noise ratio of the interferometer. Measurements of vibration velocity are made under computer control over a frequency range of 25 Hz to 2.0 kHz in 25 Hz frequency increments. The electrical input applied to the acoustic transducer is maintained constant. After the cochlear measurements have been completed the bone is reoriented and malleus vibrations are measured. Sound pressure acting on the ear is also measured with a probe microphone.

At the end of the experiment the cochleas are fixed for histological examination.

Measurements

TUNING CURVE OF THE OUTER HAIR CELL REGION

The tuning curve of the OHC region measured in the 3rd turn is shown in Figure 1. The solid line shows vibration amplitude as a function of frequency for constant electrical input applied to the acoustic transducer. The frequency response of the transducer is flat at these low frequencies, therefore the tuning curve can also be considered as vibration amplitude for constant sound pressure level. The response of the OHC region is sharply tuned with a peak at 700 Hz. For comparison, the tuning curve of the receptor potential for an outer hair cell measured in the same cochlear turn is shown with a dotted line (Dallos, 1985). The receptor potential curve shown was measured at low sound pressure levels (15 dB SPL).

Although the mechanical tuning was observed in an excised cochlea its sharpness is comparable to the tuning of the receptor potential measured in a living animal.

The mechanical tuning curve of the OHC region measued in the 4th turn is shown in Figure 2. The vibration amplitude was measured for the same constant electrical input to the acoustic transducer. The response was measured with good signal to noise ratio and was repeatable. The peak of the response in the 4th turn occurs at a lower frequency (220 Hz). The vibration amplitude at the peak is 4×10^{-7} m.

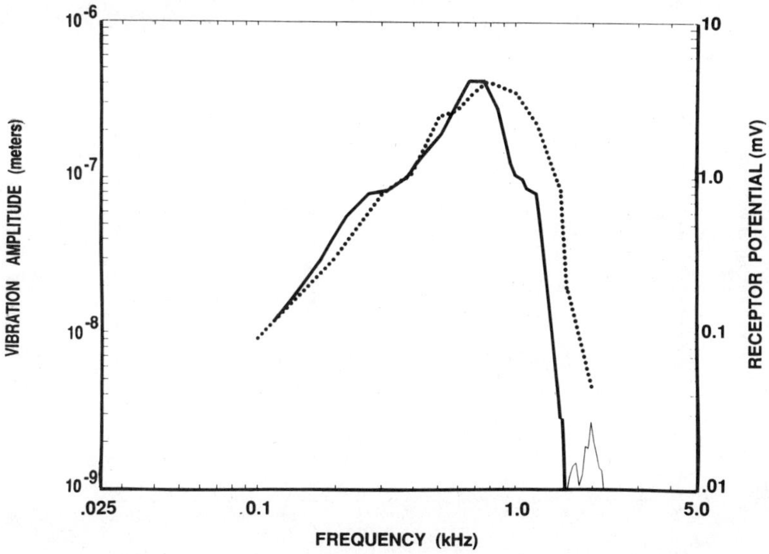

Figure 1. Solid line shows the vibration amplitude of the outer hair cell region measured in the 3rd turn as a function of frequency. The receptor potential tuning curve (dotted line) measured by Dallos is shown for comparison.

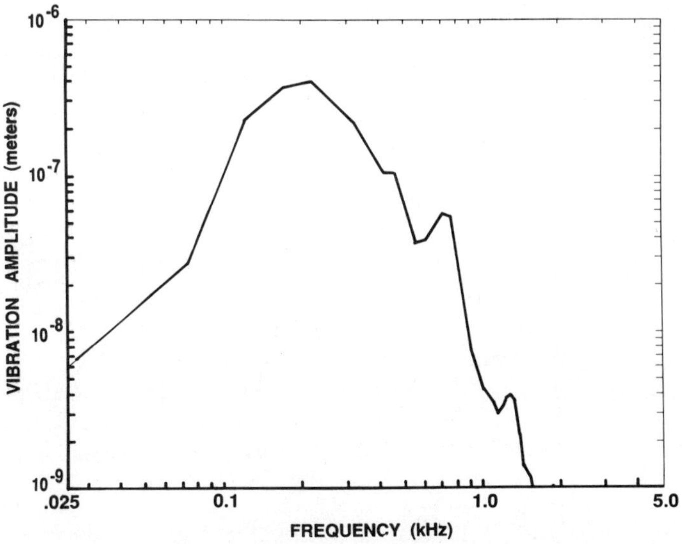

Figure 2. Vibration amplitude of the outer hair cell region measured in the 4th turn as a function of frequency for constant input voltage applied to the acoustic transducer.

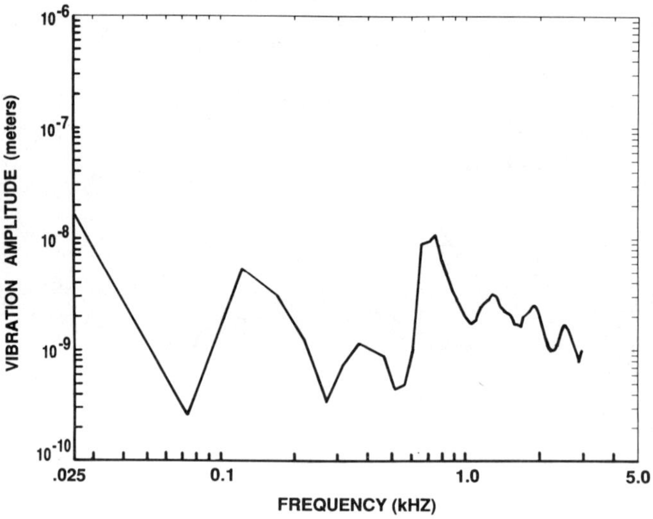

Figure 3. Vibration amplitude of the bony wall of the cochlea measured in the same cochlea and under the same acoustical conditions as the previous curve.

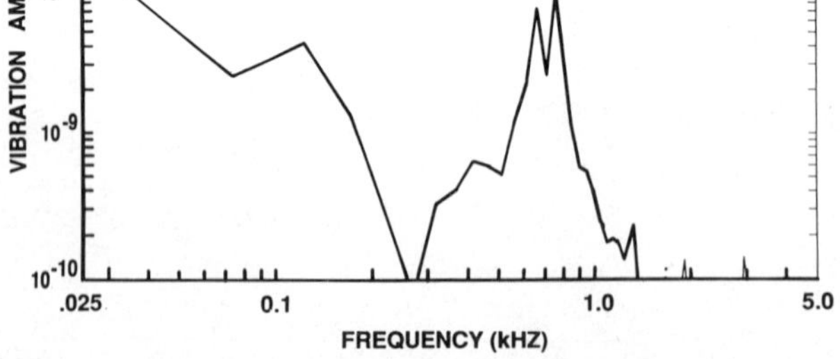

Figure 4. Vibration amplitude of the basilar membrane region measured in the same cochlea and under the same conditions as the previous two curves.

Both the low and high frequency slopes of the tuning curve are shallower as compared to the response obtained in the 3rd turn. The magnitude of the response was found to vary approximately linearly with the voltage applied to the acoustic transducer, therefore the shape of the tuning curve was independent of the stimulus level. The sound pressure level used in these experiments was about 94 dB.

MECHANICAL RESPONSE OF THE BONY COCHLEAR WALL

Mechanical vibrations of the bony wall were also measured in the same cochlea in the 4th turn radially from the point of measurement in the OHC region. Identical input stimulus was used. The optical signal from the bone was strong and carrier to noise ratio at the detector was high. The lower limit of vibration measurement was therefore determined by the demodulator noise. The vibrations of the bony wall (Figure 3) vary between 10^{-8} and 3×10^{-10} meters. These measurements are close to the detection threshold at low frequencies and therefore noisy. Similar observations were made in other experiments on the osseus spiral lamina. The important conclusion is that the vibrations of the bony partitions are at a level much lower than that of the OHC region.

MECHANICAL RESPONSE OF THE BASILAR MEMBRANE

In the 4th turn nearly half of the basilar membrane lies between the edge of the Hensen cells and the spiral ligament. Claudius cells overlie the basilar membrane in this region. Measurements of the Claudius cell-basilar membrane complex were made adjacent to the Hensen cells, or roughly in the center of the basilar membrane. The longitudinal position was along the same radial axis at which OHC vibration measurements shown in Figure 2 were made. The same electrical input to the acoustic transducer was used as in the previous measurements. The vibration levels mesured are comparable to those seen at the bony wall. No tuned response is seen in the 220 Hz region, and the vibration amplitude of the basilar membrane at 220 Hz is 2×10^{-10} m.

Discussion

The basilar membrane vibrations may be low because the bony cap on the apical turn was removed to gain access to the cochlea, and the scala vestibuli was open to the fluid. Because the basilar membrane response was lower than the OHC response by a factor of at least 100:1, it is safe to say that the basilar membrane was not contributing to the tuned response seen in the OHC region.

The presence of a sharply tuned OHC region response which is comparable to the receptor potential response measured in the outer hair cells suggests that the organ of Corti in our experimental preparation has an independent mechanical tuning mechanism. This experimental evidence provides further support to our original suggestion that the sharply tuned component of the mechanical response does not represent the basilar membrane tuning (Khanna & Leonard, 1986).

Acknowledgement

This research was supported by NINCDS and NSF Grants.

References

Dallos, P. (1985): Response characteristics of mammalian cochlear hair cells. J. Neurosci. 5(6); 1591-1608.

Khanna, S.M. and Leonard, D.G.B. (1986): Relationship between basilar membrane tuning and hair cell condition. Hearing Res. 23: 55-70.

Koester, C.J. (1980): Scanning mirror microscope with optical sectioning characteristics: Applications in ophthalmology. Applied Optics 19(11): 1749-1757.

Willemin, J-F., Dandliker, R. and Khanna, S.M. (1988): Heterodyne interferometer for submicroscopic vibration measurements in the inner ear. J. Acoust. Soc. Am. 83(2): 787-795.

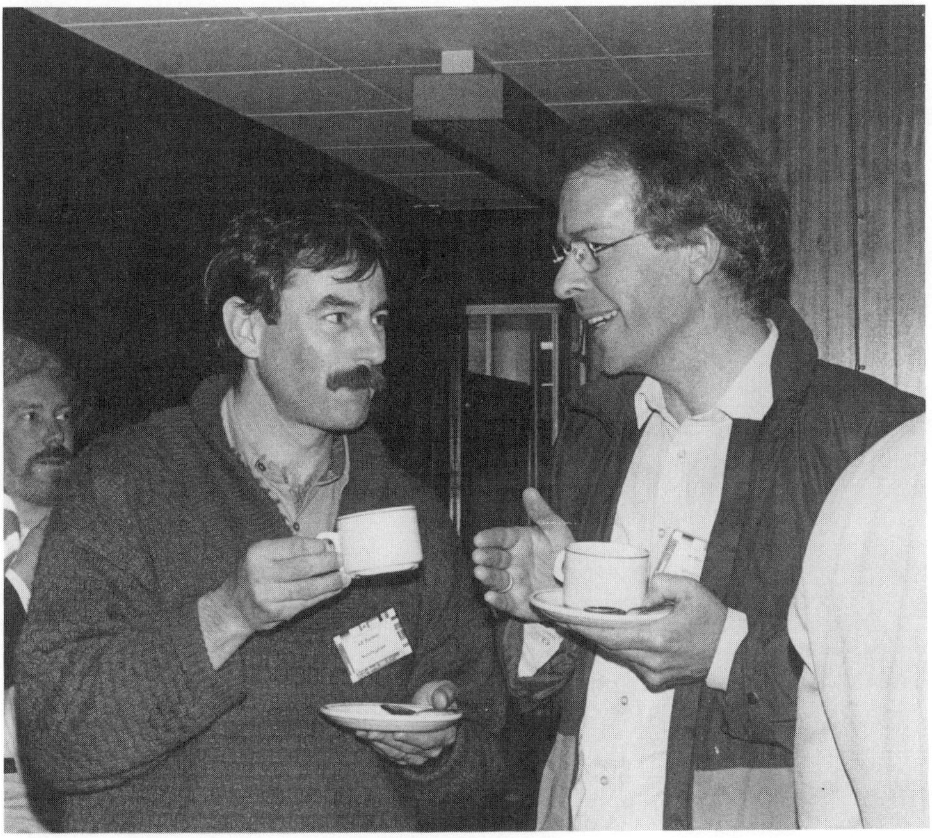

D.C. Mountain, A.R. Palmer and H. Duifhuis

7. NONLINEAR MODELS

POWER-LAW NONLINEARITIES: A REVIEW OF SOME LESS FAMILIAR PROPERTIES

H. Duifhuis

Biophysics Department, Rijksuniversiteit Groningen

Introduction

At this point I assume that nonlinear behaviour of the auditory system is a generally accepted, although not completely understood, experimental fact. In order to explore the underlying mechanisms I take a biophysical approach, viz. I try to describe the processes in terms of useful, efficient, mathematical physics. Of course this approach is by no means new. Even worse, the applied mathematical content of this paper is dated. However, the relevant literature and the major results appear to be fairly inaccessible for many colleagues (e.g. Fahey & Allen, 1988). In this paper I will first (re-)present some general, primarily mathematical results. In the last part the implication for auditory research will be discussed. For a historical review of the analysis of auditory nonlinearity the reader is referred to, e.g. Zwicker (1955), Goldstein (1967), Smoorenburg (1972,1974), Hall (1972), Schroeder (1975), Duifhuis (1976).

Description of the nonlinearity

The auditory nonlinearity is assumed to be time-independent, i.e. constant on the time grid of interest, with steps of say 10 microseconds. Any time-invariant nonlinear transfer characteristic g, $y = g(x)$, can be devided into an even part g_e and an odd part g_o, where $g = g_e + g_o$, and $g_e(x)=g_e(-x)$, while $g_o(x) = -g_o(-x)$. These two components have quite different and independent effects.

It is well known that any nonlinearity can be approximated by a Taylor expansion. Note, however, that this expansion consists of even and odd terms which for the general case are not independent. Note also that all terms except the constant have a power ≥ 1. Thus all terms beyond the linear have an *expansive* shape. The auditory nonlinearity is undoubtedly of the *compressive* type. It is known that expansive and compressive nonlinearities have entirely different properties, e.g. with respect to phase there can be a 180 degrees difference. Thus, the individual elements of the Taylor expansion carry no useful information. Only the sum of the infinite series formally does that. It is an interesting exercise to look at Taylor's expansion for the log function for

$x >> 1$.

Almost forgotten is the more efficient approximation of continuous functions according to Bernstein (1922). His statement implies that any such function, over any arbitrary bounded interval can be approximated arbitrarily closely by a linear combination of functions of the set of power functions in x $\{1, x^{p1}, x^{p2},..., x^{K}\}$ where $0<p1<p2...<K$. Taylor's expansion (Weierstrass' theorem) is just a special case for which the p's are the integers.

Analysis of responses of the general power-law device

INTRODUCTION

The responses of half-wave power rectifiers with characteristic:

$$y_+ = c(s - b)^p \qquad s > b,\ p > 0$$
$$= 0 \qquad s < b \tag{1}$$

to tonal and narrow-band stimuli have been studied extensively in electrical engineering (Bennett, e.g.1933; Rice, 1945; Middleton, 1948,1960; Sternberg, Kaufman, Shipman, and Thurnston, 1953,1954,1955; Feuerstein, 1957). A general result is that the response to the complex time function

$$s(t) = \sum_{i=0}^{N} A_i \cos(\omega_i t + \phi_i) \tag{2}$$

can be written as

$$y_+(t) = cA_0^p \sum_{m_0=0}^{\infty} \cdots \sum_{m_N=0}^{\infty} \tfrac{1}{2}\ A^{(p)}_{m_0 m_1 \ldots m_N}(h,k_1,k_2 \ldots k_N) \prod_{i=0}^{N} \varepsilon_i \cos m_i(\omega_i t + \phi_i) \tag{3}$$

In this equation ε is the Neumann factor: $\varepsilon_0=1$, $\varepsilon_i=2$ for all $i \geq 1$, and the stimulus components have been ordered, so that $A_0 = A_{max} = \max_i\{A_0, \ldots A_N\}$. Hence, the factors $k_i = A_i/A_{max}$, the normalized amplitudes, are less than 1; $h = b/A_{max}$ is the normalized bias of the rectifier. Sternberg *et al.* introduced the term "Bennett Function" for the amplitude factors A in the multiple Fourier series, for several of which tables have been published. The Bennett functions have been expressed in terms of contour integrals (Rice and Bennett) and in hypergeometric functions (e.g. Middleton, 1960). Neither of these two presentations relates to familiar funtions, so that preference is determined by the simplicity of numerical evaluation.

The present study is limited to the analysis of a nonlinearity without bias (h=0), and the arbitrary factor c will be set equal to 1. I will deal in some detail with the results for one- and two-tone stimuli, but it should be noted that this analysis can be extended "straightforwardly." Note that the one-tone, or narrow-band case, has been treated in detail by Davenport and Root (1958, Ch.13). In the special case that p is an integer, the highest order terms will vanish, as will be shown in the next subsection.

The Bennett functions can be decomposed into two terms, one giving the major stimulus amplitude dependence, and a second that depends only weekly on the level. For this second term I have proposed the term "modified Bennett function" **B** (unpublished IPO-report M267II, 1975), which for all i is asymptotically constant if k_i approaches 0. In formula

$$A^{(p)}_{m_0 m_1 \ldots m_N}(h, k_1, k_2 \ldots k_N) = \mathbf{B}^{(p)}_{m_0 m_1 \ldots m_N}(h, k_1, k_2 \ldots k_N) \prod_{i=1}^{N} k_i^{m_i} . \tag{4}$$

RESPONSE TO A SINGLE TONE

The response $y_+(t)$ of the half-wave p-law unbiased rectifier to the stimulus $s(t) = A \cos(\omega t + \phi)$ is

$$y_+(t) = \tfrac{1}{2} A^p \sum_{m=0}^{\infty} \varepsilon_m \mathbf{B}^{(p)}_m \cos m(\omega t + \phi) \tag{5}$$

as follows directly from Eqs. 3 and 4 with N = 0. The responses $y_o(t)$ and $y_e(t)$ for the odd and even full-wave nonlinearities follow directly from the appropriate summation of two half-wave rectifier responses, yielding:

$$y_o(t) = 2\; A^p \sum_{m=0}^{\infty} \mathbf{B}^{(p)}_{2m+1} \cos\{(2m+1)(\omega t + \phi)\} \tag{6}$$

which contains odd harmonics only, and

$$y_e(t) = A^p \sum_{m=0}^{\infty} \varepsilon_{2m} \mathbf{B}^{(p)}_{2m} \cos\{2m(\omega t + \phi)\} \tag{7}$$

containing only even harmonics.

For the amplitude factor **B** one finds (Davenport and Root, 1958):

$$\mathbf{B}^{(p)}_m = \frac{\Gamma(p+1)}{2^p \cdot \Gamma(1 + \frac{p+m}{2}) \Gamma(1 + \frac{p-m}{2})} \tag{8}$$

(which also can be written as a beta function). Note that the gamma function $\Gamma\{1+(p-m)/2\}$ plays an important role in the behaviour of **B**. For negative arguments the sign of the gamma function switches at each integer value; $\Gamma(x)$ approaches ± infinity as x approaches an integer value ≤ 0, so that **B** then approaches zero. For full wave even or odd powers, the natural elements in a Taylor expansion, this restricts the number of relevant terms in the expansion considerably. The values of **B** have a relative maximum when the argument x

defined above equals $\frac{1}{2} - n$ for $n \geq 0$, or if $m \approx 2n + 1 + p$, but this happens only for half-wave rectifiers (more generally: for nonlinearities with neither odd symmetry, nor even symmetry). It is generally true that **B** is smaller than 1 for all $p > 0$ *and* $m \geq 0$ (Braaksma, pers.comm.). The DC-response for the even nonlinearity is equal to the average response of $|y_o|$ for the odd nonlinearity:

$$<|y_o(t)|>_{av} = <y_e(t)>_{av} = A^p \mathbf{B}_0^{(p)} = \pi^{-1} A^p \mathrm{B}(\tfrac{1}{2}, \tfrac{1}{2}+p/2). \tag{9}$$

where B is the beta function.

RESPONSE TO TWO TONES

The response of the half-wave rectifier to the sum of two tones

$$s(t) = A_1 \cos(\omega_1 t + \phi_1) + A_2 \cos(\omega_2 t + \phi_2) \tag{10}$$

is given by

$$y_+(t) = \tfrac{1}{2} A_1^p \sum_{m_1=0}^{\infty} \sum_{m_2=0}^{\infty} k^{m_2} \varepsilon_{m_1} \varepsilon_{m_2} \mathbf{B}_{m_1 m_2}^{(p)}(k) \cos m_1(\omega_1 t + \phi_1) \cos m_2(\omega_2 t + \phi_2) \tag{11}$$

where $k = A_2/A_1 < 1$. The Bennett function for the two-tone case becomes

$$\mathbf{B}_{m_1 m_2}^{(p)}(k) = \frac{2^{-p} \Gamma(1+p)\, {}_2F_1\{\tfrac{1}{2}(m_1+m_2-p), \tfrac{1}{2}(-m_1+m_2-p); m_2+1; k^2\}}{\Gamma\{1-\tfrac{1}{2}(m_1+m_2-p)\}\, \Gamma\{1-\tfrac{1}{2}(-m_1+m_2-p)\}} \tag{12}$$

where ${}_2F_1$ is a hypergeometric function, which under all circumstances appoaches 1 as $k \to 0$. Obviously, $\mathbf{B}_{m0}{}^{(p)}(0) = \mathbf{B}_m{}^{(p)}$. The response of the full-wave odd nonlinearity, or the response fraction due to the odd component in the general nonlinearity, follows directly from Eq.11 (cf. the relation between Eqs. 6 and 5). The factor $\frac{1}{2}$ drops and only odd combinations of m_1+m_2 occur, implying, e.g., no DC, no even harmonics, no difference tones. Likewise, the even nonlinearity (nonlinear fraction) contains only the even combinations of m_1+m_2.

Conclusion

The above result has several other straightforward implications that are relevant in hearing research:

1: Equations 11 and 12 show that the response is not symmetrical in m_1 and m_2. Instead it depends strongly on which of the two amplitude, A_1 and A_2, is the largest. It is clear that the larger one determines the overall behaviour, the smaller only has a ratio-dependent (k) effect (cf. Table A1). Equation 11 gives the result for $A_1 > A_2$. For $A_1 < A_2$ the response is obtained by permutation of the indices. For $A_1 = A_2$ (k=1), despite possible formal

problems about convergence, the two responses can be continued analytically, showing a smooth transition.
2: Equation 11 shows single amplitude terms for the products $\cos m_1(\omega_1 t + \phi_1) \cos m_2(\omega_2 t + \phi_2)$. Since these can be rewritten as $\frac{1}{2}[\cos\{m_1(\omega_1 t + \phi_1) + m_2(\omega_2 t + \phi_2)\} + \cos\{m_1(\omega_1 t + \phi_1) - m_2(\omega_2 t + \phi_2)\}]$, it follows that the distortion products at $m_1\omega_1 + m_2\omega_2$ (e.g., $2f_1+f_2$) and $m_1\omega_1 - m_2\omega_2$ ($2f_1-f_2$) have the same amplitude term. It is also clear that the amplitudes of $2f_1-f_2$ and $2f_2-f_1$ will be different, except when $A_1 = A_2$.
3: As in the single tone response, sign (polarity) changes in **B** can occur if the arguments of the gamma functions in Eq.12 cross an integer value ≤ 0. This can occur if dominance of one term in the Bennett expansion is transferred to another. Where such changes have been reported in experimental data, these can be interpreted to imply that the underlying nonlinearity can not be approximated closely by a single term in Bennett's expansion.
4: The (modified) Bennett functions of different order are related through Gauss' recurrence relations for hypergeometric functions. Some examples are given in the appendix. For the odd nonlinearity all higher order terms can be expressed in terms of the amplitudes at f_1 and f_2. In case of a harmonic relation between f_1 and f_2 there is a complication because many higher order

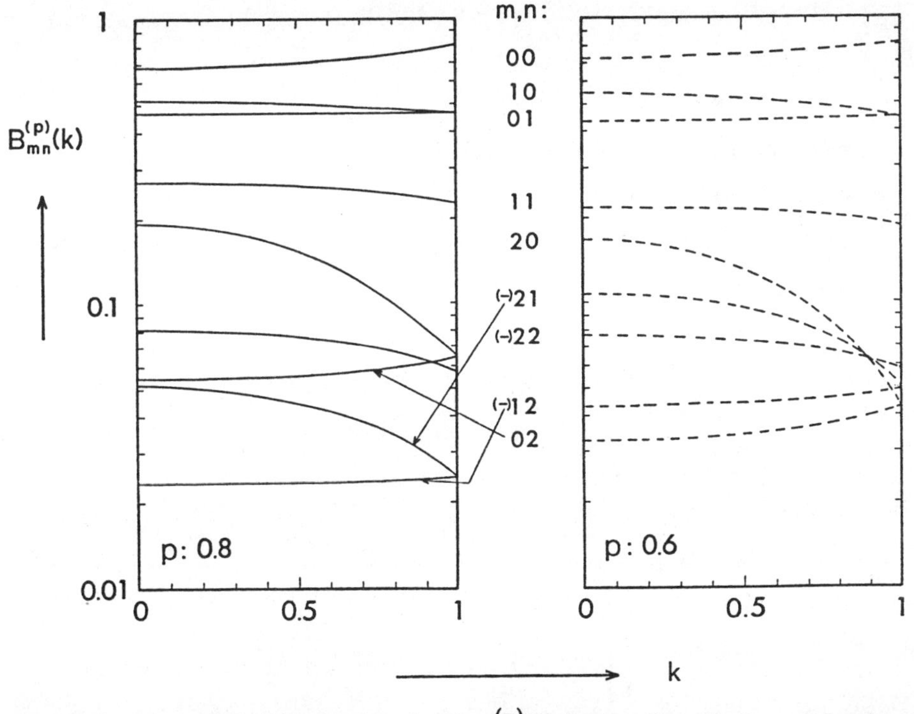

FIGURE 1. The modified Bennett function $B_{mn}^{(p)}(k)$ as a function of k, for p=0.8 and p=0.6 and low order m and n. The minus signs in the m,n-column imply that the corresponding functions are negative. Note that $B_m^{(p)}$, being equal to $B_{m0}^{(p)}(0)$, can be read from the appropriate intersections with the k = 0 axis.

intermodulation products will be generated at the same frequency. If, e.g., $4f_1 = 3f_2$, then $2f_1-f_2 = (2+4n)f_1-(1+3n)f_2$. In this case there is an interference of odd and even distortion products, because e.g., $6f_1-4f_2$ is an even term. If the nonlinearity is entirely odd, than the next term at $2f_1-f_2$ is $10f_1-7f_2$, or high enough to have only a small effect.

In Fig.1 I have plotted values of some lower order odd and even **B**s for the powers 0.8 and 0.6. The lowest order **B**s are clearly dominant. For the higher order terms the response order does not seem to be completely straightforward.

APPENDIX

Some recurrence relations for the modified Bennett function, based on Gauss' recurrence relations for hypergeometric functions (in this section the explicit description with argument k and power p is omitted):

$$(\mathrm{m-n+p+2})\mathbf{B}_{\mathrm{m+1,n-1}} \equiv -(\mathrm{m+n-p-2})\mathbf{B}_{\mathrm{m-1,n-1}} - 2\mathrm{m}k^2\mathbf{B}_{\mathrm{m,n}} \quad \text{(A1)}$$

$$(\mathrm{m+n+p})\mathbf{B}_{\mathrm{m,n}} \equiv -(\mathrm{m-n-p-2})\mathbf{B}_{\mathrm{m-2,n}} - 2(\mathrm{m}-1)\mathbf{B}_{\mathrm{m-1,n-1}} \quad \text{(A2)}$$

$$(\mathrm{m+-n+p})\mathbf{B}_{\mathrm{m,n}} \equiv -(\mathrm{-m+n-p-2})\mathbf{B}_{\mathrm{m,n-2}} - 2(\mathrm{n}-1)k^{-2}\mathbf{B}_{\mathrm{m-1,n-1}} \quad \text{(A3)}$$

$$(\mathrm{-m+n+p+2})\mathbf{B}_{\mathrm{m-1,n+1}} \equiv -(\mathrm{m+n-p-2})k^{-2}\mathbf{B}_{\mathrm{m-1,n-1}} - 2\mathrm{m}k^{-2}\mathbf{B}_{\mathrm{m,n}}. \quad \text{(A4)}$$

Hence:

$$\mathbf{B}_{10} \equiv {}_2F_1\{\tfrac{1}{2}(1-\mathrm{p}),\tfrac{1}{2}(-1-\mathrm{p});1;k^2\}\cdot\mathbf{B}_1 \quad \text{(A5)}$$

$$\mathbf{B}_{01} \equiv \tfrac{1}{2}(1+\mathrm{p})\,{}_2F_1\{\tfrac{1}{2}(1-\mathrm{p}),\tfrac{1}{2}(-1-\mathrm{p});1;k^2\}\cdot\mathbf{B}_1 \quad \text{(A6)}$$

$$(3+\mathrm{p})\mathbf{B}_{21} \equiv (\mathrm{p}+1)\mathbf{B}_{01} - 2\mathbf{B}_{10} \quad \text{(A7)}$$

$$(3+\mathrm{p})\mathbf{B}_{12} \equiv -2k^2\mathbf{B}_{01} + (\mathrm{p}+3)k^2\mathbf{B}_{10} \quad \text{(A8)}$$

$$(5+\mathrm{p})\mathbf{B}_{32} \equiv (\mathrm{p}+1)\mathbf{B}_{12} - 4\mathbf{B}_{21} \quad \text{etc.} \quad \text{(A9)}$$

Table 1: Amplitudes for lower order odd components in the 2-tone response of a full-wave odd nonlinearity. Note that the overall level of every component increases with power p, so that the ratio between the components is independent of the overall level.

	$A_1 > A_2$ ($k=A_2/A_1$)	$A_1 < A_2$ ($k=A_1/A_2$)
f_1	$2A_1^{\mathrm{p}}\,\mathbf{B}_{10}$	$2A_1A_2^{\mathrm{p}-1}\,\mathbf{B}_{01}$
f_2	$2A_1^{\mathrm{p}-1}A_2\,\mathbf{B}_{01}$	$2A_2^{\mathrm{p}}\,\mathbf{B}_{10}$
$2f_1-f_2$	$2A_1^{\mathrm{p}-1}A_2\,\mathbf{B}_{21}$	$2A_1^2A_2^{\mathrm{p}-2}\,\mathbf{B}_{12}$
$2f_2-f_1$	$2A_1^{\mathrm{p}-2}A_2^2\,\mathbf{B}_{12}$	$2A_1A_2^{\mathrm{p}-1}\,\mathbf{B}_{21}$
$3f_1-2f_2$	$2A_1^{\mathrm{p}-2}A_2^2\,\mathbf{B}_{32}$	$2A_1^3A_2^{\mathrm{p}-3}\,\mathbf{B}_{23}$
$3f_2-2f_1$	$2A_1^{\mathrm{p}-3}A_2^3\,\mathbf{B}_{23}$	$2A_1^2A_2^{\mathrm{p}-2}\,\mathbf{B}_{32}$

References

Bennett, W.R. (1933) New results in the calculation of modulation products. Bell System Tech. J. 12, 228-243.

Bernstein, S.N. (1922) Sur l'ordre de la meilleure approximation des functions continues par des polynomes. Académie Royale de Belgique, Classe de Sciences, Mémoires, Deuxième Série, Tome IV, 1-103.

Braaksma, B.L.J. (1988) Math.Dept.,R.U.Groningen, pers.communication.

Davenport, W.B. and Root, W.L. (1958) Random signals and noise. McGraw-Hill, New York.

Duifhuis, H. (1976) Cochlear nonlinearity and second filter; possible mechanism and implications. J. Acoust. Soc. Am. 59, 408-423.

Fahey, P.F. and Allen, J.B. (1988) Power law features of acoustic distortion product emissions. In: Basic Issues in Hearing (Eds. Duifhuis, H., Horst, J.W. and Wit, H.P.) Academic, London (in press).

Feuerstein, E. (1957) Intermodulation products for ν-law biased wave rectifiers for multiple frequency input. Quart. Appl. Math. 15, 183-192.

Goldstein, J.L. (1967) Auditory nonlinearity. J. Acoust. Soc. Am. 41, 676-689.

Hall, J.L. (1972) Auditory distortion products f_2-f_1 and $2f_1$-f_2. J. Acoust. Soc. Am. 51, 1863-1871.

Middleton, D. (1948) Some general results in the theory of noise through non-linear devices. Quart. Appl. Math. 5, 445-498.

Middleton, D. (1960) An Introduction to Statistical Communication Theory. McGraw-Hill, New York.

Rice, S.O. (1945) Mathematical analysis of random noise. IV. Noise through non-linear devices. Bell System Tech. J. 24, 115-162.

Schroeder, M.R. (1975) Amplitude behavior of the cubic difference tone. J. Acoust. Soc. Am. 58, 728-732.

Smoorenburg, G.F. (1972) Combination tones and their origin. J. Acoust. Soc. Am. 52, 615-632.

Smoorenburg, G.F. (1974) On the mechanism of combination tones and lateral suppression in hearing. In: Facts and Models in Hearing (Eds. Zwicker, E. and Terhardt, E.) Springer, Berlin, pp. 332-342.

Sternberg, R.L. and Kaufman, H. (1953) A general solution of the two-frequency modulation product problem.I. J. Math. & Phys. 32, 233-242.

Sternberg, R.L. (1954) A general solution of the two-frequency modulation product problem.II. Tables of the functions $A_{mn}(h,k)$. J. Math. & Phys. 33, 68-79.

Sternberg, R.L., Shipman, J.S. and Thurston, W.B. (1954) Tables of Bennett functions for the two-frequency modulation product problem for the half-wave linear rectifier. Quart. J. Appl. Math. 7, 505-511.

Sternberg, R.L., Shipman, J.S. and Kaufman, H. (1955) Tables of Bennett functions for the two-frequency modulation product problem for the half-wave square-law rectifier. Quart. J. Appl. Math. 8, 457-467.

Zwicker, E. (1955) Der ungewöhnliche Amplitudengang der nichtlinearen Verzerrung des Ohres. Acustica 5, 67-74.

FAHEY

This paper shows that if one varies the amplitudes of both input tones together (A_1=k, A_2=A) that the amplitude of the distortion product (DP) grows to the p-th power ($p < 1$) of A. This is consistent with the psychophysical DP data only if one assumes that the cancellation tone used to measure the DP mixes with and cancels the DP at the site of the nonlinearity (Smoorenburg, 1972). It is otherwise inconsistent with the psychophysical data which generally increases linearly with A under condition when the p-th law would predict increase with the p-th power. Furthermore, since the DP's measured in animal ear canals are not measured with cancellation tones, the predictions of the p-th power law nonlinearity do not describe the animal DP's when both input tones are varied together (e.g. Brown, 1988; Fahey and Allen, 1986; Weiderhold, et al., 1986).

The predictions of the p-th law nonlinearity that do fit the animal and the psychophysical data are the predictions in Table 1 when $A_1 > A_2$ when A1 is held constant and when $A_1 < A_2$ and A_2 is held constant. But under these conditions several (and probably all) monotonically saturating nonlinearities give the same predictions. Indeed, M. Schroeder has pointed out in a comment to the paper by Fahey and Allen (1988) that even an infinite peak clipper will show this scaling. It is a simple exercise to use Bennett's method (1933) to express the output of an infinite peak clipper in a power series in k ($=A_1/A_2$ or A_2/A_1) that does show the proper scaling.

When one amplitude is held constant the regime where the p-th law nonlinearity differs from the nonlinearities that show much harder saturation, such as infinite and finite peak clippers, the hyperbolic tangent and certain hyperbolic nonlinearities is in the behaviour of the DP when the swept amplitude is greater than the fixed amplitude. Here, for instance in the $2f_1$-f_2 DP with A_1 p-th law nonlinearity and as the inverse of A_2 for the harder saturating nonlinearities if the fixed level is high enough.[2]

Brown, A.M. (1987) "Acoustic distortion from rodent ears: A comparison of responses from rats, guinea pigs and gerbils", Hearing Research, 31, 25-38.

Fahey, P.F. and Allen, J.B. (1986) "Characterization of cubic intermodulation distortion products in the cat external auditory meatus", In: Peripheral Auditory Mechanisms, eds. J.B. Allen, J.L. Hall, A. Hubbard, S.T. Neely, and A. Tubis (Springer-Verlag, Berlin), 314-321.

Weiderhold, M.L., Mahoney, J.W., and Kellogg, D.L. (1986) "Acoustic overstimulation reduces $2f_1$-f_2 cochlear emissions at all levels in cat", Peripheral Auditory Mechanisms, eds. J.B. Allen, J.L. Hall, A. Hubbard, S.T. Neely, and A. Tubis (Springer-Verlag, Berlin), 322-329.

DUIFHUIS

Thank you for your remarks. With respect to your second paragraph, I agree with your point that a significant part of the data is insensitive to the value of the power p, although the remaining part is. I want to emphasize, however, that even when amplitude behaviour is independent of p, phase data may be informative. In fact Smoorenburg's (1974) and Schroeder's (1975) conclusion that $2f_1$-f_2 is generated by a compressive nonlinearity, strongly relies on the phase data.

With respect to your first paragraph I want to emphasize that my interpretation of psychophysical and neurophysiological literature data deviates from your formulation. Combination tone data and two-tone suppression data, at least at levels over about 30dB SL, show compressive nonlinear behaviour (e.g. Duifhuis, 1976, 1980).

Duifhuis, H. (1980) Level effects in psychophysical two-tone suppression, J. Acoust. Soc. Am., 67, 914-927.

MATTHEWS

I would like to repeat our warning from the Boston meeting (Matthews and Molnar, 1986). It is difficult to interpret nonlinearities seen in a distributed cochlear mechanical model in terms of the "nonlinear generator" located in the cochlear partition. We showed that a *quadratic nonlinear element* (which in isolation could not produce odd-order distortion), produced the "cubic difference tone" ($2f_1 - f_2$) in our model by secondary interactions, e.g., between f_1 and ($f_2 - f_1$).

Matthews, J.W., and Molnar, C.E. (1986) Modeling intracochlear and ear canal distortion product ($2f_1$-f_2) In: Peripheral Auditory Mechanisms (Eds: Allen, J.B., Hall, J.L., Hubbard, A.E., Neely, S.T. and Tubis, A.) Springer Verlag, Berlin, pp. 258-265.

DUIFHUIS

You raise a serious point. It does play an important role in distributed models with an even nonlinearity and an odd(-order) stimulus, where the even interaction of an odd + an even term can generate an odd product. Formally: n.even + m.odd = odd iff m = odd, irrespective of the sum n + m. In your example $f_2 - f_1$ is even, but the fundamental f_1 (or f_2) is odd, hence you can have a result that is odd. However, in distributed models with an odd nonlinearity this problem does not arise. There, both fundamentals and distortion products are odd. Since n.odd + m.odd = odd iff n + m = odd, which is the case for all nonlinear interactions, the distributed odd nonlinearity does not suffer from the confounding problem which you have pointed out for the even nonlinearity. That is to say, the odd distributed model will not be able to generate even distortion.

This paper was presented as a poster during the meeting and was not therefore subject to general discussion.

DISTORTION PRODUCT RESPONSES OF SATURATING NONLINEARITIES

Paul F. Fahey

Dept. of Physics/Electronics Engineering
University of Scranton
Scranton, PA 18510 USA

Introduction

Saturating nonlinearities (Figure 1) show several amplitude scaling relationships that are common to this class of nonlinearity. Here we examine the output of distortion products (DP's) at the DP frequencies $f_d = 2f_1-f_2$ and at $f_d = 3f_1-2f_2$. The nonlinearities are both (a) hard satu-

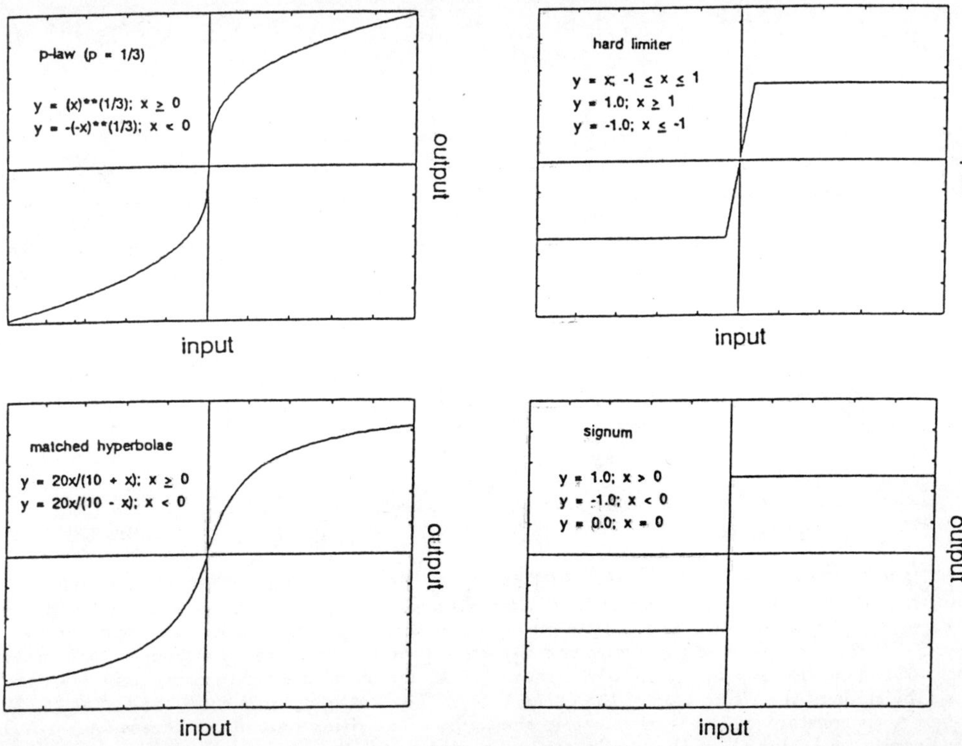

FIGURE 1. The input-output curves of the nonlinearities used in this study are displayed along with their governing equations.

rating, i.e., at high enough amplitude the output of the nonlinearity is a waveform of constant amplitude and (b) soft saturating, i.e., the output of the nonlinearity has no maximum amplitude. We find an amplitude scaling behavior that is common both. There are also scaling relationships that vary with the details of the nonlinearity.

The following saturating nonlinearities have been examined in this study: the p-law nonlinearity ($p < 1$) (see Duifhuis (1988) in these proceedings); the infinite peak clipper (or signum); the hard limiter (finite peak clipper); and matched rectangular hyperbolae ($y = a1*x/(a1 + x)$ $x \geq 0$; $y = a2*x/(a2 - x)$ $x < 0$). If $a1 = a2$ this nonlinearity is odd, otherwise this nonlinearity has both odd and even terms and is the only nonlinearity in this study with any even symmetry.) The odd order matched hyperbolae is a good model of the outer hair cell response function in vivo and the matched hyperolae with some even symmetry can be a good approximation the response function of the inner hair cell in vivo and hair cells in vitro.

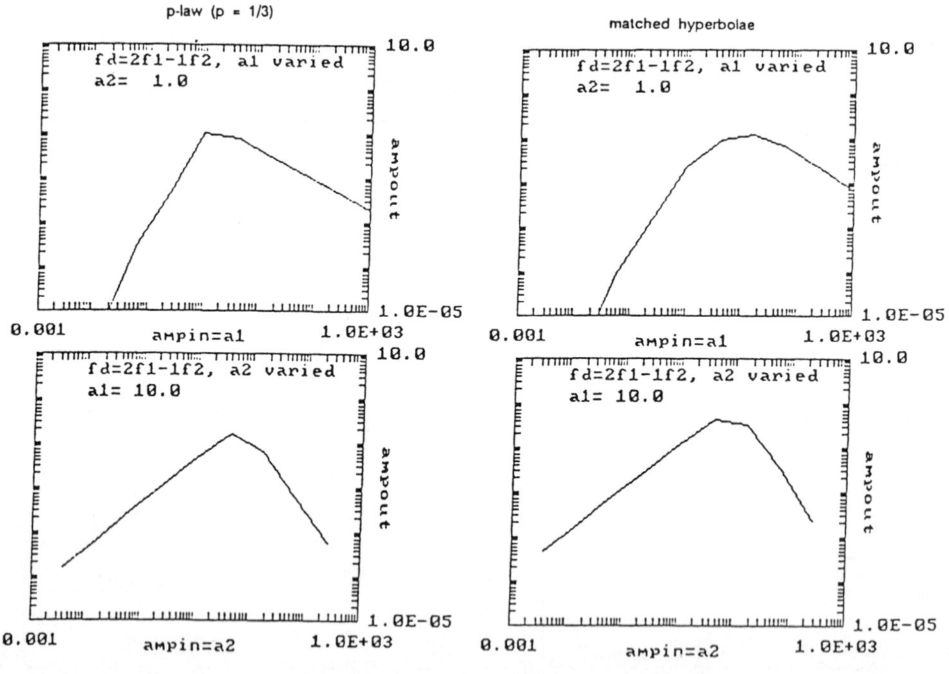

FIGURE 2. The distortion product (DP) at $2f_1-f_2$ when A_2 is held constant is shown as a function of the level of A_1 (ampin) in the top panels. The level of A_2 is also shown in the figure. In all cases the DP is a maximum in the region where A_1 and A_2 are approximately equal. In the top panels of this figure the distortion product amplitudes (ampout) in the rising part of the curves ($A_1 < A_2$) go as the square of A_1 for all of these saturating nonlinearities. I.e., the slope of the rising part of the curve is two. The bottom panels show the DP at $2f_1-f_2$ when A_1 is constant at the level shown in the figure. The rising part of the curves ($A_2 < A_1$) go linearly in A_2 for all of the nonlinearities studied here. In this figure both the p-law (left column) and the matched hyperbolae (right column) are displayed. The descending slopes of the p-law are -2/3 in the top panel and -5/3 in the bottom in agreement with Table 1 of Duifhuis (1988).

The distortion product output of both types of matched hyperbolae are qualitatively the same and only the odd order case will be presented here. The response of the nonlinearities to two pure tone inputs will be examined through the study of both third order and fifth order distortion products. These responses have been determined by implementing the nonlinearities in software and determining the Fourier amplitudes in the output waveform. Both the p-law nonlinearity and the infinite peak clipper have been checked using Bennett's method (1933). See Duifhuis (1988) for the p-law response and for the signum response (i.e., p = 0).

Results

ONE AMPLITUDE VARIED

Figure 1 shows the nonlinearities under study. Only the p-law nonlinearity has a response that grows without bound as the input amplitude grows. The p-law nonlinearity is the only example here of the class of soft saturating nonlinearities. Duifhuis (1988) in his Table 1 for the p-law nonlinearity driven by two sine waves, one at amplitude A_1 with frequency f_1 and the other at amplitude A_2 with frequency f_2, shows some

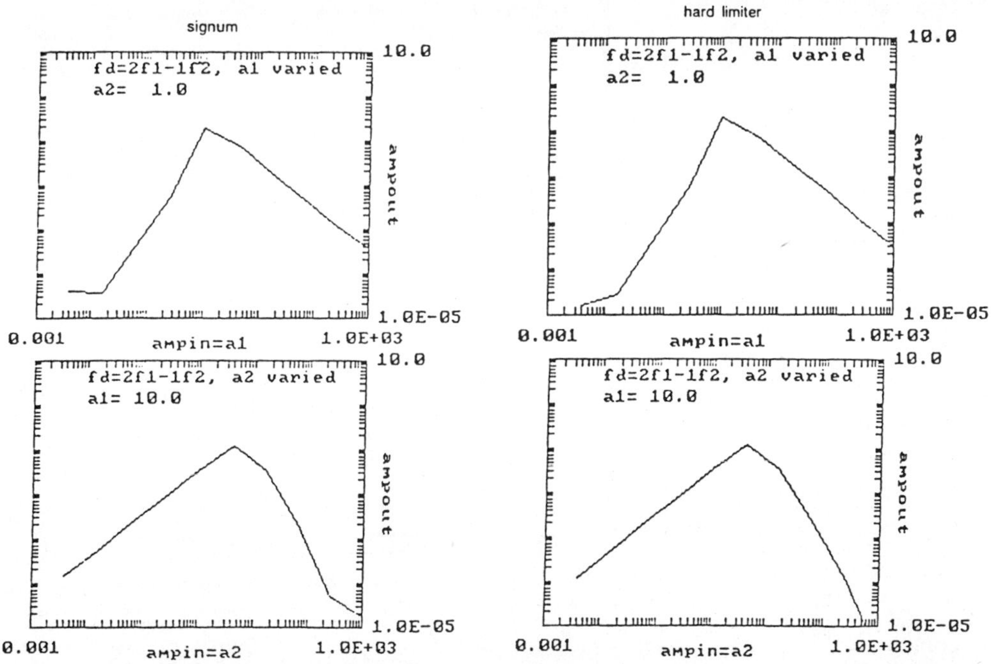

FIGURE 3. Same as Figure 2 but with the signum and the hard-limiter displayed. For the hard-limiter the clipping level is a factor of ten below the level of the fixed tone in each case. When the clipping level is greater than the level of the fixed tone the hard-limiter does not show the simple scaling that is shown here. The descending slopes are as predicted using Bennett's method (1933) and are -1 in the top panels and -2 in the bottom.

scaling of the distortion products with input amplitude that is common to all of the saturating nonlinearities. Namely, if A_1 is constant and greater than A_2 then the DP at $2f_1$-f_1 grows linearly with A_2; the DP at $2f_2$-f_1 grows as A_2 squared; the DP at $3f_1$-$2f_2$ grows as A_2 squared and the DP at $3f_2$-$2f_1$ grows as A_2 cubed. Now if A_2 is held constant and is greater than A_1 then the following complementary set of relationships hold: the DP at $2f_1$-f_2 scales as A_1 squared; the DP at $2f_2$-f_1 is linear in A_1; the DP at $3f_1$-$2f_2$ scales as A_1 cubed and the DP at $3f_2$-$2f_1$ grows as A_1 squared. These scaling relationships for the p-law nonlinearity are the same as the scaling relationships for all of the other nonlinearities examined here. Figures 2 and 3 show the scaling for $2f_1$-f_2 in the p-law with p=1/3, the signum output, the hard limiter output, and the output of the odd symmetry matched hyperbolae. Note that the rising slopes are the same for all of these nonlinearities when A_2 is constant and again when A_1 is constant. Figures 4 and 5 show the output at $3f_1$-$2f_2$ for the p-law (p=1/2), for the signum, for the hard limiter, and the matched hyperbolae and here also the rising slopes are the same for all of these nonlinearities when a given amplitude is constant.

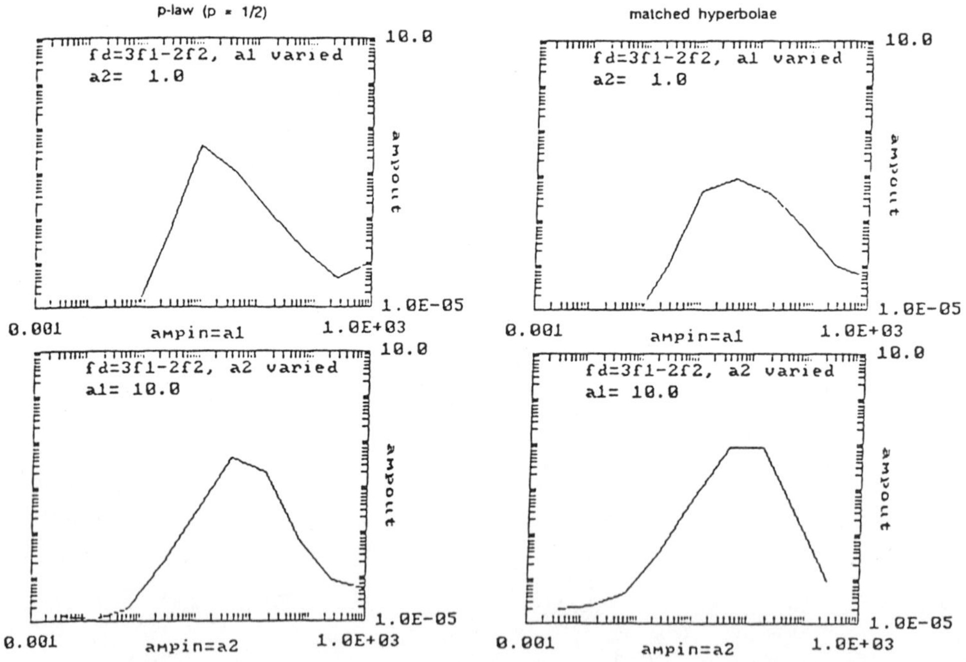

FIGURE 4. The DP at $3f_1$-$2f_2$ when A_2 is held constant is shown as a function of the level of A_1 in the top panels. In the top panels the distortion product amplitudes (ampout) in the rising part of the curves ($A_1 < A_2$) go as the cube of A_1 for all of these saturating nonlinearities. I.e., the slope of the rising part of the curve is three. The bottom panels show the DP at $3f_1$-$2f_2$ when A_1 is constant at the level shown. The rising part of the curves ($A_2 < A_1$) goes quadratically in A_2 for all of the nonlinearities studied here. In this figure both the p-law and the matched hyperbolae are displayed. The descending slopes of the p-law are -3/2 in the top panel and -5/2 in the bottom in agreement with Table 1 of Duifhuis (1988).

Where the hard saturating nonlinearities differ from the p-law nonlinearities is in the falling slope. The p-law predictions are in Table 1 of Duifhuis (and in Figures 2 and 4) and these differ from the falling slopes of the hard saturating nonlinearites. For instance, for the signum, we see that for $2f_1$-f_2 when A_1 is constant but A_2 is greater than A_1 that the DP falls off as the inverse of A_2 squared; and for the DP at $3f_1$-$2f_2$ falls off as A_2 cubed. At high enough levels of the fixed tone all of the hard saturating nonlinearities look enough like a signum to have response like the signum response. In hard saturation all of the amplitude information is lost at high levels and the only information passing the nonlinearity is the zero crossings.

TWO AMPLITUDES VARIED

In Figure 6 are the results of varing both A_1 and A_2 together (A_1 = A_2 = A). Each of the nonlinearites shows quite different response in the $2f_1$-f_2 intermodulation distortion products. The $3f_1$-$2f_2$ distortion products (not shown) show responses similar to the $2f_1$-f_2 responses. Notice that in none of the outputs does the DP at $2f_1$-f_2 show pure cubic scaling (slope

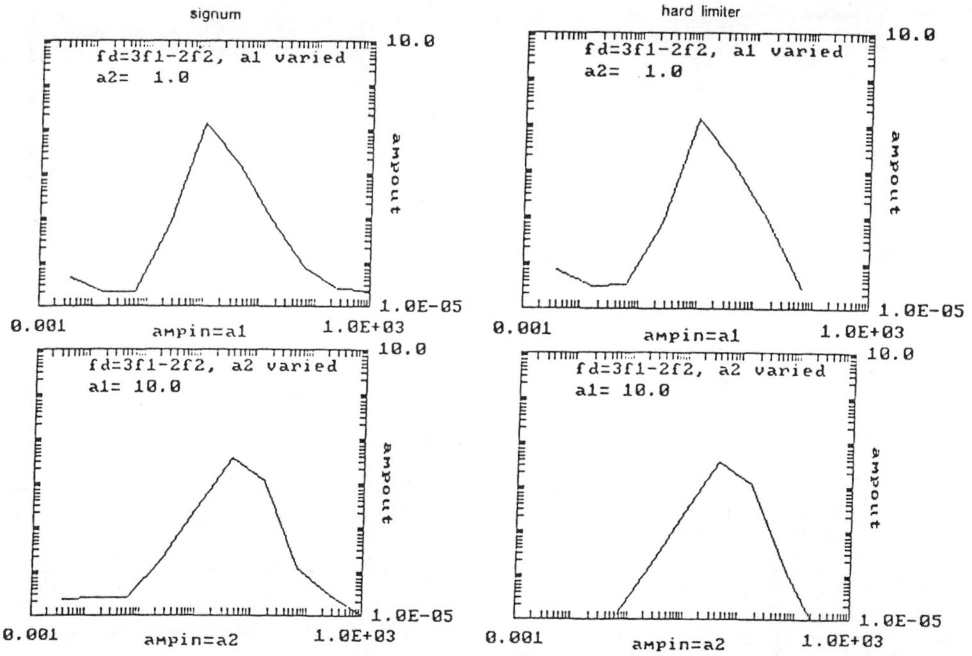

FIGURE 5. Same as Figure 4 except in this figure both the signum and the hard-limiter are displayed. For the hard-limiter the clipping level is a factor of ten below the level of the fixed tone in each case. When the clipping level is greater than the level of the fixed tone the hard-limiter does not show the simple scaling that is shown here. The descending slopes are as predicted using Bennett's method (1933), i.e., in the top panels the descending slope are -2 and in the bottom panels they are -3.

of 3) nor does the DP at $3f_1$-$2f_2$ show pure quintic scaling (slope of 5). It is apparent that the signum function shows very substantial distortion at all levels as is expected. The p-law nonlinearity shows substantial distortion at low levels. This because the slope of the p-law nonlinearity is infinite at zero and the nonlinearity is an effective amplifier at these low levels. At low levels the hard-limiter shows no distortion because the input is in the linear region. As the input gets into the nonlinear region the hard-limiter begins to look like the signum.

Finally, in Figure 7 is the output of a nonlinearity similar to that suggested by Johnstone et.al. (1986) in their Figure 5. This response function shows saturating amplification at low levels and becomes linear at high levels. (A response function discussed by Allen (1988) in these proceedings.) This response function shows many of the features already discussed. As A_1 and A_2 are varied together the response at very high levels is less than the responses of the hard saturating nonlinearities.

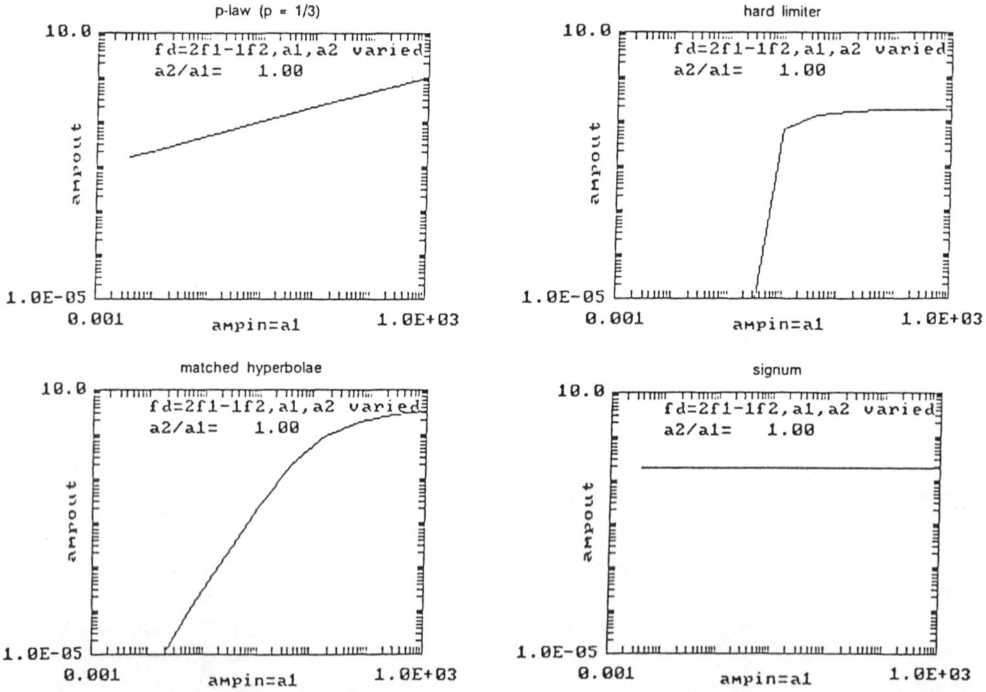

FIGURE 6. The DP at $2f_1$-f_2 (ampout) when both A_1 and A_2 are varied together and are equal is plotted against the level of A_1 for four nonlinearities. For the p-law (p = 1/3) the rising slope is 1/3; for the matched hyperbolas the rising slope is 2 before going into saturation; for the signum the slope is zero; for the hard limiter there is no DP until the sum of the two amplitude is great enough to take the input into the peak clipping part of the nonlinearity.

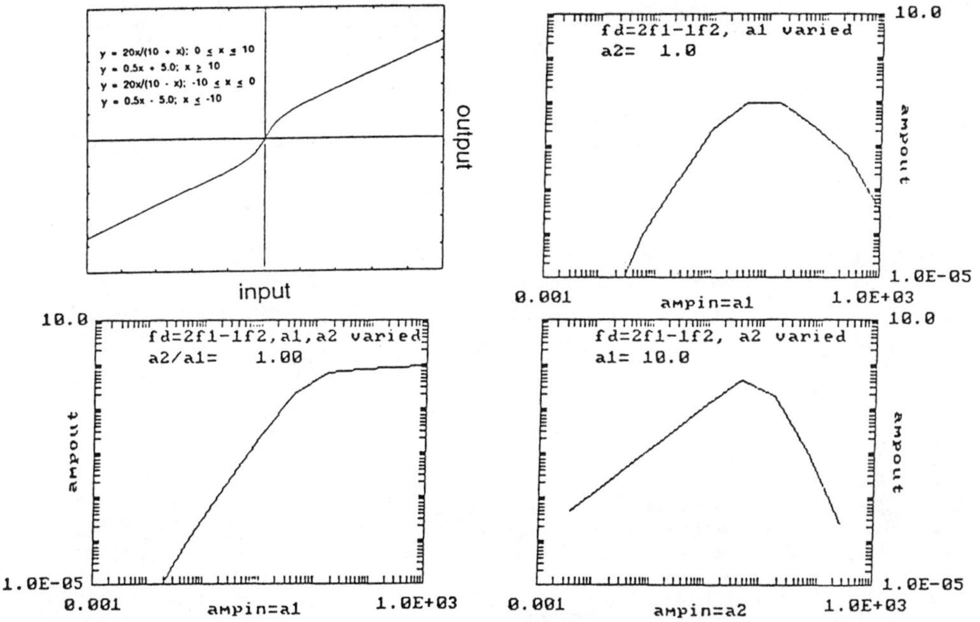

FIGURE 7. The response of the input-output curve shown in the upper left panel is shown in the other three panels. The function is linear at high levels and is nonlinear at low levels. It's response differs from the response of the matched hyperbolas only at very high levels.

Conclusion

I. For one amplitude fixed and one amplitude varied (with the exception of the hard-limiter when the fixed amplitude is near or below the clipping amplitude) all of the saturating nonlinearities show the same rising slopes for distortion product production for any given distortion product. Here one can not distinguish a signum from a p-law, etc.. This is the point of Figures 2,3,4, and 5.

II. For one amplitude fixed and one amplitude varied the descending slopes are different across the saturating nonlinearities. Although at high enough levels of the fixed tone all of the hard saturations are asymptotically the same and effectively look like the signum. This is the other point of Figures 2,3,4, and 5. Notice that the change from rising slope to descending slope occurs in the region where A_1 is approximately equal to A_2.

III. When both amplitudes are varied together the rate of distortion product increase is very different across the nonlinearities. This is the point of Figure 6. In the psycophysical data the interpretation of the distortion product data is not necessarily straightforward (Smoorenburg, 1972). Distortion products measured in animal ear canals (for example

Fahey and Allen (1986); Brown (1987); Weiderhold et al. (1986)) seem to be the product of a nonlinearity akin to the matched hyperbolae. Since the animal distortion products are the vector sum of waves generated at a continuum of nonlinear sites along the basilar membrane the nonlinearity can be determined only by deconvoling from the response. This problem has not yet been solved.

References

Allen, J.B. (1988) Is BM tuning the same as neural tuning - where do we stand? Mechanics of Hearing 1988 Preprints.

Bennett, W.R. (1933) New results in the calculation of modulation products. Bell System Technical Journal, 12, 228-243.

Brown, A.M. (1987) Acoustic distortion from rodent ears: A comparison of responses from rats, guinea pigs and gerbils. Hearing Research, 31, 25-38.

Duifhuis, H. (1988) Power-law nonlinearities: A review of some less familiar properties. Mechanics of Hearing 1988 Preprints.

Fahey, P.F. and Allen, J.B. (1986) Characterization of cubic intermodulation distortion products in the cat external auditory meatus. In: Peripheral Auditory Mechanisms (Eds. J.B. Allen, J.L. Hall, A. Hubbard, S.T. Neely, and A. Tubis) Springer-Verlag, Berlin, pp. 314-321.

Johnstone, B.M., Patuzzi, R., and Yates, G.K. (1986) Basilar membrane measurements and the travelling wave. Hearing Research, 22, 147-153.

Smoorenburg, G.F. (1972) Combination tone and their origin. J. Acoust. Soc. Am. 52, 615-632.

Weiderhold, M.L., Mahoney, J.W., and Kellogg, D.L. (1986) Acoustic over, stimulation reduces 2f1-f2 cochlear emissions at all levels in cat. In: Peripheral Auditory Mechanisms (Eds. J.B. Allen, J.L. Hall, A. Hubbard, S.T. Neely, and A. Tubis) Springer-Verlag, Berlin, pp. 322-329.

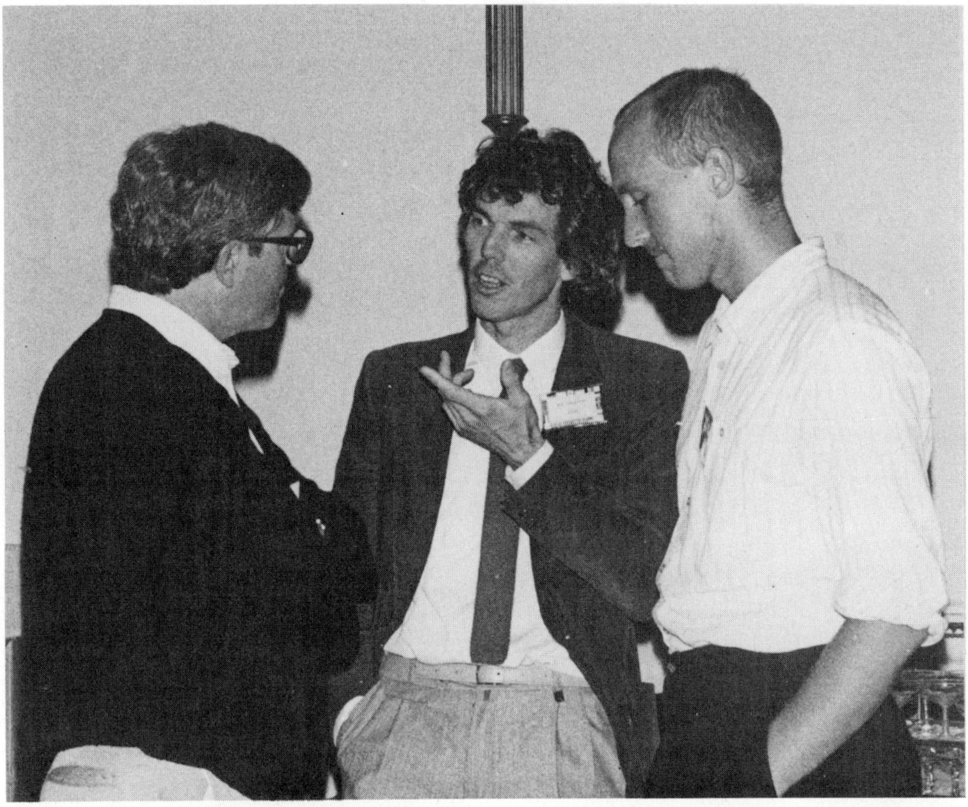

P.F. Fahey, M.A. Viergever and P.J. Kolston

8. COCHLEAR MODELS

REALISTIC BASILAR MEMBRANE TUNING DOES NOT REQUIRE ACTIVE PROCESSES

Paul J. Kolston [1] and Max A. Viergever [2]

Faculty of Mathematics and Informatics, Delft University of Technology, Delft, The Netherlands
Current affiliations:
1. Department of Electrical and Electronic Engineering University of Canterbury, Christchurch, New Zealand
2. Department of Radiology and Nuclear Medicine University Hospital Utrecht, The Netherlands

Abstract

This paper describes two versions of a cochlear model (called the OHCAP model), both of which exhibit mechanical response tuning very similar to that recently measured in the real cochlea. Two assumptions made in the formulation of the model, that make it different from previous cochlear models, are that the basilar membrane has two radial modes of vibration (corresponding to division into its arcuate and pectinate zones), and that the outer hair cells (OHCs) greatly modify the mechanics of the arcuate zone. The two versions of the OHCAP model presented here have different models for the OHCs. Both versions exhibit very realistic tuning, and so it remains to be determined which is more acceptable in terms of physiological justifiability. However, both versions of the OHCAP model are passive, which shows that active processes are not necessary to explain the cochlea's sharp tuning.

Introduction

The description and analysis of cochlear models is one method by which the operation of the real cochlea can be better understood. For this insight to be worthwhile, a cochlear model should satisfy three criteria: its response should agree with experimental measurements of basilar membrane (BM) vibration; the model should conform with cochlear anatomy/physiology; and the model should be the simplest possible, which means that it cannot be simplified without loss of essential properties.

The cochlea is an extremely small and delicate system and, because of this, accurate measurements of its response are very difficult. The sharpness of the mechanical response is very susceptible to trauma and therefore, as surgical techniques have improved, so has the correlation between mechanical and neural tuning sharpness. It now seems likely that the very sharp tuning exhibited by nerve fibre action potentials is also present in the BM response (Sellick et al., 1983; Robles et al., 1986).

Most investigators have found that active processes are necessary in cochlear models in order for them to exhibit sharp BM tuning. However, in the formulation of these models, it has always been assumed that the BM has only one mode of vibration in the radial direction. This assumption is supported neither by the BM's anatomical structure, nor by the radial position of the organ of Corti (positioned on top of the arcuate zone of the BM). This paper describes a passive cochlear model that exhibits realistic tuning, by allowing two radial modes of vibration in the BM.

The OHCAP model

The model is called the OHCAP model, to emphasize the importance of the OHCs and the Arcuate and Pectinate zones of the BM. The usual macromechanical assumptions are made in the formulation of the OHCAP model (see Viergever (1986) for a review). The fluid flow within the scalae is assumed to be one-dimensional, meaning that all pertinent dependent variables depend only on one independent variable, the longitudinal coordinate. A schematic of one section of the cochlear partition appears in Fig. 1, which shows the two zones of the BM and the organ of Corti. Vertical motion of the arcuate zone causes shear motion in the subtectorial space. The OHC stereocilia present an impedance to subtectorial shear motion, and hence alter the impedance of the arcuate zone.

Fig. 2 shows a simplified schematic of the section drawn in Fig. 1. The complete OHCAP model is formed by cascading a number of these sections. The fluid mass between the sections is represented by M_f. The BM is divided into its arcuate and pectinate zones, with the components M_a, C_a and R_a representing the mass, compliance and resistance respectively in the arcuate zone, and similarly for M_p, C_p and R_p in the pectinate zone. The additional impedance in the arcuate zone, due to the bending impedance of the OHC stereocilia, is represented by Z_o. The frequency dependence of Z_o determines the low frequency response shape (in the arcuate zone).

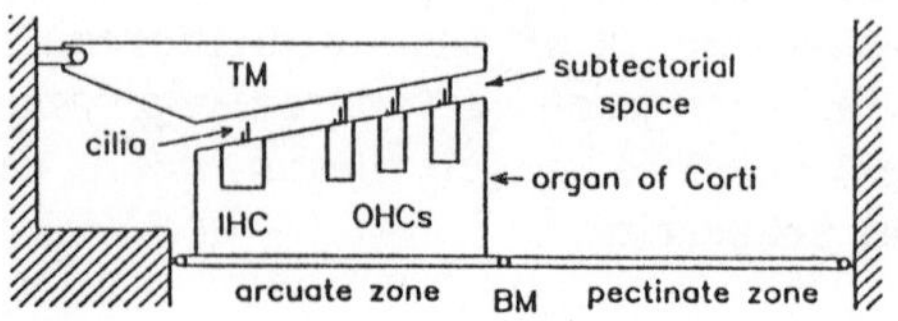

Fig. 1: Cross section schematic of the cochlear partition. The basilar membrane is divided into its two zones. The OHC stereocilia alter the impedance of the arcuate zone.

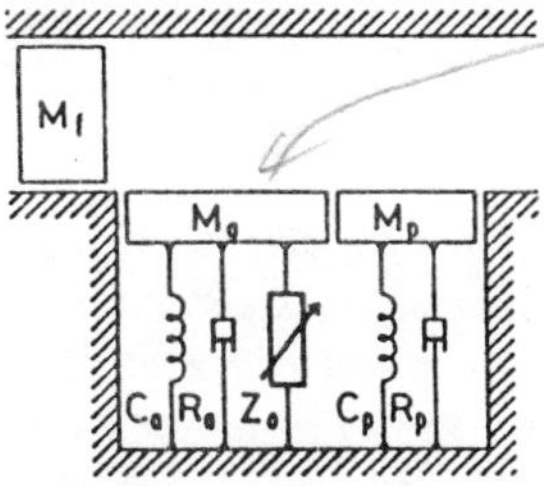

Fig. 2: Simplified partition schematic, with lumped elements representing the arcuate and pectinate zones (subscript a and p respectively). The OHC stereocilia impedance is represented by Z_o, the frequency dependence of which determines the shape of the arcuate zone response.

The OHCAP model, as first described in Kolston (1988a), had two major shortcomings. Firstly, Z_o was prescribed functionally and was not justified physiologically. Secondly, it was assumed in the formulation of the model that the presence of the OHCs increased the impedance of the arcuate zone. Any malfunction in the operation of the OHCs would result in an increase in response sensitivity, and this does not agree with experimental observations of traumatised cochleae.

In the OHCAP model described in this paper the OHCs decrease the net arcuate impedance. It is assumed that in the dead cochlea the impedance of the BM is much greater in the arcuate zone than in the pectinate zone. This is consistent with two features of cochlear anatomy. Firstly, in the arcuate zone the BM fibres form a close-meshed mat, while in the pectinate zone the fibres lie in distinct bundles (Iurato, 1962). Secondly, the arches of Corti have a high torsional stiffness (due to connections between the arch heads) and this would further increase the arcuate impedance (Miller, 1985).

The two versions of the OHCAP model presented here include different models for the OHCs. The first version (called the DOHCAP model ("D" for Deiters' cells)) has been described elsewhere (in two slightly different forms: Kolston, 1988b; Kolston et al., 1989). In this model the signal that controls the frequency dependence of the Z_o is derived from the difference in motion between two adjacent sections of the pectinate zone. In the second version (called the FOHCAP model ("F" for Filtering - by the OHCs)) the signal that controls Z_o is derived from within the OHC itself. The FOHCAP model makes fewer assumptions concerning the anatomy of the organ of Corti, but it requires a more complicated filtering process to be performed by the OHCs.

The DOHCAP model

Fig. 3 shows the geometric arrangement of the OHCs, the Deiters' cells and their phalangeal processes. The base of each OHC is supported by the top of a Deiters' cell, while the top of each OHC is in close proximity to a phalangeal process from an adjacent Deiters' cell (Voldrich, 1983). The Deiters' cells sit on the edge of the pectinate zone. It is postulated that the top of the OHC senses the velocity of the adjacent (basal) Deiters' cell (v_b), while the bottom of the OHC senses the velocity of its supporting Deiters' cell (v_a).

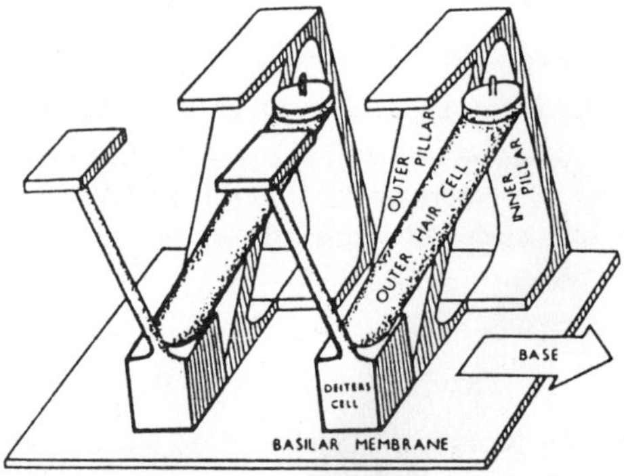

Fig. 3: Drawing of the geometric arrangement of the supporting cells and the outer hair cells (OHCs) in the organ of Corti (after Voldrich, 1983). In the DOHCAP model each OHC is assumed to control its stereocilia bending impedance using stimuli received from adjacent sections of the pectinate zone.

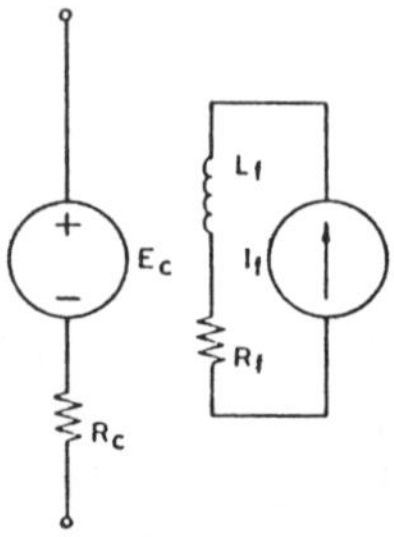

Fig. 4: The DOHCAP OHC stereocilia bending impedance is determined by a controlled voltage source (E_c) in series with a resistance R_c. E_c is controlled by the potential difference across the current source I_f. The elements with subscript f represent the filtering action of the OHC.

Fig. 4 shows an electrical circuit representation of the DOHC model, the mechanical equivalent of which replaces the element Z_o in Fig. 2. The correct frequency dependence for Z_o is obtained by deriving a controlling signal for E_c from the motion of two adjacent sections of the pectinate zone.

For the purpose of this discussion the pectinate signals v_b and v_a are represented by voltages V_b and V_a, respectively. The current source in Fig. 4 is described by $I_f = K_f \,.\, V_a$. The potential difference developed across I_f is V_f. The voltage source is described by $E_c = K_c \,.\, (V_f - V_b)$ and this, in series with R_c, determines the stereocilia bending impedance. The parameters K_f, L_f and R_f are chosen so that, for stimulus frequencies much less than the CF, V_f and V_b have very similar magnitude and phase. Therefore, the magnitude of E_c is very small. When the stimulus frequency nears the CF of both v_a and v_b, the phase of V_f deviates from that of V_b, and so E_c increases in magnitude. The phase of E_c is imaginary and positive, and so the increase in magnitude has the effect of reducing the net arcuate zone stiffness. Therefore, the arcuate motion increases, producing realistic mechanical tuning.

The FOHCAP model

In this version of the OHCAP model it is assumed that an OHC is a one-port device, in that Z_o is determined solely by the filtering action of the OHC. In order to achieve realistic tuning the OHC is modelled by a fourth order network. The FOHC model, in electrical network form, is shown in Fig. 5.

The voltage sources are described by: $E_c = -K_c V_C$ and $E_f = -K_f V_L$; where V_C is the potential difference across C_c and V_L is the potential difference across L_f. The impedance function for this network (ignoring R_f and assuming that L_b is much smaller than L_f) is given by:

$$Z_o = i/[wC_c/K_c + (w_b^2/w^3)(1 - w^2/w_f^2)]$$

where $w_f^2 = 1/(L_f C_f)$ and $w_b^2 = w_f^2/(K_f L_b)$

Inclusion of R_f means that L_f is multiplied by $R_f /(R_f + iwL_f)$.

For all stimulus frequencies (w) less than the CF, Z_o is imaginary and positive, and so the net arcuate impedance is reduced from that due to the BM alone (since below the CF the BM impedance is imaginary and negative). The amount of impedance reduction is dependent on the magnitude of Z_o. For low frequencies the magnitude is small compared to the BM impedance, and hence the presence of the OHCs has little effect on the response. For stimulus frequencies near the CF Z_o is approximately equal to the BM impedance, which results in a large response peak. For intermediate frequencies the arcuate zone response closely follows the frequency dependence of Z_o. Therefore, the OHC network (Fig. 5) parameters are chosen so as to obtain realistic tuning.

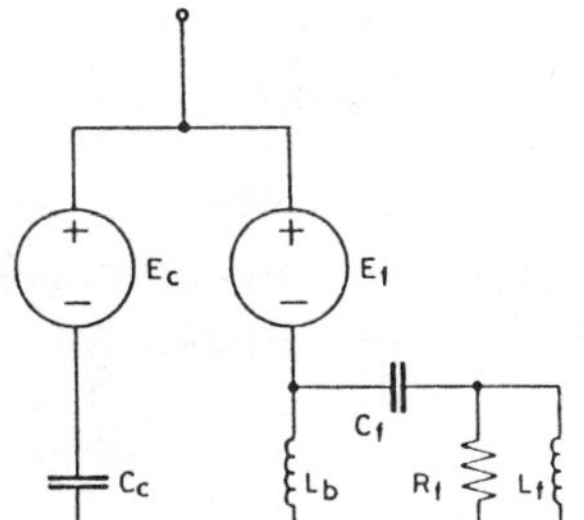

Fig. 5: The FOHCAP OHC stereocilia bending impedance is determined by two controlled voltage sources connected to a fourth order network. E_c and E_f are controlled by the potential differences across C_c and L_f, respectively.

Response of the OHCAP model

The OHCAP model was numerically analysed in the frequency domain, using 50 sections (Fig. 2) per mm. Both versions used the same set of BM parameters. The (mechanical) parameters used are listed below (all dimensions are in cgs units. Δ = fractional distance from stapes).

scala width = 0.16
scala height = 0.08
arcuate width = pectinate width = 0.0275
fluid density = 1.0

$M_{a,p} = 3.2 \times 10^{-3}$
$R_{a,p} = 1.4 \times 10^{1}$
$C_a = 2.3 \times 10^{-12}\, e^{5\Delta}$
$C_p = 2.3 \times 10^{-8}\, e^{5\Delta}$

FOHCAP model:
$M_b = 3.5 \times 10^{-5}$
$M_f = 8.0 \times 10^{-3}$
$C_c = 2.3 \times 10^{-8}\, e^{5\Delta}$
$C_f = 2.3 \times 10^{-8}\, e^{5\Delta}$
$R_f = 8.8 \times 10^{3}$
$K_c = 1.0 \times 10^{4}$
$K_f = 1.0 \times 10^{8}$

DOHCAP model:
$M_f = 1.8 \times 10^{-4}$
$R_c = 1.0 \times 10^{1}$
$R_f = 1.8 \times 10^{1}$
$K_c = 5.0 \times 10^{7}$
$K_f = 9.1 \times 10^{-5}$

The response (in the arcuate zone) of both versions is compared to that measured by Robles et al. (1986) in the chinchilla. Their data were selected since they appear to be very difficult to match using passive cochlear models (Diependaal et al., 1987). The response measured in animal M044 is used for comparison with the OHCAP model responses, since it has a very high peak-to-tail ratio making it the most difficult to match. The data of Robles et al. have the form of BM motion relative to pressure at the eardrum, and so a middle ear model - that of Neely and Kim (1986), with the same parameters - was added to the OHCAP model.

Fig. 6 shows the magnitude and phase of the BM velocity response, relative to sound pressure at the eardrum. Positive phase sense is motion in the direction of the scala tympani, for rarefaction at the eardrum. The dots, dashed line and solid line show the measured data, the DOHCAP model response and the FOHCAP model response, respectively. It should be noted that a comparison of the OHCAP model response with the data of Robles et al. (1986) for other animals would reveal smaller discrepancies, and so Fig. 6 presents the worst-case comparison.

The phase data features a low frequency phase jump which is not exhibited by the OHCAP model. The phase jump is approximately π radians, which implies that the BM impedance is mass dominated for low frequencies, and stiffness dominated for frequencies above the jump. The phase response in both versions of the OHCAP model is very similar. This is as expected since the phase is determined mainly by the pectinate zone impedance (Kolston, 1988a).

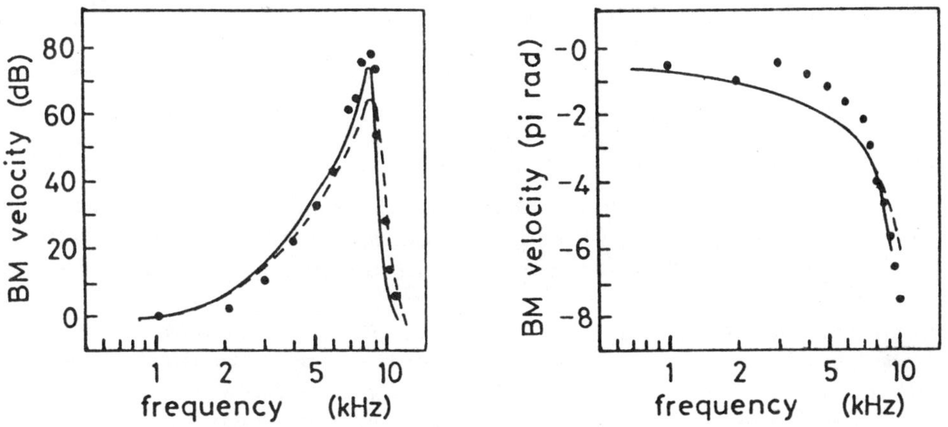

Fig. 6: Comparison of OHCAP model response with that measured by Robles et al. (1986) in animal M044. The dots, dashed line and solid line show the measured data, the DOHCAP model response and the FOHCAP model response, respectively. The measured phase jump is not simulated in the OHCAP model, but apart from this discrepancy the responses are very similar.

Robles et al. (1986) found that the measured sensitivity (particularly at CF) is reduced due to trauma. In the OHCAP model this can be simulated by assuming that the source gain coefficients (K_a, K_c, K_f) are physiologically vulnerable, in that they are reduced in the presence of trauma. In the model animal death can be simulated by setting the gain parameters to zero, in which case the calculated response is very similar to that measured in post-mortem cochleae.

Discussion

This paper describes two versions of a new type of cochlear model. The purpose of presenting both F- and D- versions of the OHCAP model is to show that a cochlear model, with different micromechanical mechanisms, can produce realistic mechanical tuning without the use of active processes.

For the responses shown in the paper, the real part of the OHC bending impedance (Z_o) is positive for all stimulus frequencies. Hence, in the terminology of network theory, the OHCAP model is passive. Since the model exhibits very realistic tuning, the hypothesis "that active (energy-producing) processes are responsible for sharp BM tuning" must be reassessed.

There can be little doubt that the OHCAP model is solidly based on features of cochlear anatomy. However, with the present knowledge of OHC and organ of Corti physiology, it is difficult to determine the validity of the DOHCAP and FOHCAP models. In the formulation of the DOHCAP model a number of assumptions are made concerning the organ of Corti microstructure, particularly with respect to the stiffness of the Deiters' cells' phalangeal processes, and the geometric relationship between the cells' phalangeal processes, and the geometric relationship between the Deiters' cells and the OHCs. Furthermore, it is assumed in the DOHCAP model that the OHCs can receive stimuli from their outer surfaces. The validity of these proposed mechanisms is unknown.

The FOHCAP model relies less on the microstructure of the organ of Corti, but requires the OHCs to perform a more complicated filtering function. All recent active cochlear models attribute some sort of filtering function to the OHCs, and so it remains to be determined what complexity of filter is physiologically justifiable. The filtering performed by the OHCs can take many forms, only one of which is presented in this paper. The complexity of OHC filter required in the FOHCAP model is determined by the shape of response being simulated. Responses with smaller peak-to-tail ratios (e.g. Sellick et al., 1983) can be achieved with a lower order filter.

Further experimental measurements should be made to determine the accuracy of the assumptions made in the formulation of the OHCAP model. Measurements of the relative sensitivity and selectivity between the arcuate and pectinate zones of the BM would be very useful in determining this.

References

Diependaal, R.J., de Boer, E. and Viergever, M.A. (1987). Cochlear power flux as an indication of mechanical activity. J. Acoust. Soc. Am., 82, 917-926.

Iurato, S. (1962). Functional implications of the nature and submicroscopic structure of the tectorial and basilar membranes. J. Acoust. Soc. Am., 34, 1386-1395.

Kolston, P.J. (1988a). Sharp mechanical tuning in a cochlear model without negative damping. J. Acoust. Soc. Am., 83, 1481-1487.

Kolston, P.J. (1988b). Micromechanics remove the need for active processes in cochlear tuning. In Basic Issues in Hearing, edited by H. Duifhuis, J.W. Horst and H.P. Wit (Academic Press, London).

Kolston, P.J., Viergever, M.A., de Boer, E. and Diependaal, R.J. (1989). Realistic mechanical tuning in a micromechanical cochlear model. Submitted for publication in J. Acoust. Soc. Am.

Miller, C.E. (1985). Structural implications of basilar membrane compliance measurements. J. Acoust. Soc. Am., 77, 1465-1474.

Neely, S.T. and Kim, D.O. (1986). A model for active elements in cochlear biomechanics. J. Acoust. Soc. Am., 79, 1472-1480.

Robles, L., Ruggero, M.A. and Rich, N.C. (1986). Basilar membrane mechanics at the base of the chinchilla cochlea. I. Input-output functions, tuning curves, and response phases. J. Acoust. Soc. Am., 80, 1364-1374.

Sellick, P.M., Patuzzi, R. and Johnstone, B.M. (1983). Comparison between the tuning properties of inner hair cells and basilar membrane motion. Hearing Research, 10, 93-100.

Viergever, M.A. (1986). Cochlear macromechanics - a review. In Peripheral Auditory Mechanisms, edited by J.B. Allen, J.L. Hall, A. Hubbard, S.T. Neely and A. Tubis. Springer, Munich, pp 63-72.

Voldrich, L. (1983). Experimental and topographic morphology in cochlear mechanics. In Mechanics of Hearing, edited by E. de Boer and M.A. Viergever. Delft University Press, pp 163-168.

Comments and Discussion

WILSON

Wilson and Bruns (1983) found phase differences between the pars tecta and pars pectinata which appeared to be due to a model of this type (see Comment of Wilson following Allen's paper). Vector subtraction of these components however did not support this interpretation. Although Kolston is correct in supposing that the pars tecta motion would not have been measured accurately by the capacitive probe, owing to spatial averaging, if pars tacta motion had been very small, the response was sufficiently localised to have indicationed this, if it had been the case.

Wilson, J.P. and Bruns, V. (1983) Basilar membrane tuning properties in the specialised cochlea of the CF-bat, Rhinoloplus ferrumequinun. Hear. Res. 10, 15-35.

NEELY

Your OHCAP models assume the presence of controlled sources of mechanical force which are inside the organ of Corti. From the standpoint of mechanical analysis, these sources represent active elements. It may be that realistic basilar membrane responses do not require active processes, but it appears to me that your OHCAP models do.

KOLSTON and VIERGEVER

If the term "active process" signifies that the mechanical energy content of the cochlea is increased (which is the generally accepted interpretation), the OHCAP model does not contain an active process. We suggest that the term "cochlear amplifier" should be used for the enhancement of BM motion by the OHCs. This enhancement is not necessarily due to an active process.

A MODEL FOR PERIPHERAL AUDITORY PREPROCESSING

D. Michel

Lehrstuhl f. allgemeine Elektrotechnik und Akustik
Ruhr Univ. Bochum
D-4630 Bochum, F.R.G.

Introduction

Speech recognition systems as well as models of the binaural system as e.g. described by Blauert (1983) use to require the input signals to be treated in some kind of way before they are processed in higher processing stages. In both applications mentioned above, properties of the auditory system are simulated in one or the other aspect. Thus, it seems reasonable to process the input signals according to the properties of the peripheral auditory system and so, hopefully preserve and even enhance most of the relevant cues the higher processing stages need despite not knowing their very character.

The structure of a complete auditory preprocessing chain is depicted in Fig.1. The first elements of the chain contain models of the outer and the middle ear.

Concerning a model of peripheral auditory preprocessing the influences of outer and middle ear may, except at high levels, be described by linear filtering with a sufficient precision. Confining oneself to headphone presentation of all signals all signal processing up to the oval window may well be described by a transfer function or the corresponding impulse response which the input signals are to be convoluted with.

A more sophisticated task, however, is to model the functional mechanisms of the inner ear. One of the reasons is that due to the vulnerability and small size of the cochlea and the organ of Corti even today not all the underlying mechanisms have been totally explored. The other reason is the fact that even a very coarse model of the cochlea leads to quite unpleasant mathematical implications which do not allow a neat solution of the problem. As a consequence, a lot of models have been presented during the past decades which differ with respect to their mathematical complexity, accuracy in detail and method of solution.

Modeling the cochlea

Compared to the simulation of the outer and middle ear an adequate model of the cochlea and the subsequent signal processing stages appears to be the most difficult task.

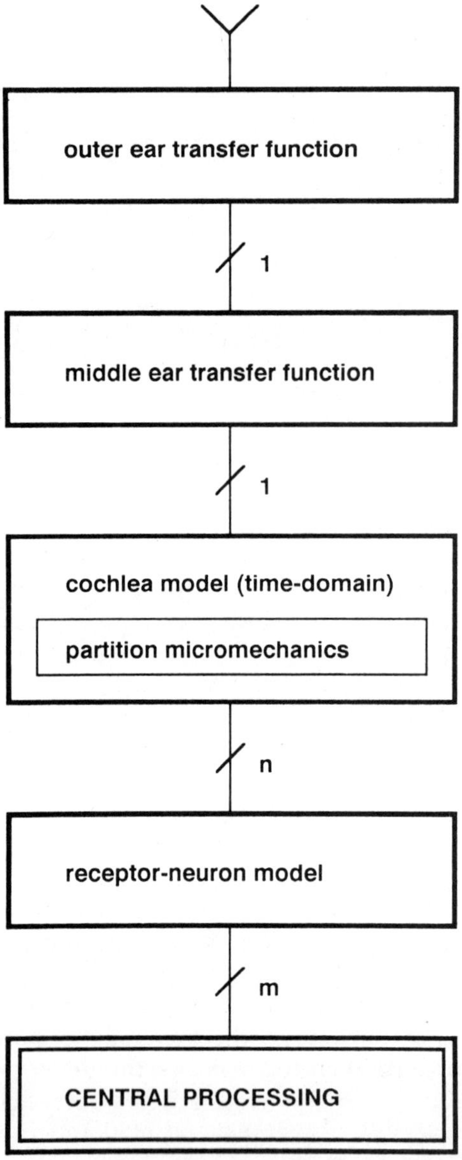

Fig. 1: Block structure of a model of peripheral auditory preprocessing. Note that there is a one-channel input but multiple (m, n) channel output structure.

Even a short survey of the literature on these topics makes clear that one has to confine oneself to a model of reduced complexity to maintain a chance of bearable effort for the numerical solution, despite not giving up modeling the relevant mechanism of data resp. irrelevance reduction of the peripheral auditory system. This predominantly involves modeling the active and nonlinear properties of the cochlear partition as well as the masking and/or suppression mechanisms and the micromechanics of the organ of Corti. Since the whole model will be designed to perform signal processing, a numerical solution in the time domain is required although especially time- domain solutions are known to be quite time-consuming.

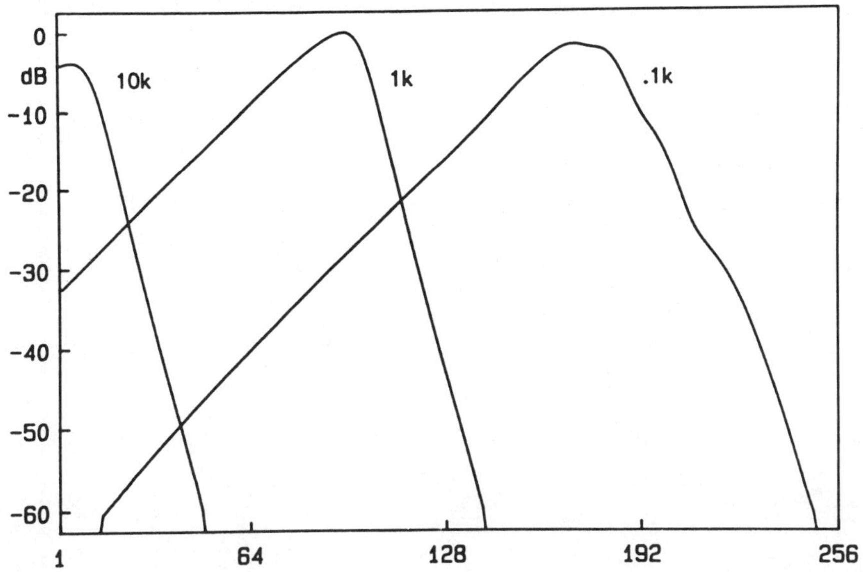

FIGURE 2. Envelopes of partition for sinusoidal stapes velocity vs. discrete distance from base and three input frequencies (100Hz, 1kHz, 10kHz) in the macromechanical model.

As a conclusion, the properties of the cochlear model have to be:
- the solution has to be performed in the time domain.
- the solution algorithm must be efficient with respect to computing time.
- the model must not be too complex in order to reduce computational effort.
- important features of the inner ear should be modeled at least optionally.
- modularity of the model is desired to be able to fit the complexity of the model to the specific task.
- all features should be covered by one model, there should not be any specialisation to model only partial aspects.

The solution method originates in a suggestion by a former coworker, Schlichthaerle (1980), and in principle applies methods of digital filter design to the problem.

We chose to use a simple one-dimensional model with its inherent constraints similar to the one described by Viergever (1980) so as to reduce the mathematical complexity to a minimum without giving up the basic functional principles. For our application some of the constraints of the one-dimensional model are compensated by the freedom of choosing modified mechanical model parameters which is more efficient than solving models of higher dimensionality. The solution algorithm is described in detail in Michel (1988) so that a short list of the features may suffice. Basically, the partial differential equation is transformed into a digital filter algorithm which is different from wave-digital

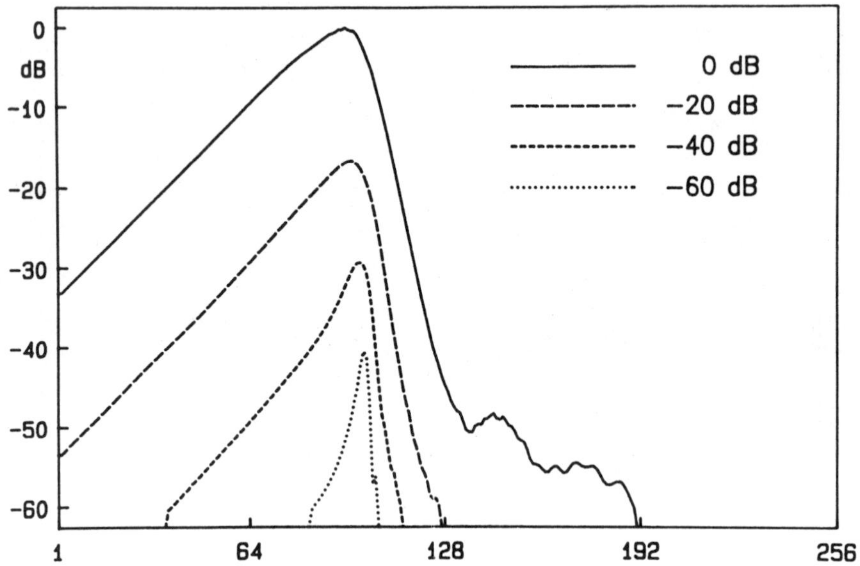

Fig.3. Level dependent mechanical tuning curves for sinusoidal input in the macromechanical model.

filter solutions as e.g. described by Strube (1985). The advantages of the algorithm mainly are:

- the algorithm solves the differential equation and does not consist of chained digital filters. Thus, waves travelling back and forth on the basilar membrane can be taken into account.
- the structure of the algorithm is very close to solutions in the frequency domain.
- like most digital filter algorithms it works very fast compared to the classical numerical integration schemes.
- the sampling frequency can be chosen relatively low compared to the frequency range used.
- nonlinear mechanisms can be taken into account like in every time-domain solution.
- stability of the digital system can be verified easily for the linear models.
- the algorithm may easily be extended to incorporate cochlear micromechanics and active processes without changing the program structure.
- the numerical solution contains a large percentage of vector operations which allow a significant speed increase using vector processors.

Results

Starting with the simple transmission line model, we get results similar to von Bekesy's data as depicted in Fig.2. Fig.2 shows the envelopes of partition velo-

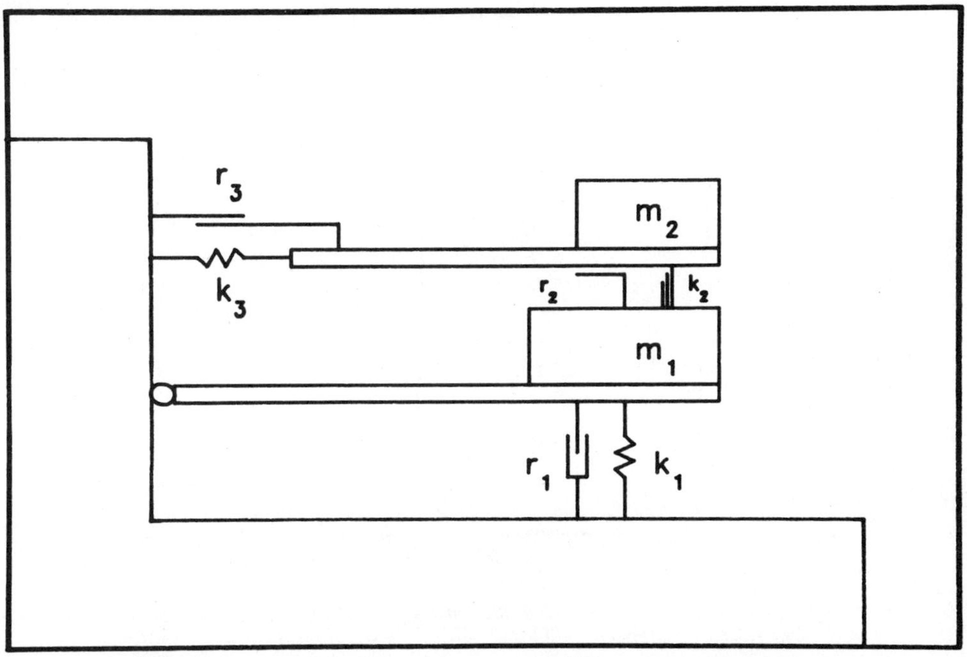

Fig.4. Simplified model for a cross-sectional element of the cochlear partition.

city on a logarithmic scale integrated over a predefined time. This sometimes, e.g. in the 100Hz curve, results in a fainted ripple in the mechanical tuning curves for low frequencies when the integration time covers only a few periods.

For these simulations, the unrolled cochlea was divided into 265 spatial discretization steps which represent the length of the cochlea from the 10 kHz region near the apex up to the helicotrema. With parameters for the properties of the cochlear partition found in literature the sampling frequency of the discrete-time model algorithm was set to 50 kHz.

Active and nonlinear mechanisms

The mechanical tuning curves shown in Fig.2 can obviously no longer be considered to reflect the real conditions of cochlear physiology. Nonlinear and apparently also active features can be found in the mechanical motion of the cochlear partition and should also influence models of cochlear function since they may well contribute to irrelevance reduction and data compression within the auditory system.

A first order approach to the modeling of the active and nonlinear process consists of a phenomenological model of the properties of the cochlear partition in that the resistive part of the partition point-impedance is thought to be modified in a nonlinear way by active process of whatever nature.

With this appproach active and nonlinear models are often designed to vary partition resistance dependent on the partition velocity or displacement. Zwick-

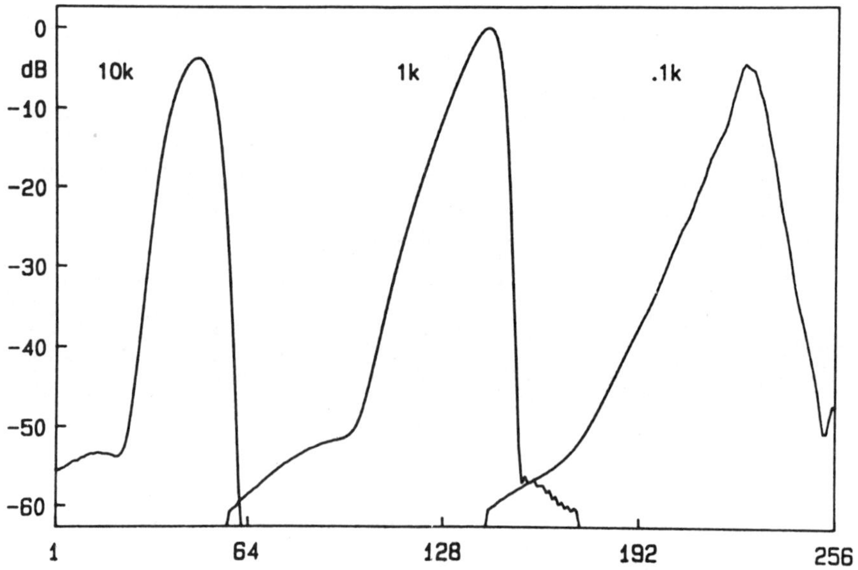

FIGURE 5. Envelopes of partition velocity for sinusoidal stapes velocity vs. discrete distance from base and three input frequencies (100kHz, 10kHz) in the micromechanical model.

er (1986), for example, uses a hardware transmission line model of the cochlea to incorporate active processes by adding amplifiers with nonlinear feedback loops which can, after Lumer (1985), actually be described by conductances switched in parallel to the conductance of the basilar membrane yielding a velocity-dependent effective partition resistance.

Using frequency domain models this mechanism is difficult to incorporate except when the input signals are not too complex as shown by Lumer (1985). Since our model works in the discrete-time domain, active and nonlinear properties can be integrated more easily by modifying the corresponding mechanical model parameters dependent on the actual partition velocity according to an appropriate control function.

As pointed out by Strube (1985), consistency problems are to be expected since the actual partition resistance has to be computed from the actual partition velocity which can obviously not be done simultaneously. So, usually, one has to let the model algorithm work in a piecewise linear way and compute the new partition resistance from the partition velocity of the previous sample period.

After having modified the model algorithm appropriately it delivers input level dependent mechanical tuning curves as depicted in Fig.3 which can similarly be found in the work of Zwicker (1986).

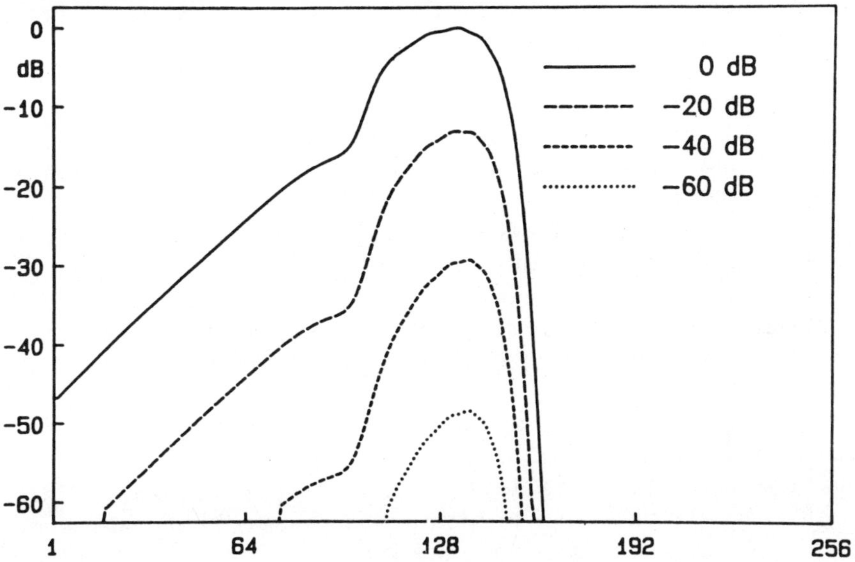

Fig.6. Level dependent mechanical tuning curves for sinusoidal input in the micromechanical model.

Cochlear micromechanics

Recent in vivo measurements have revealed that in contrast to the previous assumptions mechanical tuning of the cochlear partition is similar to the neural tuning thus sparing the need for a second filter structure. Especially, the difference between in vivo and post mortem data consists of a sharply tuned peak in the mechanical tuning curve of almost 40 dB in magnitude above post mortem level which can be removed by means of chemical or physical influence.

De Boer (1983) could show mathematically that a cochlea model can only exhibit mechanical tuning curves with these qualities when the partition resistance is allowed to become negative at least in confined regions. It is, however, impossible to simulate these properties using a macromechanical model since it would lead to oscillations in regions of negative partition resistance.

Thus, models have been presented in the past which incorporate the fine structure of the organ of Corti as e.g. depicted in Fig.4 in a simplified form. Usually, the tectorial membrane adds an additional mechanical degree of freedom to the system, which is able to sharpen mechanical partition tuning and allows active energy sources to be incorporated. At present, the function of amplifying cochlear response tends to be assigned to the outer hair cells (OHC), which are suspected to be able to add mechanical energy to the cochlear partition by means of the motility of their ciliae or their cell bodies. A cochlear model which is intended to work close to auditory, especially cochlear, physiology has to incorporate active and nonlinear cochlear micromechanics to deliver realistic responses.

A model which combines the micromechanical structure of the organ of Corti with the description of the function of the outer hair cells is the model presented by Neely & Kim (1986) which we decided to use exemplarily to create a fast time-domain simulation of cochlear function which is quite close to cochlear physiology.

The model algorithm allows to include partition micromechanics without really changing the structure of the program in that only a modified term for the partition point-impedance has to be used for the numerical solution. Almost the only changes concerns the fact that additional degrees of freedom will be modeled at the expense of additional memory and the handling of more mechanical parameters.

Neely & Kim especially have introduced an OHC-gain variable y which is defined in their work to describe the global changes in outer hair cell activity and is very suited to formulate a nonlinear micromechanical model of the cochlea. Setting the value of y to 1, we get mechanical tuning curves as depicted in Fig.5 which is comparable to Fig.2 with respect to scaling and the quantities displayed. Note that levels are plotted relative to an arbitrary 0 dB margin since for our applications absolute values are not of direct interest.

To create a nonlinear model, we chose to treat the OHC-Gain parameter as a vector an let it be locally dependent on the partition velocity according to a control function in a similar way as in the macromechanical case. This procedure results in an input-level dependance of the mechanical tuning-curves as depicted in Fig.6 which is quite similar to the behaviour shown in Fig.3.

Note that both in the macromechanical and micromechanical model mechanical tuning becomes more sensitive for low-level input and thus enables both models to simulate suppression effects as described by Zwicker (1986). Suppression effects shown by our model are discussed further in Michel (1988) who also takes nonsimultaneous effects into account.

References

Blauert, J. (1983) Spatial Hearing. The MIT Press, Cambridge, Mass.

Boer, E. de (1983) On active and passive cochlear models - towards a generalized analysis. J. Acoust. Soc. Am. 73, 574-579.

Lumer, G. (1985) Nachbildung nichtlinearer simultaner Verdeckungseffekte bei schmalbandigen Schallen mit einem Rechnermodell. Doct. Diss., München.

Michel, D. (1988) Time-domain simulation of an active cochlea model with nonlinear partition micromechanics. In preparation.

Neely, S.T. und Kim, D.O. (1986) A model for active elements in cochlear biomechanics. J. Acoust. Soc. Am. 79, 1472-1480.

Schlichthaerle, D. (1980) Modelle des Hörens. Doct. Dissertation, Bochum.

Strube, H.W. (1985) A compotetionally efficient basilar membrane model. Acustica, 58, 207-214.

Viergever, M. (1980) Mechanics of the inner ear. Doct. Dissertation, Delft.

Zwicker, E. (1986) A hardware cochlear nonlinear preprocessing model with active feedback. J. Acoust. Soc. Am. 80, 146.

Appendix

The partial differential equation used for the model simulations depicted in this paper reads in its frequency domain formulation:

$$\frac{\partial^2}{\partial x^2} P_d(x,\omega) = \frac{2\rho j\omega}{h Z_p(x,\omega)} P_d(x,\omega) \quad (1)$$

ω being the frequency variable, h the height of the scala, ρ the fluid density, $P_d(x,\omega)$ the pressure difference across the cochlear partition and x the locus along the partition.

The mechanical properties of the partition are described by the point-impedance function $Z_p(x,\omega)$:

$$Z_p(x,\omega) = j\omega m(x) + r(x) + k(x)/j\omega \quad (2)$$

where $k(x)$ denotes the stiffness, $r(x)$ the damping and $m(x)$ the mass per unit area.

Fluid mass moving with the partition has already been lumped into $m(x)$. In the same way variations in channel or partition geometry may be taken account of.

The boundary conditions at the basal resp. apical end of the cochlea are:

$$\frac{\partial}{\partial x} P_d(x,\omega)\Big|_{x=0} = j\omega\rho v_{Stapes} \quad (3)$$

$$\frac{\partial}{\partial x} P_d(x,\omega)\Big|_{x=L} = 0 \quad (4)$$

Eq.4 may additionally be modified to represent the hydrodynamical properties of the helicotrema.

A fast time-domain simulation is easily established using the Laplace-transform of the time-domain formulation of Eq.1, s being the complex frequency variable:

$$\frac{\partial^2}{\partial x^2} P_d(x,s) = H_c(x,s)\, P_d(x,s) \quad (5)$$

with

$$H_c(x,s) = \frac{2\rho}{h}\left(\frac{s}{m(x)s + r(x) + k(x)/s}\right) \quad (6)$$

where $H_c(x,s)$ denotes the transfer function between trans-membrane pressure and its second spatial derivative.

Replacing the continuous variable x by its discrete counterpart i, we get:

$$P_d(i-1,s) - 2P_d(i,s) + P_d(i+1,s) = H_d(i,s)\, P_d(i,s) \quad (7)$$

with: $H_d(i,s) = H_c\, \Lambda^2$ (8)

and: $\Lambda = L/(N-1)$; L := length of the cochlea

N := number of grid points

To transform Eq.7 into the discrete time domain we use the bilinear transform technique with the transform $s \rightarrow \frac{2}{T}\frac{z-1}{z+1}$, T being the sampling period of the discrete-time system.
Using the standard form of Eq. 8:

$$H_d(i,s) = \frac{2\rho\Lambda^2}{h} \frac{A_2(i)s^2}{B_0(i) + B_1(i)s + B_2(i)s^2} \tag{9}$$

$A_2(i) = 1$

$B_0(i) = k(i)/m(i)$

$B_1(i) = r(i)/m(i)$

$B_2(i) = 1$

bilinear transform yields:

$$H(i,z) = K \frac{a_0(i) + a_1(i)z + a_2(i)z^2}{1 + b_1(i)z + b_2(i)z^2} \; ; \qquad K = \frac{2\rho\Lambda^2}{h} \tag{10}$$

$a_0(i) = 1$ $\qquad N(i) = T^2 + B_1(i)T + B_0(i)$

$a_1(i) = -2$ $\qquad b_1(i) = (2B_0(i) - 2T^2)/N(i)$

$a\ (i) = 1$ $\qquad b\ (i) = (T^2 - B\ (i)T + B\ (i))/N(i)$

Eq.7 transformed into the z-domain and H(i,z) substituted reads:

$$\begin{aligned} P_d(i-1,z) - (2 + Ka_0(i))\,P_d(i,z) + P_d(i-1,z) = & \\ & [a_1(i)z^{-1} + a_2(i)z^{-2}]\,P_d(i,z) \\ & - b_1(i)z^{-1}\,[\,P_d(i-1,z) - 2P_d(i,z) + P_d(i+1,z)\,] \\ & - b_2(i)z^{-2}\,[\,P_d(i-1,z) - 2P_d(i,z) + P_d(i+1,z)\,] \end{aligned} \tag{11}$$

Transforming Eq. 11 into the discrete-time domain yields:

$$\begin{aligned} P_d(i-1,k) - (2 + Ka_0(i))\,P_d(i,k) + P_d(i+1,k) = & \\ & a_1(i)\,P_d(i,k-1) + a_2(i)P_d(i,k-2) \\ & - b_1(i)\,[\,P_d(i-1,k) - 2P_d(i,k) + P_d(i+1,k)\,] \\ & - b_2(i)\,[\,P_d(i-1,k) - 2P_d(i,k) + P_d(i+1,k)\,] \end{aligned} \tag{12}$$

where k denotes the discrete time variable.
Eq. 12 describes a recursive digital filter algorithm which provides a fast time-domain solution. Using appropriate boundary and initial conditions, each new time-step requires the computation of the right-hand side of Eq.12 from already known values and the diagonalization of the tridiagonal matrix on the right-hand side of Eq.12. To compute partition acceleration the relationship

$$\frac{\partial^2}{\partial x^2} P_d(x,\omega) = \frac{2\rho j\omega}{h} v_p(x,\omega) \tag{13}$$

may be used.
Since the model is still linear, subsequent integration of the model output for computing partition velocity or displacement may equally well be performed on the stapes acceleration so as to reduce computational effort.

Comments and Discussion

DIEPENDAAL, VIERGEVER, KOLSTON

Q1. You state that it is impossible to simulate in a macromechanical model active processes which are present in a confined region of the BM, since these would lead to oscillations in regions of negative partition impedance. This is incorrect. If the negative damping is not too large, the added energy will be transported by the travelling wave to regions of positive resistance and will be absorbed there.

Q2. A numerical method satisfying the conditions mentioned in your paper has already been published (Diependaal et al. 1987). It is not clear in which respect the method proposed by you might show improved performance.

Diependaal, R.J., Duifhuis, H., Hoogstraten, H.W., Viergever, M.A. (1987) Numberical methods for solving one-dimensional cochlear models in the time domain, J. Acoust. Soc. Am. 82, 1655-1666.

MICHEL

1. In the passage in my paper you refer to, I do not actually state that it is impossible to have a macromechanical model that exhibits any active regions.

Referring to the work of de Boer (1983) I did state that it would be impossible to have a macromechanical cochlear model which would exhibit the referenced properties of neural-like tuning, almost 40dB extra gain above post-mortem level and have regions of negative partition resistance.

For this reason, active and nonlinear micromechanical models have been presented in the recent years by various workers, e.g. Neely and Kim (1986). Nevertheless, I agree that it is impossible to have a macromechanical model that exhibits active regions on the BM, but it would not exhibit the other features claimed.

2. I appreciate very much the work of R.J. Diependaal, H. Duifhuis, H.W. Hoogstraten and M.A. Viergever and especially of R.J. Diependaal in developing numerical solution algorithms for 1-D, 2-D and 3-D cochlear models.

Nevertheless, I consider the algorithm presented in my paper to be rather adequate for signal processing since it replaces classical integration schemes like e.g. the Runge-Kutta method by simple sampling-period delays.

To do so is a very common procedure in the field of digital signal processing and is used e.g. to implement digital filters where classical quadrature formulae are avoided to increase computation speed. Thus, I would suspect the algorithm presented in my paper to be more efficient with respect to computation speed than an algorithm that uses the Runge-Kutta integration method.

However, I do not claim to present a numerical method that delivers results more precise with respect to the physical and physiological properties of the cochlea it models. This, because the algorithm is intentionally confined to simulate a 1-D method of the cochlea.

Another quite useful property of the algorithm presented is that it allows a quite simple inclusion of cochlear micromechanics with very little changes in program structure as long as the properties of the cochlear partition can be described by a point-impedance function.

This only requires to use the paint-impedance function modified in terms of cochlear micromechanics when computing the filter coefficients used in the simulation.

Boer, E. de (1983) "On active and passive cochlear models - towards a generalized analysis". J. Acoust. Soc. Am., 73, 574-579.

Neely, S.T. and Kim. D.O. "A model for active elements in cochlear biomechanics". J. Acoust. Soc. Am., 79, 1472-1480.

ON THE STABILITY OF COCHLEAR MECHANICAL MODELS

John W. Matthews and Charles E. Molnar

Institute for Biomedical Computing
Washington University, St. Louis, MO 63130, USA

Introduction

We have found that the introduction of nonlinear damping into stable computational simulations of active cochlear mechanical models generally made the simulations unstable in the sense that unbounded or oscillatory responses were obtained. This paper reports preliminary results of our efforts to determine what combinations of several possible causes might be responsible.

One possibility is that such behavior is a fundamental property of the cochlea and therefore *should* be a property of cochlear models. If this is the case then what are the essential structural features of the cochlea that make it so and what are appropriate parameter values? There is evidence in the literature indicating this possibility: cochlear emissions (e.g., Kemp, 1978); threshold microstructure (e.g., Long, 1984); and the correlation of both emissions and threshold microstructure to pathology (e.g., Long, et al., 1986).

A second possibility is that such behavior is an artifact of model structure and/or discretization. Some examples of this second possibility: the form of the differential equations; the way in which the model is discretized in space, particularly along the length of the cochlea; the way in which the model is discretized in time; the number of degrees of freedom used to represent the cochlear partion (micro-mechanics).

A third possibility is the effect of computational artifacts, i.e., the computed solutions do not represent the behavior of even the discretized model. Some possible causes of this could be computational algorithms that are unstable or inadequate numerical precision used in computations.

Nonlinear dynamical systems theory (NLDS) provides tools that give insight into these questions (Hirsch and Smale, 1974; Guckenheimer and Holmes, 1986; Boyce and DiPrima, 1969; Cook, 1986; Kubicek and Marek, 1983; Percival and Richards, 1982). Computer programs that aid in applying this theory to the analysis of specific dynamical systems models are available (Doedel, 1981). We present preliminary results that have been obtained from our studies of cochlear mechanical models that are similar in form to the models that we have previously studied using computational simulation, but with the number of spatial positions in the model greatly reduced to make the analysis practical with the available tools.

The Cochlear Mechanical Model

Our cochlear model consists of a fluid-filled box divided into two symmetric scalae by a locally reactive partition. The box has n pistons representing positions along the cochlear partition. At each piston, the partition is represented by a two-degrees-of-freedom (2-DOF) mechanical system (Neely, 1981). As a starting point for partition parameters, we used Neely's parameter set B (PSB). We refer to this as a starting point because Neely's PSB specifies a *linear* (though active) cochlear partition. In our NLDS studies we use a nonlinear coupling damping to be given in equation 6 below. Previously, we had used Neely's PSB as a starting point in *computational simulations* that became unstable whenever we included nonlinearities of the type shown in equation 6. However, our NLDS analysis indicates that our *mathematical model* is *stable* for these parameter values!

Our model has a pressure source at the stapes and a rigid wall at the apex. All the properties of the stapes, bony walls, *linear* fluid, and partition mass are modeled by a Green's function method, which was first applied to cochlear modeling by Lien and Cox (1974, Lien 1973) and was first solved by Allen (1977). The particular formulation used here was developed by Neely (1979) and is available in Matthews (1980). Because the Green's function method we use requires partition mass not to vary with position; we set parameters "M_{1E}" and "M_{2E}" from Neely's PSB to zero.

NOTATION

Matrices are indicated by bold symbols; for example, "**G**" represents our Green's function matrix. Underlined symbols represent vectors of piston variables and, if subscripted, the subscript refers to the DOF; for example, "$\underline{P}$" represents the vector of piston pressures and "$\underline{d_1}$" represents the vector of the displacements of the first DOF. The first subscript (j = 1,2) of the symbols: M; R; K; d; v; and a, refers to the DOF (degree of freedom) and the second subscript refers to piston number:

$d_{ji} \equiv$ displacement of jth DOF at piston i	$M_{ji} \equiv$ mass of jth DOF at piston i
$v_{ji} \equiv$ velocity of jth DOF at piston i	$R_{ji} \equiv$ damping of jth DOF at piston i
$a_{ji} \equiv$ acceleration of jth DOF at piston i	$K_{ji} \equiv$ stiffness of jth DOF at piston i

Note that the symbols R_{3i} and K_{3i} represent coupling between the 1st and 2nd DOF.

MODEL EQUATIONS

We assume a linear relationship (fluid constraint) between the pressure at a piston (we consider only trans-partition pressure) and the acceleration of the first DOF at the n pistons of our fluid-filled box:

$$P_1 = f_{11}a_{11} + f_{12}a_{12} + \cdots + f_{1n}a_{1n}\,; \tag{1.1}$$

$$\cdots$$

$$P_i = f_{i1}a_{11} + f_{i2}a_{12} + \cdots + f_{in}a_{1n}\,; \tag{1.i}$$

$$\cdots$$

$$P_n = f_{n1}a_{11} + f_{n2}a_{12} + \cdots + f_{nn}a_{1n}\,; \tag{1.n}$$

or

$$\underline{P} = \mathbf{F}\,\underline{a_1}\,. \tag{2}$$

Solving for $\underline{a_1}$ yields

$$\underline{a_1} = \mathbf{F}^{-1}\,\underline{P}\,. \tag{3}$$

In our 2-DOF model, a fourth-order mechanical system relates the pressure and state variables (partition constraint) at each piston (Neely, 1981):

$$P_i = M_{1i}a_{1i} + (R_{1i} + R_{3i})v_{1i} + (K_{1i} + K_{3i})d_{1i} - R_{3i}v_{2i} - K_{3i}d_{2i} \; ; \qquad (4.i)$$

$$0 = M_{2i}a_{2i} + (R_{2i} + R_{3i})v_{2i} + (K_{2i} + K_{3i})d_{2i} - R_{3i}v_{1i} - K_{3i}d_{1i} \; . \qquad (5.i)$$

However, our model is nonlinear because we assume that the instantaneous value of the coupling damping depends on velocity:

$$R_{3i}(t) = R_{30}\, e^{R_{3E}x_i} + (v_{2i}(t) - v_{1i}(t))^2 , \qquad (6.i)$$

where x_i indicates the position along the length, L, of the cochlea

$$x_i = (i - ½)\frac{L}{n} \, . \qquad (7.i)$$

DYNAMICAL SYSTEM EQUATIONS

Combining equations 1.i and 4.i, we get

$$f_{i1}a_{11} + \cdots + f_{ii}a_{1i} + \cdots + f_{in}a_{1n} =$$
$$M_{1i}a_{1i} + (R_{1i} + R_{3i})v_{1i} + (K_{1i} + K_{3i})d_{1i} - R_{3i}v_{2i} - K_{3i}d_{2i} \; . \qquad (8.i)$$

Collecting acceleration on the left yields

$$f_{i1}a_{11} + \cdots + (f_{ii} - M_{1i})a_{1i} + \cdots + f_{in}a_{1n} =$$
$$(R_{1i} + R_{3i})v_{1i} + (K_{1i} + K_{3i})d_{1i} - R_{3i}v_{2i} - K_{3i}d_{2i} \; , \qquad (9.i)$$

or

$$\mathbf{F}'\underline{a_1} = \underline{X} \, , \qquad (10)$$

where an element of $\underline{X}$ is

$$X_i = (R_{1i} + R_{3i})v_{1i} + (K_{1i} + K_{3i})d_{1i} - R_{3i}v_{2i} - K_{3i}d_{2i} \; . \qquad (11.i)$$

Solving for acceleration, we get:

$$\underline{a_1} = \mathbf{G}\,\underline{X} \, , \qquad (12)$$

where

$$\mathbf{G} = (\mathbf{F}')^{-1} \qquad (13)$$

is our Green's function matrix. Solving equation 5.i for acceleration gives

$$\underline{a_2} = \underline{Y} \, , \qquad (14)$$

where an element of $\underline{Y}$ is

$$Y_i = -\frac{R_{2i} + R_{3i}}{M_{2i}}v_{2i} - \frac{K_{2i} + K_{3i}}{M_{2i}}d_{2i} + \frac{R_{3i}}{M_{2i}}v_{1i} + \frac{K_{3i}}{M_{2i}}d_{1i} \; . \qquad (15.i)$$

Finally, in the canonic form of NLDS representation, our system equations are:

$$\underline{\dot{d}_1} = \underline{v_1} \; ;$$

$$\underline{\dot{v}_1} = \mathbf{G}\,\underline{X} \; ;$$

$$\underline{\dot{d}_2} = \underline{v_2} \; ;$$

and

$$\underline{\dot{v}_2} = \underline{Y} \, . \qquad (16)$$

Note that we are solving a homogeneous set of equations; there is no external stimulus or driving function.

AUTO Applied to Our Cochlear Model

"AUTO" is a software package for continuation and bifurcation analysis of nonlinear dynamical systems (Doedel, 1986, 1984). We have recently used AUTO to gain insight into the behavior of our nonlinear and active cochlear mechanical model.

A 2-PISTON MODEL

Figure 1 shows a bifurcation diagram given by AUTO for a 2-piston nonlinear cochlear model. A bifurcation diagram illustrates what type of solutions (fixed-point or periodic) exist at different parameter values and also indicates the stability (or not) of these solutions. The figure shows the type of solution and stability versus the R_{30} parameter of the model. For our cochlear model, the system variables are the velocities and displacements of each DOF at each piston; i.e., for this 2-piston cochlea the system is 8-dimensional.

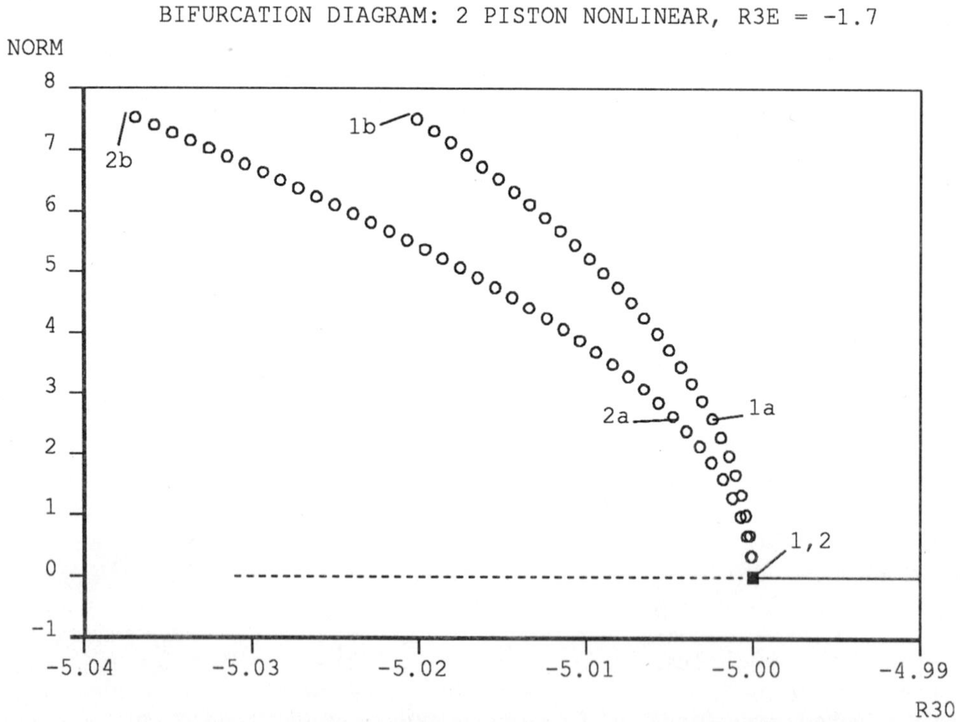

Figure 1. Bifurcation diagram for a 2-piston nonlinear cochlear model. In all figures shown, partition velocity is in units of $10^{-2}\,cm/s$ and partition displacement is in units of $10^{-6}\,cm$. In the bifurcation diagrams, the ordinate is the standard Euclidean norm of all system variables for stationary solutions (fixed points) and is a periodic norm for periodic solutions. These norms are selected such that at a Hopf bifurcation point, the norm is the same whether the point is considered a stationary solution or a periodic solution (see Doedel, 1986). In bifurcation diagrams: solid lines trace branches of stable stationary solutions; dashed lines trace branches of unstable stationary solutions; filled squares indicate Hopf bifurcations points; filled circles trace branches of stable periodic solutions; open circles trace branches of unstable periodic solutions.

The bifurcation parameter, R_{30}, is varied between -4.99 and -5.04 in the diagram; for comparison, Neely's PSB has $R_{30} = -4.96$ (off scale to the right).

The bifurcation diagram shows that this 2-piston nonlinear cochlear model has a stable fixed-point solution at zero (indicated by the solid line) for all values of R_{30} more positive than -5.0. A fixed-point solution is a point in state space at which the time derivatives of all state variables are zero. The fixed-point solution shown has a Euclidean norm equal to zero; this implies that each of the state variables must be equal to zero. For more negative values of R_{30} the fixed-point solution at zero is unstable (dashed line). This means that if the system was disturbed from the zero state it would not return to the zero state, but would diverge or oscillate.

At $R_{30} = -5.0$ there are 2 Hopf bifurcation points (1 and 2). A Hopf bifurcation occurs where a fixed-point solution branch gives rise to a periodic solution branch. Emanating from these Hopf bifurcation points are two branches of unstable periodic solutions (open circles). A periodic solution is a closed trajectory in state space. A stable periodic solution would attract all state trajectories originating in some neighborhood of the periodic solution, while trajectories originating in any neighborhood of an unstable periodic solution would be repelled.

Multiple (or degenerate) bifurcation points are difficult to deal with and in fact manual intervention was necessary to produce both branches of periodic solutions shown in figure 1. For Neely's PSB, there will be as many Hopf bifurcations at $R_{30} = -5.0$ as there are pistons. To separate the Hopf bifurcation points, we made a slight change in R_{3E}. For figure 1, $R_{3E} = -1.7$ (Neely's value); in the next model we used $R_{3E} = -1.705$. (We also increased the number of pistons to three.)

A MODIFIED 3-PISTON MODEL

The bifurcation diagram in figure 2 shows that this 3-piston nonlinear cochlear model has a stable fixed point at zero (indicated by the solid line) for all values of R_{30} more positive than approximately -5.01. For more negative values of R_{30} the fixed point at zero is unstable (dashed line).

Hopf bifurcations occur at $R_{30} = -5.00938$, -5.0282 and, -5.047 (labels 1, 2, and 3 respectively). Emanating from these Hopf bifurcation points are branches of periodic solutions (filled and open circles). Note that the only stable periodic solutions (also called "limit cycles") are on the branch emanating from label 1 (filled circles). The frequencies of the periodic solution along the three branches (near the bifurcation points) are approximately 7.2, 2.3, and 0.7 kHz, respectively. These frequencies are equal to the resonant frequencies of the second DOF at pistons 1, 2, and 3, respectively, and the R_{30} values of the Hopf bifurcation points are those needed to cause $R_{3i} = -R_{2i}$ at each of the pistons. (The reason that the 2-piston cochlea of figure 1 had a multiple Hopf bifurcation was that for all i, $R_{3i} = -R_{2i}$ when $R_{30} = -5.0$.)

Panels a to c of figure 3 show three phase-plane diagrams. Each phase-plane diagram shows trajectories of pairs of velocities for labeled points along the periodic solution branches shown in the bifurcation diagram of figure 2 (which is repeated in panel 3d for convenience). Panel a shows the velocities of the 1st and 2nd DOF in piston 1. Note that only periodic solution branch 1 shows significant velocity in the 2nd DOF. Panel b shows velocities of the 1st DOF for pistons 1 and 2. Here there is some motion of both pistons for all three solution branches. Panel c shows velocities of the 2nd DOF for pistons 1 and 2. Note here that only solution branch 1 shows significant velocity in piston 1 and only solution branch 2 shows significant velocity in piston 2; note also that 3a is a point at the center of the plot.

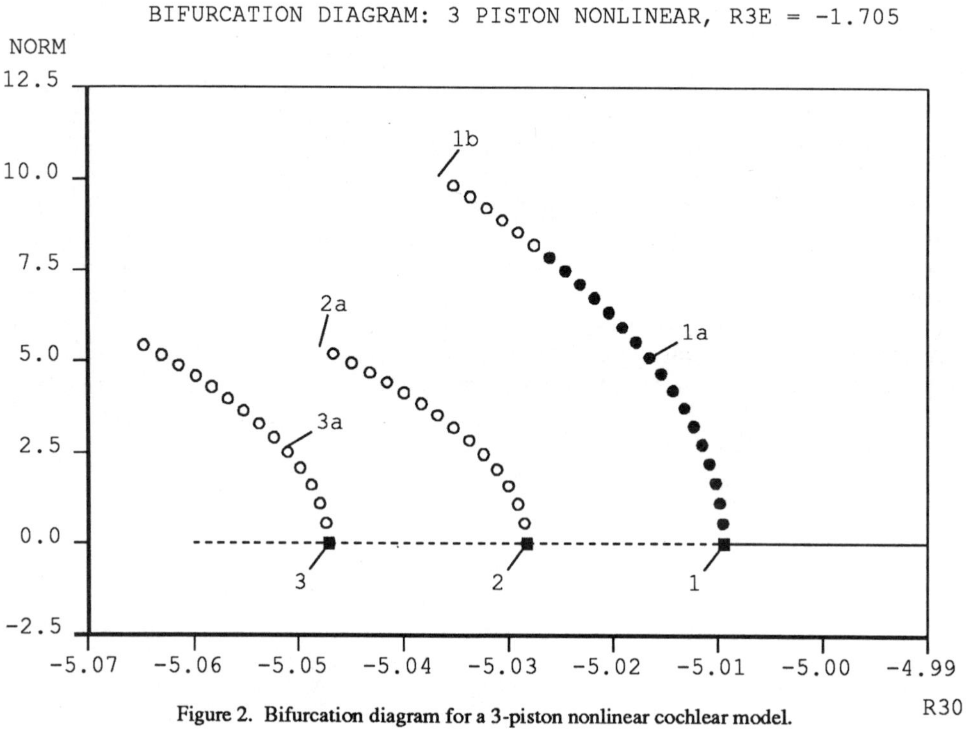

Figure 2. Bifurcation diagram for a 3-piston nonlinear cochlear model.

Discussion and Conclusions

We have found the concepts of NLDS to be useful in studying the stability properties of simplified nonlinear and active cochlear models. The program AUTO was helpful in applying these concepts to our specific 2- and 3-piston models.

For the 3-piston model of figure 2, as the value of the negative coupling damping coefficient R_{30} is varied, Hopf bifurcations occur along the axis at points at which $R_{3i} = -R_{2i}$ for each piston in turn. For R_{30} values more positive than the value for the rightmost Hopf bifurcation (label 1) the system has a *stable* fixed point with all state variables equal to zero. For R_{30} more negative than this value, the system has an *unstable* fixed point with all state variables equal to zero. At values of R_{30} between the two rightmost Hopf bifurcations (labels 1 and 2), the system also has a *stable periodic solution.* For values of R_{30} to the left of the Hopf bifurcation labeled 2, there are multiple *unstable periodic solutions.* We do not yet know what all the branches of such a system can be; there may be additional unconnected branches that have not been found by our analysis.

We conjecture that the above conclusions extend to systems with a large number of pistons, such as the 240 pistons for which we have previously obtained computational simulations. If this conjecture is correct, then we must attribute the unstable behavior of our earlier simulations to some artifact of the computation, since our simulations were *unstable* with values of R_{30} well within the stable fixed point region of the bifurcation diagrams; the value we used, $R_{30} = -4.96$ would be off the right side of the page of figure 1. (The computational simulations we have done correspond more closely to the parameters of the model presented in figure 1 than that of figure 2.)

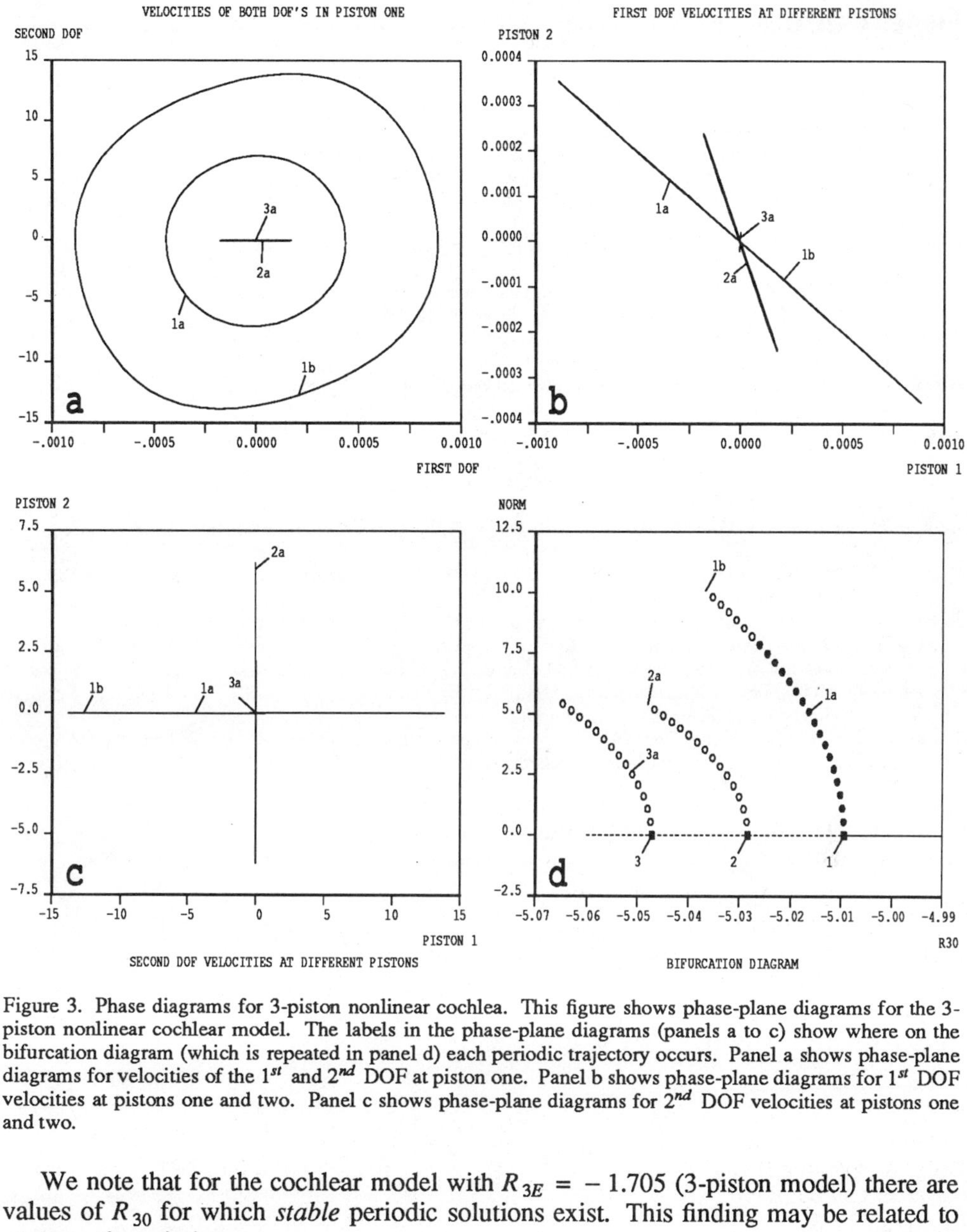

Figure 3. Phase diagrams for 3-piston nonlinear cochlea. This figure shows phase-plane diagrams for the 3-piston nonlinear cochlear model. The labels in the phase-plane diagrams (panels a to c) show where on the bifurcation diagram (which is repeated in panel d) each periodic trajectory occurs. Panel a shows phase-plane diagrams for velocities of the 1st and 2nd DOF at piston one. Panel b shows phase-plane diagrams for 1st DOF velocities at pistons one and two. Panel c shows phase-plane diagrams for 2nd DOF velocities at pistons one and two.

We note that for the cochlear model with $R_{3E} = -1.705$ (3-piston model) there are values of R_{30} for which *stable* periodic solutions exist. This finding may be related to otoacoustic emissions.

Acknowledgements

The task of learning to use AUTO was greatly facilitated by the generous help of its author Eusebius Doedel. The authors thank Walter Bosch, Jim McNally, Don Ronken, Fred Rosenberger, and Rai Winslow for helpful comments and Walter Bosch for assistance in figure preparation. This work was supported by US NIH grants NS-21592 and RR-01379.

References

Allen, J.B. (1977) Two-dimensional cochlear fluid model: New results. J. Acoust. Soc. Am. 61, 110-119.

Boyce, W.E. and DiPrima, R.C. (1969) Elementary Differential Equations and Boundary Value Problems. John Wiley and Sons, Inc., New York.

Cook, P.A. (1986) Nonlinear Dynamical Systems. Prentice Hall International, Englewood Cliffs, New Jersey.

Doedel, E.J. (1981) AUTO: A program for the automatic bifurcation analysis of autonomous systems. Cong. Num. 30, 265-284. (Proc. 10th Manitoba Conf. on Num. Math. and Computing, Winnepeg, Canada, October 1980)

Doedel, E.J. (1984) The computer-aided bifurcation analysis of predator-prey models. J. Math. Biology 20, 1-14.

Doedel, E.J. (1986) AUTO: Software for Continuation and Bifurcation Problems in Ordinary Differential Equations. California Institute of Technology, Pasadena, Calif.

Guckenheimer, J. and Holmes, J.P. (1986) Nonlinear Oscillations, Dynamical Systems, and Bifurcations of Vector Fields. Springer-Verlag, New York.

Hirsch, M.W. and Smale, S. (1974) Differential Equations, Dynamical Systems and Linear Algebra. Academic Press, New York.

Kemp, D.T. (1978) Stimulated acoustic emissions from within the human auditory system. J. Acoust. Soc. Am. 64, 1386-1391.

Kubicek, M. and Marek, M. (1983) Computational Methods in Bifurcation Theory and Dissipative Structures. Springer-Verlag, New York.

Lien, M.D. and Cox, J.R. (1974) A mathematical model of the mechanics of the cochlea. J. Acoust. Soc. Am. 55, 432(A).

Lien, M.D. (1973) A mathematical model of the mechanics of the cochlea. D.Sc. dissertation, Washington University, St. Louis.

Long, G.R. (1984) The microstructure of quiet and masked thresholds. Hearing Res. 15, 73-87.

Long, G.R., Tubis, A. and Jones, K.L. (1986) Changes in spontaneous and evoked otoacoustic emissions and the corresponding psychoacoustic threshold microstructure induced by aspirin consumption. In: Peripheral Auditory Mechanisms (Eds: Allen, J.B., Hall, J.L., Hubbard, A.E., Neely, S.T. and Tubis, A.) Springer Verlag, Berlin, pp. 213-218.

Matthews, J.W. (1980) Mechanical Modeling of Nonlinear Phenomena Observed in the Peripheral Auditory System. D.Sc. dissertation, Washington University, St. Louis.

Neely, S.T. (1979) Research on cochlear mechanics -- spring 1979. (unpublished manuscript).

Neely, S.T. (1981) Fourth-Order Partition Dynamics for a Two-Dimensional Model of the Cochlea. D.Sc. dissertation, Washington University, St. Louis.

Percival, I. and Richards, D. (1982) Introduction to Dynamics. Cambridge University Press, Cambridge.

TIME-DOMAIN SOLUTIONS FOR 1D, 2D AND 3D COCHLEAR MODELS

Rob J. Diependaal

Faculty of Mathematics and Informatics
Delft University of Technology
P.O. Box 356
2600 AJ Delft, The Netherlands

Introduction

The field of mathematical modeling of cochlear mechanics has shifted its focus towards nonlinear and active processes. Arguments for modeling the cochlea as a nonlinear system have been given by recent observations of the presence of nonlinear behavior at a mechanical level [13, 14, 12, 16, 15]. The inclusion of active features in descriptions of cochlear functioning is motivated by measurements of acoustic emissions (pioneered by Kemp [9]), which are shown to be the result of an (unstable) active filtering process rather than being filtered noise [2]. Moreover, calculations on cochlear models [1, 17, 3] strongly suggest that this activity is responsible for the sharp tuning of the recently measured basilar membrane (BM) vibration data [10, 16, 15]. However, the presence of activity at the BM level has not been proven beyond all doubt [18, 11].

Since the underlying mechanisms of the nonlinear and active behavior are hardly known, it is useful to test and compare different types of cochlear models. For this purpose robust and efficient solution methods are constructed, with which responses of such models to various types of input signals can be computed in the time domain. In the present paper numerical solution methods for one-, two-, and three-dimensional (1D, 2D, 3D) models are presented, which makes it possible to study the effect of the dimensionality of the fluid flow on the motion of the BM. Results of numerical calculations in a modified Van der Pol oscillators model are shown.

The integral equation for the 3D model

The 1D, 2D, and 3D descriptions of cochlear mechanics to be discussed in this paper all derive from the same model geometry. The model consists of two identical rectangular channels, filled with an incompressible, inviscid fluid that behaves linearly. The channels are separated by the cochlear partition, the plane $z=0$. The BM has a width β; it occupies a fraction of the width b of the partition. The system is considered to be driven in push-pull; the component p of the fluid pressure that induces a travelling wave along the BM is, consequently, antisymmetric with respect to the plane $z=0$. Hence we can confine ourselves to events occuring in the upper channel.

Owing to the assumptions made about the fluid filling the model, the fluid pressure must satisfy Laplace's equation for potential flow. This Laplace's equation is subject to six boundary conditions; see *e.g.* [6] for a presentation of the 3D model equations. In order to obtain a numerical solution we might directly discretize the model equations. However, this involves discretization in three spatial variables and the time variable, which costs a lot of computer storage and computer time. In this paper another procedure is followed. The first step in the procedure is the conversion of the model equation to an integral equation in only one spatial variable (and time) for the acceleration of the center line of the BM. We skip the derivation here (it can be found in [6]) and give the resulting integral equation:

$$\frac{16\rho}{\pi^2 b}\int_0^L \beta(\xi)G^{3D}(x,\xi)\ddot{u}_1(\xi,t)d\xi - m(x)\ddot{u}_1(x,t) = g(x,t) + \frac{8\rho A_s \ddot{u}_s(t)}{\pi b h}(L-x), \tag{1}$$

with

$$G^{3D}(x,\xi) = \sum_{n=0}^{\infty}\{\frac{\cos(n\pi b_1(x)/b)+\cos(n\pi b_2(x)/b)}{b^2-n^2\beta^2(x)}G_n(x,\xi)\}, \tag{2}$$

$$g(x,t) = r(x,t)\dot{u}_1(x,t) + s(x,t)u_1(x,t), \tag{3}$$

where a means differentiation with respect to time, t the time variable, x the coordinate along the BM from stapes to apex, ρ is the density of the fluid, b and h the width and height of the cochlear channels, L the length of the BM, β the BM width, b_1, b_2 the edges of the BM, A_s the area of the stapes, m, r, and s the mass, resistance, and stiffness of the BM per unit of area, u_1 the displacement of the BM center line, u_s the displacement of the stapes. Furthermore, G_n is given by

$$G_n(x,\xi) = -\frac{b^4[\cos(n\pi b_1(\xi)/b)+\cos(n\pi b_2(\xi)/b)]}{\delta_n L[b^2-n^2\beta^2(\xi)]}\times$$

$$\sum_{k=0}^{\infty}\{\frac{\coth(\gamma_{n,k}h)}{\gamma_{n,k}}\cos[(k+\tfrac{1}{2})\pi x/L]\cos[(k+\tfrac{1}{2})\pi\xi/L]\},\ \delta_n = \begin{cases}2, & n=0\\ 1, & n\geq 1.\end{cases} \tag{4}$$

with

$$\gamma_{n,k}^2 = [(k+\tfrac{1}{2})\pi/L]^2 + (n\pi/b)^2. \tag{5}$$

It should be noted that in the derivation of the integral equation the three-dimensional character of the fluid flow is not affected. Furthermore, r and s may depend on t; in particular, r and s are allowed to be functions of u_1 and $\dot{u}_1$, thus rendering the model nonlinear. The input signal of the model is a prescribed stapes vibration u_s, but the model may as well be driven by a prescribed pressure at the eardrum. In that case a set of equations representing the middle-ear are included in the model description. The analysis and numerical treatment of the model equations is described in detail in [5], and will not be repeated here.

The corresponding 2D and 1D models

In the preceding section an integral equation for the motion of the BM in a 3D model has been presented. The corresponding 2D and 1D descriptions can be obtained by averaging the pressure over the channel width and the channel cross-section, respectively. This results in integral equation of the form of eq. (1), but with simplified kernels G^{2D}, G^{1D}, respectively, instead of G^{3D}. The kernel for the 2D model reads

$$G^{2D}(x,\xi)=-\frac{2}{\pi}\sum_{k=0}^{\infty}\{\frac{\coth[(k+½)\pi h/L]}{k+½}\cos[(k+½)\pi x/L]\cos[(k+½)\pi\xi/L]\}. \tag{6}$$

The series in eq. (6) can summed analytically with the aid of a very accurate approximation [5]. The kernel for the 1D model is

$$G^{1D}(x,\xi)=\frac{4}{hL}[\max(x,\xi)-L]. \tag{7}$$

An equivalent integral formulation for the 1D model has been presented by Jones *et al.* [8]; the resulting equation has been solved numerically. However, in the 1D case a numerically more efficient method can be constructed by discretizing the 1D model equations directly [4].

Numerical results

In order to obtain numerical solutions, we have to render the integral equation discrete. The interval $[0,L]$ is divided into n subintervals by a set of $n+1$ equidistant nodal points. The integral is evaluated using the trapezium rule; special attention is paid to the logarithmic singularity at $x=\xi$. The result of the discretization in the spatial variable is a system of ordinary differential equations in time, that is subsequently solved with the aid of a fourth-order Runge-Kutta scheme. To obtain solutions in the 1D case the more efficient method as described in [4] is used.

We have calculated responses on a pure tone in a nonlinear active model, a modified Van der Pol oscillators model [7; see also 6]. In Fig. 1A we show the results (after Fourier transformation) for a 1 *kHz* tone stimulus at the eardrum of relatively low level. Presented is the amplitude of the fundamental of the response for the 1D, 2D, and 3D models. The graphs show that for this low input level there is entrainment only in the region of the 1 *kHz* characteristic place. Furthermore, there is not much difference between the 2D and 3D model responses, but the 1D model response is clearly deviant. The multidimensional model responses show

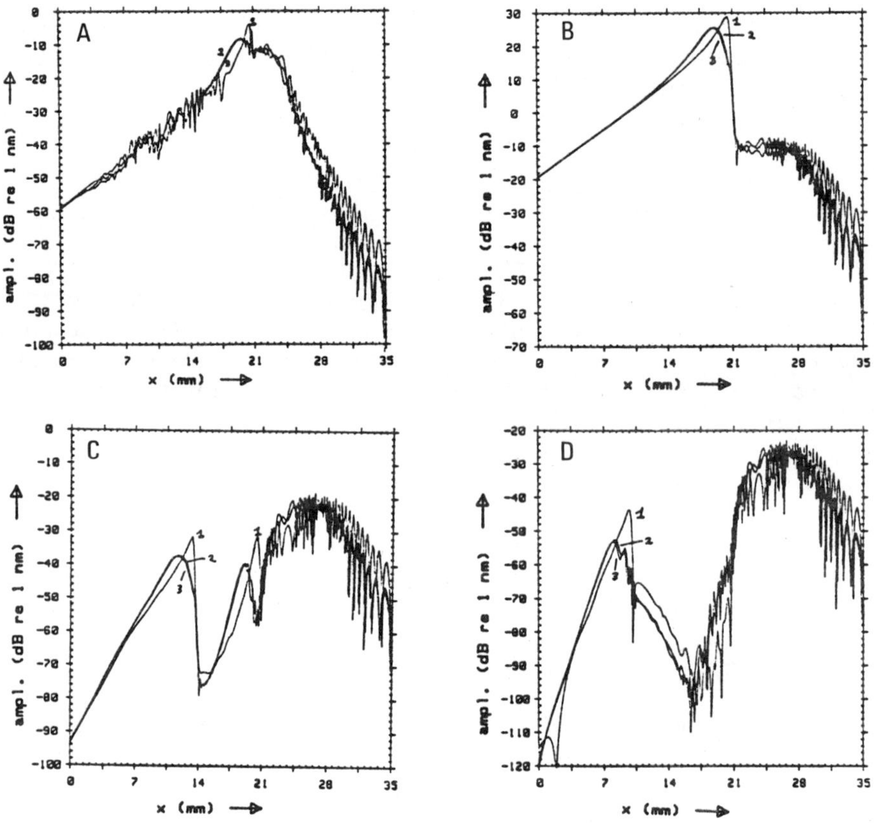

FIGURE 1 **Amplitudes of the BM displacement in the modified Van der Pol oscillators model for a low (panel A) and for a high (panel B, C, and D) input.** Panel A and B: Amplitudes of the fundamental Fourier components of the responses. Panel C and D: Amplitudes of the third and fifth Fourier components, respectively. Curves labeled 1, 2, 3: 1D, 2D, 3D model responses. Parameters as in [6]. Stimulus: a sinusoidal pressure at the eardrum with amplitude $3.16 \times 10^{-7}\ mg/(mm\ ms^2)$ (panel A) or with amplitude $3.16 \times 10^{-5}\ mg/(mm\ ms^2)$ (panel B, C, D). The BM has been divided into 256 elements of equal size.

two amplitude peaks: a narrow one at the place of the amplitude peak of the 1D model response and a broader one slightly basalwards.

In Fig. 1B, C, D the amplitudes of the responses (after Fourier transformation) are shown for a 1 *kHz* stimulus at the eardrum of relatively high level. The high level stimulus entrains the oscillators over a wide range, and uneven higher harmonics are clearly present in the response (fig. 1C). The third harmonic shows two peaks, at the characteristic places of a 1 *kHz* tone and of a 3 *kHz* tone. The fifth harmonic shows only a clear amplitude peak at its own characteristic place. It can also be seen that again there is hardly any difference between the 2D and 3D model responses, but that the 1D model response is quite different from the others. The amplitude peak of the fundamental as well as those of the higher uneven harmonics are sharper and higher (a few *dB* for the fundamental, about 10 *dB* for the fifth harmonic) in the 1D case than in the 2D or 3D case.

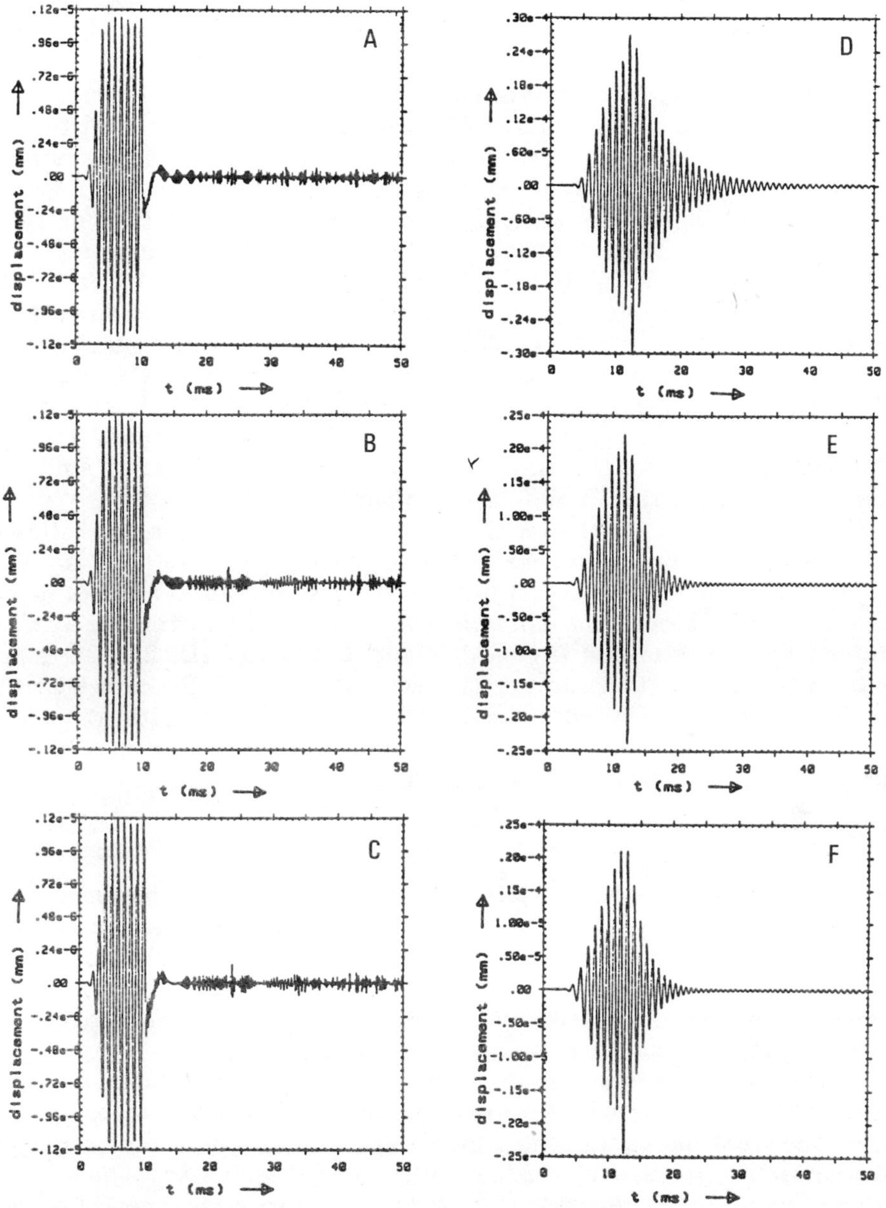

FIGURE 2 Model responses of the modified Van der Pol oscillators model on a tone burst. Panel A, B, C: BM displacement at $x/L = 29$ % in the 1D, 2D, 3D model, respectively. Panel D: BM displacement at $x/L = 58$ % in the 1D model. Panel E, F: BM displacement at $x/L = 54$ % in the 2D, 3D model. Parameter values as in figure 1. Stimulus: a 1 kHz tone burst of ten cycles with amplitude 3.16×10^{-5} $mg/(mm\ ms^2)$ (pressure at the eardrum).

We have also computed the responses of the modified Van der Pol oscillators model on a tone burst. The stimulus at the eardrum is a 1 *kHz* tone of 10 *ms* duration and of relatively high level.

In fig. 2 the first 50*ms* of the responses are shown at two different places: at the characteristic place of a 20 *kHz* tone, and at the characteristic place of a 1 *kHz* tone. At both places the reponses show a time delay (smaller at the more basal place) of a few *ms* corresponding to the time the BM wave needs for travelling to the place of observation. After the time delay the response function at the more basal place shows a quick rise to its maximum amplitude and the BM oscillates with the input frequency 1 *kHz*. When the input is switched off, the amplitude of the oscillation falls down to the limit cycle amplitude of the modified Van der Pol oscillator and the BM starts to vibrate in a quasi chaotic way with a frequency of about 20 *kHz*. At the more apical place the response function rises gradually to reach its maximum and then slowly decreases to the limit cycle amplitude. The slope of the amplitude rise is the same for all dimensions, the rate of amplitude decrease is greater in the 2D and 3D case than in the 1D case.

In the last figure (3) the results of fig. 2 are replotted in the following way: The BM response at the characteristic place of a 1 *kHz* tone is plotted as a function of the response just basal to it. The first 10—15 cycles there is a strong positive correlation between the two oscillators because both are entrained by the stimulus (fig. 3A, B and C for the 1D, 2D, 3D model, respectively). After the stimulus has been switched off, the correlation has been lost, because then both oscillators are vibrating with their own, (slightly) different, limit cycle frequencies (see figs. 3D-F, which are enlarged pictures of the middle parts of figs. 3A-C).

Conclusions

A robust numerical method to solve 3D cochlear models in the time domain has been presented. With this method, the response of models equipped with nonlinear and active features can be calculated for a variety of stimuli, such as pure tones, two tones, noise, and clicks. The method thus makes it possible to evaluate models with different types of nonlinearity and activity. Furthermore, the present numerical method can be used as a frame of reference in order to assess the accuracy of asymptotic methods, which generally need less computer time than numerical methods.

We have calculated responses on a pure tone and on a tone burst in a nonlinear, active model, the modified Van der Pol oscillators model [7]. In all these cases, the 2D response is close to the 3D solution; the 1D solution deviates considerably from the multidimensional solutions. However, from simulation studies in linear, passive models we learn that for realistic values of the parameters the 2D model response may deviate significantly from the 3D response [6]. So, the appropriate dimensionality of a cochlear model depends on how much information one wants to obtain from the simulation studies. If one is only interested in the global behavior of the model, a 1D approach is often satisfactory. For a more detailed evaluation of the

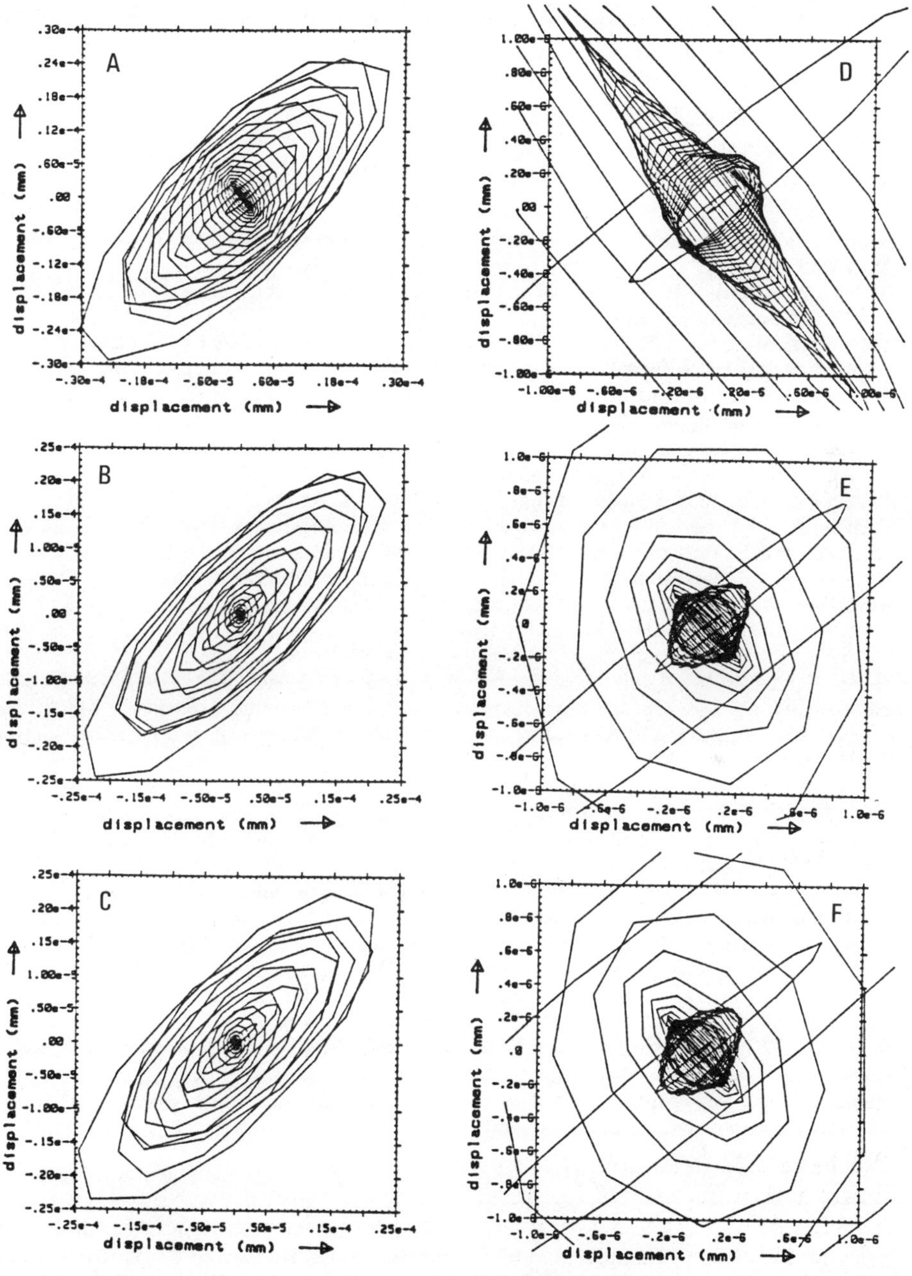

FIGURE 3 Displacement of one section of the modified Van der Pol oscillator model as a function of the displacement of its adjacent section. Panel A: BM displacement in sections 150 and 151 in the 1D model. Panel B, C: BM displacement in sections 140 and 141 in the 2D, 3D model, respectively. Parameter values and stimulus condition as in figure 2.

cochlear model a 2D, sometimes even a 3D, approach is necessary. Furthermore, a 3D approach seems mandatory in case the radial direction plays a more important role in the model examples [11] than in the model example presented in this paper.

References

[1] Boer, E, de (1983). No sharpening? A challenge for cochlear mechanics. J. Acoust. Soc. Am. 73, 567-573.

[2] Bialek, W.S. and Wit, H.P. (1984). Quantum limits to oscillator stability: theory and experiments on acoustic emissions from the human ear. Phys. Lett. 104A, 173-178.

[3] Diependaal, R.J., Boer, E. de, and Viergever, M.A. (1987a). Cochlear power flux as an indicator of mechanical activity. J. Acoust. Soc. Am. 82, 917-926.

[4] Diependaal, R.J., Duifhuis, H., Hoogstraten, H.W. and Viergever, M.A. (1987b). Numerical methods for solving one-dimensional cochlear models in the time domain. J. Acoust. Soc. Am. 82, 1655-1666

[5] Diependaal, R.J. and Viergever, M.A. (1988a). Nonlinear and active two-dimensional cochlear models: time-domain solution. Submitted to J. Acoust. Soc. Am.

[6] Diependaal, R.J. and Viergever, M.A. (1988b). Nonlinear and active three-dimensional cochlear models: time-domain solution. Submitted to J. Acoust. Soc. Am.

[7] Duifhuis, H., Hoogstraten, H.W., Netten, S.M. van, Diependaal, R.J. and Bialek, W. (1986). Modelling the cochlear partition with coupled Van der Pol oscillators. In: Peripheral Auditory Mechanisms, pp. 290-297. Editors: J.B. Allen, J.L. Hall, A. Hubbard, S.T. Neely, and A. Tubis. Springer Verlag, Berlin, Heidelberg, New York.

[8] Jones, K., Tubis, A., Long, G.R., Burns, E.M., and Strickland, E.A. (1986). Interactions among multiple spontaneous otoacoustic emissions. In: Peripheral Auditory Mechanisms, pp. 266-273. Editors: J.B. Allen, J.L. Hall, A. Hubbard, S.T. Neely, and A. Tubis. Springer Verlag, Berlin, Heidelberg, New York.

[9] Kemp, D.T. (1978). Stimulated acoustic emissions from within the human auditory system. J. Acoust. Soc. Am. 64, 1386-1391.

[10] Khanna, S.M. and Leonard, D.G.B. (1982). Basilar membrane tuning in the cat cochlea. Science 215, 305-306.

[11] Kolston, P.J. (1988). Sharp mechanical tuning in a cochlear model without negative damping. To appear in J. Acoust. Soc. Am.

[12] LePage, E.L. and Johnstone, B.M. (1980). Nonlinear mechanical behaviour of the basilar membrane in the basal turn of the guinea pig cochlea. Hearing Res. 2, 183-189.

[13] Rhode, W.S. (1971). Observations of the vibration of the basilar membrane in squirrel monkeys using the Mossbauer technique. J. Acoust. Soc. Am. 49, 1218-1231.

[14] Rhode, W.S. (1978). Some observations on cochlear mechanics. J. Acoust. Soc. Am. 64, 158-176.

[15] Robles, L., Ruggero, M.A. and Rich, N.C. (1986). Basilar membrane mechanics at the base of the chinchilla cochlea. I.Input-output functions, tuning curves, and response phases. J. Acoust. Soc. Am. 80, 1364-1374.

[16] Sellick, P.M., Patuzzi, R. and Johnstone, B.M. (1982). Measurement of basilar membrane motion in the guinea pig using the Mossbauer technique. J. Acoust. Soc. Am. 72, 131-141.

[17] Viergever, M.A. and Diependaal, R.J. (1986). Quantitative validation of cochlear models using the Liouville-Green approximation. Hearing Res. 21, 1-15.

[18] Wickesberg, R.E. and Geisler, C.D. (1986). Longitudinal stiffness coupling in a 1-dimensional model of the peripheral ear. In: Peripheral Auditory Mechanisms, pp. 113-120. Editors: J.B. Allen, J.L. Hall, A. Hubbard, S.T. Neely, and A. Tubis. Springer Verlag, Berlin, Heidelberg, New York.

IS BASILAR MEMBRANE TUNING THE SAME AS NEURAL TUNING -- WHERE DO WE STAND?

Jont B. Allen

Acoustics Research Dept.
AT&T Bell Laboratories, Room 2D530
600 Mountain Ave.
Murray Hill NJ, 07090, USA

Introduction

One of the most important problems which still remains unsolved in cochlear theory is explaining the sharpness of tuning of the neurally measured response in the base of the cochlea. To solve this problem we must answer the following questions:

Should the compressive and frequency dependent basilar membrane nonlinearity be viewed as a gain at low levels, or is it an attenuation at high levels? Over what frequency and amplitude range is the basilar membrane nonlinear? How are these cochlear nonlinearities related to the 'cochlear amplifier' as described by Davis (1983) and by Neely and Kim (1983)? Is the basilar membrane response the same as the hair cell excitation (the tectorial membrane to reticular lamina shear), or are they separate by a mechanical degree of freedom. To what extent is the neural tuning entwined with cochlear nonlinearities, as seen in basilar membrane input-output functions and in hair cell input-output functions?

It is my intention to review the data and try to summarize some of the relevant issues in an objective manner. I shall then ask what conclusions may be reached from neural phase data as a function of place, frequency, and level? Finally I will review the models of tuning and discuss the relative merits of each model.

A Nonlinear Paradox

It is interesting to reflect on a paradox that results from combining the fluid mechanical law of mass conservation with the nonlinear motion as measured by Rhode (1971 & 1978). {Rhode observed a nonlinear compressive basilar membrane input/output displacement (or velocity) response near the best frequency (CF), and found the response to be linear at frequencies away from CF. One popular interpretation of this nonlinear effect is that of a level dependent gain for frequencies near CF, with increasing gain at lower levels.}

First, the mass conservation law says that the net fluid volume displacement of the basilar membrane must equal the stapes volume displacement at every instant of time. Second, Rhode observed that the basilar membrane displacement is not proportional to the stapes displacement, and therefore appears to have excess gain, relative to a linear motion, at low levels near the best frequency (CF). From the conservation law and the nonlinear observation, it would appear that the traveling wave pattern must change its distribution along the basilar membrane length as a function of the stapes input level. *This in turn would imply that the neural phase would change with sound level, which in general is not found in the region defined, namely for frequencies below 4 kHz and amplitudes below 65 dB-SPL (Allen, 1983).* Rhode found the phase to vary with level, which is consistent with this argument (Geisler and Rhode, 1982). It is hard to imagine how the basilar membrane phase could change with level and not effect the neural phase.

One possible way out of this paradox is to add an extra degree of freedom between basilar membrane motion and hair cell excitation. This approach may not actually resolve the paradox, but may only frustrate a conclusion. A second more promising approach is to note that the experimental evidence for the nonlinear excess gain is above 4 kHz. *This opens the possibility that the excess gain (the cochlear nonlinearity) is not present to the same degree in the apex of the cochlea for levels below 65 dB-SPL, namely that region where the neural phase data has been found to be linear.* A conclusion of this kind would have a great impact on cochlear theory as applied to speech processing and hearing impairment, since this is an important level and frequency region for speech signals. Furthermore, if the basilar membrane were linear in this region, then it would impact the long-standing question of the difference between the basilar membrane and the transduction (neural and hair cell) tuning.

Discussion

In question here is not the existence of cochlea nonlinearity, but the range of frequencies and levels over which the nonlinearity is present, and the degree of the excess gain (a convenient measure of the magnitude of the nonlinearity effect) as a function of frequency and level. The amount of excess gain, as a function of frequency, seen by Rhode and others who have measured the mechanical response (e.g. 35 dB at 7 kHz), seems to agree qualitatively with the amount of suppression seen in the tip of tuning curves as measured neurally (e.g. 40 dB), again as a function of frequency (Allen and Fahey, 1983; Fahey and Allen, 1985). The question being raised here is the strong frequency dependence of these effects.

The amplitude-frequency plane may be bisected twice, once in frequency, and once in amplitude, defining several regions. The low frequency phase locked region below 4 kHz, and the high frequency non-phase locked region create one bisection, while the amplitude bisection is frequency dependent, but is roughly at 65 dB-SPL. Below 800 Hz the level of the amplitude bisection may have higher levels. In the phase locked region at the lower levels, the neural phase was found to be linear. These various regions seem correlated with features of two tone suppression as measured neurally. Constalupes, Rich, and Ruggero (1987) divided the suppression slopes into two frequency regions, with the transition at the CF. Delgutte (1986) found the slopes of suppression to be frequency dependent in a more graded manner, with the suppression slopes depending on both frequency and CF. He found suppression slopes to decrease above 5 kHz for units having CF's above that frequency. Allen and Fahey (1983) and Fahey and Allen (1985) found a threshold effect which defined a locus of suppressor threshold levels as a function of frequency, above which suppression was present, and below which it was not present. In their case the measure was suppression to spontaneous activity rather than a measurable drop in the driven rate (Sachs and Kiang, 1968), or a shift in the rate level curve (Javel, 1985; Delgutte, 1986; Constalupes et al. (1987)).

Other related experimental correlates are the high lability in the base of the cochlea, the change in characteristic shape of the FTC's with CF, and the variation of the rate-level slopes re CF vs. CF.

Basilar Membrane vs. Hair Cell and Neural Tuning

While two-dimensional models have brought the model calculations and transduction data into agreement on the high frequency side of the tuning curve, they have not improved the match on the low frequency side. This mismatch of model and experiment is compounded by the fact that most experimental mechanical measurements show a 15-20 dB difference between basilar membrane responses and transduction responses on the low frequency side of the tuning curve.

The receptor potential in the inner hair cell was first measured by Russell and Sellick (1978) and is tuned like a neuron. When these measurements were first made, there was no question that the hair cell had neural-like tuning. This should be contrasted to the situation that has existed for the last 30 years between mechanical measures of tuning and neural tuning where the match has been less convincing. In Fig. 10 of Sellick et al. (1982) they show tuning responses of the basilar membrane compared to a transduction (hair cell) measure, where the responses differ by about 10 to 20 dB on the low frequency side of the response. In a later paper, Sellick et al. (1983) show much more detail, as seen in their Figs. 1,2,3 and 4. These results consistently show a difference on the low frequency side of the characteristic frequency. In the summary of their 1983 paper they stated: "*In conclusion, a demonstration of inner hair cell tuning at the level of the basilar membrane continues to elude us.*"

Robles et al. (1986) have also compared basilar membrane tuning to a transduction measure. Their summary result is shown in Fig. 11 of their paper. Again on the low frequency side of the tuning curve they find a difference, but in their case, the difference is in the form of a large variance, which they indicate by error bars (note the displacement response at 2.8 kHz). It is interesting to note that in the frequency region near 1.75 kHz the neural measure is less sharply tuned than either of the mechanical measures, *an observation unique to all such experiments.*

The measurements of basilar membrane motion by Khanna and Leonard (1982) are not direct comparisons to transduction measures. Furthermore they have not observed the nonlinear compression as seen by Rhode (1971,1978), Russell and Sellick (1978), Sellick et al. (1982,1983) and Robles et al. (1986). As a result of the ear canal pressure standing wave they report (Khanna and Leonard, 1986), which was used to normalize the basilar membrane data, their data do not appear to be a useful test of this question.

Are the observed differences between basilar membrane and transduction measures significant, or are they an artifact of some experimental technique? Unfortunately, we still cannot be sure of the answer to this important question. At present the Neely and Kim (1983) model fits neural tuning threshold data best for CF's above 5 kHz. This model assumes that basilar membrane tuning is equal to neural tuning. The Allen model (1980a,b;1985) describes neural threshold data for frequencies below 5 kHz, but in that model, neural and mechanical tuning differ by about 20 dB one half octave or so below the best frequency, as a result of the resonant tectorial membrane transduction filter that has been applied. Thus two micromechanical models which make quite different assumptions have been shown to approximately fit tuning data in different frequency regions. Until the experimental questions are resolved, it seems that this theoretical question is likely to remain open. Meanwhile, micromechanical models of the transduction process will provide insight in exploring these questions.

Micromechanical Models

We next discuss the two classes of theories which attempt to model the experimentally observed frequency selectivity. The *first* is based on the idea that the tectorial membrane vibrates at its own resonant frequency, near the resonant frequency of the basilar membrane. In 1980, different versions of this resonant tectorial membrane approach were independently proposed by Zwislocki and Kletsky (1980), Zwislocki (1980), and Allen (1980 a,b). The *second* is the theory of Neely and Kim (1983), which calls on the idea of an active, or negative resistance, basilar membrane. More recently, Neely and Kim (1986) have published a more comprehensive theory in which they merge the resonant tectorial membrane model of Allen (1980) with their active basilar membrane theory.

The most commonly accepted description of the motion of the organ of Corti was proposed by ter Kuile in 1900. A simple analysis of this model reveals that the vertical motion (the y direction) of the basilar membrane is linearly related to the radial shearing motion (the z direction) seen by the cilia of the inner hair cells, which are known to be the transducers which sense the motions of the basilar membrane. This use of *radial* refers to the direction tangent to the reticular membrane surface. Thus the model of ter Kuile is equivalent to a lever or transformer which linearly converts the vertical basilar membrane motion into radial shearing motions appropriate for the excitation of the inner hair cells. (The word "motion" is used in order to avoid the important question of whether velocity or displacement is the actual inner hair cell excitatory stimulus). It was hoped that a simple modification of the ter Kuile model might unify the various theories and the experimental data. There have been no direct observations to confirm the ter Kuile model due to the inherent difficulty in making observations of such small motions in such difficult places.

ZWISLOCKI'S TECTORIAL MEMBRANE MODELS

Zwislocki has proposed a number of tectorial membrane models for sharpening the basilar membrane response. In 1979 he and Kletsky proposed a model for sharpening based on longitudinal smoothing by the tectorial membrane (a spatial low pass filter), which they modeled by assuming longitudinal mechanical coupling of the tectorial membrane, followed by a difference which resulted from the usual ter Kuile shearing motion at the inner hair cells (Zwislocki and Kletsky, 1979). With some simple analysis, one may show that this model is similar in its effect to the spatial difference model proposed by Hall in 1977 {see the discussion in Hall, (1981)} and acts as a spatial high pass filter. This model is not a resonant tectorial membrane model.

In 1980, Zwislocki and Kletsky proposed two new approaches to this problem (1980) which they called models I and II. Model I is a resonant reed that is mass loaded. The resonant system is meant to represent the tectorial membrane mass and the sterocilia stiffness.

This model differs distinctly from the model of ter Kuile, since there is no analogue of the spiral limbus-tectorial membrane coupling. Their model differs from that of Allen (1980 a,b) in exactly this way, since in Allen's model, the radial stiffness of the tectorial membrane was specifically taken into account in a functionally significant way. Without the limbus coupling it is hard to understand how the vertical motion of the basilar membrane can excite or couple to the radial motion of the tectorial membrane. The reticular lamina is set at an angle relative to the basilar membrane, so there would be a small inertial (mass) component of the force in the vertical motion in the radial direction, parallel to the reticular lamina. However it seems likely that viscous forces would dominate the equations of motion of such a system, thereby greatly reducing the magnitude of excitation to the inner hair cells.

In Allen's model, the relatively stiff limbus-tectorial membrane coupling element plays a critical role in the excitation of the inner hair cell cilia. As a result, the characteristics of the frequency response due to the radial resonance in (Allen, 1980a,b) is quite different from that measured by Zwislocki and Kletsky (1980) (compare their Fig. 2 vs. Fig. 19c of Allen (1985)). In summary, these two systems are <u>not</u> isomorphic.

Zwislocki and Kletsky's model-II (1980) seems to be a partial joining of the spatial smoothing model (1979) and model-I described above. This model consists of a parallel bank of resonating reeds tuned to slightly different frequencies. The reeds are connected together, along the longitudinal axis, with a nonlinear elastic medium which mechanically couples them. Again, as in model-I, this system has no spiral limbus analogue. The model system is shown in a photograph in the original paper, along with some experimental results showing the suppression effects they saw of one tone on a second. Both models I and II are described as nonlinear models, but only the first is a sharpening model.

ALLEN'S TECTORIAL MEMBRANE MODEL

Fig. 7 of (Allen, 1980) shows a model extension of the ter Kuile model where the tectorial membrane is given a new degree of freedom to vibrate in the radial direction, depicted there as the z-direction. There are two effects that result from the added degree of freedom on the transfer function between the basilar membrane displacement and the shear displacement, a pole and a zero. The zero has its effect on the low frequency side of the tuning curve and causes a partial cancellation of the shear motion at the site of the inner hair cells, relative to the up-down motion of the basilar membrane. This cancellation is a result of the elastic tectorial membrane element labeled k_T and might account for the difference frequently observed between basilar membrane motion and neural response below the characteristic frequency in both magnitude and phase. Fig. 18a of (Allen, 1985) shows cat neural tuning data for several neural units, and Fig. 18b shows the model result using a linear two-dimensional macromechanical model coupled to the resonant tectorial membrane micromechanical model (Allen, 1980,1985). In the model calculation we have held the model output constant, and plotted the required input pressure in the ear canal. The phase measurements of Kim, Siegel and Molnar (1979) using the population technique are also in agreement with this model. Kim found a π phase shift at a place about 1.5 octaves basal to the CF. The pole of the model transfer function was set above the CF, and therefore had little effect on the model response. However the pole could be useful to obtain gain at CF for the basal region of the cochlea. This option has not yet been explored by this author. Intermediate model results for the cochlear input impedance and the cochlear microphonic for this model also agreed with experimentally observed results.

Shown in Fig. 19 of Allen (1985) are four measures from the model as a function of position along the basilar membrane, for six different input frequencies : In (a) we see the model neural output, given constant input pressure in the model ear canal. In (b) we showed the model neural phase. In (c) we showed the model transfer function magnitude relating the basilar membrane to hair cell displacement, which results from the resonant tectorial membrane model, and in (d) we see the forth order basilar membrane impedance magnitude for the resonant tectorial membrane model, which is required when calculating the basilar membrane velocity using the macromechanical model.

From these figures it is clear that the model does a reasonable, but hardly perfect, job of describing the neural data in the apex region of the cochlea. For example, a significant error in bandwidth is evident for the low frequency model tuning curves. Note that the resonant tectorial membrane transfer function (Fig. 19c) has a 20 dB "sharpening" effect on the response for frequencies below the cutoff frequency, which is close to the difference observed by Sellick et al. (1983) as seen in his Figs. 1,2,3 and 4. Our model effort has not yet attempted to specifically account for the Sellick et al. data.

All of the Allen models are linear models, and therefore cannot describe the nonlinear input-output data seen in the basilar membrane and in transduction data.

NEELY AND KIM'S NEGATIVE RESISTANCE MODEL

A second and alternative approach to account for sharp neural tuning has been proposed by Neely and Kim (1983), and was first worked out in some detail by Neely (1981) in his Ph. D. thesis. This model calls upon the concept of negative damping, or resistance, in the basilar membrane. This model distinguishes itself from the resonant tectorial membrane models due to one of its basic assumptions, namely the model assumes that the neural and the basilar membrane response are identical. *Therefore the original ter Kuile model was used unmodified in Neely's theory* [the tectorial membrane was assumed to be rigid in the radial direction (Neeley and Kim, 1983, Fig. 2)]. This model is a linear model.

One serious drawback with this model is the lack of a clear relationship between the model parameters and the cochlear anatomy.

The results of Neely and Kim (1983) shown in their Fig. 5 are a very impressive match to a high frequency neural tuning curve, both magnitude and phase, where phase data is available. In general, the higher the characteristic frequency of the neural data being matched, the better the model fit.

In a recent paper, Neely and Kim (1986) join the resonant tectorial membrane model of Allen (1980 a,b) with an active source which represents active outer hair cells. This model gives the best fit to tuning curve data to date for any of the models, if the entire 100 Hz to 30 kHz hearing range is considered. This paper also improves on the earlier paper (Neely and Kim, 1983) by having a better correspondence between many of the model parameters and the cochlea anatomy. However the active pressure source still does not have a defined frame of reference (it has nothing to push against).

The source of the proposed negative damping is still unknown. In 1985 Brownell et al. (1985) found that isolated outer hair cells change their length when placed in an electric field. This has lead to the speculation that outer hair cells act as linear motors directly driving the basilar membrane. According to this line of reasoning, the length change of the hair cells might be a function of the outer hair cell receptor potential, which in turn is modulated by both the position of the basilar membrane (forming a tight feedback loop), or by the efferent neurons that are connected to the outer hair cells (forming a very slow feedback loop). In 1988 Santos-Sacchi and Dilger showed that the length change is proportional to the receptor potential (as opposed to some ion specific hair cell current), with a sensitivity of 15 nm/mv. The details of this possibility are the topic of present day research. The work of Liberman and Dodd (1984) may give some important constraints on how this system might work. In their Fig. 14 one may see the complex relationships that exist between the mechanical state of the inner and outer hair cells, and the neurally measured frequency response. Perhaps an improved understanding of this interaction will lead to the breakthrough that we need in describing the cochlear frequency selectivity and the nonlinear characteristics of the basilar membrane.

References

Allen, J. B. (1980a). "Cochlear micromechanics - A physical model of transduction," J. Acoust. Soc. Am. 68, 1660-1670.

Allen, J. B. (1980b). "A Cochlear Micromechanic Model of Transduction," in Psychophysical Physiological and Behavioural Studies in Hearing, Ed. by G. Van den Brink, and F. A. Bilsen, Delft University Press, 85-93.

Allen, J. B., and Fahey, P. F. (1983). "Nonlinear Behavior at Threshold Determined in the Auditory Canal and on the Auditory Nerve," In Hearing-Physiological Bases and Psychophysics, Ed. by R. Klinke and R. Hartmann, Springer-Verlag, New York, pp. 128-133.

Allen, J. B. (1983). "Magnitude and phase frequency response to single tones in the auditory nerve," J. Acoust. Soc. Am. 73, 2071-2092.

Allen, J. B. (1985). "Cochlear Modeling," IEEE ASSP Magazine 2, #1, January, 3-29.

Brownell, W.E., Bader, C. R., Bertrand, D., and de Ribaupierre, Y. (1985). "Evoked Mechanical Responses of Isolated Cochlear Outer Hair Cells," Science 227, 194-196.

Constalupes, J.A, Rich, N.C., and Ruggero, M.A. (1987). "Effects of excitatory and non-excitatory suppressor tones on two-tone rate suppression in auditory nerve fibers," Hearing Research, 26, 155-164.

Delgutte, B. (1986). Ninth ARO Midwinter Meeting , Abstract p. 65.

Davis, H. (1983). "An Active process in cochlear mechanics," Hearing Research 9, 79-90.

Fahey, P. F. and Allen, J. B. (1985). "Nonlinear phenomena as observed in the ear canal and at the auditory nerve," J. Acoust. Soc. Am 77, 599-612.

Geisler, C. D., and Rhode, W. S. (1982). "The Phases of basilar-membrane vibrations," J. Acoust. Soc. Am. 71, 1201-1203.

Hall, J. L. (1981). "Observations on a nonlinear model for motion of the basilar membrane," in Hearing Research and Theory I, Academic Press, New York, 1-61.

Javel, E., Geisler, D.C., Ravindran, A. (1978). "Two-tone suppression in auditory nerve of the cat: Rate-intensity and temporal analyses," J. Acoust. Soc. Am. 63, 1093-1104.

Khanna S. M., and Leonard, D. (1982), "Basilar membrane tuning in the cat cochlea." Science 215, 305-306.

Khanna, S. M., and Leonard, D. G. B. (1986), "Relationship between basilar membrane tuning and hair cell condition," Hearing Research 23, 55-70.

Kuile, E. ter. (1900). "Die Uebertragung der Energie von der Grundmanbran auf die Haazellen," Pflueg. Arch. ges Physiol. 79, 146-157.

Liberman, M. C., and Dodds, L. W. (1984). "Single-neuron labeling and chronic cochlear pathology. III. Sterocilia damage and alterations of threshold tuning curves," Hearing Research 16, 55-74

Neely, S. T. (1981). "Fourth-order partition dynamics of a two-dimensional model of the cochlea," Doctoral dissertation, Washington Univ., St. Louis, MO.

Neely, S. T., and Kim, D. O. (1983). "An active cochlear model showing sharp tuning and high sensitivity," Hearing Research 9, 123-130.

Neely, S. T., and Kim, D. O. (1986). "A model for active elements in cochlear biomechanics " J. Acoust. Soc. Am. 79, 1472-1480.

Rhode, W. (1971). "Observations of the vibrations of the basilar membrane in squirrel monkeys using the Mossbauer technique," J. Acoust. Soc. Am. 49, 1218-1231.

Rhode, W. (1978). "Some observations on cochlear mechanics," J. Acoust. Soc. Am. 64, 158-176.

Robles, L., Ruggero, M. A., Rich, N. C. (1986). "Basilar membrane mechanics at the base of the chinchilla cochlea. I. Input-output functions, tuning curves, and response phases," J. Acoustical Soc. Am. 80, 1364-1374.

Russell, I. and Sellick, P. (1978). "Intracellular studies of hair cells in the mammalian cochlea," J. Physiol. 284, 261-290.

Sachs, M. B., and Kiang, Y. S. (1968). " Two-Tone inhibition in auditory-nerve fibers," J. Acoust. Soc. Am. 43, 1120-1128.

Santos-Sacchi, J. and Dilger, J.P. (1988). "Electrically induced mechanical response of outer hair cells is membrane potential dependent," submitted to Hearing Research. Also see 11th ARO Midwinter Meeting 1988, p. 171.

Sellick, P. M., Patuzzi, R., and Johnstone, B. M. (1982). "Measurement of basilar membrane motion in the guinea pig using the Mossbauer technique," J. Acoustical Soc. Am. 72, 131-141.

Sellick, P. M., Patuzzi, R., and Johnstone, B. M. (1983). "Comparison between the tuning properties of inner haircells and basilar membrane motion," Hearing Research 10, 93-100.

Zwislocki, J. J., and Kletsky, E. J. (1979). "Tectorial Membrane: A Possible Effect on Frequency Analysis in the Cochlea," Science 204, 639-641.

Zwislocki, J. J. (1980). "Five Decades of Research on Cochlear Mechanics," J. Acoust. Soc. Am. 67, 1679-1685.

Zwislocki, J. J., and Kletsky, E. J. (1980). "Micromechanics in the theory of cochlear mechanics," Hearing Research 2, 505-512.

Comments and Discussion

ZWISLOCKI

In this article Allen has not clarified the relation of what he calls "Allen's Tectorial Membrane Model" to what he calls "Zwislocki's Tectorial Membrane Model". Allen has claimed since 1980 that the two models were independently conceived and that his is sufficiently different from mine to to warrant a different name.

In 1979, together with Kletzky who implemented my model in terms of an electronic network, I published an article in Science (Vol. 204, 639-641) under the title "Tectorial Membrane: A Possible Effect on Frequency Analysis in the Cochlea". The most revolutionary idea in the model was that the tectorial membrane was no longer considered as practically rigid but was allowed to oscillate roughly parallel to the surface of the reticular lamina. I recently had the opportunity to demonstrate experimentally that the tectorial membrane was indeed highly flexible. The new model accounted for several but not all the relevant phenomena.

The partial success with the first "tectorial-membrane model", evidence derived from MIT experiments on the alligator lizard auditory papilla, and observations of response phases of auditory-nerve fibers innervating normal and pathological cochleas led me to postulate that the tectorial membrane was capable not only of oscillating radially but also of resonating in this plane. The resonance was assumed to occur as a result of interaction between the mass of the tectorial membrane and the stiffness of the OHC stereocilia embedded in it. This fundamental idea was presented in the Spring of 1979 within a symposium I chaired at the 50th anniversary meeting of the Acoustical Society of America (Zwislocki, 1980).

J.B. Allen claimed in the discussion at that symposium that the cochlear damping was too high for the tectorial membrane resonance to work. Since he was exposed to my model at this meeting, I cannot consider his subsequent publications, in which he promoted the idea of my model without reference, as independent.

Allen's comments concerning my reed models are not relevant here because the models were developed for didactic purposes in a different context.

I reject entirely the notion that J.B. Allen contributed in any way to my concept of tectorial membrane resonance. What he seems to have contributed to the model resulting from my concept is the following: (1) First published formal drawings of the mechanical and electrical analogs of the model, although incomplete; (2) First computational implementation of the model, although incomplete and superficial; (3) Inclusion of the series resonance of the tectorial membrane, which results from its elastic attachment to the spiral limbus. I explicitly omitted this resonance in my original proposal as negligible. (It cannot enhance the radial vibration magnitude of the tectorial membrane beyond that of the reticular lamina and occurs well below BF.)

ALLEN

In 1977, I published a paper (Allen, 1977) on a cancellation method of forming a tuning curve. This method was based on the idea of subtracting pressure from displacement. The method gave a nice cancellation on the low frequency side of the basilar membrane response, and transformed the basilar membrane response into a neural like response. The failure of this model was that it had no physical realization. Thus from 1977 to 1979, my goal was to find a physical realization of a micromechanical model that would introduce a zero into the transfer function between the basial membrane response and the inner hair cell excitation. My approach was to try to find a simple modification of the widely accepted ter Kuile model (I did not know about ter Kuile at the time, but I did know his model) that would give this zero. I was not trying to introduce a pole or use resonance. My paper that introduced these results (Allen, 1980) was received by JASA on January 1, 1980. I had found a model that would give the zero I was looking for, but as is required by network theory, since the model was physically realizable, this model also had a pole. I was aware that the pole could be useful in giving improved sensitivity for high frequency CF's, but I was more interested in modelling tuning below 5 kHz, because of the applications (speech and telephone) that I was interested in. Thus I used the pole to model the bump on the high frequency side of low frequency neural tuning curves (see Evan's paper, this meeting). Therefore, although I was driven by modelling a zero in the transfer function, I ended up with a resonant model because I was searching for a physically realizable network for which a pole must come with a zero according the theorems of network theory.

The comment that I made at the 1979 ASA meeting that Professor Zwislocki is referring to was just that a single cilia standing in fluid will be greatly damped by the viscosity of the fluid. Tom Weiss stood up after my comment and agreed with me, as I remember.

Allen, J.B. (1977) "Cochlear Micromechanics - A Mechanism for Transforming Mechanical to Neural Tuning within the Cochlea", JASA, 62, 930-939.

Allen, J.B. (1980) "Cochlear Micromechanics - A Physical Model of Transduction", JASA, 68, 1660-1670.

WILSON

I do not wish to act as arbiter in this dispute but I think that it *is* important to get history correct. I should like to add that I believe I may have planted the seed of these models in my paper at the Keele meeting in 1977 (Wilson, 1977) although I would not be surprised if the same suggestion had been made earlier.

In order to explain ".. phase differences between the inner, PT, and outer, PP, segments of the (greater horseshoe bat) basilar membrane (I) suggest(ed) the possibility of *radial* vibration of structures on the scala media side of the basilar membrane. ... a radial vibration would give strong hair cell shearing even though the amplitude of basilar membrane vibration may not be great at this point. It is further suggested that such a vibration may be a feature of all cochleas ... although various ... structures ... are possible sites for such a resonator it could equally well be a property of the tectorial membrane. In either case a graded mechanical tuning over the whole frequency range would be required." In fact, further analysis of these data (Wilson and Bruns, 1983) did not support this interpretation. It is, however, interesting that the preliminary results of Khanna et al (this meeting) showing very little motion of the basilar membrane compared to the sharply-tuned motion in the outer hair cell region in apical guinea pig cochlea would appear to require a mechanism of this type.

Wilson, J.P. (1977) Towards a model for cochlear frequency analysis. In: Psychophysics and Physiology of Hearing. Eds. E.F. Evans and J.P. Wilson. Academic Press, London, pp. 115-124.
Wilson, J.P. and Bruns, V. (1983) Basilar membrane tuning properties in the specialised cochlea of the CF-bat, Rhinolophus ferrumequinum. Hearing Res., 10, 15-35.

ROBLES AND RUGGERO

Our data on chinchilla basilar membrane tuning (Robles et al., 1986) show a close match with the corresponding neural data (Fig. 11). Contrary to Allen's impression, variability of basilar membrane across well-tuned preparations was not large. In particular, standard deviations indicated in Fig. 11 for our five most sensitive cochleas were 2.5, 5.0, 3.8, 10.0 (at 2.8 kHz) and 6.0 dB. Other standard deviations (not shown in Fig. 11) ranged from 1.3dB to 6.0dB. The mean standard deviation for 20 frequencies between 200Hz and 11kHz was 4.0dB.

In regard to the comparison between neural and mechanical tuning curves, it is worth emphasizing that Fig. 11 of Robles et al. (1986) summarizes neural results for as many as 46 cochlear afferents with characteristic frequencies between 7 and 11 kHz. In contrast, individual ganglion-cell, cochlear-fiber or inner-hair-cell tuning curves were used in the comparisons of Sellick et al. (1982 and 1983) for the guinea pig and of Khanna and Leonard (1982) for the cat.

NEELY

Your criticism that "the active pressure source still ... has nothing to push against" in the model described by Neely and Kim (1986) is misleading. Given the level of simplification in this model, I see nothing wrong with having this force push against the inertial reference frame. The problem is that we don't really know how outer hair cell forces are coupled to the rest of Corti's organ.

KIM

I am in favour of your approach of subdividing the frequency-SPL space into nonlinear and linear regions. You estimate that the nonlinear-linear boundary is about 65-70 dB SPL. I suggest that the criterion of a phase shift in the pure tone response with increasing SPL is rather insensitive. The auditory nerve population data of Kim et al (1980) showed that propagated distortion products were absent at 24 dB SPL of two-tone stimuli and were present at 34 dB SPL. From this, I estimate that the boundary between nonlinear and linear behaviour of basilar membrane motion is about 30 dB SPL.

ON THE NATURE OF COCHLEAR RESONANCE

E. de Boer

Rm. D2-210, Academic Medical Centre, Amsterdam (Neth.)

Introduction - a stylized response

In this paper attention is paid to details of the shape of the response peak in cochlear models, in particular, the relation between response amplitude and phase. This is done for several types of cochlear model and the results are to be compared with experimental data on basilar membrane (BM) motion. The models used will be linear because a linear filter describes well the fundamental elements of cochlear filtering. As a matter of fact, for stimuli comprising a multitude of components, the cochlear response can be well predicted by a model containing a linear filter as its main frequency-selective element (de Boer and de Jongh, 1978).

Cochlear responses are well comparable to responses of filters that have a number of coincident pole pairs. This is true for neural responses (de Boer, 1979) and the same may be true for mechanical responses. The transfer function of a filter with n coincident pole pairs reads

$$F(x) = \frac{1}{(1 + i\epsilon x)^n} + \frac{1}{(1 + i\epsilon x + 2i\epsilon x_0)^n} \qquad (1)$$

where x is taken as a variable expressing the deviation from the point x_0 of maximum response. In a cochlear model x would be measured along the longitudinal direction of the basilar membrane (BM), the parameter ϵ expresses the scaling in the x domain. When in the complex-frequency plane the poles are close to the imaginary axis, we may retain only the first term of eq. (1) and so obtain a stylized response function. Defining the phase ϕ_0 by $\tan\phi_0 = \epsilon x$ and noting that the phase $\phi(x)$ of F(x) is -n times ϕ_0, we arrive at the following relation between the relative magnitude A(x) of F(x) and the phase $\phi(x)$:

$$\log A(x) = n \log \cos [\phi(x)/n] \qquad (2)$$

With the help of this relation we will be able to judge how well a measured response matches that of a filter with (the first term of) eq. (1) as its transfer function.

The type of response considered here was used by the author as a generalized descriptor of the cochlear response (de Boer, 1983). It was found that this response could only be realized by an active cochlear model in which the real part of the BM impedance Z(x) is negative over a certain region of x, basal to the point of maximal response. Quite apart from the (theoretical) question of activity, it is of interest to study whether this stylized response is in harmony with an actual cochlear model and with experimental data.

RESONANCE IN A SHORT-WAVE COCHLEAR MODEL

The cochlear model to be considered is the simplest possible short-wave model that exhibits a response peak. The dynamics of the BM will be described by a point-impedance function Z(x). In the present case Z(x) contains a constant real part R_o and a stiffness component that depends exponentially on x. The influence of BM mass will be neglected (cf. Steele and Taber, 1979-a,b). For constant frequency Z(x) is written as:

$$Z(x) = R_o - iX_o \exp(-\alpha x) \qquad (3)$$

where X_o is the stiffness reactance at x=o and α is the space constant of stiffness variation. For convenience we will place the response peak at x=0, hence X_o describes the magnitude of the reactance at the peak point. When we express R_o as a fraction δ of X_o, only two parameters remain, X_o and δ, and they have a simple interpretation.

The equation for short waves travelling in the direction of increasing x reads:

$$\frac{d}{dx} p(x) + [2wD / Z(x)]\, p(x) = 0 \qquad (4)$$

where p(x) is the fluid pressure at the BM, w the radian frequency and D the density of the cochlear fluid. The solution to eq. (4) is of the form:

$$p(x) = p_o \exp\left[-\int_0^x 2wD / Z(a)\, da\right] \qquad (5)$$

and we assume that this expression, with eq. (3) substituted for Z(x), contains only waves going in one direction. For the present case the integral can be evaluated analytically. The solution for the velocity v(x) of the BM can then be written in the form:

$$\log [v(x)/v_o] = -(N_o+1) \log (1+i\,\delta u) + \alpha x \qquad (6)$$

where v_o is introduced as a reference value, and N_o and u are given by $N_o=2wD/(\alpha X_o \delta)$ and $u=\exp(\alpha x)$. Equation (6) describes the course of the BM velocity in simple terms: for large and negative values of x the second term dominates and causes the response to increase with increasing x, whereas for large and positive x the first term dominates and the response decreases but this occurs at a much faster rate since N_o is generally much larger than 1. In between these extremes the velocity attains a maximum. A simple algebraic exercise reveals that the following relation must be obeyed when v(x) reaches its largest magnitude at x=0 (or, equivalently, u=1):

$$N_0 \delta^2 = 1 \quad (7)$$

In this way we are left with only one descriptor of the response, either N_0 or δ.

A peculiar feature of the solution given by eq. (6) is that the phase $\theta(x)$ of the response is $-(N_0+1)$ times the phase of $(1+i\,\delta u)$. Therefore, if we define $i\theta_0$ by $\tan i\theta_0 = \delta u$, and call the relative magnitude A(u), eq. (6) can be rewritten in a form that is similar to eq. (2):

$$\log A(u) = (N_0+1) \log \cos \theta_0 + \log \tan \theta_0 - \log \delta \quad (8)$$

It is clear that (N_0+1) plays the part of "the number of pole pairs" n in the equivalent response. The difference with eq. (2) resides in the second term.

In order to assess the importance of this difference, relation (8) is presented in graphical form in Fig. 1. The abscissa depicts the phase $\theta(u)$ of the response, with respect to the value at the peak point. Values of $x<0$ $(u>1)$ project to the left half of the figure. The ordinate shows A(u) on a decibel scale, normalized to 0 dB at the peak. The parameter of the curves is N_0, in view of relation (7) the values chosen are rather high, corresponding to acceptable values of the damping coefficient δ. Fig. 1 can be compared to later figures in this paper in which dashed lines are drawn that represent relation (2) for the stylized response. It can be concluded that the curve sets are indeed similar, that the influence of the asymmetry in Fig. 1 is only small and that, consequently, the stylized response is a reasonably good simulator of the response of a short-wave cochlear model. The agreement would be even better had we used a more elaborate model (e.g., one with BM mass included). Incidentally, we observe that the fundamental response properties of passive and active models are the same as well. That means that the physics is not fundamentally different.

TREATMENT OF EXPERIMENAL DATA

The use of the stylized response of eq. (1) was prompted by the properties of reverse-correlation (revcor) functions obtained from auditory-nerve responses to a noise stimulus. Fig. 2 gives an example, it refers to a fibre with a characteristic frequency (CF) of 2.5 kHz. The figure shows the relation between the magnitude and the phase of the spectrum associated with the revcor function. The layout of Fig. 2 is similar to that of Fig. 1 (frequency now plays the part formerly given to x or u). Note that the raw data are corrected for a delay that includes both the travelling time in the cochlea and the synaptic delay in the initiation of a nerve impulse. The dashed lines illustrate relation (2), for several values of n. The revcor data are seen to agree with the dashed curves for $n=4$ or higher. There is evidence that for fibres with higher CFs the equivalent value of n would be larger, up to 10.

The next step is to consider results of mechanical measurements of BM movements, especially the most recent ones (Sellick et al, 1983; Robles et al, 1986). This presents considerable problems, however. Due to experimental limitations data do not come in a form that can uniquely be interpreted or easily confronted with theory. As the elaborations of

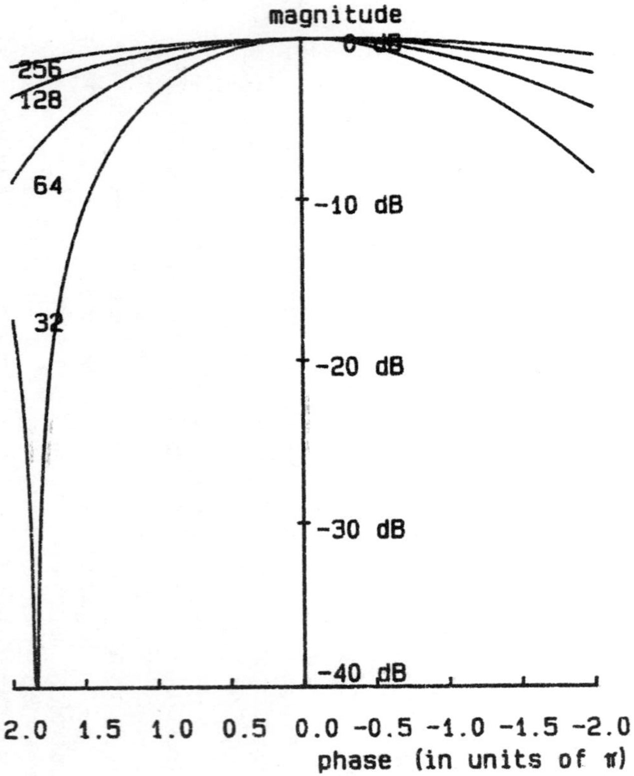

Fig. 1. Magnitude-phase relation for a mass-less short-wave model of the cochlea. Parameter: N_o.

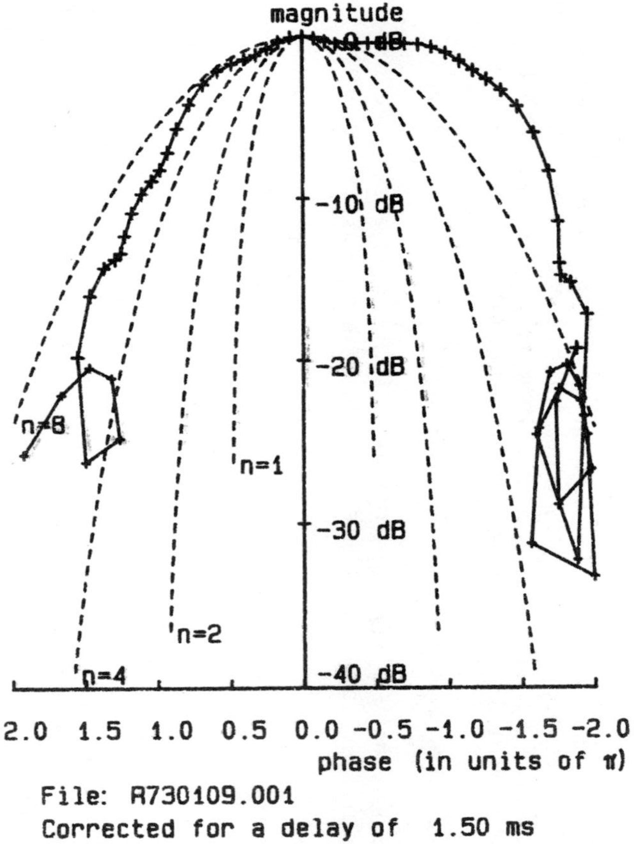

Fig. 2. Magnitude-phase relation for a revcor function.

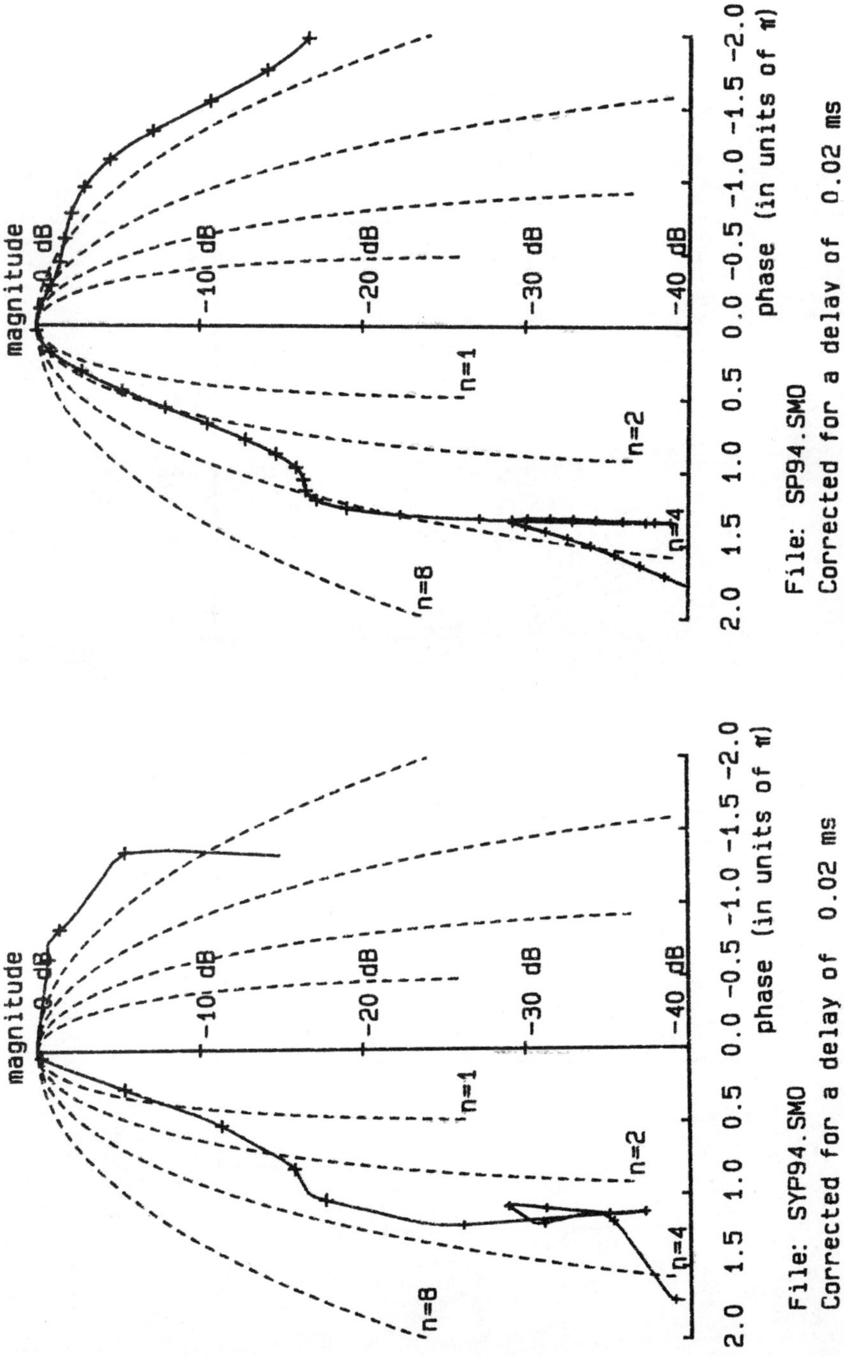

Fig. 3. Magnitude-phase relation for BM response data (see text). a (left): moderately smoothed. b (right): smoothed.

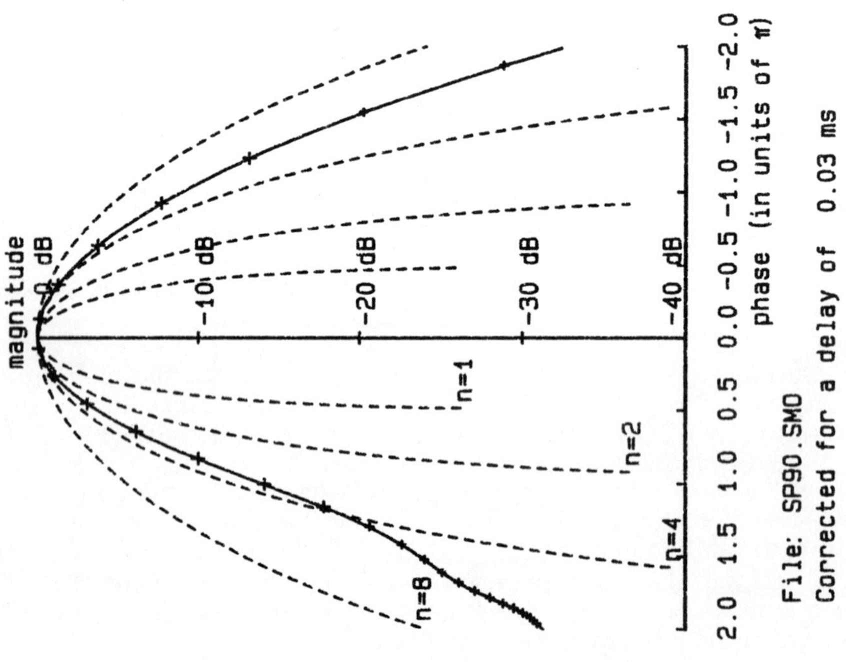

Fig. 4. Magnitude-phase relation for a BM response data set.

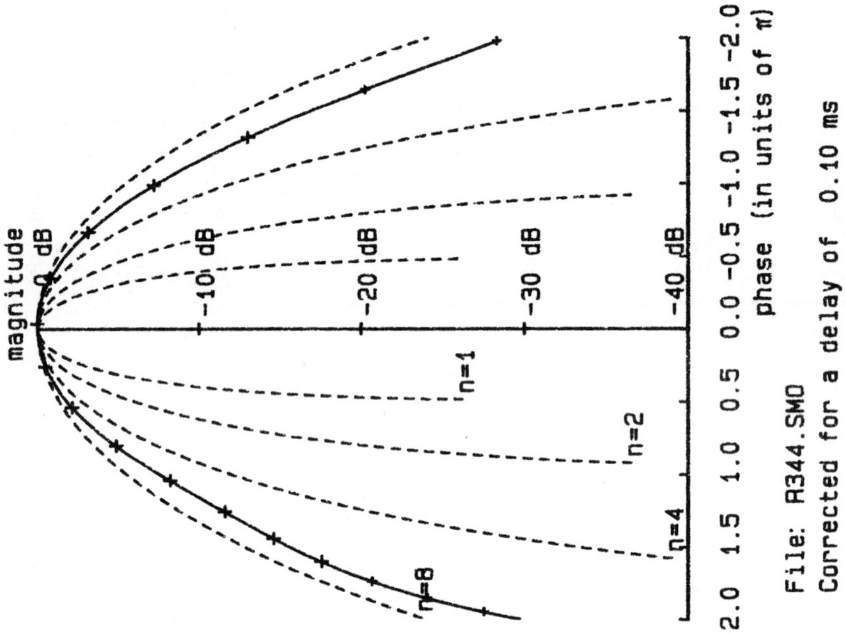

Fig. 5. Magnitude-phase relation for a BM response data set.

Diependaal et al. (1986, 1987) have shown, the data have to be interpolated and smoothed before they can be put to a useful purpose. First we present one example from the Sellick, Yates and Patuzzi paper (1983), these data are obtained in guinea pigs. Fig. 3-a shows the data in a moderately smoothed form so that the character of the original data points is retained. As before the figure only illustrates the peak region. Data are interpolated linearly (log amplitude and phase) and converted to complex numbers. A minute amount of smoothing is applied to the complex data values so as to remove sharp angles. As in the case of the revcor function, a correction is applied for a delay, this time only for a travelling-wave delay. Choosing a smaller delay produces a "wider" curve, a larger delay makes the shape of the curve unacceptable. In the form shown, about the largest value of the curvature at the top is obtained. If we allow for a lateral shift of the peak point, the equivalent n is of the order of 4. Fig. 3-b shows the same data but processed according to the cross-validation/smoothing method described by Diependaal et al. (1987). This method produces a very smooth set of data, this corresponds, however, to an impulse response with a shorter decay time than the original data which suggests that in the process the equivalent amount of damping has increased. Nevertheless, the magnitude-phase plot of Fig. 3-b shows clearly that the equivalent n has not decreased. The same property was found in all available and suitable data sets processed in this way. Fig. 4 shows a further example from results obtained in guinea pigs. Since smoothed and unsmoothed data yield comparable results only the former ones are presented. Fig. 5, finally, shows one result from the Robles, Ruggero and Rich (1986) paper. These data pertain to a lower frequency range and a different animal (the chinchilla). Despite the lower frequency range, the data also suggest a value of n of 4 or higher (up to 6).

Discussion - physical aspects

In this paper I have chosen to describe the peak region of cochlear response by a short-wave model without BM mass. A short-wave model is a logical choice in view of the local value of the wavelength, the only point is that it represents an extreme case. On the other hand, a long-wave model would not be possible without the inclusion of BM mass. In this respect it would not really be simpler.

The choice of a short-wave model has peculiar consequences when it comes to the physics of the structure. In the model treated the occurrence of a response peak is not connected with physical resonance in the BM. The response peak results from an interplay between the stiffness of the BM and the (distributed) mass involved in the propagating fluid wave. The nature of this interplay becomes clearer when we let the damping δ become smaller and go to zero. At each location the impulse response will then show an oscillation with a pronounced dispersion. This can be verified by taking the limit of eq. (6) for $\delta \to 0$ -- note that N_0 depends on δ too! Making δ nonzero produces a repartition along the BM so that a local response maximum arises.

Interpreted in a different way, this means that a fairly great deal of the movement pattern along the BM is involved in the formation of a peak. By the same token, it would be impossible to derive the parameters of a cochlear model in a unique way when the response is given. Difficulties on this point were experienced by Diependaal et al. (1986, 1987). In the present context we encounter another expression of the same issue: the stylized response of eq. (1) would indicate an active model (de Boer, 1983) whereas the reponse of a passive model is found to lead to a most similar relation between amplitude and phase (see Fig.1).

Acknowledgements

The author is greatly indebted to Rob J. Diependaal who provided the smoothed data used in the figures and to Max A. Viergever for help in many discussions.

References

De Boer, E. (1979). Travelling waves and cochlear resonance. In: Models of the Auditory System and Related Signal Processing Techniques (Eds: Hoke, M. and De Boer, E.) Scand. Audiol. Suppl. 9, pp. 17-33.

De Boer, E. (1983). No sharpening? A challenge for cochlear mechanics. J. Acoust. Soc. Am. 73, 567-573.

De Boer, E. and de Jongh, H.R. (1978). On cochlear encoding: Potentialities and limitations of the reverse-correlation technique. J. Acoust. Soc. Am. 63, 115-135.

Diependaal, R.J., Viergever, M.A. and De Boer, E. (1986). Are active elements necessary in the basilar membrane impedance? J. Acoust. Soc. Am. 80, 124-132.

Diependaal R.J., De Boer, E. and Viergever, M.A. (1987). Cochlear power flux as an indicator of mechanical activity. J. Acoust. Soc. Am. 82, 917-926.

Robles, L., Ruggero, M.A. and Rich, N.C. (1986). Mössbauer measurements of the mechanical response to single-tone and two-tone stimuli at the base of the chinchilla cochlea. In: Peripheral Auditory Mechanisms (Eds: Allen, J.B., Hall, J.L., Hubbard, A., Neely, S.T. and Tubis, A.) Springer Berlin, pp. 121-128.

Sellick, P.M., Yates, G.K. and Patuzzi, R. (1983). The influence of Mössbauer source size and position on phase and amplitude measurements of the guinea pig basilar membrane. Hear. Res. 10, 101-108.

Steele, C.R. and Taber, L.A. (1979-a). Comparison of WKB and finite difference calculations for a two-dimensional cochlear model. J. Acoust. Soc. Am. 65, 1001-1006.

Steele, C.R. and Taber, L.A. (1979-b). Three-dimensional model calculations for guinea pig cochlea. J. Acoust. Soc. Am. 65, 1007-1111.

Comments and Discussion

LEWIS

When frequency plays the part given to x, the left-hand term of Equation 1 has an interesting similarity to the model proposed by Fuortes and Hodgkin (1964) to account for temporal responses of invertebrate photoreceptors. In that case, the putative transfer function was given 8 to 10 coincident poles on the negative real axis. Shifting the poles away from the origin provided a reasonably accurate description of the effects of light adaptation. Because the only energy storage elements they invoked were capacitance-like (Lewis, 1988), Fuortes and Hodgkin were forced to include active processes in the model. Elementary network synthesis (Guillemin, 1957) tells us that passive processes involving only resistance-like (dissipative) elements and capacitance-like elements must exhibit *simple poles* (no two poles can occur at the same point). The same thing is true of passive processes involving capacitance-like elements and inertia-like elements but no dissipative elements, the only difference being that the simple poles of the latter must lie on the imaginary axis rather than the negative real axis. In both cases, the poles can be squeezed arbitrarily close to one another (short of coincidence) by means of arbitrarily large impedance mismatches. Passive processes involving all three kinds of elements can have any number of coincident poles, the only restriction being that any poles squarely on the imaginary axis still must be simple (the critically-damped second-order system provides an example of coincident poles on the negative real axis). Thus, by itself, the fact that a response seems to be reproduced by a transfer function with coincident poles bears no implication regarding the presence of active processes. On the other hand, conventional definitions of passivity aside, the second law of thermodynamics implies that even simple poles, squarely on the imaginary axis, can be realized only with augmentation of signal energy by active elements. It may be interesting to note that a passive model with an infinite number of poles (a uniform diffusion process of finite length) provided a better fit to both the temporal responses and light adaptation in Fuortes and Hodgkin's photoreceptor.

Fuortes, M.G.F. and Hodgkin, A.L. (1964) Changes in time scale and sensitivity in the ommatidia of Limulus. J. Physiol. 172: 239-263.

Guillemin, E.A. (1957) Network Synthesis. Wiley, N.Y. Table 1, p. 66.

Lewis, E.R. (1988) Tuning in the bullfrog ear. Biophys. J. 53: 441-447.

DE BOER

Let me stress (once more) that we have to distinguish well between a (linear) electrical network in general and a network designed to simulate a model of the cochlea. The elaborations of Dr. Lewis apply first of all to general networks, and they don't solve any of our present problems. In short, given the response of a realizable network, that network can be synthesized from passive elements or from a combination of passive and active elements. There is nothing in the given response that dictates the choice.

For 'cochlear-model networks' this is quite different. Certain responses cannot be realized by a cochlear-model network with only passive elements. (Note: I am restricting myself to the type of model described in the paper.) For instance, a response corresponding to eq. (1) leads to a locally active model. A slightly different response, however, may very well correspond to a passive model. I show in the paper that a strictly passive model leads to a (A, O) plot that is of the same class as that of a locally active model. I could not have expected that processing of BM response data should lead to the choice between a passive and a locally active model.

EVANS

I agree, from my Revcor data, that gammatones may be a good approximation for Revcors for cochlear fibres with CFs above 1 kHz. Do you agree that these, however, cannot be good appoximations for fibres of CFs of about 0.5 kHz and below (Evans, this volume)?

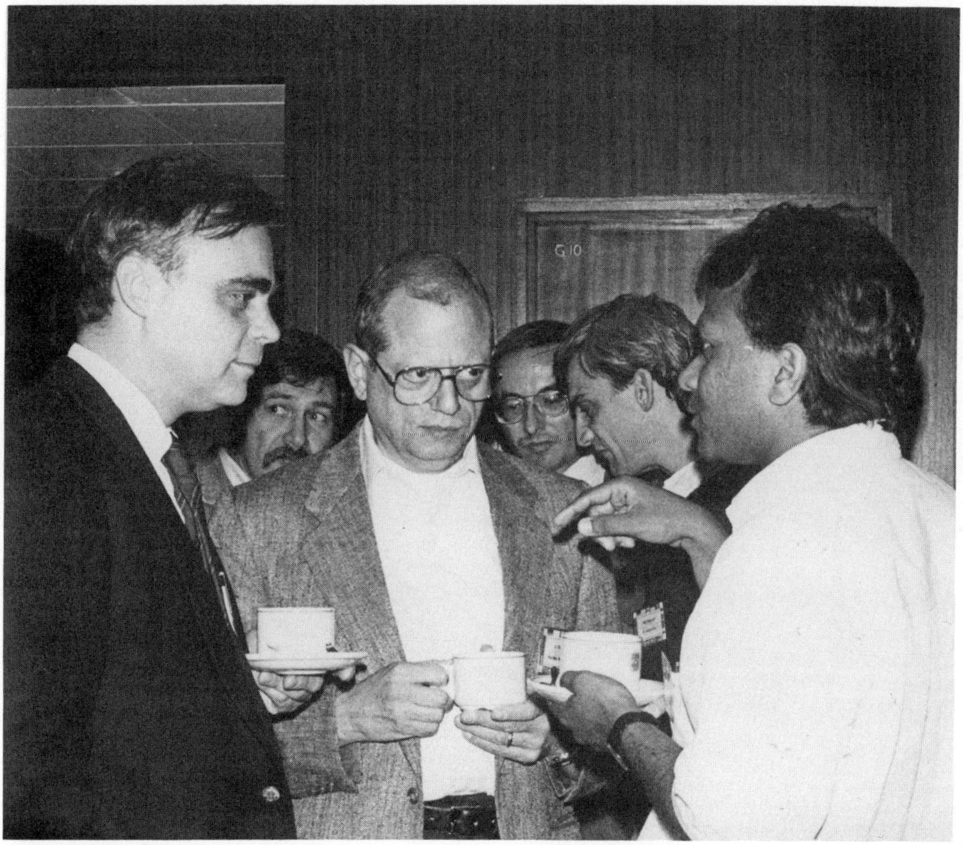

J.B. Allen, P. Dallos, A. Tubis, I.J. Russell, R.B. Patuzzi and S. Puria

9. DISCUSSION SESSION II

DISCUSSION SESSION II

Chairman - Sir James Lighthill

This tape transcript has not been checked by all contributors. Whilst all speakers knew that the workshop was being recorded, the decision to publish the discussion sessions came after the meeting. In view of this, and the spontaneous nature of the discussion, the dialogues reported below may not represent the actual or considered or final view of the named participants on any matter. The editors thank the participants for supporting (or at least tolerating) the publication of this debate, and apologise for any inaccuracies in transcription.

LIGHTHILL We now begin our general discussion of mathematical modelling. Those of you that are not in the subject, may feel that the mathematical modellers are all fighting each other. You may feel like asking "What are they doing for us experimentalists and physiologists?" But with respect, we have to argue that it *is* in the interests of the entire community working in this field that we develop some mathematical models because inevitably the amount of sound knowledge of *in vivo* mechanical properties is limited. There is always, at any point in time, too small a knowledge of these properties. Also the number of positions in the cochlea where the Mössbauer sources can be placed, and the number of other types of observations that can be carried out, means there is a limited amount of knowledge of *in vivo* response to pure tones. Somehow we have to extrapolate and it helps to have mathematical models to guide you in making that extrapolation.

I'd like to make another point. It's an old one. An aweful lot of superficially different models give a superficially good account of tuning curves. I think this is something that has struck all of us for over a decade. I did an analysis and discovered that the models which do give a superficially good account of tuning curves, all have one property in common, and that is what I call "critical layer absorbtion" which is just jargon for saying that the energy travels along, and then comes to a halt, at the best place and the oscillation then goes into quite a large amplitude!

I believe energy considerations are of great value [in helping us determine the form of the travelling wave envelope]. Obviously mass is conserved too [and Jont Allen in his presentation, used the principle of conservation of mass, to make some deductions about the phase changes in the travelling wave envelope, that must be associated with changes in travelling wave peak vibration. An upward deflection of the basilar membrane at one place involves a displacement of incompressible fluid which must then be balanced by a downward displacement elsewhere. The effect of nonlinearity at the peak must then be associated with modifications of the travelling wave at other places even though vibration there might be linear. The problem with depending on the "conservation of mass" principle here, is that it's not so awefully useful when you've got the basilar membrane going into such a "wavy" state [i.e., many very short waves within the peak envelope] because the integrated mass can still be conserved [within the peak, without adjustments to the wave elsewhere] even though you have a large [displacement] amplitude.

But energy, of course, has to be conserved in a passive system and energy flow may be very valuable in a model like - for instance - Kim and Neely's. What he is potentially saying is that instead of energy being dissipated by viscosity the active process is producing a sort of negative resistance which cancels that out.

If you want to have a simple interpretation of the [travelling wave pattern] in terms of energy flow, you want to use the concept of energy per unit length - of course the energy is half kinetic energy and half the potential energy of the displacement of the membrane. You can say that

the energy per unit length is **E**
and it is flowing with velocity **U = dw/dk** (keeping **x** constant)
where **w** is the the frequency and **k** the wavenumber
the rate of energy flowing towards the apex is then **UE** per second

It is this velocity, **U**, that is slowing down as the energy goes along slower and slower, and piles up more and more energy into unit length at the best place. So you can say that the rate of change of energy depends on the local damping coeficient, **D**, so that the rate of dissipation of vibrational energy per unit length of the cochlea will be **DE**.

We know the value of **D** very accurately because it's all produced in thin boundary layers which are about 10μm in thickness, near the basilar membrane itself, and any other membrane that's vibrating.

Equations based on this can be easily solved. We have

$$d(UE)/dx = -DE$$

$$\text{giving} \quad E(x) = \frac{U(0)E(0)}{U(x)} \exp[-\int_0^x Ddx/U]$$

That integral has a simple interpretation, because **dx/U** is the time taken for the energy to travel a distance **dx**. During that time the proportion of energy lost is **D** times **dx/U**.

In all these problems with critical layer absorption, the energy propagation velocity [graph against position] comes into the axis tangentially. It falls to zero rather steeply, and of course that's what causes the amplitude to rise. The energy goes up like **1/U** and comes to a peak at the best place. The peak is finite because the integral of the exponential increases without limit, as you go along: the integral of **Ddx/U** increases as **U** tends to zero. So **E** initially increases steeply but finally plumets to zero. That is true in all the models that produce good tuning curves, whether they are one dimensional, or two dimensional, or three dimensional. Dr Diependaal said that he preferred to do an accurate calculation in the cochlea, but he was producing results that were very close to those produced by short wave asymptotics, high frequency asymptotic. Charles Steele has shown how you can do high frequency asymptotics very efficiently for a one, two, or three dimensional model.

We want good "local bridging" between *in vivo* mechanical properties and *in vivo* responses to pure tones. For example, we want to distinguish between the arcuate and pectinate zone of the basilar membranes. We want to take into account what's happening in the neighbourhood of the outer hair cells. So at first sight, energy flow is a useful concept for these one degree-of-freedom models. I think that would include Kim and Neely's type of model - it's just that the **D** instead of being relatively large - i.e., although the absolute value may be small it's not small enough to prevent the peak being somewhat limited in its height - **D** is reduced in these models by the active process in a nonlinear way so as to allow the peak to be higher. I think it's a reasonable interpretation of any one degree-of-freedom model - so I'm just saying again - energy *can* be a useful conserved quantity for modelling.

However, the moment you go to a model like Dr Kolston's and Max Viergever's, energy conservation is not sufficient because everything depends on how much energy there is in the arcuate zone and how much in the pectinate zone, and the same will be true if you have resonating tectorial membranes - i.e., you can't be satisfied with a *single* energy, you've got to consider the separate energies in the two main modes of your model.

I'm trying to use, in terms of simple physical concepts, an analysis of how we can deal with modelling in the future. I believe that with one dimensional models one can easily classify them in the way I've described. For example, you can express the energy flow as a group velocity - the slope of the curve of wave velocity against wavenumber - and you can analyse that term in terms of a frequency which depends on the partition inertia and the fluid inertia, and take into account that the fluid inertia gets less and less in those "little bits" of the waves near short waves, where less and less of the fluid is actually taking part in the wave motion. The fluid inertia becomes less, and that's what causes the dependancy of frequency against wave number to curve over, and the group velocity to tend to zero. All that is feasible either for a linear model as deBoer showed us in his short wave asymmptotic model, or a nonlinear one, which is simply modifying the behaviour of the damping coefficient. But one needs to go to a more complicated analysis if one is to have a two degree-of-freedom model involving tectorial membrane, or a separate treatment of the two parts of the basilar membrane.

These are just a few thoughts, and I wonder what the rest of the meeting feels. And what about the future? Prof Steele has done more than anyone else to look at the local, complex three dimensional model.

STEELE I would say that even in those cases, there is still one propagated wave. Because the wavelength is getting short, then the mode in cross section changes, but still because there is one wave, the notion of the energy propagation is still a useful concept.

LIGHTHILL Yes. But then the amount of build up of amplitude *is* limited because whatever other mechanisms of damping there are, viscosity is always there, and it does produce a limit to the peak doesn't it?

STEELE Yes it does, but then even if you take zero for the viscosity, you will not get an infinite response! Instead you get a slow decay wave; short waves, but a slow decay. So I would not quite agree with the statement that it's *only* the viscosity which is a limit.

LIGHTHILL No, but nevertheless viscosity is *a* limit to how high the peak can be, and to that extent, Neely and Kim's suggestion that the nonlinear mechanism produces an effective reduction in the damping, is an attractive one. But I know there are several others who say the nonlinear element is *not* applied to the damping - the real part of the impedance - but is applied partly to the imaginary part. What do you think about that?

STEELE Well, I've been very much concerned about what the outer hair cell could be doing [see Discussion Session I]. I think the phase is very crucial. What is the phase of the force imparted by the outer hair cell, and it's relation to the input force on the stereocilia? This phase will make a difference whether it's positive damping, negative damping, or a change in stiffness. As a speculation, I think this mode will change along the cochlea.

PATUZZI We know that there *is* a contractile process of some sort but we don't yet have any estimate of what the phase delay is. As to the frequency governing that process - there are at least three sites where phase shifts could occur, but we are not in a position to make any statment about what causes that role-off with frequency.

LIGHTHILL No, indeed.

KOLSTON Is it a good time to tidy up some definitions? In our paper we said the OCAP model "did not have active processes" and used the term active to mean energy production by the cochlea. But other people use "active process" to mean hair cell motility. The problem there is that it's not true in the theoretical sense. So perhaps when we talk about the outer hair cell increasing the motion, we should use a term like "cochlear amplifier" as did Hallowell Davis, and reserve the term active process for when the force generation actually reduces the amount of damping.

PATUZZI The problem with that definition is that the tuned circuit would also be an amplifier!

KOLSTON That's right. So cochlear amplifier is probably not the best term.

LIGHTHILL Just the fact that the outer hair cell is vibrating doesn't mean it's active at all! I mean it could be vibrating passively in response to something. We know this isn't true, but the fact that it's vibrating is not an argument for calling it active.

KOLSTON That's right, but generally I think most people here would accept as fact, that the inclusion of the outer hair cell *does* increase the motion [of the basilar membrane]. To call that an active process is to presume that the increased motion is caused by the decrease in the resistive part of the impedance. That is not necessarily the case - so is there a better term than "active"?

PATUZZI To a physiologist that's not too much of a problem because we know that if you shut off the metabolic supply, the thing goes dead! That's pretty active to a physiologist.

EVANS Yes. We called it a "second filter" some time ago! And if I might say we had in mind the mechanisms that are being considered here. I think many people have not understood that. If you look at Evans and Wilson (1973) you will see that our favoured mechanism *was* positive feedback and we had a little evidence for it.

LIGHTHILL Well now, if a child is on a swing, and is getting herself going, then no doubt the impedance she is putting in, has an imaginary part and a negative real part, but nobody cares *what* the imaginary part is - it doesn't really get the swing going at all. It's only the negative resistance which gets the swing moving, and that may well be true of the outer hair cells also.

ALLEN As far as this term "active system" - my understanding of the use of the term active would imply that in Davis's model of the hair cell, where you have a parametric change in the electrical conductance at the top of the cell - well in my book that's an active process! The negative [mechanical] resistance of a hair cell is active also. I think they are all active processes and it's an OK term to use. The problem is, it is not very specific.

KOLSTON Then if you assume that it's the conductance of the cell that changes, to get energy....

ALLEN No, [I wasn't bringing in energy yet], this is for an *inner* hair cell. Just to change the electrical conductance parametrically with displacement - that's an active process.

KIM But Jont, mechanical real part is the point at issue - the hair cell *may* change it's electrical conductance as a result of hair bundle displacement but if it does not do anything to mechanical impedance, then the mechanical system would remain a passive system.

ALLEN But it's still an active process!

VIERGEVER Well let's suppose that we have membrane motion in some jelly substance with a high viscosity, instead of the perilymph, this also influences the motion but I wouldn't call that an active process!

ALLEN Well I think that's a linear process, whereas I think this other is a nonlinear process where a parameter in a system changes with another parameter. If you wrote down an electrical network of that thing, you would have to have a controlled source to represent that element, and once you put in a controlled source, then it's an active process!

KOLSTON Well that's not true because you can replace postive resistance by an active source so long as there is a correct phase relationship between the velocity and the force produced by that active source, and it still absorbs energy - it doesn't generate energy. Force generation is not the same as energy generation.

NEELY If you put sources in the model, that makes it an active model!

KOLSTON OK, but that's *your* definition of active. It's not the network definition.

DEBOER This discussion leads nowhere. In one case we have state variables in the network and we have parameters. If parameters depend on state network parameters, then we have a nonlinear system like the one Allen has been refering to. If we are talking about active, then in fact what we are thinking is that we have state variables which depend on other state variables. Then you can have a linear system which contains active elements but is as a whole, passive. It does not oscillate spontaneously.

LIGHTHILL Well obviously it's possible for the outer hair cells to be exerting forces at phases in the cycle where they do no work. In practice they will probably be expending energy, although to no effect, as far as getting the oscillation going, is concerned.

ALLEN You can take a negative resistor and put a positive resistor of a greater value in series with it and it's still an active system, right? It won't do anything interesting, but it's still an active system.

DEBOER You can still separate it into an active and a passive system, but when you are looking at the outside - you can't distinguish!

PATUZZI But in terms of the physiology that we're interested in, you can distinguish between them.

DEBOER Yes, so you have to talk about locally active systems, which on the whole are passive, or you might talk about other systems which are, what I call "pan-active" - containing active and unstable elements everywhere.

LIGHTHILL Well I deliberately suggested that we talk about *one* degree of freedom systems, and I think we've done that to some effect. I think we understand a bit about the different types of active process that can apply in a one degree-of-freedom system. But do we want now to talk about the different types of two degree-of-freedom systems, including the ones involving a separate tectorial membrane vibration, or a separate vibration to different parts of the basilar membrane? There's a suggestion there, that there is an exchange of energy between the two modes. This of course is typical in the mechanics of systems with two degrees-of-freedom - with nonlinear processes acting with an exchange of energy between the two modes. Specifically, there is the proposal that the main basilar membrane mode, in the case of the tectorial membrane theories, or the pectinate mode in the case of the Kolston-Viergever theory - that the main mode is what builds up initially, and then it feeds energy through the stereocilia of the outer hair cells into the other mode, which then goes into a sharper resonance at the expense of the main mode. I think I'm right in saying that that is characteristic of both those two degree-of-freedom theories. I wonder if there are any comments on that?

KOLSTON Yes, I agree that the OCAP model is really the type of second filter that Ted Evans was talking about. Instead of being a mechanical to neural second filter, it is a mechanical to mechanical filter with broad tuning of the pectinate zone [feeding] to the sharp tuning on the arcuate zone. Of course it might turn out to be complete nonesense - but I think it's something that's worth looking at.

LIGHTHILL Yes, and I think similarly, with the tectorial membrane models, although we don't have Joe Zwislocki with us, to comment on that.

ALLEN Well could I just say that - everybody's going around making these incredible statements that with a passive system you can't match tuning curves and you can't match threshold sensitivities - and they're just ignoring the fact that I've done it! I only did it at 4kHz and it needs a lot more work, and it does match some bandwidths..... I'm not happy with it and I don't think you should be either, but it *is* a passive system with a resonant tectorial membrane, and it does a reasonable job of matching tuning curves!

VIERGEVER Right - but not matching the mechanical displacement...

KOLSTON ... which is the hardest thing to match!

ALLEN It doesn't match the sheering displacement, but I'm trying to match *neural* data.

ASHMORE I must say I am a little bit confused about the discussion of the number of degrees-of-freedom. As a physiologist, it seems there is an infinite number of implimentations of a three-dimensional model - I mean when you start peering down at the cochlea, *everything* is wobbling about! Why should we draw the line at *two* degrees-of-freedom? One idle thought is that one of the features of many of the illustrative diagrams, that have surfaced during this workshop, to describe cochlear mechanics, have quite obviously been just radial sections of the organ of Corti. It strikes me that an important dimension that is being ignored is what's coming *out* of the flat plain of the figures. For example outer hair cells aren't necessarily in a radial plain they're at a tilt. I came here to some extend expecting the cochlear modellers to tell me what happens up and down the length of the organ of Corti.

LIGHTHILL Well can we just clarify your first point, Dr Ashmore. The fact that everything is wobbling about, is not incompatible with there being just one degree of freedom. [The question is] - is everything wobbling about in phase - that's what you'd expect with one degree-of-freedom - or are different parts of the cochlear partition wobbling about in an apparently independent way? - *that* would be more than one degree-of-freedom.

ASHMORE Well that's a question which can be addressed experimentally, and to which Zenner's group has addressed itself. The rapid answer is that I don't think we know at present, what are the actual modes of vibration of the organ of Corti. But even if modellers could direct us into thinking what *might be* the critical modes - then that would be a very constructive thing to do.

LIGHTHILL Absolutely - and Dr Khanna's paper was really suggesting that the pectinate zone of the basilar membrane is not vibrating very much near the characteristic frequency, whilst the outer hair cells are - and this is encouraging to people who would like to interpret cochlear mechanics in terms of more than one-degree-of-freedom models. But as I pointed out to Dr Kolston, it's not sufficient to just say that these two halves are vibrating completely independently because they *are* connected, so whatever the *true* pair of modes are - if he is going to use two modes - one of them will involve mainly the pectinate zone, but with some modest motion of the arcuate zone, and the other mode the other way round. So if one's going to two modes, then they ought at least to be mechanically feasible modes, of a structure which certainly is "all joined up". Does Prof Steele have any views on that?

STEELE I agree with you!

KOLSTON I think that what this whole discussion shows, is that we really don't know what's going on in the cochlea at all! ... I hear some people are disagreeing with me, but there *are* a lot of things we don't know, and we shouldn't take the active process as an energy production process [as proved].

LIGHTHILL We would still argue that we need models all the more if the data are insufficient - that at least is a credible argument isn't it?

KOLSTON We should do more experiments!

LIGHTHILL That's right, we need both, but there are limitations, as we keep hearing, to the experiments that can be done, and you've got to make progress on both fronts haven't you - which is probably why we shall argue in the business meeting that we shall need another meeting pretty soon!

VIERGEVER Well, what I think should come out of models, is suggestions for experiments which disprove certain model hypotheses, rather than experiments which support them.

KOLSTON There should be more liaison between modellers and those who do experimental work.

LIGHTHILL Yes - I've always thought, as a theoretical fluid dynamicist, that the most valuable thing I could do was, to put up plausible theories which the experimentalists would be tempted to try to shoot down, and very often they produced their best work then. I think theoreticians must be conscious that this is one of their very valuable qualities. It's more interesting to put all your energy into an experiment if you shoot down, say the famous Jont Allen theory or something!

MOUNTAIN I would like to add something to that - as someone who sort of straddles both domains. I think that the biggest problem that the mathematical modellers have, is that they rarely put their work in a form that's easily intelligible to physiologists!

SEVERAL PARTICIPANTS Here! here!

EVANS I would like to go a little bit further and say that it would be enormously helpful if the modellers would point out the weak points in their models, as well as always plugging the strong points!

KOLSTON That's human nature, unfortunately!

ALLEN I wish that the experimentalists would [also point out the weaknesses of their results]!!!

EVANS Ah! Well that's more easily done!

KOLSTON Yes, and there's so few weak points anyway!!!

PICKLES Well, I just wish modellers would come together and say at least, what they agree on. If they said, "Well at least that's water under the bridge, and now we'll start worrying about the rest" then at least the physiologists would have something to build on!

LIGHTHILL Well let's just see if there *is* anything we agree on! Don't we all agree now, that there is *something* nonlinear in the data?

ALLEN Yes, and I thought we all agreed on conservation of mass!

LIGHTHILL Yes we all agree on that too, and as you put it yourself, that's a case of a certain integral at the oval window being equal to a certain integral over the basilar membrane, and I think none of us doubt that - it's just that an integral of a linear quantity can be quite small, even when the [localised] amplitude of vibration is large, because the integration is over many wavelengths.

PATUZZI Following Jonathan Ashmore's point about the longitudinal direction, we've now got quite a bit of experimental evidence supporting the view that if there is an active [un]damping process it should be limited over a certain region. First off, it shouldn't be a point process - that doesn't seem consistent with the suppression contours we come up with. Secondly, from Rob Diependaal's work and others, it doesn't look from the model, that the vibration should be that critically dependent on just exactly where you get this negative damping process, if it exists. So I think what we'll be having in the next few years, is a series of experiments to see if we can narrow down the range of where this supposed active process really exists, and in view of this, there is an old experiment in our laboratory - it's known as the "poke" experiment, which is quite relevant to this. I think it was Bredberg, Johnstone, Cody, and Robertson opened up cochleas - poked a needle though the basilar membrane into the organ of Corti, to make a very punctate lesion, then sewed the animals up to let them recover, and then went and recorded the compound action potential. They found it had very punctate loss of threshold. Moreover, the punctate loss of threshold seemed to match very well the place-frequency map that we know of. So it didn't look as though they were knocking out a negative damping location that was much displaced from the place for that frequency. Certainly some of the models that I've found most useful over the past few years, address specifically the issue - if there is a negative damping function - where is it along the length of the cochlea?

LIGHTHILL That's for a particular frequency? I mean when we are listening to sound - it must be applying everywhere mustn't it? - because it's applying in the places for all the different frequencies.

NEELY I think what Rob is refering to - and not everyone agrees with it - is a model of the active process where the energy put in, not only compensates for the viscous damping, but actually over-compensates over some region.

LIGHTHILL You mean at a fixed point - independent of frequency?

NEELY No, not independent, it's dependent on frequency.

LIGHTHILL I see, frequency dependent, so at any one time, when you're listening to *all* frequencies as we are at the moment, its applying all along.

KIM That's correct.

LIGHTHILL I thought Pujol's paper was very interesting - that when you concentrate on a visual task, the active process switches off! What do you think of that?

PATUZZI It may be so, but the idea that these irregularies and where the spontaneous [otoacoustic] emission comes in, is also very important from an observational point of view. It also ties in well with Dr Zwicker's models. His point was that - the point at which you get oscillation may not be the place where you have the irregularity. I think the important point though is that we still don't know if it should be a frequency limit, or a place limit, or a nonlinear limit [to the active process]. I think the best information we'll get will come from nonlinear active models.

LIGHTHILL Well I have to point out that if you take a point where the energy is whizzing past very fast, then changing the damping makes very little difference. I mean changing the damping is most important fairly near the best place isn't it?

KOLSTON Yes, because otherwise it's the stiffness part of the basilar membrane which dominates.

PATUZZI It may dominate but that does mean that you can get energy in...

LIGHTHILL It's not so easy to get it in [there] when the energy is whizzing by - it's much easier when the energy is slowing down and the system is much more responsive to the negative damping.

PARTICIPNT You mentioned Pujol's observations - I don't think they're all that suprising because the work in the 1960's showed that there's probably a very strong innervation of the cochlear nucleus, by the reticular activated system. So you are probably affecting the overall feedback loop, and it's probably a level-of-arousal thing.

LIGHTHILL I suppose so, yes..

EVANS I think that's a very dangerous [assumption to make]. The 1960's stuff has been largely discredited in relation to the turning of the animal's head, and I think you are rather overstating Remy Pujol's position on this, in that the active mechanism isn't "cut off". And don't forget that in the sharp tuning measurements most of us make, the animal certainly is not attending to *us*; its patently asleep, and the active processes are still very active!

PARTICIPANT Well the experiment I was referring to, was where they put in a radioactive glycogen that's taken up, but not metabolised, so that you can look [at the activity level]. They electrically stimulated the reticular activating system, sacrificed the animal very quickly, and they found out that the metabolism was much greater in the cochlear nucleus. That doesn't depend on head angle.

LIGHTHILL Right, now if we can put the question back from the modellers to the experimenters - it seems to me, it would be enormously helpful if more centres would measure the mechanical properties of the tectorial membrane. I found this was one of the things which is most in dispute at this meeting. There are those who would swear that that it's almost like rubber and marvellously elastic and resonant, and those who would swear it's a gel-like, wishy-washy thing with enormously high [internal] damping to its movements. Wouldn't it be an enormous help, to getting an understanding, if we could get a definitive answer to that question?

ALLEN Yes!!!

MOUNTAIN Can I ask a question with my physiologist's hat on for a moment, but still using the terminology of mathematics and engineering? In terms of modelling the current measurements of basilar membrane displacement, it seems to me that there must be a consensus, even though people have used different models, that the point impedance of the basilar membrane must be modelled at least by a three or fourth order system, no matter how you bring about that higher order system. Would you say that's a consensus?

SEVERAL PARTICIPANTS Yes!

MOUNTAIN OK, so that's our task - the physiologist's task - of going through the various ways of getting a higher order system, and I guess what I'd like to see next [from the modellers] is a little summary. We've heard about the resonant tectorial membrane theory, the [arcuate-pectinate theory].....

LIGHTHILL Yes. When you say a higher order system - do you mean what I was referring to as "more degrees-of-freedom"....?

MOUNTAIN Well you don't necessarily have to have more *mechanical* degrees of freedom - it may be electrical.

LIGHTHILL No, quite, they are all degrees-of-freedom.

MOUNTAIN ..so I'm thinking of the order of the system in the context that normally you would think of - a transfer function for the impedance. Perhaps even a third order system, which is not the kind of thing people think about when they talk about two resonant systems, might be enough. We may only need one more order, and not two more, which would give a fourth order system.

ALLEN Dave, when you say this, are you saying that the basilar membrane and neural responses are the same or different?

MOUNTAIN I chose my words carefully! I'm only concerned at this stage about the basilar membrane. It seems though, that people are saying that it's easier to model neural tuning curves than the basilar membrane..

ALLEN But these system are going to behave very differently, I believe.

MOUNTAIN - that's why I chose my words carefully. I think the basilar membrane is something that is a step before the neural tuning curve, and already at the level of the basilar membrane, if we need a third or fourth order point impedance, in order to accurately model the data, then that's an important concensus for those people who are trying to model the mechanics of the basilar membrane.

VIERGEVER But not in a one degree-of-freedom system ...

LIGHTHILL No, if you're allowed to put in a little bit of negative resistance, and so on, I think you can get away with a second-order system.

MOUNTAIN But Steve Neely had to make the negative resistance, frequency dependent, and so that's adding another order to the system!

NEELY Yes, in the negative resistance model, you need the other degree of freedom to make the place frequency-dependent.

KOLSTON But, is what you're saying David, that we need perhaps a two and a half degree-of-freedom model - so we shouldn't go and opt for two, in terms of orders of magnitude..?

MOUNTAIN Yes, one of those degrees of freedom might be the voltage in a hair cell, which you can't get out mechanically, and so [the order of the system] is not necessarily going to be in even numbers.

LIGHTHILL Now some of this discussion should be about otoacoustic emissions, and really they ought to be tied in with the nonlinear modelling. Surely it's quite clear that the same models ought to be producing evoked otoacoustic emissions shouldn't they David?

KEMP Well, my feelings are that the main contribution of otoacoustic emissions has been to show that there is something in there that can produce energy, and that point was made a long time ago. I don't like to see modellers trying [at this stage of cochlear modelling] to produce delayed emissions of [say] a particular latency, because they're dependent on [system irregularities] - they are going to be the icing on the cake of the perfect model! I don't feel it's necessary to bring them in [yet].

LIGHTHILL Yes, but at least you're invoking the evoked emissions to show there's something active there?

KEMP Well I'm not sure you finally prove that point, except when the whole system's oscillating, and even then that didn't convince Jont!

EVANS Presumably Kolston's model can't cope with spontaneous emissions?

KOLSTON What I'm saying is that there is a distinction between the way the cochlea behaves, for the formulation of the travelling wave and the tuning, and how it behaves for the generation of otoacoustic emissions. I accept that the generation of emissions proves that there is energy being added but I'm also saying that we shouldn't right now tie that directly into the activity that is involved in the formation of the tuning curve.

LIGHTHILL But the emissions require a physiologically active system don't they, so there must be something being generated....

VIERGEVER Sure - at least locally!

NEELY ...and lets' not forget the lesson we learned from Prof Gold - that it makes a lot of sense to put an amplifier before your detector.

LIGHTHILL Absolutely!

KOLSTON You see, one of the big problems with active models, in terms of energy producing models, is one of stability....

PATUZZI Maybe that's why we've got an efferent system!

SEVERAL SPEAKERS [Express discontent with this statement].

WIT In combination with a nonlinearity, it's no problem at all!

SEVERAL SPEAKERS I don't see what you mean!

KOLSTON I don't either!

ALLEN But Kolston doesn't have a nonlinear model.

WIT Well that's his problem!

LIGHTHILL ...and then physiologically we are never seeing a breakdown of stability, even with a spontaneous emission, or is this a counter example?

KEMP Well [the generation of spontaneous emissions] represents a movement to a state with a degree of instability, but eventually it stabilises - the system doesn't explode like a computer model!

LIGHTHILL No, it doesn't explode...

JONES ...it's a stable periodic state.

KOLSTON But perhaps, if there is a direct correlation between these irregularities - in terms of the number of rows of outer hair cells - and the generation of the emissions, then that means that we shouldn't use the emissions as justification for their involvement in activity, to produce cochlear tuning.

LIGHTHILL No, exactly, and I think David Kemp emphasises irregularities as being very important for the generation of emissions, don't you?

KEMP Yes, for the evoked stimulus frequency emissions, irregularity seems to play a part, but for distortion product emissions [that's not the case] but [then] they don't say anything about the active process.

LIGHTHILL Well I believe David has developed a device for detecting and analysing emissions, which is available to clinicians, to get click generated otoacoustic emissions as a guide to diagnosis..... is it irregularities?

KEMP Well the proposition is that all human ears have active processes *and* irregularities. [The test detects mechanical activity...]

LIGHTHILL ...and that has diagnostic value, right?

KEMP Yes that's right, but I don't expect to sell too many to theoreticians!

LIGHTHILL Well I think the theoreticians have just about had their say for this meeting! I'm sure we are all looking forward to the next time we meet. Thank you all very much.

Local Organising Committee

D.N. Furness (25), *Treasurer*, University of Keele
M. Souter (34), *Comments and Discussion Co-ordinator*, Institute of Laryngology and Otology, London
R.J. Baker (4), *Travel Information*, University of Keele
J. Harrison (22), *Photographer*, University of Keele
J.B. Ruscoe, *Projectionist and Technician*, University of Keele
P.S. Steyger (65), *Poster Session Co-ordinator*, University of Keele
M.L. Whitehead (11), *Recordist*, University of Keele
M.J. Broad, *Secretary*, University of Keele
M. Hodgson, *Secretary*, University of Keele

Session Chairmen

R. Pujol
A.J. Hudspeth
J.J. Zwislocki
E.F. Evans
E. de Boer
P. Dallos
E. Zwicker
D.T. Kemp
E.A.G. Shaw
Sir James Lighthill

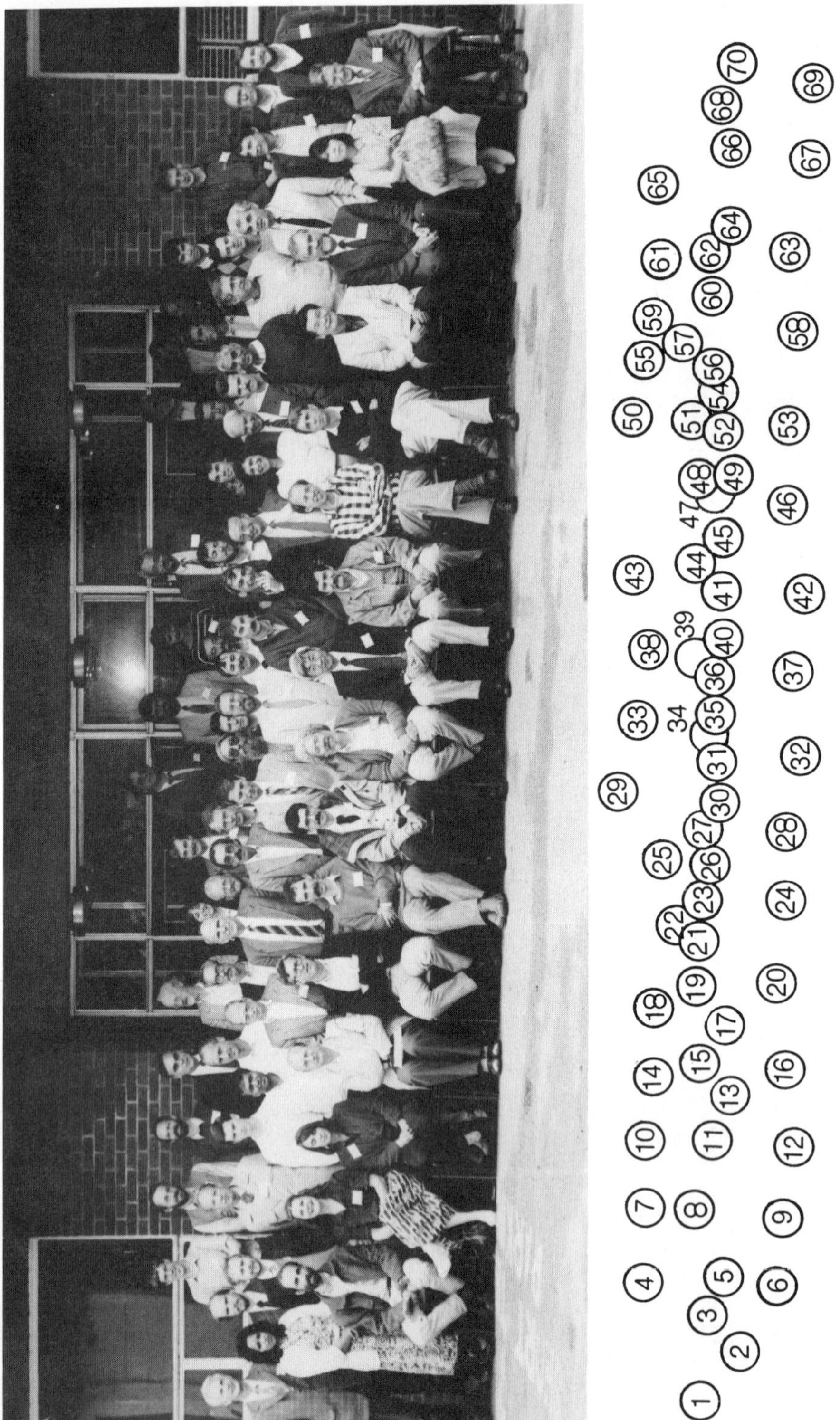

1
2
3
4
5
6
7
8
9
10
11
12
13
14
15
16
17
18
19
20
21
22
23
24
25
26
27
28
29
30
31
32
33
34
35
36
37
38
39
40
41
42
43
44
45
46
47
48
49
50
51
52
53
54
55
56
57
58
59
60
61
62
63
64
65
66
67
68
69
70

Participants (*number indicates position in photograph*)

J.B. Allen (14), AT&T Bell Labs, Murray Hill, NJ 07974-2070, USA

J.F. Ashmore (6), Dept of Physiology, University of Bristol, The Medical School, Bristol BS8 1TD, UK

E. de Boer (18), Academic Medical Centre, Meibergdreef 9, 1105 AZ Amsterdam, Netherlands

A.M. Brown (12), Dept. of Psychology, School of Biology, University of Sussex, Falmer, Sussex BN1 9QG, UK

L. Carlisle, Institute of Laryngology and Otology, 330-332 Gray's Inn Road, London, WC1X 8EE, UK

Y. Cazals, Institut National de la Santé, et de la Recherche Médicale Unité 229, Hôpital Pellegrin, Place Amélie Raba Léon, 33076 Bordeaux, France

D. Cotanche (70), Departments of Biomedical Enginnering and Otolaryngology, Boston University, Boston, MA 02115, USA

A.W. Crawford (16), Physiology Lab, University of Cambridge, Cambridge CB2 3EG, UK

P. Dallos (42), Auditory Physiology Laboratory, Frances Searle Building, Northwestern University, 2299 Sheridan Road, Evanston Il 60201, USA

A. Dancer (68), Groupe Physiologie, Institut Franco-Allemand de Recherches de St Louis, ISL, F-68301 St Louis, France

L. Décory (61), Groupe Physiologie, Institut Franco-Allemand de Recherches de St Louis, ISL, F-68301 St Louis, France

W. Denk, Department of Physics, Clark Hall, Cornell University, Ithaca, NY 14853, USA

R.J. Diependaal (44), Faculty of Mathematics, Delft University of Technology, PO Box 356, 2600 AJ Delft, Netherlands

H. Duifhuis (27), Biophsyics Dept, Lab. Gen. Physics, RUG Westersingel 34, 9718 CM Groningen, Netherlands

E.F. Evans (55), Dept of Communication & Neuroscience, University of Keele, Staffs ST5 5BG, UK

P.F. Fahey (20), Dept of Physics/EE, University of Scranton, Scranton, Pennsylvania 18510.2192, USA

R. Fettiplace (59), Physiological Lab, University of Cambridge, Cambridge CB2 3EG, UK

A. Forge (66), Institute of Laryngology and Otology, 330-332 Gray's Inn Road, London WC1X 8EE, UK

C.D. Geisler (19), Dept of Neurophysiology, 283 Medical Science Building, University of Wisconsin, Madison, Wisconsin 53705, USA

T. Gold, Center for Radiophysics and Space Science, Cornell University, Ithaca, NY 14853, USA

A.W. Gummer (7), Research School of Biological Sciences, The Australian National University, Department of Developmental Neurobiology, Box 475, Canberra A.C.T. 2601, Australia

C.M. Hackney (9), Dept of Communication & Neuroscience, University of Keele, Staffs ST5 5BG, UK

K.R. Henry (35), Department of Psychology, University of California, Davis, CA 95616, USA

M. Holley (62), Department of Physiology, University of Bristol, The Medical School, Bristol BS8 1TD, UK

K.C. Horner, Institut National de la Santé et de la Recherche Médicale, Hôpital Pellegrin, Place Amélie Raba Léon, 33076 Bordeaux, France

J.W. Horst (24), Institute of Audiology, Post Box 30 001, 9700 RB Groningen, Netherlands

A.J. Hudspeth (50), Dept of Physiology, School of Medicine, University of California, San Francisco, California 94143-0444, USA

B. Ince (49), Cerrahpasa Medical School, Istambul University, Turkey

K.L. Jones (33), School of Medicine, Division of Otolaryngology Head and Neck Surgery, University of Connecticut, Farmington, Connecticut 06032, USA

D.T. Kemp (5), Institute of Laryngology and Otology, 330-332 Gray's Inn Road, London WC1X 8EE, UK

S.M. Khanna (56), Dept of Otolaryngology, Columbia University, College of Physicians & Surgeons, 630 West 168th Street, New York, NY 10032, USA

D.O. Kim (37), School of Medicine, Division of Otolaryngology, Head and Neck Surgery, University of Connecticut, Farmington, Connecticut 06032, USA

B. Kollmeier (3), Drittes Physikalisches Institut, Universität Göttingen, Bürgerstr. 42-44, D-3400 Göttingen 1, FRG

P.J. Kolston (15), Delft University of Technology, PO Box 356, 2600 AJ Delft, Netherlands

M. Kössl, Ethology and Neurophysiology Group, School of Biology, University of Sussex, Brighton, Sussex, UK

A.B.A. Kroese (57), Department of Medical Physics, University of Amsterdam, Academic Medical Centre, Meibergdreef 15, 1105 AZ Amsterdam, Netherlands

C.J. Kros (46), Physiology Lab, University of Cambridge, Cambridge CB2 3EG, UK

E.R. Lewis (30), Dept of EECS, University of California, Berkeley, CA 94720, USA

Sir James Lightill, The Provost, University College, Gower St, London, UK

D.J. Lim (58), Otological Research Labs, Dept of Otolaryngology, Ohio State University College of Medicine, Columbus, Ohio OH 43210, USA

G.A. Manley (39), Institut für Zoologie, Technische Univ München, Lichtenbergstrasse 4, D-8046 Garching, FRG

J.W. Matthews (36), Computer Systems Laboratory, 724 S. Euclid Ave, St Louis, MO 63110, USA

D. Michel (54), Ruhr-Universität Bochum, Lehrstuhl für allgemeine Elektrotechnik und Akustik, Universitätsstr. 150, D-4630 Bochum 1, FRG

D.C. Mountain (32), Depts of Biomedical Engineering & Otolaryngology, Boston University, Boston, MA 02115, USA

S.T. Neely (28), Boys Town National Institute, 555 North 30th Street, Omaha, Nebraska 68131, USA

S.M. van Netten (51), Department of Otolaryngology, Columbia University, College of Physicians & Surgeons, 630 West 168th Street, New York, NY 10032, USA

A.R. Palmer (40), Institute of Hearing Research, Nottingham Medical School, Notts, UK

R.B. Patuzzi (41), Dept of Physiology, University of Western Australia, Nedlands, Australia

J.O. Pickles (43), Dept of Physiology, University of Birmingham, Birmingham B15 2TJ, UK

R. Pujol (64), INSERM U.254, Laboratorie de Neurobiologie de l'Audition, CHR Hôpital St Charles, 34059 Montpellier, France

S. Puria (13), Dept. of Electrical Engineering, The City College of New York, NY, USA

G. Reuter (29), Universitätsklinik und Poliklinik, für Hals-Nasen-Ohrenkranke, Universität Würzburg, D-8700 Würzburg, FRG

L. Robles (26), Departamento di Fisiologia y Biofisica, Facultad de Medicina, Universidad de Chile, Cassilla 70055-Correo 7, Santiago, Chile

M.A. Ruggero (31), Dept of Otolaryngology, Medical Research East, University of Minnesota, Minneapolis, MN55414, USA

I.J. Russell (45), Ethology & Neurophysiology Group, School of Biology, University of Sussex, Brighton, Sussex, UK

J.C. Saunders (60), Dept of Otolaryngology and Human Communication, University of Pennsylvania, 3400 Spruce Street, Philadelphia PA 19014-4283, USA

E.A.G. Shaw (69), Researcher Emeritus, Division of Physics, National Research Council Canada, Ottawa K1A 0R6, Canada

S. Sivaramakrishnan (2), Dept Physics, Purdue University, West Lafayette, IN 47907, USA

J.W.T. Smolders (10), Zentrum der Physiologie, J W Goethe-Universität, Theodor-Stern-Kai 7, D-6000 Frankfurt 70, FRG

M. Sneary (23), 145 Cory Hall, Dept. of Electrical Engineering and Computer Science, University of California, Berkeley CA 94720, USA

C.R. Steele (63), Division of Applied Mechanics, Stanford University, Stanford, CA 94305, USA

A. Tubis (17), Dept. Physics, Purdue University, West Lafayette, IN 47907, USA

B.T. Ulrich, Technische Universität München, D-8000 München 2, FRG

M. Vater (47), Zoologisches Instit. der Universität München, Luisenstrass 14, 8 München 2, FRG

M.A. Viergever (48), Dept. of Mathematics & Informatics, Delft University of Technology, PO Box 356, 2600 AJ Delft, Netherlands

J.P. Wilson (1), Dept. of Communication & Neuroscience, University of Keele, Staffs ST5 5BG, UK

H.P. Wit (53), Institute of Audiology, Post Box 30 001, 9700 RB Groningen, Netherlands

E. **Zwicker** (8), Institut für Electroakustik, Technische Universität München, Arcisstr. 21, D-8000 München 2, FRG

J.J. **Zwislocki** (52), Institute for Sensory Research, Syracuse University, Merrill Lane, Syracuse, NY 13210, USA

Author Index

(Pages of **Main Papers**, *Comments and Discussion*)

Subject Index

(First pages of papers and discussions)